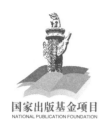

National Key Book Publishing Planning Project of the 13th Five-Year Plan

"十三五"国家重点图书出版规划项目

International Clinical Medicine Series Based on the Belt and Road Initiative

"一带一路"背景下国际化临床医学丛书

国家出版基金项目
NATIONAL PUBLICATION FOUNDATION

Pathologic Anatomy

病理解剖学

Chief Editor　Chen Kuisheng　Liang Li　Li Mincai　Pan Yun
主编　陈奎生　梁　莉　李敏才　潘　云

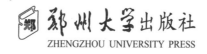

郑州大学出版社
ZHENGZHOU UNIVERSITY PRESS

图书在版编目(CIP)数据

病理解剖学 = Pathologic Anatomy：英文／陈奎生等主编. — 郑州：郑州大学出版社，2020. 12

("一带一路"背景下国际化临床医学丛书)

ISBN 978-7-5645-5993-9

Ⅰ. ①病…　Ⅱ. ①陈…　Ⅲ. ①病理解剖学 – 英文　Ⅳ. ①R361

中国版本图书馆 CIP 数据核字(2019)第 006072 号

病理解剖学 = Pathologic Anatomy：英文

项目负责人	孙保营　杨秦予		策 划 编 辑	杨秦予
责 任 编 辑	苗瑞敏		装 帧 设 计	苏永生
责 任 校 对	张彦勤		责 任 监 制	凌　青　李瑞卿

出版发行	郑州大学出版社有限公司		地　　　址	郑州市大学路 40 号(450052)
出 版 人	孙保营		网　　　址	http://www. zzup. cn
经　　销	全国新华书店		发行电话	0371-66966070
印　　刷	河南文华印务有限公司			
开　　本	850 mm×1 168 mm　1／16			
印　　张	29		字　　数	1119 千字
版　　次	2020 年 12 月第 1 版		印　　次	2020 年 12 月第 1 次印刷

书　　号	ISBN 978-7-5645-5993-9		定　　价	129.00 元

Staff of Expert Steering Committee

Chairmen

Zhong Shizhen   Li Sijin   Lü Chuanzhu

Vice Chairmen

Bai Yuting	Chen Xu	Cui Wen	Huang Gang	Huang Yuanhua
Jiang Zhisheng	Li Yumin	Liu Zhangsuo	Luo Baojun	Lü Yi
Tang Shiying				

Committee Member

An Dongping	Bai Xiaochun	Cao Shanying	Chen Jun	Chen Yijiu
Chen Zhesheng	Chen Zhihong	Chen Zhiqiao	Ding Yueming	Du Hua
Duan Zhongping	Guan Chengnong	Huang Xufeng	Jian Jie	Jiang Yaochuan
Jiao Xiaomin	Li Cairui	Li Guoxin	Li Guoming	Li Jiabin
Li Ling	Li Zhijie	Liu Hongmin	Liu Huifan	Liu Kangdong
Song Weiqun	Tang Chunzhi	Wang Huamin	Wang Huixin	Wang Jiahong
Wang Jiangang	Wang Wenjun	Wang Yuan	Wei Jia	Wen Xiaojun
Wu Jun	Wu Weidong	Wu Xuedong	Xie Xieju	Xue Qing
Yan Wenhai	Yan Xinming	Yang Donghua	Yu Feng	Yu Xiyong
Zhang Lirong	Zhang Mao	Zhang Ming	Zhang Yu'an	Zhang Junjian
Zhao Song	Zhao Yumin	Zheng Weiyang	Zhu Lin	

专家指导委员会

主 任 委 员

钟世镇　李思进　吕传柱

副主任委员 （以姓氏汉语拼音为序）

白育庭　陈　旭　崔　文　黄　钢　黄元华　姜志胜

李玉民　刘章锁　雒保军　吕　毅　唐世英

委　　　员 （以姓氏汉语拼音为序）

安东平　白晓春　曹山鹰　陈　君　陈忆九　陈哲生

陈志宏　陈志桥　丁跃明　杜　华　段钟平　官成浓

黄旭枫　简　洁　蒋尧传　焦小民　李才锐　李国新

李果明　李家斌　李　玲　李志杰　刘宏民　刘会范

刘康栋　宋为群　唐纯志　王华民　王慧欣　王家宏

王建刚　王文军　王　渊　韦　嘉　温小军　吴　军

吴卫东　吴学东　谢协驹　薛　青　鄢文海　闫新明

杨冬华　余　峰　余细勇　张莉蓉　张　茂　张　明

张玉安　章军建　赵　松　赵玉敏　郑维扬　朱　林

Staff of Editor Steering Committee

Chairmen

Cao Xuetao   Liang Guiyou   Wu Jiliang

Vice Chairmen

Chen Pingyan   Chen Yuguo   Huang Wenhua   Li Yaming   Wang Heng

Xu Zuojun   Yao Ke   Yao Libo   Yu Xuezhong   Zhao Xiaodong

Committee Member

Cao Hong   Chen Guangjie   Chen Kuisheng   Chen Xiaolan   Dong Hongmei

Du Jian   Du Ying   Fei Xiaowen   Gao Jianbo   Gao Yu

Guan Ying   Guo Xiuhua   Han Liping   Han Xingmin   He Fanggang

He Wei   Huang Yan   Huang Yong   Jiang Haishan   Jin Chengyun

Jin Qing   Jin Runming   Li Lin   Li Ling   Li Mincai

Li Naichang   Li Qiuming   Li Wei   Li Xiaodan   Li Youhui

Liang Li   Lin Jun   Liu Fen   Liu Hong   Liu Hui

Lu Jing   Lü Bin   Lü Quanjun   Ma Qingyong   Ma Wang

Mei Wuxuan   Nie Dongfeng   Peng Biwen   Peng Hongjuan   Qiu Xinguang

Song Chuanjun   Tan Dongfeng   Tu Jiancheng   Wang Lin   Wang Huijun

Wang Peng   Wang Rongfu   Wang Shusen   Wang Chongjian   Xia Chaoming

Xiao Zheman   Xie Xiaodong   Xu Falin   Xu Xia   Xu Jitian

Xue Fuzhong   Yang Aimin   Yang Xuesong   Yi Lan   Yin Kai

Yu Zujiang   Yu Hong   Yue Baohong   Zeng Qingbing   Zhang Hui

Zhang Lin   Zhang Lu   Zhang Yanru   Zhao Dong   Zhao Hongshan

Zhao Wen   Zheng Yanfang   Zhou Huaiyu   Zhu Changju   Zhu Lifang

编审委员会

Editorial Staff

Chief Editors

Chen Kuisheng	Zhengzhou University
Liang Li	Southern Medical University
Li Mincai	Hubei University of Science and Technology
Pan Yun	Dali University

Vice Chief Editors

Liu Yueping	Hebei Medical University
Zhang Xu	Lanzhou University
Xu Zhengshun	Henan University of Science and Technology
Wang Miao	Capital Medical University
Ma Liqin	Zhejiang University
Zheng Jing	Hainan Medical University

Editorial Staff

Ai Hongwei	Henan University of Science and Technology
Cui Jing	Xinxiang Medical University
Gan Yaping	Hubei University of Science and Technology
Hou Xiaomin	Shanxi Medical University
Hou Zhiping	Chengde Medical University
Jia Huijie	Xinxiang Medical University
Ma Yihui	Zhengzhou University
Niu Baohua	Henan University
Niu Haiyan	Hainan Medical University
Qin Xiaojiang	Shanxi Medical University
Sun Miaomiao	Zhengzhou University
Wang Haijun	Xinxiang Medical University
Wang Ye	Sichuan University
Wei Na	Zhengzhou University
Wu Suxia	Henan University
Xu Jingjing	Zhengzhou University
Yang Wenjuan	Dali University

Yang Zhihong   Kunming Medical University

Zhang Chenli   Lanzhou University

Zhang Yingying   Kunming Medical University

Zhong Jiateng   Xinxiang Medical University

Zhou Rui   Southern Medical University

作者名单

主　编

　　陈奎生　　郑州大学

　　梁　莉　　南方医科大学

　　李敏才　　湖北科技学院

　　潘　云　　大理大学

副主编

　　刘月平　　河北医科大学

　　张　煦　　兰州大学

　　徐正顺　　河南科技大学

　　王　苗　　首都医科大学

　　马丽琴　　浙江大学

　　郑　晶　　海南医学院

编　委（以姓氏汉语拼音为序）

　　艾红伟　　河南科技大学

　　崔　静　　新乡医学院

　　甘亚平　　湖北科技学院

　　侯晓敏　　山西医科大学

　　侯志平　　承德医学院

　　贾慧婕　　新乡医学院

　　马怡晖　　郑州大学

　　牛保华　　河南大学

　　牛海艳　　海南医学院

　　秦小江　　山西医科大学

　　孙淼淼　　郑州大学

　　王海军　　新乡医学院

　　王　晔　　四川大学

　　韦　娜　　郑州大学（兼秘书）

　　吴素霞　　河南大学

　　许晶晶　　郑州大学

　　杨雯娟　　大理大学

杨志鸿　昆明医科大学
张晨丽　兰州大学
张荧荧　昆明医科大学
钟加滕　新乡医学院
周　蕊　南方医科大学

Preface

At the Second Belt and Road Summit Forum on International Cooperation in 2019 and the Seventy-third World Health Assembly in 2020, General Secretary Xi Jinping stated the importance for promoting the construction of the "Belt and Road" and jointly build a community for human health. Countries and regions along the "Belt and Road" have a large number of overseas Chinese communities, and shared close geographic proximity, similarities in culture, disease profiles and medical habits. They also shared a profound mass base with ample space for cooperation and exchange in Clinical Medicine. The publication of the International Clinical Medicine series for clinical researchers, medical teachers and students in countries along the "Belt and Road" is a concrete measure to promote the exchange of Chinese and foreign medical science and technology with mutual appreciation and reciprocity.

Zhengzhou University Press coordinated more than 600 medical experts from over 160 renowned medical research institutes, medical schools and clinical hospitals across China. It produced this set of medical tools in English to serve the needs for the construction of the "Belt and Road". It comprehensively coversaspects in the theoretical framework and clinical practicesin Clinical Medicine, including basic science, multiple clinical specialities and social medicine. It reflects the latest academic and technological developments, and the international frontiers of academic advancements in Clinical Medicine. It shared with the world China's latest diagnosis and therapeutic approaches, clinical techniques, and experiences in prescription and medication. It has an important role in disseminating contemporary Chinese medical science and technology innovations, demonstrating the achievements of modern China's economic and social development, and promoting the unique charm of Chinese culture to the world.

The series is the first set of medical tools written in English by Chinese medical experts to serve the needs of the "Belt and Road" construction. It systematically and comprehensively reflects the Chinese characteristics in Clinical Medicine. Also, it presents a landmark achievement in the implementation of the "Belt and Road" initiative in promoting exchanges in medical science and technology. This series is theoretical in nature, with each volume built on the mainlines in traditional disciplines but at the same time introducing contemporary theories that guide clinical practices, diagnosis and treatment methods, echoing the latest research findings in Clinical Medicine.

As the disciplines in Clinical Medicine rapidly advances, different views on knowledge, inclusiveness, and medical ethics may arise. We hope this work will facilitate the exchange of ideas, build common ground while allowing differences, and contribute to the building of a community for human health in a broad spectrum of disciplines and research focuses.

Nick Lemoine

Foreign Academician of the Chinese Academy of Engineering

Dean, Academy of Medical Sciences of Zhengzhou University

Director, Barts Cancer Institute, London, UK

6th August, 2020

Foreword

In the context of international medical personnel training in the "One Belt One Road" initiative, we write this *Pathologic Anatomy* that has been designed for medical undergraduates and foreign students. I am honored to write the preface for this book.

Pathology occupies an important position in medical education and serves as a bridge between basic medicine and clinical medicine. William Osler, a famous medical educator in Canada, once said "As is our pathology, so is our medicine". In order to integrate medical education with international practice and enhance the pathological communication between China and foreign countries, we write the book.

Pathologic Anatomy consists of 18 chapters, including 6 general pathology and 12 systematic chapters. The general pathology includes Adaptation and Injury of Cells and Tissues, Tissues Repair, Regional Hemodynamic Disorders, Inflammation, Neoplasm and Environmental and Nutritional Diseases. The systematic pathology includes The Blood Vessel and Heart, Respiratory Diseases, Digestive System Diseases, The Disease of Hematopoietic and Lymphoid System, Diseases of the Immune System, Diseases of the Urinary System, Female Genital System and Breast, Endocrine System Diseases, Diseases of Nervous System, Infectious disease and deep mycosis, Parasitosis and Pathological Techniques.

This book has been edited by 32 pathologists from 16 Medical Universities. The editors of this book have taken time out of their busy teaching and clinical work to write carefully and revise repeatedly. Here, I would like to thank the editorial committees for their hard work. At the same time, I would like to thank Hainan Medical University for providing a platform for the compilation of this book.

There must be some shortcomings in this compilation. Readers and peer experts are invited to criticize and give suggestions.

Authors

Contents

Chapter 1

Adaptation and Injury of Cells and Tissues

❯ Introduction

Cells and tissues can make a reactive adjustment of different forms, functions and metabolism to stimulate the environment in vitro and *in vivo*. When the physiological load is too much or too little or when a mild and sustained pathological stimulus is encountered, the cells, tissues and organs can make adaptive changes. If the stimulation exceeds the tolerance and adaptation of cells, tissues and organs, the damage changes the morphology, function and metabolism will occur. Most of the mild damage to cells is reversible, but irreversible injury-cell death can occur in serious case. Normal cells, adaptive cells, reversibly damaged cells and irreversibly damaged cells are continuous processes morphologically. Under certain conditions, they can transform each other, and the boundaries between them are sometimes not clear. A specific stimulus can induce adaptation, reversible injury or irreversible injury. But which one it induces is not only determined by the nature and intensity of stimulation, but also related to the susceptibility, differentiation, blood supply, nutrition and past state of the involved cells. Adaptation and damage change are basic pathological changes in the development of most diseases.

1.1 Adaptation

Adaptation is a noninvasive response to various unfavorable factors and the continuous stimulation of the cells, tissues and organs in the internal and external environment. Adaptation includes two aspects of functional, metabolism and morphological structure, its objective is to avoid injury of cells and tissue, which reflects adjustment and response ability to a certain extent. Adaptation is generally shown as atrophy, hypertrophy, hyperplasia and metaplasia, including changes in number, volume and differentiation of cell. Adaptive response mechanism includes up-regulation or down-regulation of cell-specific receptor function, synthesis of new proteins, transformation of one protein to another protein or an overdose of some original protein. Therefore, the adaptive response of cells and tissues can occur in any of the following aspects, such as gene expression and regulation, signal transduction combined with the receptor, protein transcription, transport and output.

Adaptation is essentially the result of the adjustment of cell growth and differentiation. It can be considered as a state between normal and damage. A new balance of metabolism, function and morphology in the internal and external environment can form through a series of adaptive changes. In general, most of the adaptive cells can be gradually restored to normal after the removal of the cause.

1.1.1 Atrophy

Atrophy is the reduction in the volume of normal cells, tissues or organs. In this condition, cell synthesis and metabolism decreases, energy demand and the original function also decreases. The atrophy of tissues and organs can also be accompanied by a decrease in the number of parenchymal cells in addition to the reduction in the volume of the substance in its parenchymal cells due to the loss of substance in the cells. The non-development or development remove the other organ and addtissues is not in the category of atrophy.

1.1.1.1 Types of Atrophy

Atrophy can be divided into two types: physiological and pathological atrophy

(1) Physiological Atrophy

It is often shown as thymus atrophy at puberty, postmenopausal atrophy of the ovary and the uterus and the atrophy of the testis in the female and male reproductive system respectively. In most atrophy, the decrease in the number of cells is achieved through cell apoptosis.

(2) Pathological Atrophy

According to the causes, it can be divided into:

Atrophy due to inadequate nutrition: It can be caused by insufficient protein intake, excessive consumption of steroids and other drugs. It can be divided in to: ①systemic malnutrition atrophy, for example, when the patient has diabetes, tuberculosis and cancer and other chronic wasting diseases, long-term malnutrition can cause muscle atrophy, called cachexia. ②local malnutrition atrophy, for example, after cerebral arteriosclerosis, the thickening of the vascular wall, the narrowing of the lumen, and the lack of sufficient blood supply in the brain can cause brain atrophy. The cells and organs of the affected cells adjust the cell volume, quantity and function, in order to adapt to the reduced supply of blood and nourishment.

Atrophy due to pressure: It is caused by long-term compression of tissues and organs. The mechanism is the hypoxia and ischemia. The atrophy of adjacent normal tissues can be caused by push and oppression of tumor in liver, brain or lung. When there is urinary tract obstruction, the hydronephrosis pressure surrounding renal tissue, causes the atrophy of renal cortex and medulla (Figure 1-1). When the right ventricular function is not complete, the central vein of the hepatic lobule and blood sinus become congested, this congestion also cause the adjacent hepatocytes to atrophy due to compression.

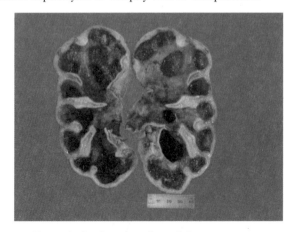

Figure 1-1   **Atrophy of renal due to pressure**

Hydronephrosis and dilation causes atrophy of renal due to pressure

Atrophy due to decreased workload: It can be caused by the decrease of long-term working load of organ tissues and low function. For example, if patients are bedridden over a prolonged period of time after limb fracture, limb muscle atrophy and osteoporosis may occur. As the limb resumes normal activity, the corresponding skeletal muscle cells will return to normal size and function.

Atrophy due to loss of innervation: It is caused by atrophy of a motoneuron or axon causing an effector to atrophy, such as muscle atrophy caused by a brain or spinal cord injury. The mechanism is the loss of neural regulation of muscle movement, as well as reduced activity and acceleration of skeletal muscle cell catabolism.

Atrophy due to loss of endocrine stimulation: Due to the decline of endocrine gland function, the target organ cells atrophy occurs. For example, pituitary ischemic necrosis in the thalamus cause the decrease of adrenocortical hormone, which then causes the atrophy of adrenal cortex. The hypofunction of the anterior pituitary can cause atrophy in the thyroid gland, the adrenal gland, the gonadal gland, etc. In addition, the tumor cells can also atrophy. For example, the prostate cancer cells can atrophy when given estrogen treatment.

Atrophy due to aging and injury: The atrophy of brain and muscle cells are the main causes of aging in brain and heart. In addition, chronic inflammation caused by viruses and bacteria is also a common cause of cell, tissue or organ atrophy. For example, the gastric mucosa may atrophy during chronic gastritis and small intestine mucous villi atrophy during chronic enteritis. Apoptosis also induces atrophy of tissues and organs. For example, the brain atrophy with Alzheimer disease(AD) is caused by apoptosis of many nerve cells.

In clinical casese, some kind of atrophy can be caused by a variety of factors. For example, muscular atrophy after fracture may be the result of various factors like nerve, nutrition, decreased workload, or even pressure factors; But atrophy of the heart or brain caused by aging could be caused by both physiological and pathological atrophy.

1.1.1.2   Pathological Change

The volume is reduced, the weight is reduced, and the color and lustre become deeper in the atrophied cell, tissues and organs. lipofuscin granules of cytoplasm can occur in the atrophy cells of myocardial cells and liver cell. lipofuscin is a membrane-covered organelle rich in phospholipids that are not completely digested in the cell. In the atrophied cells, the protein synthesis decreases, the decomposition increases, and the organelle is greatly degraded. The functions of atrophied cells, tissues and organs are mostly decreased. By reducing cell volume, quantity and reducing functional metabolism, a new balance has been reached between nutrition, hormones, growth factors and neurotransmitters. After removing the cause, the cells with mild pathological atrophy may recover to the normal state. But the cells with persistent atrophy can eventually die.

1.1.2   Hypertrophy

hypertrophy is defined as volume enlargement of the cells, tissues, or organs due to the increase of function and high metabolism. The hypertrophy in tissues or organs is often caused by volume enlargement of parenchymal cells, but also may be accompanied by an increase in the number of parenchymal cells.

1.1.2.1   Types of Hypertrophy

In nature, hypertrophy can be divided into two kinds: physiological hypertrophy or pathological hypertrophy. The causes can be divided into compensatory hypertrophy and endocrine hypertrophy. It is called endocrine hypertrophy or hormonal hypertrophy due to the excessive effect of endocrine hormones on the effector.

(1)Physiological Hypertrophy

Compensatory hypertrophy: For example, in the physiological state, the skeletal muscle of the upper limb in the weightlifter is thickened and hypertrophied. Exuberant demand and increasing load are the most common reasons.

Endocrine hypertrophy: During pregnancy, due to the action of estrogen, progesterone and its receptors, the smooth muscle cells of the uterus are hypertrophic and the number of cells increases. The uterus is thickened from 0.4 cm to 5 cm, and become heaver from 100 g to 1,000 g.

(2)Pathological Hypertrophy

Compensatory hypertrophy: Left ventricular hypertrophy can be caused by increased cardiac output when hypertension or functional compensation of normal myocardial function occurs after left ventricular partial necrosis(Figure 1-2). Organ hypertrophy can also be a response after. For example, when unilateral nephrectomy or unilateral renal artery occlusion, which causes lose of renal function, occur, the contralateral kidney can realize compensatory by hypertrophy.

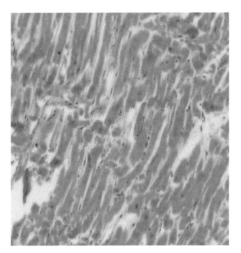

Figure 1-2   Myocardial hypertrophy(HE, low power)
Part of the myocardial cell thicken, the nuclei are irregular and
hyperchromatic, presenting a compensatory hypertrophy state

Endocrine hypertrophy: Hyperthyroidism increases the secretion of thyroxine, causing hypertrophy of thyroid follicle epithelial cells; Hypophysis eosinophil adenoma increases the secretion of the adrenocorticotropic hormone, resulting in hypertrophy of the adrenocortical cells.

1.1.2.2   Pathological Changes of Hypertrophy

The volume of hypertrophied cells increases, the nucleus hypertrophies and anachronisms, uniform enlargement in hypertrophies tissues and organs can be seen. The activation of many pro-oncogenes in cells with hypertrophy result in increased DNA content and organelles, active structural protein synthesis, and enhanced cell function. But the function of compensatory hypertrophy cells make is limited. For example, in myocardial hypertrophy, blood supply of myocardial cells is relatively lacking; the normal contraction protein in myocardial cells, also due to activation of embryonic genes, transforms into naive contractile protein whose contraction efficiency is poor; the myocardial fiber contraction component even dissolves or disappears, leading to reversing injury. Those changes eventually lead to myocardial overload, induces dysfunction(decompensation).

In condition of certain pathological factors, during the atrophy of parenchymal cells, interstitial adipocytes can proliferate to maintain the original volume of organs and even increase the volume of organs and tissues. This is called pseudohypertrophy.

1.1.3   Hyperplasia

Hyperplasia is defined as the phenomenon that results in the number of cells of tissues and organs increase, caused by active mitosis. It is oftencauses the volume to increase and the function active in tissues or organs. It is often caused by excessive stimulation of cell and overexpression of growth factor and its receptor, and may also be related to inhibition of cell apoptosis. It is usually finely regulated by proliferating genes, apoptotic genes, hormones and various peptide growth factors and their receptors.

1.1.3.1   Types of Hyperplasia

According to its nature, hyperplasia can be divided into two type of physiological hyperplasia and pathological hypertrophy. According to the causes, it can be divided into compensatory hyperplasia and endocrine hypertrophy, or called hormonal hyperplasia.

(1) Physiological Hyperplasia

Compensatory hyperplasia: For example, the hyperplasia of residual hepatocyte after partial liver resection. Because the oxygen content in air at high altitude is low, the bone marrow erythrocyte precursor cells and peripheral blood erythrocyte increase in compensation.

Endocrine hypertrophy: For example, the hyperplasia of lobular gland epithelium in the normal female during puberty and endometrium glands in the menstrual cycle.

(2) Pathological Hypertrophy

Compensatory hyperplasia: In the process of wound healing after tissue injury, fibroblasts and capillary endothelial cells are often proliferated because of increased growth factor stimulation; Also a chronic or long exposure to physical and chemical factors often cause the proliferation of tissue cells, especially the skin and some organ coated cells.

Endocrine hyperplasia: The most common cause of pathological hyperplasia is excessive hormone or excessive growth factor. The absolute or relative increase of estrogen may cause the hyperplasia of the endometrium glands to grow too long, resulting in functional uterine bleeding.

Hyperplasia is an important adaptable response of the interstitium. For example, fibroblasts and capillary endothelial cells can achieve the purpose of repair by hyperplasia; Inflammation and the hyperplasia of tumor interstitial fibroblasts are important histologically and cytological manifestation of anti-inflammatory and anti-tumor mechanisms of the body. The hyperplasia of parenchymal cells and interstitial cells is not uncommon. For example, the estrogen metabolite two dihydrotestosterone, can cause hyperplasia of prostate gland and interstitial fibrous tissue in men; excessive estrogen secretion can cause hyperplasia in women's mammary terminal ducts, acinus epithelium and interstitial fibrous tissue.

1.1.3.2   Pathological Changes of Hyperplasia

The number of cells increases, the form of cell and cell nucleus is normal or enlarge slightly. Hyperplasia of cell can be divided into diffuse or limited hyperplasia, It is characterized by a proliferation of tissue, a homogeneous and diffuse enlargement of the organ, or a single or multiple proliferative nodules in the tissues and organs. Most pathological (such as inflammation) cell hyperplasia can stop due to the removal of the trigger factor. If cell hyperplasia is uncontrolled, it may become a neoplastic hyperplasia.

1.1.3.3   The Relationship Between Hypertrophy and Hyperplasia

Although hypertrophy and hyperplasia are two different pathological processes, the causes of hypertrophy and hyperplasia of cells, tissues and organs are similar. So they often go hand in hand. For example, when cell mitosisis blocked in G2 phase, it will have hypertrophic polyploid cells but not divided. If the cells are successively entered into subsequent phases, the process of splitting and multiplying is completed. In general, the proliferation of cells themselves (permanent cells, stable cells, unstable cells) determines whether it is simple hypertrophy or hyperplasia. For organs that are active in cell division and proliferation like the uterus, mammary gland, its hypertrophy can be the result of both cell volume increase and cell number increase. However, in the myocardium and skeletal muscle, which have low cell division and proliferation ability, the enlargement of the tissues or organs is only caused by cell hypertrophy.

1.1.4 Metaplasia

Metaplasia is defined as a process in which one kind of mature differentiated cell types are replaced by another kind of mature differentiated cell types, which is only in the cell with more active splitting and proliferation ability. It is not caused by directly transforming from mature cells in the original, but is the result of transdifferentiation of the stem cells with the and capacity of proliferation and multidirectional differentiation such as immature differentiated cells and reserve cells, which are (trans-differentiation) the product of some gene activation or inhibition and cell reprogramming expression caused by environmental factors. That is the morphological expression of histomorphological cell change in differentiation and growth regulation. This process may be reached by methylation and demethylation of certain gene DNA.

1.1.4.1 Types of Metaplasia

Metaplasia has many types, which usually occurs in homologous cells, namely in Epithelial or mesenchymal cells. It is usually preformed as cell types with higher specificity replacing cell type with lower specificity. The metaplasia of the epithelial tissue may recover after the causes eliminated, but the metaplasia of the mesenchymal tissue is mostly irreversible.

(1) The Metaplasia of the Epithelial Tissue

Squamous metaplasia: Squamous metaplasia is the most common metaplasia of covering epithelia. For example, the bronchial pseudostratified ciliated columnar epithelium is prone to squamous metaplasia (Figure 1–3); When salivary glands, pancreas, pelvis, bladder, liver and gallbladder produce stones or vitamin A is insufficient, columnar epithelium, cuboidal epithelium or transitional epithelium can be turned into the squamous epithelium.

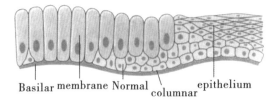

Basilar membrane Normal columnar epithelium

Figure 1–3　Squamous metaplasia of columnar epithelium
Reserve cells in columnar epithelial cells proliferate. Differentiating and forming stratified squamous epithelium

Metaplasia of columnar epithelium: The metaplasia of the epithelial tissue of the gland is also more common. When chronic gastritis occurs, Metaplasia of gastric mucosal epithelial, small intestine or colon epithelial tissue with Paneth cells or goblet cells may occur, which is called intestinal epithelial metaplasia; if gastric gland of antrum and body are replaced by pyloric glands, it is called pseudopylori gland metaplasia. In the case of chronic reflux esophagitis, the squamous epithelium of the lower esophageal segment can also be transformed into a gastric or intestinal columnar epithelium. In the case of chronic cervicitis, the squamous epithelium of the cervix is replaced by the columnar epithelium of the cervix mucosa, forming the cervical erosion in the naked eye.

(2) Metaplasia of Mesenchymal Tissue

The infantile fibroblasts in the mesenchymal tissue can be transformed into osteoblasts or chondrocytes after injury. It is called bone or cartilaginous metaplasia. This type of metaplasia is mostly seen in damaged soft tissues such as ossifying myositis, and also in the interstitium of some tumors.

1.1.4.2   The Significance of the Metaplasia

The biological meaning of metaplasia have both the pros and cons. For example, epidermal epithelium of respiratory mucosa is formed by epidermal metaplasia on the scale, local resistance to external stimulation can be enhanced due to the increase and thicken of cell layers. But because the surface of the squamous epithelium has no ciliary structure like columnar epithelium, the self-purification ability of mucosa may be weakened. In addition, if the factors that cause the metaplasia continue to exist, malignancy may occur. For example, bronchial squamous metaplasia and intestinal metaplasia of the gastric mucosa are related to the occurrence of squamous cell carcinoma of the lung and gastric adenocarcinoma. Columnar metaplasia is the histologic source of certain esophageal adenocarcinoma when chronic reflux esophagitis occurs. In this sense, some metaplasia is a precancerous lesion associated with the evolution of multistep tumor cells.

1.1.4.3   Epithelial-mesenchymal Transition

Epithelial-mesenchymal transition (EMT) mainly refers to the biological process of epithelial cells transforming into specific mesenchymal cells. It plays an important role in embryonic development, tissue reconstruction, chronic inflammation, tumor growth and metastasis, and various fibrotic diseases.

The transformation of epithelial cells into interstitial cells is characterized with gradual loss of epithelialphenotype, such as the decrease of E-cadherin and cytoskeletal keratin expression, and the expression of interstitial cell phenotypes, such as vimentin, fibronectin and N-cadherin. When EMT in epithelial malignant tumor occurs, epithelial cell polarity and basement membrane connection is lost, migration and invasion ability increase, making tumor cells to infiltrate growth to peripheral tissues easily, and making it easier to move to distant sites by blood flow to form metastases sites. Tyrosine kinase receptor signaling pathway, the integrin signaling pathway, Wnt signaling pathway, NF signaling pathway and TGF-β signaling pathway, may be involved in the regulation of EMT.

1.2   The Cause and Mechanism of Cell Tissue Damage

When the changes of outside environment of body exceed the tissue and cell adaptability, metabolism, histochemistry, ultrastructure, even microscope and abnormal changes visible may occur in damaged cells and stromal cells, which is called the injury. The way and result of injury depend not only on the nature, duration and intensity of the injury factors, but also on the type, status, adaptability and heredity of the damaged cells.

1.2.1   The Causes of Injury in Cell and Tissue

All the causes of the disease are also the main causes of cellular tissue damage. It can be divided into the biophysical, chemistry, nutrition, immune-neuroendocrine, genetic variation congenital internal factors such as age, gender, and social psychological behavior and iatrogenic external, pathogenic factors such as social psychological factors.

1.2.1.1   Hypoxia

Hypoxia and ischemia are the most common reasons leading to injury of cells and tissue. Cardiorespiratory failure makes arterial oxygenation insufficient, the blood oxygen carrying capacityis decreased caused by anemia and carbon monoxide poisoning, or blocked blood vessels may decrease oxygen supply. All those changes above can lead to the reduced supply of oxygen and nutrition to cells and tissues, causing damage of structure and loss of function in cell and tissue.

1.2.1.2   Biological Factors

Biological factors are the most common reason for cell injury, including all kinds of pathogenic organisms, like bacteria, viruses, Rickettsia, mycoplasma, spirals, fungi, protozoa and worms. Pathogenic organisms invade the body, cause mechanical injury, induce allergy, release internal and external toxins or secrete certain enzymes, which may damage the structure and function of cells and tissues.

1.2.1.3   Physical Factors

When various physical factors in the environment go beyond the physiological tolerance of the body, cell damage can be caused. For example; high temperature and high radiation can cause heatstroke, scalding or radiation damage, cold causes frostbite, the strong electrical current impact causes electrical injury, mechanical damage can cause trauma, fracture and so on.

1.2.1.4   Chemical Factors

Chemical factors including exogenous substances, such as acid, alkali, lead, mercury and other inorganic toxicants; organic phosphorus, cyanide and other organic toxicants, venom, muscarine and other biological toxins; endogenous substances, some metabolites such as decomposition products of cell necrosis, urea, free radicals, can cause injury to cells. Drugs, health agents, etc. can not only treat and prevent some cell damage, but also have side effects on cells.

1.2.1.5   Nutritional Imbalance

Insufficient or excessive intake of nutrients can cause corresponding lesions to body. For example, lack of vitamin D, protein and iodine lead to rickets, malnutrition and endemic goiter respectively; lack of iron, selenium and other trace elements cause developmental disorders of red blood cells and brain cells; long-term intake of high calorie and high fat is an important cause of obesity, hepatic steatosis and atherosclerosis.

1.2.1.6   Neuroendocrine Factors

Primary hypertension and peptic ulcer have a relationship with excessive excitability of vagus; when hyperthyroidism occurs, the body cells and tissues become more sensitive to infection and poisoning. The secretion of insulin makes the body prone to, especially the subcutaneous tissues, complications by bacterial infection.

1.2.1.7   Immune Factors

The body cells react exceedingly to some antigen, allergic or hypersensitivity reactions such as asthma and allergic shock may occur; self-antigen can cause tissue injury, such as systemic lupus erythematosus, rheumatoid arthritis; immunodeficiency diseases such as AIDS, can cause damage of immune function and damage of lymphocyte.

1.2.1.8   Hereditary Defect

The role of gene damage is mainly reflected in two aspects: one is the gene mutation or chromosomal aberrations, directly causing progeny genetic diseases such as Down syndrome, hemophilia, acute hemolytic anemia; the other is a genetic defect that makes the offspring tend to be prone to certain (genetic susceptibility).

1.2.1.9 Social Psychological Factors

Coronary heart disease, primary hypertension, peptic ulcer and even some tumors are closely related to social psychological factors. They are called psychosomatic diseases. For medical workers, it is necessary to prevent iatrogenic injury caused by improper health services, such as hospital-acquired infection, drug-induced injury.

1.2.2 The Injury Mechanism of Cells and Tissues

The mechanism of cell damage is mainly in the cell membrane damage, reactive oxygen species and increased increased cystolic free calcium, hypoxia-ischemia, chemical toxicity and genetic mutation, interact with each other or are reciprocal causation, causing the occurrence and development of cell injury.

1.2.2.1 Injury of Cell Membrane

The direct effect of mechanical stress, enzyme dissolution, hypoxia-ischemia, reactive oxygen species, bacterial toxins, complement components, ion pump and ion channel chemical damage, can destroy the permeability and integrity of cell membrane structure, affect functions such as membrane information and material exchange, immune response, cell division and differentiation. The early change is a selective loss of membrane permeability and eventually obvious cell membrane damage. The important mechanism of cell membrane damage is the formation of free radicals and the secondary lipid peroxidation, resulting in the progressive decrease of membrane phospholipids, accumulation of phospholipid degradation, production of cytotoxicity. The cell membrane is separated from the cytoskeleton, and the cell membrane is vulnerable to tension damage.

Morphologically, the damage of cell membrane structure causes the cells and mitochondria, endoplasmic reticulum and other organelles to become swollen, the microvilli on the surface of the cells disappear, and the vesicles form. The lipid of cell membrane and organelle membrane degenerates, curl like a spiral or concentric round Figures, forming myelin Figures. Lysosome membrane is broken, releasing a large amount of acid hydrolase, causing cell dissolution. Most of the cell necrosis starts with the dysfunction of cell membrane permeability, and ends with the loss of cell membrane integrity. Therefore, cell membrane destruction is often the key link of cell injury, especially the irreversible damage at the early stage of cell.

1.2.2.2 Mitochondrial Damage

Mitochondria are the main sites of intracellular oxidative phosphorylation and ATP production, and they are also involved in some processes such as cell growth and differentiation, information transmission and cell apoptosis. After the mitochondrial damage, the mitochondria is swollen and vacuolated, the mitochondrial crista becomes shorter, sparse or even disappeares, and the calcium amorphous dense body appears in the matrix. Mitochondrial ATP production decreases and consumption increase, resulting in dysfunction of cell membrane sodium pump and calcium pump. Transmembrane transport protein and lipid synthesis decreased, phospholipid deacylation and reacylation stops. Mitochondrial damage is often accompanied by the infiltration of mitochondrial pigments into the cytoplasm, which can initiate cell apoptosis. When the ATP energy supply reduces to $5\% - 10\%$, the cell will have a significant damage effect. After the suspension of mitochondrial oxidative phosphorylation, cell acidosis may occur, eventually cell necrosis occurs. Mitochondrial damage is an important early marker of irreversible cell injury.

1.2.2.3 Damage of Activated Oxygen Species

Activated oxygen species(AOS), also named as reactive oxygen species, including oxygen in the free radical state(such as O^{2-}), $OCl_3 \cdot$, $NO \cdot$, and H_2O_2 which is hydrogen peroxide that does not belong to the free radicals. Free radical is a group formed by the loss of an electron of an atom in the outer layer of the atom, it has strong oxidation activity. It can be activated by a copper-containing enzyme. AOS can be the product of normal metabolism of cells, and can also be produced by exogenous factors. It is very easy for it to react with the surrounding molecules, release energy and cause cell damage. It also causes the surrounding molecules to produce toxic free radicals to form a chain amplification reaction and further cause cell damage.

There is a system that produces AOS in the cell and the antioxidant system that is resistant to its formation. Normal small amounts of AOS generated will be cleared by intracellular antioxidants such as superoxide dismutase, glutathione peroxidase, catalase and vitamin E. During the process of hypoxia-ischemia, cell phagocytosis, chemical radiation injury, inflammation and aging, AOS production increases. lipid, protein and DNA peroxide. By several target points such as the membrane lipid peroxidation, non oxidative mitochondrial damage, DNA damage and protein cross-linking, changes in lipid and carbohydrate, protein, nucleic acid molecular structure may occur, the stability of membrane lipid bilayer structure decrease, DNA single-strand damage and breaks, which promotes mutual crosslinking of sulfur-containing protein and can directly cause the polypeptide broke into pieces. The strong oxidation of AOS is the basic link of cell damage.

1.2.2.4　Damage of Intracellular Free Calcium in the Cytoplasm

Phospholipids, proteins, ATP and DNA will be degraded by phospholipase, protease, ATP enzyme and nuclease in the cytoplasm. This process requires the activation of free calcium. Normally, intracellular calcium is combined with intracellular calcium transporters and stored in calcium pools, such as calcium pools endoplasmic reticulum and mitochondria. The cell membrane ATP calcium pump and calcium channel are involved in the regulation of low free calcium concentration in the cytoplasm. When cells are anoxic and poisoned, ATP decreases, and Ca^{2+} exchange proteins are activated directly or indirectly. The cell membrane's permeability to calcium increases, the calcium pumping from cells decreases, the calcium intracellular flows increases, and mitochondria and endoplasmic reticulum release calcium repeatedly, resulting in the increase of intracellular free calcium(intracellular calcium overload), which promotes the activation of these enzymes and damages the cells. The intracellular calcium concentration is often related to the degree of functional damage of the cell structure, especially the mitochondria. A large number of intracellular free calcium is a terminal link of many factors that damage cells, and it is a potential mediating agent for cell death, biochemical and morphological changes.

1.2.2.5　The Injury of is Chemic Anoxia

Ischemia is defined as insufficiency of the arterial blood supply in local cell tissue. Ischemia can cause nutrients and oxygen supply disorders, the former is known as malnutrition, and the latter is known as hypoxia. Anoxia means that cells cannot get enough oxygen or there is oxygen utilization barriers. According to the reasons, it can be divided into: ①hypotonic hypoxia, oxygen partial pressure or airway breathing disorders; ②hematologic anoxia, the quality and quantity of hemoglobin is abnormal; ③circulatory hypoxia, cardiopulmonary failure or local ischemia; ④histogenous hypoxia, mitochondrial biological oxidation, especially oxidative phosphorylation, and other internal respiratory dysfunction. In this significance, ischemia is one reason for the anoxia.

Cell hypoxia-ischemia leads to inhibition of mitochondrial oxidative phosphorylation, decrease of ATP formation, activation of phosphofructokinase and phosphorylase. The function of the sodium and potassium pump in the cell membrane becomes low, and the sodium-calcium ion accumulates in the cell and increases with the water molecules. After that, protein synthesis and fat transport disorders occur in the cytoplasm, anaerobic glycolysis increases, cell acidosis may occur, lysosomal membrane ruptures, DNA chain may be damaged and nuclear chromosome may be agglutinated. Ischemic anoxia also causes the increase of reactive oxygen species, causing lipid disintegration and destruction of cytoskeleton. Blood flow blocking is the most common cause of ischemia and hypoxia. Usually, ischemia causes more rapid and severe for tissue damage. Anaerobic glycolysis can continue during anoxia, but it stops during ischemia. Mild anoxia can cause cell edema and fatty change; mild continuous hypoxia can lead to cell apoptosis; severe continuous anoxia can lead to cell necrosis. In some cases, the recovery of blood flow after ischemia can cause the peroxidation of living tissue, aggravating the tissue damage, which is called ischemia-reperfusion injury, and commonly seen after myocardial infarction and cerebral infarction. Ischemic and anoxia is the most common and important central link in cell injury.

1.2.2.6   Chemical Damage

Many chemicals, including drugs, can cause cell damage. Chemical damage can be systemic like chloride poisoning or local damage like damage of the skin and mucous membrane due to exposure to strong acid and strong alkali. The effects of some chemicals may also be organ specific, such as the liver damage caused by CCl4. The ways in which chemical damage occur are: ①the chemical substance itself has the direct cytotoxic effect. For example, cyanide can quickly seal the cytochrome oxidase system of the mitochondria and cause sudden death. During mercury poisoning, mercury binds with sulfur containing protein in cell membrane, damaging ATP enzyme dependent membrane transport function. Chemical antitumor drugs and antibiotics can also hurt cells by similar direct effects; ②the cytotoxic effects of metabolites on target cells. The liver, kidney, bone marrow and myocardium are the target organs of toxic metabolites, and cytochrome P450 complex function enzyme plays an important role in the metabolic process. If CCl4 itself is not active, it will be transformed into toxic free radicals CCl3 in liver cells, which will cause swelling of the smooth endoplasmic reticulum and lipid metabolism disorder. ③It will induce immune injury such as anaphylaxis. For example, penicillin leads to type Ⅰ allergy; ④It will induce DNA damage. The degree, speed and location of chemical injury are affected by the dosage of chemical substances and drugs, the time of action, the location of absorption, accumulation and the individual difference of metabolic rate.

1.2.2.7   Genetic Variation

The damage of genetic variation may occur by congenital heredity or during embryogenesis, and can also occur after birth. Chemical substances and drugs, viruses, rays, and so on, can damage the DNA in the nucleus, induce gene mutation and chromosome aberration, and cause cell genetic variation. Those changes are caused by: ①the low synthesis of protein structure, and lack of the essential protein in cells; ②prevention of nuclear division in important functional cell; ③the synthesis of abnormal growth regulator; ④inducing enzyme synthesis disorders of congenital or acquired, cell dies due to lack of necessary metabolism mechanism for life.

1.3   Reversible Injury

Reversible injury, whose morphological change is called denaturation, refers to the phenomenon that causes the accumulation of normal substances or appearance of abnormal substances in cells or intercellular interstitial due to metabolic disorders after being damaged, usually accompanied by low cell function. The accumulation is caused by excessive or too fast production of these normal or abnormal substances. The cell itself lacks the corresponding mechanism of metabolism, clearance or transport and makes them accumulate in organelles, cytoplasm, nuclear or intercellular substance. After removing the cause, most of these injuries can be restored to normal. Therefore, it is a nonfatal and reversible damage.

All the harmful factors play their role at the molecular level first. It can identify cellular adaptation, reversible injury or irreversible damage and other morphological changes, which depend on the nature of cell lesions and the sensitivity of observation methods. But in general, the affected cells show biochemical metabolic changes, and histochemical and ultrastructural organization (such as a few minutes to dozens of minutes after ischemia), and the morphological changes that occurred appear visibly under the light microscope (like a few hours to a few days after ischemia). Most of the mild damage can be restored to normal after the cause is eliminated, usually called reversible damage. Serious cell damage is irreversible, directly or ultimately leading to cell death.

1.3.1 Cellular Swelling

Cellular swelling, also called hydropic degeneration is often the initial change in cell damage. It is caused by the functional decline of cell volume and cytoplasmic ion concentration regulation mechanism.

1.3.1.1 Mechanism

Due to the damage of mitochondria, the decrease of ATP production and the dysfunction of the potassium pump in the cell membrane, sodium ions accumulate excessively and a large amount of water is attracted into the cell to make intracellular and extracellular ion isosmotic. After that, the accumulation of the metabolites of inorganic phosphate, lactic acid and purine nucleotides can increase the osmotic pressure and further aggravate the edema of the cells. Any damage that can cause changes in cell fluid and ionic homeostasis can lead to cell edema, which is commonly seen in the parenchymal cells of liver, kidney, heart and other organs during hypoxia, infection and poisoning.

1.3.1.2 Pathological Changes of Cellular Swelling

At the beginning of the lesion, the mitochondria and the endoplasmic reticulum become swollen and forms a red-dyed granular substance that appear in the cytoplasm under microscope. If water and sodium accumulate further, the cells will be swollen obviously. The cytoplasm is highly porous and vacuolar, and the nucleus can also be swollen. There are vesicles on the surface of plasma membrane, and the microvilli disappear. It is called ballooning variant in fastigium (Figure 1-4). Sometimes the changes in cell edema are not easily identified by microscopy, but the changes in the whole organ may be more obvious. The volume of the affected organs increases can be seen by the naked eye, the envelope is tense, the cut surface is valgus, and the color becomes pale.

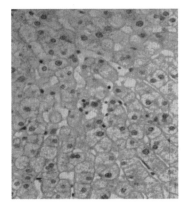

Figure 1-4   swelling of hepatocyte (HE, low power)

The liver cells are significantly swollen, the cytoplasm is light dying, and some of the hepatocytes are swollen like balloon samples

1.3.2 Fatty Change

Steatosis is defined as phenomenon in which triglycerides accumulate in the cytoplasm of cells that are not adipocytes. It occurs mostly in hepatocytes, cardiomyocytes, renal tubular epithelial cells, skeletal muscle cells and so on, which are related to infection, alcoholism, poisoning, hypoxia, malnutrition, diabetes and obesity.

1.3.2.1   The Pathology of Fatty Change

There is no obvious change in the organs with slight fatty change when observed with the naked eye. With the aggravation of the lesion, the volume of the fat change organs increases, its color is yellow, the edge is blunt and the section is greasy sense. Under the electron microscope, the fat in the cytoplasm aggregate into the fat corpuscle and then fuse into the lipid droplets. Under the microscope, there are different sizes of spherical lipid droplets in the cytoplasm of fatty change. The large one can fill the whole cell and squeeze the nucleus to one side. In the paraffin section, the fat is vacuolated as the fat is dissolved in organic solvents(Figure 1-5). In frozen section, the special dyeing of Sultan Ⅲ and Sultan Ⅳ can distinguish the fat from other substances.

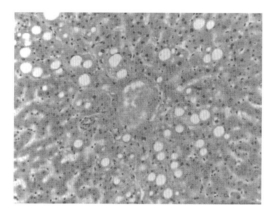

Figure 1 – 5   fatty changes of hepatocyte
(HE, low power)

In the cytoplasm of the liver, the vacuoles of different sizes are seen as lipid droplets. Some of the nuclei are partial to one side

Hepatocyte is an important place for fat metabolism, in which fatty changes most often occurs, but mild hepatic steatosis usually does not cause morphological changes and dysfunction of the liver. The distribution of fat in the lobule of the liver has a certain relationship with the cause of the disease. For example, during chronic liver congestion, centrilobular hypoxia is serious, so the fat first occurs in centrilobular sites; during phosphorus poisoning, peripheral lobular liver cells are more sensitive to phosphorus poisoning, so peripheral lobular liver cell is involved more obviously; during severe poisoning and infectious disease, fatty change often involves the entire liver cell. Significant diffuse hepatic steatosis is called fatty liver, and severe hepatic steatosis may develop to liver necrosis and cirrhosis.

Chronic alcoholism or anoxia can cause myocardial steatosis, often involves the left ventricular endocardium and papillary muscles. Myocardialsteatosis is yellow. It is between the dark red of the normal myocardium, forming the yellow red markings, which is called tigroid heart. Sometimes the adipose tissue of the epicardial hyperplasia can extend between the human cardiac myocytes. It is called myocardial fatty infiltration, but not the degeneration of the myocardium. Severe myocardial fatty infiltration can cause rupture of the heart, causing sudden death.

The renal tubular epithelial cells can also undergo steatosis. Under the light microscope, lipid droplets are mainly located in the proximal part of renal tubular cells, which are excessive reabsorption of lipoproteins in the original urine, and those of severe cases can involve the distal renal tubule cells.

1.3.2.2 The Mechanism of Hepatic Steatosis

The mechanism of hepatic steatosis is as follows: ①Liver cytoplasmic fatty acid increases: as high-fat diet or malnutrition, fat tissue in vivo is decomposed. Excess free fatty acids enter into live by blood flow; a large number of lactic acid turn into fatty acid oxidation in liver cells due to hypoxia; obstacles of oxidation decrease fatty acid utilization, fatty acid increase relatively; ②triglyceride synthesis increases; for example, excessive drinking can change function of mitochondria and smooth endoplasmic reticulum, promote synthesis of a new triglyceride; ③the lipoprotein and apolipoprotein decrease: when Ischemic, anoxia, poisoning or malnutrition occur, lipoprotein and apolipoprotein synthesis in liver cells decrease, fat output is blocked and accumulates in the cell.

In addition, when atherosclerosis or hyperlipidemia syndrome occurs, excess cholesterol and cholesterol can exist in some non-adipocytes, such as macrophages and smooth muscle cells. which can be regarded as a special type of intracellular lipid accumulation. When the macrophages are significantly increased and gathered in subcutaneous tissue, It is called yellowish tumors.

1.3.3　Hyaline Change

The accumulation of translucent protein in cells or interstitial cells is called hyaline change, or hyaline degeneration, HE staining presents eosinophilic homogenization. Hyaline change is a group of lesion which has morphologically similar physical properties, but its chemical composition and pathogenesis are different.

1.3.3.1 Mechanism of Hyaline Change

The mechanism of it may be the congenital genetic disorder of protein synthesis or the acquired defect of protein folding, which makes the third level structure and amino acid sequence of some proteins mutate, resulting in the accumulation of denatured collagen, plasma protein and immunoglobulin.

1.3.3.2 Pathological Changes of Hyaline Change

According to the lesion sites, it can be divided into.

The hyaline changes in the cells: they are usually rounded corpuscles of homogeneous red dye, located in the cytoplasm. For example, there are wicking vesicles in the renal tubular epithelial cells, which re-absorp the urine protein, fuse with lysosomes, forming hyaline droplets; immunoglobulin in the rough endoplasmic reticulum of plasmocyte cytoplasm accumulates, forming Rusell bodies; alcoholic liver disease. Degeneration of the intermediate filaments prekeratin of the cells in the cytoplasm of the hepatocyte occurs, forming Mallory body.

Hyaline changes in the fibrous connective tissue: it occurs in the physiological and pathological connective tissue proliferation, which is a manifestation of the aging fibers tissues. It is characterized by collagen cross-linking, denaturation and fusion. The collagen fibers proliferate and thicken, and there are few vascular and fibroblast cells. Grossly, it is gray and white, and its quality is tough and translucent. It can be seen in the atrophic uterus and breast stromal, scar tissue, atherosclerotic fibrous plaque, and the organization of various necrotic tissues.

Arterioles hyalinization: also known as arteriolosclerosis, is common in fine arterial wall of the kidney, brain, spleen and other organs with chronic hypertension and diabetes (Figure 1−6). Due to infiltration of plasma protein and deposition of metabolism of the basement membrane, fine arterial wall thickens, the tube becomes narrow, blood pressure rises, organs become ischemic. The elasticity of the arteriole wall with hyaline change is weakened, the brittleness increases, and the dilatation, rupture and bleeding are easily secondary.

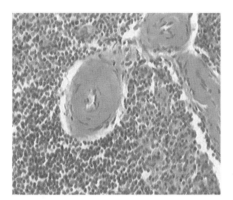

Figure 1-6   hyaline change in central arteries of spleen(HE, low power)

In the primary hypertension, the central artery wall was thickened, the lumen was relatively small, and the wall of the artery was stained with red dye, and the homogenous glass-like substance

1.3.4   Amyloid Change

Amyloidosis is accumulation of amyloid protein and sticky polysaccharide in the mesenchymal cell, named using starch dyeing characteristics. Amyloidosis is also a class of morphological and special coloring, but the changes in chemical structure and production mechanism are different.

1.3.4.1   Mechanism of Amyloid Change

The amyloid protein is derived from the light chain of immunoglobulin, peptide hormone, calcitonin precursor protein and serum amyloid A protein. The new polypeptide chain of amyloid is composed of ribosomes and can be arranged in chain α and chain β. Because the body does not contain the enzyme which can digest large molecules with β-folding structure, β-folding protein and its precursors are easy to accumulate in the tissue in the body.

1.3.4.2   Pathological Changes in Amyloid Change

Amyloidosis is mainly deposited in the cell interstitium, under the small vascular basement membrane or along the reticular fibrous scaffold. Under the microscope, HE staining is characterized by light red homogeneous substance, and shows a coloration reaction of amyloid. It is orange-red when Congo red used, it is brown when meets iodine, and turns blue when diluted sulfuric acid is added.

Amyloidosis can be divided into localized amyloidosis and systemic amyloidosis. Localized amyloidosis can be found in the skin, conjunctiva, tongue, larynx and lung. It can also be found in the interstitial tissue of Alzheimer disease brain and Hodgkin's disease, multiple myeloma, medullary thyroid carcinoma and other tumors. Systemic amyloidosis can be divided into primary and secondary amyloidosis, the former mainly originates from the serum α-immunoglobulin light chain, involving the liver, kidney, spleen, heart and other organs; the latter from unknown origin, main components are non immunoglobulin synthesis in liver(amyloid protein), it can be found in the elderly, chronic inflammation such as tuberculosis and tumor stroma.

1.3.5   Mucoid Change

Mucoid change or Mucoid degeneration is defined as the accumulation of protein(glucosaminoglycans, hyaluronic acid, etc.)in the cytoplasm, which are commonly seen in mesenchymal tissue tumors, atherosclerotic plaques, rheumatic foci, and malnourished bone marrow and adipose tissue. The characteristics under microscope are that in the loose interstitial, there are many protruding star-shaped fibrous cells, scattered in the grayish blue mucous matrix. Hyaluronidase activity is inhibited, hyaluronan mucoid substance and moisture accumulate in the skin and subcutaneous tissue, forming characteristic mucinous edema during hypothyroidism.

1.3.6   Pathological Pigmentation

The normal human body contains hemosiderin, lipofuscin, melanin, bilirubin and other endogenous pigment; carbon dust, coal dust, tattoo pigment and other exogenous pigment sometimes enter the body. In pathology, some of the above pigments will increase and accumulate inside and outside the cell, known as pathological pigmentation.

1.3.6.1   Hemoflavin

It is an aggregation of ferritin particles produced by macrophages phagocytosis and degradation of erythrocyte hemoglobin. It is a combination of Fe^{3+} and protein. It is golden or brown under microscope (Figure 1-7), and can be dyed blue by Prussian blue. The presence of hemoflavin reflects the destruction of erythrocyte and the residual of iron-containing substance systemic or local. After the rupture of macrophages, this pigment can also be seen outside the cell. In physiological conditions, a small amount of hemoflavin can be formed in the liver, spleen, lymph nodes and bone marrow. In pathological conditions, such as old bleeding and hemolytic disease, the accumulation of hemoflavin in cell tissue is found in the cell tissue.

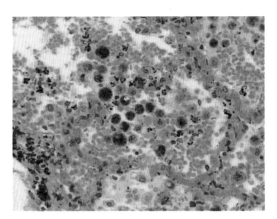

Figure 1-7   pigmentation of hemoflavin(HE, low power)

In chronic pulmonary blood stasis, a large number of macrophages in the alveolar cavity phagocyte and decompose red blood cells, and many gold or brown hemosiderin granules are formed in the cytoplasm

1.3.6.2   Lipofuscin

It is the undigested organelle debris residues in autophagy lysosomes, and is seen as brown fine granular under the microscope. Its composition is a mixture of phospholipids and proteins. It comes from peroxidation of free radical catalyzed unsaturated fatty acid peroxide with cell membrane phase structure. Normally, a small amount of lipofuscin may be seen in the epididymal epithelial cells, leydig cells and cytoplasm of ganglion cells. In elderly patients and patients with nutrient depletion, a large number of lipofuscin can be seen in atrophic myocardial cells and around hepatic nucleus, it is signs that cell has been damaged by free radical peroxidation, therefore it is known as consumptive pigment. When most cells contain lipofuscin, obvious organ atrophy usually can be seen there.

1.3.6.3　Melanin

It is a black-brown fine particle in the cytoplasm, which is produced from tyrosine by the polymerization of levodopa. Its formation is promoted by the pituitary ACTH(adrenocorticotropic hormone) and MSH (melanocytic stimulating hormone). In addition to melanocytes, melanin can also be clustered in the keratinocyte of the skin basal cells and in the macrophages of dermis. In some chronic inflammation and pigmented nevus, melanoma, and basal cell carcinoma, melanin can be locally increased. Addison's disease with low adrenocortical function can have melanosis of the whole body and mucous membrane.

1.3.6.4　Bilirubin

It is the main pigment in the bile duct, which is the product of the aging and destruction of red blood cells in the blood. It is also derived from hemoglobin, but it does not contain iron. The pigment is rough, golden and granular in the cytoplasm. When the blood bilirubin is increased, the patient has jaundice in the skin and mucous membrane.

1.3.7　Pathological Calcification

Pathological calcification is defined as solid calcium salt deposition in tissues besides the bone and teeth. It can be located within or outside the cell. The main components of calcium salts are calcium phosphate, calcium carbonate, a small amount of iron, magnesium, or other minerals.

1.3.7.1　Types of Pathological Calcification it Has Two Types

Dystrophic calcification: it is called malnutrition calcification when calcium salts are deposited in necrotic, soon necrotic tissues or foreign bodies. The metabolism of calcium and phosphorus is normal in the body. It can be seen in tuberculosis, thrombosis, atherosclerotic plaques, heart valve disease and scar tissue (Figure 1-8), which may be related to increased local alkaline phosphatase.

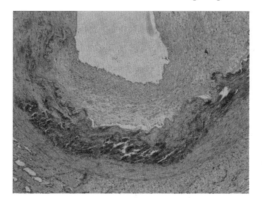

Figure 1-8　dystrophic calcification of the arterial wall(HE, low power)

　　Under low power lens, atherosclerosis occurs in the arterial wall, then secondary dystrophic calcification. Blue granulated calcium salt deposits

Metastatic calcification: it is called metastatic calcification when calcium salts deposits in normal tissue due to disorders of calcium and phosphorus metabolism(hypercalcemia), mainly in hyperparathyroidism, excessive intake of vitamin D, renal failure and some bone tumors, often occurs in interstitial tissue of blood vessel, kidney, lung and stomach.

1.3.7.2   Pathological Changes of Calcification

The pathological calcification appears blue granular to flaky under the microscope, and is fine particles or lumps grossly, feel like the sand and gravel. A large area of pathological calcification can cause deformation, sclerosis and dysfunction of tissues and organs. Another form of pathological calcification is the formation of stones made up of calcium carbonate and cholesterol in the gallbladder, bladder, renal pelvis, ureter, and pancreas.

To sum up, the accumulation of different normal or abnormal substances in the cell or in the cytoplasm can cause different types of reversible damage.

1.4   Cell Death

When the cell has fatal metabolism, structure and dysfunction, irreversible cell damage can occur, which is cell death. Cell death is the most important physiological and pathological change involving all cells. There are two main types of cell death. One is apoptosis and the other is necrosis. Apoptosis is mainly seen in the physiological death of cells, but it is also seen in some pathological processes. Necrosis is the main form of cell pathological death. Both of them have relatively different mechanisms, pathological significance, morphological and biochemical characteristics. Which way a cell dies is dependent not only on types, intensity, duration, the degree of ATP deletion in affected cells, but also on the state of programmed expression of gene in cells.

1.4.1   Necrosis

Necrosis is local cell death in vivo characterized by changes of enzyme solubility. Necrosis can be directly induced by strong pathogenic factors, but most of them develop from reversible injury. Its basic manifestations are cell swelling, disintegration of cell organelles and protein denaturation. Lysosomal enzymes release from necrotic cells and the exudative neutrophils around. It can promote the further development of necrosis and the dissolution of local parenchymal cells. So necrosis often includes many cells at the same time.

1.4.1.1   Basic Pathological Changes of Necrosis

(1) The Changes in the Nucleus

The changes in the nucleus are the main morphological markers of cell necrosis, they mainly have three forms.

Pyknosis: nuclear chromatin DNA are thickening and crinkling, making the nuclear volume reduce, basophilic increase, suggesting that DNA transcriptional synthesis stops.

Karyorrhexis: with nucleus chromatin disintegrating and nuclear membrane rupture, nuclear fragmentation occurs, making nuclear matter disperse in cytoplasm, which can also be formed from nuclear condensation to fragmentation.

Karyolysis: activation of non-specific DNA enzymes and nucleoprotein decompose nuclear DNA and nucleocapsid, decrease acidophilia of chromatin and make killing nuclei disappear within 1−2 days.

The three processes are not always progressive. Its nucleus changes are not the same in different diseases and cells.

(2) Cytoplasmic Changes

Besides the change of nucleus, the acidophilus of cytoplasmic in necrotic cells is enhanced due to the loss of ribosome, the increase of cytoplasmic denatured protein and the decrease of glycogen granules. The main ultrastructural morphology of cell irreversible injury is the formation of mitochondrial vacuoles, accumulation of amorphous calcium-dense deposits in mitochondria matrix, acid hydrolase release by lysosome to dissolve cell components.

(3) Interstitial Changes

The tolerance of interstitial cell is better than parenchymal cell, so it is later for interstitial cell to show lesion later on. After necrosis of interstitial cells, the extracellular stroma is also gradually disintegrating and liquefied, finally fused into a flaky unstructured substance.

As necrosis cell membrane permeability increases; intracellular lactate dehydrogenase, succinate dehydrogenase, creatine kinase and aspartate aminotransferase, alanine aminotransferase, amylase and its isoenzyme are released into blood, resulting in the corresponding reduction in enzyme activity in the cells and increase corresponding enzyme levels. Those can be used as a reference index for clinical diagnosis of some cell necrosis(such as liver, myocardium and pancreas the reference index of necrosis). Changes in the activity of enzymes in the cell and in the plasma can be detected at the beginning of the necrosis, which is earlier than the changes in the ultrastructure. So they are helpful to the early diagnosis of cell damage.

1.4.1.2 Types of Necrosis

Due to different positions of enzyme degradation or protein denaturation. The necrotic tissue may appear to have distinct morphological changes, usually divided into three basic types; coagulation necrosis, liquefaction necrosis and fibrinoid necrosis. In addition, caseous necrosis, fat necrosis, gangrene and other special types of necrosis can also occur. Generally speaking, after tissue necrosis, the color is pale, elasticity disappears, normal sensory and motor function is lost, blood vessels pulsation disappear, no fresh blood outflow when cut, clinically called inactivating tissue. It should be excised in time.

(1) Coagulative Necrosis

When the protein denaturation occurs and lysosomal enzyme hydrolysis is weak, the necrotic region is gray yellow, dry and qualitative, which is called coagulant necrosis. Coagulation necrosis is the most common, often seen in the heart, liver, kidney, spleen and other essential organs, often caused by ischemic anoxia, bacterial toxins, chemical corrosion agents. The limit between the necrosis and the healthy tissue is often obvious. The feature under microscope is the disappearance of the cell microstructure, and the outline of the tissue structure can still be preserved. There is congestion, bleeding and inflammatory reaction around the necrotic area. The basic outline of tissue structure can be maintained for several days. There may be a continuous acidosis caused by necrosis, which denaturate the structural protein and enzyme protein of necrotic cells, and retards the decomposition process of protein.

(2) Liquefaction Necrosis

Due to the lack of coagulable protein in the necrotic tissue, the release of a large number of hydrolytic enzymes from the necrotic cells and infiltrated neutrophils, tissue is rich in water and phospholipid, the liquefaction is prone to occur after the necrosis of the cell and tissue, which is called liquefaction necrosis. It can be found in abscesses caused by bacteria or certain fungal infections, softening of the brain caused by ischemia and anoxia, and dissolved necrosis developed from cell edema. The characteristics under microscope are that the dead cells are completely digested, and the local tissues are rapidly dissolved.

(3) Fibrinoid Necrosis

It is known as fibrinoid degeneration, is a common form of necrosis in connective tissue and small vascular walls. Filamentous, granular or small lump-like unstructured material forms in the site of the lesion. Because of its similar dyeing properties with cellulose, it is known as cellulosic necrosis. It can be seen in some allergiy diseases such as rheumatism, polyarteritis nodosa, crescentic glomerulonephritis, and accelerated hypertension, the small blood vessels at the bottom of gastric ulcer. the mechanism is related to collagen fiber swelling and disintegration caused by antigen-antibody complex, immunoglobulin deposition of connective tissue, or plasma fibrin exudation and degeneration.

(4) Caseous Necrosis

In the case of tuberculosis, the necrosis is yellow, like a cheese due to too much lipid there, which is known as caseous necrosis. It is an unstructured granular red mass under microscope. No necrotic part of the original organizational structure blur, even not nuclear debris, it is a special type of more complete necrosis. Casesic necrosis is not easy to dissolve and is not easily absorbed because the substance inhibits the activity of hydrolase in the necrotic foci. Caseous necrosis is also found in some infarcts, tumors and tuberculous leprosy and so on.

(5) Fat Necrosis

Cells release trypsin decomposing fat when acute pancreatitis, fat cell can be decomposed during breast injury, both of which can cause enzymolysis and traumatic fat necrosis, also included in liquefaction necrosis. After fat necrosis, the released fatty acids are combined with calcium ions to form a gray, white calcium soap that is visible grossly.

(6) Gangrene

Gangrene is defined as large tissue necrosis and infection secondary, it can be divided into dry gangrene, moist gangrene, and gas gangrene, in which the two formers are developed from ischemic necrosis caused by disturbance of blood circulation.

Dry gangrene: it is often seen in the terminal limb whose arteries are obstructed but veins are not. It is dry, crinkle, and black due to the loss of water (because Fe^{2+} is combined with H_2S in the corrupt tissue, forming the color of iron sulfide). It forms obvious limit with normal tissue, the corrupt changes are slight (Figure 1-9).

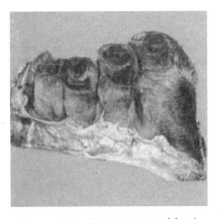

Figure 1-9   **dry gangrene of food**

When dry gangrene involves toes, the toes are black, dry, and have clear boundary with the surrounding tissue, is the ischemic necrosis caused by thromboangiitis obliterans. The toe has come off

Moist gangrene: it often occurs in the viscera interlinked with the outside such as lung, intestine, uterus, appendix and gallbladder, the same as a limb. There is a lot of water in the necrosis tissue, It is easy for bacteria to reproduce, so the swollen tissue is blue-green and the boundaries of the surrounding organization are not clear.

Gas gangrene: It also belongs to moist gangrene, is the open injury to deep muscle, combined with infection of anaerobes such as bacilli perfringens. In addition to necrosis, gas can be produced, which makes necrosis tissue feel like twisting hair.

Moist and gas gangrene are often accompanied with system poisoning symptom. In this type of necrosis, most dry gangrene belongs to coagulative necrosis, and moist gangrene can be the mix of coagulative necrosis or liquefactive necrosis.

1.4.1.3   Outcomes of Necrosis

(1) Dissolution and Absorption

Necrotic cells and neutrophils around release hydrolases, making necrotic tissue dissolved, liquefied, absorbed by lymphatic vessels or blood vessels. The fragments that cannot be absorbed are swallowed up by macrophages. When the necrotic liquefaction is large, the capsule can be formed. After the necrotic cells dissolved, the acute inflammatory response can be caused in the tissue around.

(2) Separation and Discharge

When necrotic foci are larger and not completely absorbed, the necrotic substance of epidermis can be separated and form tissue defects. The shallow is called erosion and the deep is called ulcer. Deep blind tube that only opens on the surface of skin and mucosa after tissue necrosis is called sinus. A channel-like a defect that connects two visceral organs or the organ to the body surface is known as a fistula. After liquefaction, necrosis in lung, kidney and other organs can be discharged through bronchia, ureter and other natural pipeline, the residual cavity called the hole(cavity).

(3) Organization and Encapsulation

The process that new granulation tissue takes the place of necrotic tissue, thrombus, pus, and foreign body is called organization. If the necrotic tissue is too large, granulation tissue can hardly grow into or absorb into the central part. It will be wrapped by the granulation tissue around it, which is called encapsulation. The encapsulation of granulation tissue formed by organization and encapsulation can eventually form a fibrous scar.

Calcification: If necrotic cells and cell debris are not promptly removed, the calcium salt and other mineral are easily attracted and deposit, which can cause dystrophic calcification.

1.4.1.4   The effect of Necrosis

The effect of necrosis on the body is related to the following factors:

1) the physiological importance of necrotic cells, such as the serious consequences of necrosis in the heart and brain tissue.

2) the number of necrotic cells, such as extensive necrosis of the liver cells, can cause the body to die.

3) the regeneration of similar cells around necrotic cells. For example, liver and epidermis are easy to regenerate. The structure and function of necrotic tissue are easy to recover. But neurons and cardiomyocytes can not regenerate after necrosis.

4) the reserve and compensatory capacity of necrotic organs. For example, kidney, lung and other paired organs have a strong reserve and metabolic capacity.

1.4.2 Apoptosis

Apoptosis is a manifestation of programmed cell death in single cell of local tissue in vivo. It is a way of cell death induced by internal and external factors triggering the cell death process. It is different from necrosis in morphological and biochemical characteristics. Apoptosis plays an irreplaceable role in the development of biological embryogenesis, mature cells, new and old alternation, hormone-dependent physiological degradation, atrophy and aging, as well as autoimmune diseases and tumor progression. It is not only a product of cell damage.

1.4.2.1   Morphological and Biochemical Characteristics of Apoptosis

Morphology of apoptosis(Figure 1-10) can be: ①Cell shrunken: The cytoplasm is dense, the water is reduced, the cytoplasm is highly eosinophilic, and the apoptotic cells are separated from the surrounding cells. ②Chromatins condensation, nuclear chromatin concentrate to dense clumps(pyknosis), or arrange on the inner surface of the karyotheca assembly(nuclear chromatin edge accumulation), then the nucleus split into pieces(karyorrhexis). ③The formation of apoptotic body: the cell membrane invaginates, cytoplasm buds and then fall away, forming nuclear debris and apoptotic body wrapped in the membrane of organelles. The apoptotic body is an important morphological marker of apoptosis, it can be phagocytized and degraded by the macrophage. ④Integrity of plasma membrane: because of the complete plasma membrane in the apoptotic cells, the recognition with other cells are prevented. Therefore, they neither cause inflammatory reaction nor induce proliferation and repair of surrounding cells. Eosinophilic body in the hepatocytes of viral hepatitis is the expression of hepatocyte apoptosis.

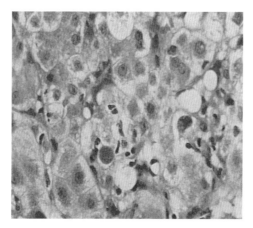

Figure 1-10   apoptosis of liver cells(HE, low power)

Under high power lens, the apoptosis of single hepatocyte can be seen in the center vision, separated from the adjacent cells, the cytoplasmic eosinophilic is obviously enhanced, the cell is solid, and the apoptosis body is formed

Biochemical characteristics of apoptosis are the activation of aspartic protease containing cysteine, Ca^{2+}/Mg^{2+} dependent endonuclease and calpain. Caspases in normal cells are zymogen, when activated it can crack many important cell protein, disrupt cytoskeleton and nuclear skeleton; and then activate restriction endonuclease. DNA degradation fragments of 180-200 dp can be seen in an early stage, characteristic DNA the ladder can be seen in agar gel electrophoresis. The apoptotic protease and endonuclease are the main executors of the program.

1.4.2.2   Mechanism of Apoptosis

Apoptosis can be divided into three stage: signal transduction, central control and structural change, in which the two former are starting stages and the last is execution stage. The signal transduction combines with the related protein Fas(CD95) and Fas ligand(Fas-L) by the exogenous(death receptor initiation) pathway, TNF-α receptor on the cell surface, introducing the apoptotic signals into the cell. Central regulation is activated by mitochondrial permeability and apoptotic molecules such as cytochrome C cytoplasm is released, it is though endogenous pathway(mitochondrial pathways). On the basis of the first two, the apoptotic protease activates the cascade reaction, and the apoptotic body appears to be morphologically changed.

The factors regulating apoptosis include inhibitory factors and inducing factors. The former includes growth factor, cell matrix, sex steroid hormone and some viral proteins and so on. The latter is growth factor deficiency, glucocorticoid, free radicals and ionizing radiation. There are dozens of genes involved in the apoptosis process. Among them. Bad\Bax\Bak\p53 and other genes have the effect of promoting apoptosis. Bcl-2\Bcl-xL\Bcl-AL and other genes have the effect of inhibiting apoptosis. C-myc and other genes may have two-way regulation, it induces proliferation when growth factor is enough, induces apoptosis when growth factor is lack.

It is necessary to point out that cell death is similar to apoptosis in the way of inducing way of cell death, morphological feature and biochemical characters. For example, pyknosis, karyorrhexis and nuclear chromatin edge accumulation can also be seen in the process of apoptosis in addition to cell death; the ladder feature of agar gel electrophoresis during apoptosis can sometimes be seen in necrotis cell.

In addition, cell death can also be caused by cell autophagy. Cell rough endoplasmic reticulum membrane without ribosomal or lysosomal membrane protrudes, engulfing, and encapsulating cells, forming autophagy bodies(autophagic vesicles), and then merges with lysosomes to form autophagic lysosomes, so as to degrade the contents wrapped, this process is called autophagy. Under physiological condition, cells can eliminate digestive, damaged, denatured, senescent and dysfunctional cell organelles and various biological macromolecules through autophagy, and achieve the recycling and utilization of cell materials, and provide raw materials for cell reconstruction and regeneration. In the pathological condition, autophagy can resist the invasion of the pathogen and protect the cells from the damage of poison. Too much or too less autophagy can cause cell death, and play an important role in the development of immunity, infection, cardiovascular diseases, neurodegenerative diseases and tumors. Autophagy has the similar stimulant factors and regulates proteins with apoptosis, but a different evoked threshold. Autophagy can cause cell death by inducing apoptosis.

1.5   Cellular Aging

Cell aging is a degenerative change that occurs with the growth of the aging body. It is the basis of the aging in individual organisms. Biological individuals and their cells must undergo growth, development, aging and death, and aging is the necessity of life development. It should be said that, the aging process has begun from the time of birth in any cell.

1.5.1   Characters of Cellular Aging

Cellular aging has some characters as follow: ①Universality: Aging can appear to vary degrees in all cells, tissues, organs and bodies. ②Progressivity and irreversibility: As time goes on, aging continues to develop. ③Endogenous: It's not the direct effect of external causes such as trauma, but the decline in the cell's inherent genetic decision. ④Harmful: When aging, cellular metabolism, adaptation and compensation and other functions are low, and lack of recovery ability, which leads to the emergence of geriatric diseases. The morbidity and mortality of other diseases are also increasing.

1.5.2 Morphology of Cellular Aging

Synthesis of structural proteins, enzyme protein and receptor protein when cells age, decreases, and the ability to absorb nutrition and repair chromosomal damage decreases. The morphology is characterized by cell volume reduction, water loss, cell and nucleus deformations, mitochondria and Golgi bodies decrease, distorts or shows vacuole-shape, cytoplasmic pigmentation (lipofuscin) can be seen. Thus, the weight of organs is reduced, interstitial hyperplasia and hardening can be seen, functional metabolism decrease, and reserve function is insufficient.

1.5.3 Mechanism of Cellular Aging

It is not clear, mainly has two types: genetic programming theory and error accumulation theory.

1.5.3.1 Genetic Programming Theory

According to the genetic programming theory, the aging of cells is determined by the genetic factors of the body, that is, the growth, development, maturation and aging of cells are completed by a certain gene in the cell gene bank expressing successively by pre-arranged procedures. The final death is the result of exhaustion of genetic information. For example, human fibroblasts in vitro stop splitting after about 50 division. The phenomenon that monozygotic twins live and die together supports the genetic programming theory. Some studies have shown that the mechanism which controls a number of cell divisions is closely related to the telomere structure at the end of the chromosomes.

Telomere is a special structure of eukaryotic cell chromosome ends. It consists of a repeated sequence of non-transcribed short segments DNA and some binding proteins. Telomere has functions of avoiding the fusion and degeneration of the chromosome ends. It plays an important role in chromosome stability, replication, protection and control of cell growth and longevity, and is closely related to apoptosis and cell immortalization.

The telomere at the ends of the chromosomes will gradually shorten with each cell division. This is because the DNA polymerase that copies DNA can not replicate the DNA at the end of the linear chromosome. Usually, the telomere shortens about 50−200 nucleotides once the cells divide until the cells are senescent and stop division, so the obviously shortened telomere is the signal of cell aging.

Telomerase is an inverse transcriptase that prolongs the shortened telomere, and is a ribonucleoprotein complex (RNP) composed of RNA and protein. It uses self RNA as a template to synthesize the telomere fragments and connect them to the telomere ends of the chromosomes, which restores and stabilizes the telomere length at the end of the chromosome. Most of the mature somatic cells do not exhibit telomerase activity. In germ cells and some stem cells need long-term replication, the telomere shortened after cell division can be recovered by the activity of telomerase in the cell and maintained in a certain length. More significant finding is in immortalized cancer cells, telomerase also shows obvious activity, which brings new hope for tumor therapy research targeting for telomerase activity.

Telomere and telomerase theory can explain the aging process of most differentiated mature cells. However, there may be other aging mechanisms for those neurons and cardiomyocytes with the low ability of division and proliferation. In addition, in the lower organisms, the degradation gene clk-1 and the mechanical sensing gene DAF-2 can change the growth rate and time of cell development process, and also play the role of genetic control of aging, but their role in mammalian animals needs to be confirmed.

1.5.3.2 Error Accumulation Theory

In addition to the procedural mechanism of cell heredity, the length of cell life is also dependent on the injury caused by metabolism and the balance between the molecular responses after injury. During cell division, damage from free radicals and other harmful substances can induce lipid peroxidation and damage the mobility, permeability and integrity of mitochondrion and so on. The DNA breakage mutation causes the mistake of its repair and replication process. When DNA is duplicated, the p53 gene with the function of cell cycle G1 detection and correction is activated, and its protein products induce the transcription enhancement of cyclin-dependent kinase inhibitor(CDKI), p21 and p16. The binding of p21 and p16 to cyclin-dependent kinase(CDK) and cyclin complexes can inhibit activity of CDK. The increase of p16 also activates the dephosphorylation of the retinoblastoma gene(Rb gene), which further impede the cell division from multiple links. There is evidence that the expression of P16 and other genes in the stem cells increases with age, and the stem cells themselves gradually lose their self-renewal capacity. At the same time, with the accumulation of errors, abnormal proteins from, the function of the original protein peptides and enzymes disappears, leading to the aging of the cells eventually.

In addition, as the age of individuals increases, lymphocytes T and B decrease, NK cell activity decreases, cytokine activity decreases, immune recognition ability is disordered. On the one hand, foreign bodies such as pathogens and tumor cells cannot be eliminated, on the other hand, it leads to autoimmune disease. Neuroendocrine disorders are also one of the important characteristics of aging. The hypothalamic-pituitary-adrenal system plays an important role in aging. When aging, neurons can also be lose to varying degrees. The release of catecholamine and other neurotransmitters are reduced, and production of sex hormones are reduced, the function of hormones receptor decrease.

To sum up, the mechanism of cell aging includes both the role of genetic programming factors and the effect of harmful factors accumulation in the intracellular and external environment. The aging of cells in the body can be carried out in accordance with the speed of genetic regulation. The natural lifespan(natural aging) can be achieved. If the harmful factors impede the metabolic function of the cell, the cell aging will be accelerated. Therefore, it can be said that in the decisive background of genetic arrangement, cell metabolic disorders are the factors contributing to the aging of cells.

Chapter 2

Tissue Repair

Repair refers to the restoration of tissue/cell architecture and function after any injury or disease. It contains two types of reactions: complete regeneration (means the injured tissues are able to replace the damaged components and essentially return to a normal state) and fibrous repair or scar formation (means the injured tissues are incapable of complete restitution, or the supporting structures of the tissue are severely damaged, repair occurs by laying down of connective tissue). After many common types of injury, both types contribute in varying degrees to the ultimate repair. Repair involves the proliferation of various cells, and close interactions between cells and the extracellular matrix (ECM). The mechanism of repairing depends on the type of inflammation, the extent of tissue necrosis, the types of cells involved and the regenerative ability of damaged parenchymal cells.

2.1 Regeneration

Regeneration can be physiological regeneration (e. g. in gut epithelium), it can also be pathological regeneration (e. g. cell and tissue injury, the replacement of lost parenchymal cells by division of adjacent surviving parenchymal cells to restore injured tissue).

2.1.1 Cell Cycle and the Regeneration Capacity of Different Types of Cell

The key processes in the proliferation of cells are DNA replication and mitosis. The cell cycle consists of the presynthetic growth phase 1 (G1), the DNA synthesis phase (S), the premitotic growth phase 2 (G2), and the mitotic phase (M). Any stimulus that initiates cell proliferation, such as exposure to growth factors. Checkpoint controls prevent DNA replication or mitosis of damaged cells and either transiently stop the cell cycle to allow for DNA repair or eliminate irreversibly damaged cells by apoptosis. Once cells enter the S phase, the DNA is replicated and the cell progresses through G2 and mitosis. The ability of cells to repair themselves is critically influenced by their intrinsic proliferative capacity. Based on this, the cells are divided into three groups.

2.1.1.1 Labile Cells (Continuously Dividing Cell)

These cells are continuously being lost and replaced by maturation from stem cells and by proliferation of mature cells. Labile cells include hematopoietic cells in the bone marrow and majority of surface epithelia, such as the stratified squamous surfaces of the skin, oral cavity, vagina, and cervix; the cuboidal epithelia of the ducts draining exocrine organs; the columnar epithelium of the gastrointestinal tract, uterus, and fallopian tubes and the transitional epithelium of the urinary tract. These tissues can readily regenerate after injury as long as the stem cells are preserved.

2.1.1.2   Stable Cells(Quiescent Cell)

These cells are quiescent and have only minimal replicative activity in their physiological state. However, they are capable of proliferating in response to injury or loss of tissue mass. Stable cells constitute the parenchyma of most solid tissues, such as liver, kidney, and pancreas. They also include endothelial cells, fibroblasts, and the proliferation of these cells is particularly important in wound healing.

2.1.1.3   Permanent Cells(Nondividing Cell)

These cells are considered to be terminally differentiated and nonproliferative in postnatal life. The majority of neurons and cardiac muscle cells belong to this category. Thus, injury to brain or heart is irreversible and results in a scar, because neurons and cardiac myocytes do not divide. Skeletal muscle is usually classified as a permanent tissue, but satellite cells attached to the endomysial sheath provide some regenerative capacity for this tissue. In permanent tissues, repair is typically dominated by scar formation.

2.1.1.4   Stem Cells

In most continuously dividing tissues the mature cells are terminally differentiated and short-lived. As mature cells die the tissue is replenished by the differentiation of cells generated from stem cells. Stem cells are characterized by two important properties; self-renewal capacity and asymmetric replication. Asymmetric replication of stem cells means that after each cell division, some progeny enter a differentiation pathway, while others remain undifferentiated, retaining their self-renewal capacity. Stem cells with the capacity to generate multiple cell lineages(pluripotent stem cells) can be isolated from embryos and are called embryonic stem(ES) cells. Stem cells are normally present in proliferative tissues and generate cell lineages specific for the tissue. However, it is now recognized that stem cells with the capacity to generate multiple lineages are present in the bone marrow and several other tissues of adult individuals. These cells are called tissue stem cells or adult stem cells.

2.1.2   Tissue Regeneration

2.1.2.1   Epithelial Regeneration

Cell renewal occurs continuously in labile cells, such as gut epithelium, skin. Damage to epithelia can be corrected by the proliferation and differentiation of stem cells. Tissue regeneration can occur in parenchymal organs with stable cell populations. Pancreas, adrenal, thyroid, and lung tissues have some regenerative capacity. Much more dramatic, however, is the regenerative response of the liver that occurs after surgical removal of hepatic tissue. As much as 40% to 60% of the liver may be removed in a procedure called living-donor transplantation, in which a portion of the liver is resected from a normal individual and is transplanted into a recipient with end-stage liver disease, or after partial hepatectomies performed for tumor removal. In all of these situations, the tissue resection triggers a proliferative response of the remaining hepatocytes(which are normally quiescent) , and the subsequent replication of hepatic nonparenchymal cells.

2.1.2.2   Regeneration of Bone and Cartilage

Injury of bone tissue is followed by rapid regeneration. In mature cartilage, the injury defects are likely to be filled with fibrous tissues or the lesion may precipitate a degeneration of adjacent cartilage. Fibroblasts from the sheath of the injured tendon and other sources proliferate, become active, and lay down orderly collagen fibers, which can restore most of the original strength of the tendon. Injury to permanent cells is always followed by connective tissues/scar formation.

2.1.2.3 Angiogenesis

Angiogenesis refers to the healing process of blood vessel at the injury sites. It begins with the degradation of the basement membrane by proteases secreted by activated endothelial cells that migrate and proliferate. This leads to the formation of endothelial cell sprouts and vascular loops; and the capillary tubes develop with formation of tight junctions and deposition of a new basement membrane (Figure 2-1). But permeability of the new capillary wall is increasing undergoing the incomplete basement membrane.

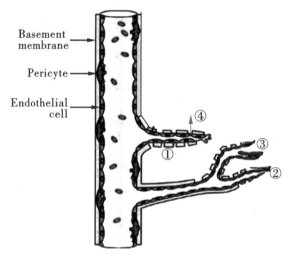

Figure 2-1   Model of angiogenesis

①degradation of the basement membrane; ②migration and
proliferation of endothelial cells; ③formation of endothelial cell
sprouts and vascular loops; ④increasing permeability

2.1.2.4 Regeneration of Peripheral Nerves

If the peripheral nerve has been transected, the axon distal to the injury site rapidly degenerates and eventually disappears. The myelin sheath and axon of the remaining intact nerve degenerates back to the next node of Ranvier. Then macrophages enter this area to remove the myelin and axonal debris. Schwan cells line up in the basement membrane tube and synthesize growth factors, inducing axonal sprouts formed at the terminal end of the proximal segment of the severed axon. The basement membrane tubes provide pathways for the regeneration axons to follow to muscles and skin (Figure 2-2). Axonal regeneration may be accompanied by recovery of function in the denervated area. If there has been severe trauma to nerve and disruption of its fascicular architecture or long distance between two ends of nerve disconnection, a fibrous scar can form and obstruct regenerated axons.

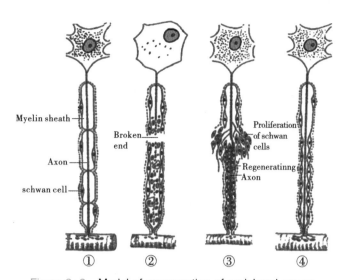

Figure 2-2   Model of regeneration of peripheral nerves

①Normal nerve fiber;②Broken nerve fiber;③Regeneration of nerve fiber;④after regeneration

2.1.3   Influence Factors of Regeneration

2.1.3.1   Growth Factors

Most growth factors have pleiotropic effects; they stimulate the cellular proliferation, migration, differentiation and contractility, and enhance the synthesis of specialized proteins (such as collagen in fibroblasts). A growth factor may act on a specific cell type or multiple cell types. They induce cell proliferation by binding to specific receptors and affecting the expression of genes whose products typically have several functions, they prevent apoptosis, and enhance the synthesis of cellular proteins in preparation for mitosis. A major activity of growth factors is to stimulate the function of growth control genes, many of which are called proto-oncogenes because mutations in them lead to unrestrained cell proliferation characteristic of cancer (oncogenesis). Some growth factors stimulate proliferation of some cells and inhibit cycling of other cells. In fact, a growth factor can have opposite effects on the same cell depending on its concentration. There is a list of mainly growth factors and their functions (Table 2-1).

Table 2-1   Growth factors involved in regeneration and wound healing

Cytokine	Source	Functions
Epidermal growth factor (EGF)	Activated macrophages, salivary glands, keratinocytes, at el	Mitogenic for keratinocytes and fibroblasts; stimulates keratinocyte migration and granulation tissue formation
Transforming growth factor a(TGF-α)	Activated macrophages, T lymphocytes, keratinocytes, at el	Similar to EGF; stimulates replication of Hepatocytes and many epithelial cells
Transforming growth factor β(TGF-β)	macrophages, endothelial cells, keratinocytes, SMCs, fibroblasts-platelets, T lymphocytes	Chemotactic for PMNs, macrophages, lymphocytes, fibroblasts, and SMCs; stimulates angiogenesis, and fibroplasia; inhibits production of MMPs and keratinocyte proliferation; regulates integrin expression and other cytokines
Vascular endothelial cell growth factor(VEGF)	Mesenchymal cells	Increases vascular permeability; mitogenic for endothelial cells

Continue to Table 2-1

Cytokine	Source	Functions
Platelet-derived growth factor(PDGF)	Platelets, macrophages, endothelial cells, keratinocytes, SMCs	Similar to TGF-β; mitogenic, for fibroblasts, endothelial cells, and SMCs; stimulates production of MMPs, fibronectin, and HA; stimulates angiogenesis and wound remodeling; regulates integrin expression
Keratinocyte growth factor(KGF)	Fibroblasts	Stimulates keratinocyte migration, proliferation, and differentiation

SMCs: Smooth muscle cells; PMNs: Polymorph nuclear neutrophils; MMPs: Matrix Metalloproteinases; HA: Hyaluronic acid

2.1.3.2 Cell Surface Receptors

Receptor proteins are generally located on the cell surface, but the ligands must be sufficiently hydrophobic to enter the cell(e. g. vitamin D, or steroid and thyroid hormones). The binding of a ligand to its cell surface receptor leads to a cascade of secondary intracellular events that culminate in transcription factor activation or repression, leading to cellular responses. These are usually transmembrane molecules with an extracellular ligand-binding domain; ligand binding causes stable dimerization with subsequent phosphorylation of the receptor subunits.

2.1.3.3 Extracellular Matrix(ECM)

Tissue repair depends not only on growth factor activity but also on interactions between cells and ECM components. By supplying a substratum for cell adhesion and serving as a reservoir for growth factors, ECM regulates the proliferation, movement, and differentiation of the cells living within it. Synthesis and degradation of ECM accompanies morphogenesis, wound healing, chronic fibrotic processes, and tumor invasion and metastasis. Its various functions include: ①Mechanical support for cell anchorage, cell migration and maintenance of cell polarity. ②Control of cell growth. ③Maintenance of cell differentiation. ④Scaffolding for tissue renewal. ⑤Establishment of tissue microenvironments. Basement membrane acts as a boundary between epithelium and underlying connective tissue and also forms part of the filtration apparatus in the kidney. ⑥Storage and presentation of regulatory molecules.

Collagen: The collagens are composed of three separate polypeptide chains braided into a ropelike triple helix. The collagen proteins are rich in hydroxyproline and hydroxylysine. About 30 collagen types have been identified, some of which are unique to specific cells and tissues. The fibrillar collagens form a major proportion of the connective tissue in healing wounds and particularly in scars. The tensile strength of the fibrillar collagens derives from their cross-linking, which is the result of covalent bonds catalyzed by the enzyme lysyl-oxidase. Genetic defects in these collagens cause diseases such as osteogenesis imperfecta and Ehlers-Danlos syndrome. Other collagens are nonfibrillar and may form basement membrane(type IV), or be components of other structures such as intervertebral discs(type IX) or dermal-epidermal junctions(type VII).

Elastin: Although tensile strength is derived from the fibrillar collagens, the ability of tissues to recoil and return to a baseline structure after physical stress is conferred by elastic tissue. This is especially important in the walls of large vessels, as well as in the uterus, skin, and ligaments. Elastins require a glycine in every third position, but they differ from collagen by having fewer cross-links. The fibrillin meshwork serves as a scaffold for the deposition of elastin and assembly of elastic fibers; defects in fibrillin synthesis lead to skeletal abnormalities and weakened aortic walls(Marfan syndrome).

Proteoglycans and Hyaluronan: Proteoglycans consist of long polysaccharides called glycosaminoglycans linked to a protein backbone. Hyaluronan, a huge molecule composed of many disaccharide repeats without a protein core, is also an important constituent of the ECM. Because of its ability to bind water, it forms a viscous, gelatin-like matrix. Besides providing compressibility to a tissue, proteoglycans also serve as reservoirs for growth factors secreted into the ECM. Proteoglycans can also be integral cell membrane proteins and have roles in cell proliferation, migration, and adhesion.

Adhesive Glycoproteins and Adhesion Receptors: Adhesive glycoproteins and adhesion receptors are structurally diverse molecules involved in cell-to-cell adhesion, the linkage between cells and ECM, and binding between ECM components. The adhesive glycoproteins include fibronectin(major component of the interstitial ECM) and laminin(major constituent of basement membrane). The adhesion receptors, also known as cell adhesion molecules(CAMs), are grouped into four families: immunoglobulins, cadherins, selectins, and integrins.

Fibronectin is a large(450kD) disulfide-linked heterodimer synthesized by a variety of cells. Fibronectin messenger RNA(mRNA) has two splice forms, which generate tissue and plasma fibronectin. Fibronectins have specific domains that bind to a wide spectrum of ECM components and can also attach to cell integrins via a tripeptide arginine-glycine-aspartic acid motif. Tissue fibronectin forms fibrillar aggregates at wound healing sites; plasma fibronectin binds to fibrin to form the provisional blood clot of a wound.

Laminin is the most abundant glycoprotein in basement membrane. It is a 820 kD cross-shaped heterotrimer that connects cells to underlying ECM components such as type Ⅳ collagen and heparin sulfate. It can also modulate the cell proliferation, differentiation, and motility.

Integrins are a family of transmembrane heterodimeric glycoproteins composed of a and b chains that are the main cellular receptors for ECM components. They bind to many ECM components through RGD motifs, initiating signaling cascades that can affect cell locomotion, proliferation, and differentiation. Their intracellular domains link to actin filaments at focal adhesion complexes, through adaptor proteins such as talin and vinculin.

2.2 Fibrous Repair

If tissue injury is severe or chronic, and results in damage to parenchymal cells and epithelia as well as the stromal framework, or if nondividing cells are injured, repair cannot be accomplished by regeneration alone. Under these conditions, repair occurs by replacement of the nonregenerated cells with connective tissue, or by a combination of regeneration of some cells and scar formation.

2.2.1 Granulation Tissue

Repair begins within 24 hours of injury by the emigration of fibroblasts and the induction of fibroblast and endothelial cell proliferation. By 3 to 5 days, a specialized type of tissue that is characteristic of healing, called granulation tissue is apparent. The term granulation tissue derives from the pink, soft, granular gross appearance, such as that seen beneath the scab of a skin wound. Its histological appearance is characterized by proliferation of fibroblasts and new thin-walled, delicate capillaries and inflammatory cells such as the macrophages, neutrophils and lymphocytes(Figure 2-3). Macrophages can secrete PDGF, FGF, TGF-β and TNF, IL-1, with the PDGF released by platelets when blood-clotting on the surface of wound, can stimulate hyperplasia of fibroblasts and capillary. Macrophages and neutrophils can engulf bacteria and tissue pieces.

Granulation tissue has some important roles in the process of tissue repair: ①anti-infection and wound protection; ②filling the wound and other defective tissues; ③organization or wrapping the necrosis, thrombosis, inflammatory exudation, and other foreign tissues.

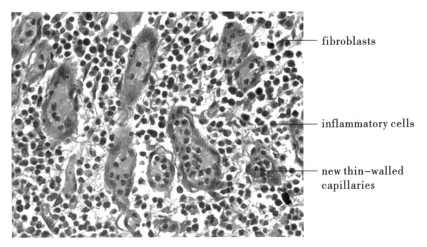

fibroblasts

inflammatory cells

new thin-walled capillaries

Figure 2-3   Granulation tissue(400×, HE stain)

2.2.2   Scar Tissue

Granulation tissue then progressively accumulates connective tissue matrix, eventually resulting in the formation of scar tissue(Figure 2-4). So scar tissue refers to the mature fibrous connective tissue redeveloped by granulation tissue. Repair by connective tissue deposition consists of four sequential processes: Formation of new blood vessels(angiogenesis); Migration and proliferation of fibroblasts; Deposition of ECM (scar formation); Maturation and reorganization of the fibrous tissue(remodeling). So the histological appearance of scar tissue is characterized by proliferation of a mass of collagen fiber and a little of fibrocytes, blood vessels. The gross appearance of scar tissue is characterized by local contraction, white or grey, translucent, strong, tough and inelastic.

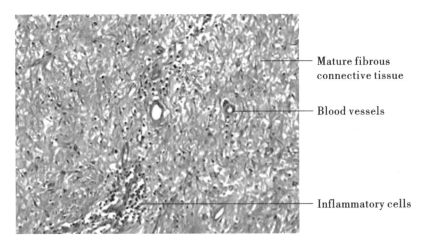

Mature fibrous connective tissue

Blood vessels

Inflammatory cells

Figure 2-4   Scar tissue(100×, HE stain)

Scar tissue has some beneficial roles in the process of tissue repair: ①filling the wound and other defective tissues, keeping the tissues integrity; ②keeping the tissues and organs strong.

But the scar tissue has also some harmful effects: ①Scar contraction, because of tough, inelastic, deformation caused by contraction, scar tissue can cause the organs dysfunction, especially for the joints and some important organs. ②Cicatricial adhesion, it often occurs between organs or organ and coelomic cavity wall, then affects the their function, such as extensive fibrosis, hyaline, sclerosis. ③Excessive hyperplasia of scar tissue, also called "hypertrophic scar". If this kind of hypertrophic scar protrude even sprawl from the skin, known as "keloid". Generally it is considered related to skin tension and physique.

2.2.3　Formation Course of Granulation Tissue and Scar

2.2.3.1　Angiogenesis

Blood vessels are assembled by two processes: vasculogenesis, in which the primitive vascular network is assembled from angioblasts(endothelial cell precursors)during embryonic development; and angiogenesis, or neovascularization, in which preexisting vessels send out capillary, sprouts to produce new vessels. Angiogenesis is a critical process in healing at sites of injury, in the development of collateral circulations at sites of ischemia, and in allowing tumors to increase in size beyond the constraints of their original blood supply. It has recently been found that endothelial precursor cells may migrate from the bone marrow to areas of injury and participate in angiogenesis at these sites.

The main steps that occur in angiogenesis from preexisting vessels are listed bellow.

1) Vasodilation in response to nitric oxide and increased permeability of the preexisting vessel induced by vascular endothelial growth factor(VEGF).

2) Migration of endothelial cells toward the area of tissue injury.

3) Proliferation of endothelial cells just behind the leading front of migrating cells

4) Inhibition of endothelial cell proliferation and remodeling into capillary tubes.

5) Recruitment of periendothelial cells(pericytes for small capillaries and smooth muscle cells for larger vessels)to form the mature vessel.

New vessels formed during angiogenesis are leaky because of incompletely formed interendothelial junctions and because VEGF increases vessel permeability. This leakiness explains why granulation tissue is often edematous, and accounts in part for the edema that may persist in healing wounds long after the acute inflammatory response has resolved. Structural ECM proteins participate in the process of vessel sprouting in angiogenesis, largely through interactions with integrin receptors in endothelial cells. Nonstructural ECM proteins contribute to angiogenesis by destabilizing cell-ECM interactions to facilitate continued cell migration or degrade the ECM to permit remodeling and in growth of vessels.

2.2.3.2　Growth Factors and Receptors Involved in Angiogenesis

Several factors induce angiogenesis, but the most important are VEGF and basic fibroblast growth factor (FGF-2). In angiogenesis originating from preexisting local vessels, VEGF stimulates both proliferation and motility of endothelial cells, thus initiating the process of capillary sprouting. VEGFs are dimeric glycoproteins with many isoforms and with different properties, such as VEGFs bind to a family of receptors(VEGFR-1, VEGFR-2, and VEGFR-3)with tyrosine kinase activity. The most important of these receptors for angiogenesis is VEGFR-2, which is restricted to endothelial cells. VEGF acts through VEGFR-2 to mobilize these cells from the bone marrow and to induce proliferation and motility of these cells at the sites of angiogenesis. Targeted mutations in this receptor result in lack of vasculogenesis. Several agents can induce VEGFs, the most important being hypoxia. Other inducers are platelet-derived growth factor(PDGF), TGF-α, and TGF-β. Regardless of the process that leads to capillary formation, new vessels need to be stabilized by the recruitment of pericytes and smooth muscle cells and by the deposition of connective tissue. Angiopoietins 1 and 2(Ang 1 and Ang 2)and PDGF, TGF-β participate in the stabilization process. In particular, Ang l interacts with a receptor on endothelial cells called Tie2 to recruit periendothelial cells. PDGF participates in the recruitment of smooth muscle cells; TGF-β enhances the production of ECM proteins. FGFs constitute a family of factors with more than 20 members. The best characterized are FGF-1 (acidic FGF) and FGF-2 (basic FGF). Released FGF can bind to heparin sulfate and be stored in the ECM. FGF-2 participates in angiogenesis mostly by stimulating the proliferation of endothelial cells. It also promotes the migration of macrophages and fibroblasts to the damaged area, and stimulates epithelial cell migration to cover epidermal wounds.

2.2.3.3　Scar Formation

Scar formation builds on the granulation tissue framework of new vessels and loose ECM that develop early at the repair site. It occurs in two steps: ①migration and proliferation of fibroblasts into the site of injury; ②deposition of ECM by these cells.

As healing progresses, the number of proliferating fibroblasts and new vessels decreases; however, the fibroblasts progressively assume a more synthetic phenotype, and hence there is increased deposition of ECM. Collagen synthesis, in particular, is critical to the development of strength in a healing wound site. Collagen synthesis by fibroblasts begins early in wound healing (days 3 to 5) and continues for several weeks, depending on the size of the wound. Ultimately, the granulation tissue scaffolding evolves into a scar composed of largely inactive, spindle-shaped fibroblasts, dense collagen, fragments of elastic tissue. As the scar matures, there is progressive vascular regression, which eventually transforms the highly vascularized granulation tissue into a pale, largely avascular scar.

(1) Growth Factors Involved in ECM Deposition and Scar Formation

Many growth factors are involved in these processes, including TGF-β, PDGF, and FGF. TGF-β belongs to a family of homologous polypeptides (TGF-β1, TGF-β2, and TGF-β3) that includes other members such as bone morphogenetic proteins, activins, and inhibins. In the context of inflammation and repair, TGF-β has two main functions: ①TGF-β is a potent fibrogenic agent. ②TGF-β inhibits lymphocyte proliferation and can have a strong anti-inflammatory effect. PDGF causes migration and proliferation of fibroblasts, smooth muscle cells, and macrophages. Cytokines may also function as growth factors and participate in ECM deposition and scar formation. IL-1 and TNF, for example, induce fibroblast proliferation and can have a fibrogenic effect. They are also chemotactic for fibroblasts and stimulate the synthesis of collagen and collagenase by these cells.

(2) ECM and Tissue Remodeling

The transition from granulation tissue to scar involves shifts in the composition of the ECM; even after its synthesis and deposition, scar ECM continues to be modified and remodeled. The outcome of the repair process is, in part, a balance between ECM synthesis and degradation. The degradation of collagens and other ECM components is accomplished by a family of matrix metalloproteinases (MMPs), which are dependent on zinc ions for their activity. MMPs include interstitial collagenases, which cleave fibrillar collagen (MMP-1, MMP-2 and MMP-3); gelatinases (MMP-2 and MMP-9), which degrade amorphous collagen and fibronectin; and stromelysins (MMP-3, 10, and-11), which degrade a variety of ECM constituents, including proteoglycans, laminin, fibronectin, and amorphous collagen. The synthesis of MMPs is inhibited by TGF-β and may be suppressed pharmacologically with steroids. In addition, activated collagenases can be rapidly inhibited by specific tissue inhibitors of metalloproteinases (TIMPs), produced by most mesenchymal cells.

2.3   Wound Healing

2.3.1   Cutaneous Wound Healing

Cutaneous wound healing has four main phases: ①inflammation; ②wounds contract; ③formation of granulation tissue and scar; ④ECM deposition and remodeling, Re-epithelialization of the wound surface. Based on the nature of the wound, the healing of cutaneous wounds can occur by first or second intention.

2.3.1.1   Healing by First Intention

One of the simplest examples of wound repair is the healing of a clean, uninfected surgical incision approximated by surgical sutures. This is referred to as primary union, or healing by first intention. The incision causes only focal disruption of epithelial basement membrane continuity and death of a relatively few epithelial and connective tissue cells. As a result, epithelial regeneration predominates over fibrosis. A small scar is formed, but there is minimal wound contraction. The narrow incisional space first fills with fibrin-clotted blood, which is rapidly invaded by granulation tissue and covered by new epithelium. Within 24 hours, neutrophils are seen at the incision margin, migrating toward the fibrin clot. Basal cells at the cut edge of the epidermis begin to show increased mitotic activity. Within 24 to 48 hours, epithelial cells from both edges have begun to migrate and proliferate along the dermis, depositing basement membrane components as they progress. By day 3, neutrophils have been largely replaced by macrophages, and granulation tissue progressively invades the incision space. Collagen fibers are now evident at the incision margins, but these are vertically oriented and do not bridge the incision. Epithelial cell proliferation continues, yielding a thickened epidermal covering layer. By day 5, neovascularization reaches its peak as granulation tissue fills the incisional space. Collagen fibrils become more abundant and begin to bridge the incision. The epidermis recovers its normal thickness as differentiation of surface cells yields a mature epidermal architecture with surface keratinization(Figure 2-5).

2.3.1.2   Healing by Second Intention

When cell or tissue loss is more extensive, such as in large wounds, abscess formation, and ulceration, the repair process is more complex. In second-intention healing, also known as healing by secondary union, the inflammatory reaction is more intense; there is abundant development of granulation tissue, and the wound contracts by the action of myofibroblasts. This is followed by accumulation of ECM and formation of a large scar. In larger wound, inflammation is more intense because large tissue defects have a greater volume of necrotic debris, exudates, and fibrin that must be removed. Consequently, large defects have a greater potential for secondary, inflammation-mediated, injury. Larger defects require a greater volume of granulation tissue to fill in the gaps and provide the underlying framework for the regrowth of tissue epithelium. A greater volume of granulation tissue generally results in a greater mass of scar tissue(Figure 2-5).

Secondary healing involves wound contraction. Within 6 weeks, for example, large skin defects maybe reduced by 5% to 10% of their original size, largely by contraction. This process has been ascribed to the presence of myofibroblasts, which are modified fibroblasts exhibiting many of the ultrastructural and functional features of contractile smooth muscle cells.

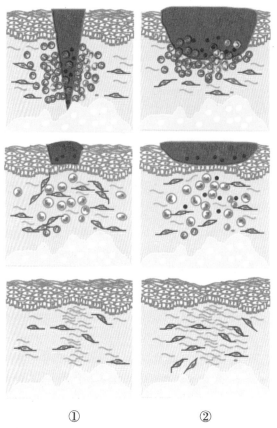

Figure 2-5　Model of wound healing

①Healing by first intention;②Healing by second intention

2.3.2　Fracture Healing

Fracture,the most common bone lesion,is defined as a break in the continuity of a bone. If the break occurs at the site of previous disease(e. g. a bone cyst,a malignant tumor),the result is a pathologic fracture. Traumatic fracture may be the result of an excessive impact,rotation,bending or other mechanical force action on previously normal bone. The repair of a fracture is a highly regulated process that can be artificially separated into overlapping histological,biochemical and biomechanical stages(Figure 2-6).

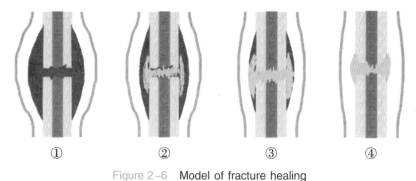

Figure 2-6　Model of fracture healing

①Hematoma;②Soft tissue callus;③Bony callus;④Bone remodeling

2.3.2.1　Hematoma

Immediately following fracture,rupture of blood vessels results in a hematoma,which fills the fracture gap and surrounds the area of bone injury. Many bone cells and other cells at the fracture site undergo necrosis as a result of physical injury ischemia. An acute inflammatory response occurs in regions of tissue injury and necrosis. Hematoma also provides a fibrin mesh, which helps seal off the fracture site and at the same time serves as a framework for the influx of inflammatory cells and ingrowths of fibroblast and capillary buds.

2.3.2.2   Soft Tissue Callus

Within a week, the involved tissue is primed for new matrix synthesis. This soft tissue callus is able to hold the ends of the fractured bone in apposition, but it is non-calcified and can not support weight bearing.

2.3.2.3   Bony Callus

Bone progenitors in the medullary cavity deposit new foci of woven bone, and activated mesenchymal cells at the fracture site differentiate into cartilage synthesizing g chondroblasts. In uncomplicated fracture, this early repair process peaks in 2−3 weeks. The newly formed cartilage acts as a nidus for endochondral ossification, recapitulating the process of bone formation in epiphyseal growth plawth plates. This bony callus bridges the fractured ends.

2.3.2.4   Bone Remodeling

Subsequent weight bearing leads to resorption of the callus and at the same time there is fortification of regions that support greater loads. This callus remodeling restores the original size and shape of the bone, including the spongy cancellous architecture of the medullary cavity.

The healing of a fracture healing process can be disrupted by many factors, such as displaced fracture, inadequate immobilization, too much motion, infection and calcium insufficiency. Generally, healing process varies tremendously among patients. Also, it is closely related to the age, health, fracture types and the bone involved.

2.3.3   Influence Factors of Repair

Wound healing may be altered by a variety of influences, frequently reducing the quality or adequacy of the reparative process. Particularly important are infections and diabetes. Variables that modify wound healing may be extrinsic(e. g. infection) or intrinsic to the injured tissue:

Infection is the single most important cause of delay in healing; it prolongs the inflammation phase of the process and potentially increases the local tissue injury. Nutrition has profound effects on wound healing; protein deficiency, for example, and particularly vitamin C deficiency, inhibits collagen synthesis and retards healing. Glucocorticoids(steroids) have well-documented anti-inflammatory effects, and their administration may result in poor wound strength due to diminished fibrosis. In some instances, however, the anti-inflammatory effects of glucocorticoids are desirable. For example, in corneal infections, glucocorticoids are sometimes prescribed(along with antibiotics) to reduce the likelihood of opacity that may result from collagen deposition. Mechanical variables such as increased local pressure or torsion may cause wounds to pull apart, or dehisce. Poor perfusion, due either to arteriosclerosis and diabetes or to obstructed venous drainage, also impairs healing. Finally, foreign bodies such as fragments of steel, glass, or even bone impede healing.

The location of the injury and the character off the tissue in which the injury occurs are also important. For example, inflammation arising in tissue spaces(e. g. pleural, peritoneal, synovial cavities) develops extensive exudates. Subsequent repair may occur by digestion of the exudates, initiated by the proteolytic enzymes of leukocytes and resorption of the liquefied exudate. This is called resolution, and in the absence of cellular necrosis, normal tissue architecture is generally restored. However, in the setting of larger accumulations, the exudates undergoes organization: granulation tissue grows into the exudates, and a fibrous scar ultimately forms.

Chapter 3

Regional Hemodynamic Disorders

❯ Introduction

The function and structure of cells and tissues require normal fluid homeostasis, which delivers oxygen and nutrients and removes wastes. Normal fluid homeostasis depends on the integrity of the vessel wall, the maintenance of intravascular pressure and the osmolarity of regional tissue. Abnormal fluid homeostasis is associated with the vascular volume or pressure, the plasma protein content, and the endothelial function, which changed by the tissue injury or disease. For example, the increased vascular volume is called hyperemia or congestion. The vessel wall integrity depends on the endothelial function and structure, which is involved in the thrombosis formation. In general, the inappropriate clotting(thrombosis) or movement of clots (embolism)can block blood supplies and cause cell or tissue infarction.

3.1   Hyperemia and Congestion

The terms hyperemia and congestion imply an increased volume of blood in a local tissue. Hyperemia usually happens in arteriolar dilation, which is an active process resulting from augmented blood flow. Congestion usually happens venously, which is a passive hyperemia resulting from impaired venous return out of a tissue, obstruction with the distal veins, venules and capillaries. The affected tissue has a red-blue color owing to the accumulation of deoxygenated hemoglobin.

Congestion might be caused by the three-factor: the pressure from the vessel wall, the obstruction in the vessel and heart failure. The left ventricular affectes the lung congestion and the right-side failure affectes the systemic organs, such as the liver, the limb. The congestive heart failure is the systemic phenomenon in the left and right ventricular failure.

Congestion of capillary beds is closely associated with the edema development, so that edema and congestion usually happen together. In long-standing congestion, called chronic passive congestion, the condition of poorly oxygenated blood results in chronic hypoxia, which could cause parenchymal cells degeneration or death, subsequently developed tissue fibrosis. A capillary rupture in chronic congestion may result in small foci of hemorrhage; phagocytosis and digestion of the erythrocyte debris can cause accumulations of hemosiderin-laden macrophages.

3.1.1   Morphology

Edema is also called congestion edema. In acute congestion, the cut surfaces of tissues and organs are excessively wet and hemorrhagic. In chronic passive congestion, the hypoxia results in the atrophy, degeneration or even death of the parenchymal cells. The deposition of microhemorrhages with hemosiderin and the formation of fibrous scarring commonly appear. These important organs, the lungs, liver and spleen develop the most obvious manifestation of chronic passive congestion.

3.1.2   Important Organs Congestion

3.1.2.1   Lungs Congestion

Lungs congestion is mainly associated with left ventricular failure, e. g. , myocardial infarction, myocarditis, cardiomyopathy, and so on. There is elevated left atrial pressure and consequent elevated pulmonary venous pressure. Microscopically, alveolar capillaries engorged with blood characterize acute pulmonary congestion; there may also be associated with alveolar septal edema or focal minuteintra-alveolar hemorrhage. In chronic pulmonary congestion, the septa become thickened and fibrotic, and numerous hemosiderin-laden macrophages("heart failure cells")(Figure 3-1)appear in the alveolar spaces. In time the fibrotic septa and together with the hemosiderin pigmentation constitute the basis for the designation brown indurations of lungs. The longtime congestion and consequent pulmonary may cause progressive thickening of the walls in the pulmonary arteries and arterioles.

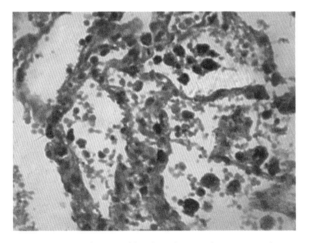

Figure 3-1   Lung with chronic passive congestion, the alveolar spaces are filled with edematous fluids and heart failure cells(hemosiderin-laden macrophages)

3.1.2.2   Liver Congestion

Acute and chronic hepatic congestion is associated with right-sided heart failure. In acute hepatic congestion, the liver is dark-red in grossly. Microscopically, the central vein and sinusoids are distended with blood. Therefore, there may even be central hepatocyte degeneration or necrosis; the periportal hepatocytes endure less severe hypoxia and may develop only fatty change. In chronic passive congestion, the hepatic lobule regions are grossly red-brown and slightly depressed(because of cell death)and are accentuated against the surrounding zones of uncongested tan, sometimes fatty, liver("nutmeg liver"; Figure 3-2). Microscopically, there is centrilobular necrosis with the hepatocyte dropout, hemorrhage, and hemosiderin-laden macrophages (Figure 3-3). In long-standing, severe hepatic congestion, the hepatic hemorrhagic fibrosis may develop. Because the central portion of the hepatic lobule is the last to receive blood. The centrilobular necrosis occurs whenever there is reduced hepatic blood flow; there need not be previous hepatic congestion.

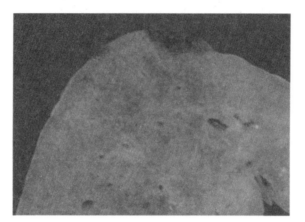

Figure 3-2   Liver with chronic passive congestion, central areas of the hepatic lobules are red-brown and slightly depressed compared with the surrounding zones viable parenchyma, forming a "nutmeg liver" pattern

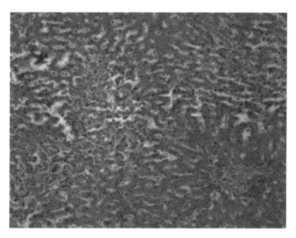

Figure 3-3   Liver with chronic passive congestion, centrilobular necrosis with degenerating hepatocytes and sinusoidal congestion

3.2   Hemorrhage

Hemorrhage means the rupture of blood vessels or the heart wall and the blood overflow from vessels or the heart wall into the extravascular space. Capillary bleeding can occur under conditions of chronic congestion. An increased tendency to hemorrhage with insignificant injury happens in a wide variety of clinical disorders collectively called hemorrhagic diathesis. However, the rupture of a large artery or vein is always due to vascular injury, including trauma, atherosclerosis, inflammatory or neoplastic erosion of the vessel wall, and results in severe hemorrhage.

Hemorrhage can be confined within a tissue or can be external; any accumulation within the tissue is referred to as hematoma. Hematomas might be relatively insignificant(as in the bruise), or might involve so much bleeding as to result in death. Minute(1–2 mm) hemorrhages into the skin, mucous membranes, or serosal surfaces are called petechiae, and the slightly larger(3–5 mm) hemorrhages are called purpura. Larger (1–2 cm in diameter) subcutaneous hematomas are called ecchymoses.

The red blood cells in local hemorrhages are phagocytosed and are degraded by macrophages; the hemoglobin(red-blue color) is enzymatically transformed to bilirubin(blue-green color) and eventually to hemosiderin(golden-brown), constituting of the characteristic color changes in the hematoma. Large accumulations of blood in the body cavities are called hemothorax, hemopericardium, hemoperitoneum, or hemarthrosis(in joints). Sometimes patients with extensive hemorrhages develop jaundice from the breakdown of massive erythrocytes and the systemic increased bilirubin.

The clinical significance of hemorrhage depends on the rate and the volume of blood loss, the site of hemorrhage. The rapid loss of as much as 20% of the blood volume, or the slow losses of larger amounts may have little impact on healthy adults; nevertheless, the greater losses can cause hemorrhagic shock. The hemorrhage site is also important; bleeding that would be trivial in the subcutaneous tissues may cause death if located in the brain or heart. The net iron loss can be great if hemorrhage occurs externally. Patients with chronic or recurrent external blood loss result in an iron deficiency anemia. In contrast, when red blood cells are retained in tissues or body cavities, the iron can be reutilized for hemoglobin synthesis.

3.3   Hemostasis and Thrombosis

3.3.1   *Normal Hemostasis*

Normal hemostasis is a consequence of regulated processes that maintain blood in a fluid, clot-free state in normal vessels while inducing the rapid formation of a localized hemostatic plug at the site of an injured vessel. The pathologic form of hemostasis is thrombosis, which involves the formation of thrombus in uninjured vessels or the thrombotic occlusion after relative injury.

After the initial injury, the arteriolar vasoconstriction occurs because of reflex neurogenic mechanisms and is augmented by the local secretion of factors such as endothelium. The effect is transient, and bleeding would resume were if not for activation of the platelet and coagulation factor. Three key contributors to hemostasis are: the vascular wall, particularly endothelium and underlying connective tissue, platelets and the coagulation cascade.

3.3.1.1   Endothelium

Endothelial cells modulate several aspects of normal hemostasis. The balance between endothelial anti thrombotic and prothrombotic activities determines whether thrombus formation, propagation, or dissolution occur.

(1) Antithrombotic Properties

①Antiplatelet effects: An intact endothelium prevents platelets from interacting with the highly thrombogenic subendothelial ECM. Endothelial prostacyclin and nitric oxides are potent vasodilators and inhibitors of platelet aggregation. ②Anticoagulant effects: Anticoagulant effects are mediated by membrane-associated, heparin-like molecules and thrombomodulin. Thrombomodulin binds to thrombin, converting it from a procoagulant to an anticoagulant capable of activating the anticoagulant protein C. ③Fibrinolytic properties: Endothelium synthesizes tissue plasminogen activator(t-PA), promoting fibrinolytic activity to clear fibrin deposits from endothelial surfaces.

(2)Prothrombotic Properties

Endothelium can become prothrombotic, with activities that affect platelets, coagulation protein, and the fibrinolytic system. The endothelial injury causes platelet adhesion to subendothelial collagen through won Willebrand factor(VWF). Loss of endothelium allows circulating VWF to bind to the basement membrane and induce platelets to adhere.

3.3.1.2　Platelets

Platelets play a critical role in normal hemostasis. After vascular injury, platelets encounter ECM constituents and undergo three reactions:

(1)Platelet Adhesion

Adhesion to ECM is mediated by interactions with VWF. Failure of the normal proteolytic processing of VWF leads to aberrant platelet aggregation in the circulation: this defect in VWF processing can cause thrombotic microangiopathies.

(2)Secretion

Secretion of both granule types occurs soon after adhesion. The release of dense body contents is especially important to platelet aggregation. Finally, platelet activation increases surface expression of phospholipid complexes and provide coagulation factors.

(3)Platelet Aggregation

Aggregation follows platelet adhesion and granule release. ADP and TXA promote the formation of the primary hemostatic plug. Thrombin converts fibrinogen to fibrin within the platelet plug to contribute to the stability of the clot. Thrombin contributes by directly stimulating neutrophil and monocyte adhesion from the cleavage of fibrinogen.

3.3.2　*The Pathogenesis of Thrombosis*

We discuss the dysregulation that underlies pathologic thrombus formation. Three primary influences predispose to thrombus formation, the so-called Virchow's triad: ①endothelial injury; ②turbulence of blood flow; ③hypercoagulability.

3.3.2.1　Endothelial Injury

The endothelial injury might lead to thrombosis. It is particularly important for thrombus formation occurring in the heart or arterial circulation, where the normal high flow rates might hamper clotting by preventing platelet adhesion or diluting coagulation factors. Thus, thrombus formation within the cardiac chambers, over ulcerated plaques in atherosclerotic arteries, or at sites of traumatic or inflammatory vascular injury(vasculitis)is largely due to endothelial injury. Regardless of the loss cause of endothelium, the end results will lead to exposure of subendothelial ECM, adhesion of platelets, the release of tissue factor, and local depletion of prostacyclin and plasminogen activator.

3.3.2.2　Turbulence of Blood Flow

Turbulence contributes to arterial and cardiac thrombosis by causing endothelial injury or dysfunction as well as by forming countercurrents and local pockets of stasis. Stasis is a major factor in the development of venous thrombi.

Normal blood flow is that the platelets flow centrally in the vessel lumen, separated from the endothelium by a slower-moving clear zone of plasma. Stasis and turbulence therefore, ①disrupt laminar flow and bring platelets into contact with the endothelium; ②prevent the dilution of activated clotting factors; ③retard the inflow of clotting factor inhibitors and permit the build-up of thrombi; and ④promote endothelial cell activation, predisposing to local thrombosis and leukocyte adhesion.

Turbulence and stasis clearly contribute to thrombosis in a number of clinical settings. Ulcerated atherosclerotic plaques expose subendothelial ECM and are sources of turbulence. Abnormal aortic and arterial dilations called aneurysms cause local stasis and are favored sites of thrombosis. myocardial infarctions have associated with endothelial injury and have regions of noncontractile myocardium, adding an element of stasis in the formation of mural thrombi. Mitral valve stenosis results in left atrial dilation.

3.3.2.3   Hypercoagulability

Hypercoagulability is an important component and contributes less to thrombotic states. The causes of hypercoagulability may be primary(genetic) and secondary(acquired) disorders.

(1) Primary Hypercoagulability

Of the inherited causes of hypercoagulability, mutations in the factor V gene and prothrombin gene are the most common. The factor V mutation substitutes a glutamine for the normal arginine residue and renders the protein resistant to cleavage by protein C. Patients with an inherited deficiency of anticoagulants present with venous thrombosis and recurrent thromboembolism in adolescence or early adult life. The mutations underlying these inherited thrombophilias may be co-inherited. and have a much higher risk than normal individuals of developing venous thrombosis.

(2) Secondary Hypercoagulability

The pathogenesis of acquired thrombotic diatheses is more complicated. Hypercoagulability is associated with the hyperestrogenic state of pregnancy, probably related to increased hepatic synthesis of coagulation factors and reduced synthesis of antithrombin Ill, the release of procoagulant tumor products predisposes to thrombosis in disseminated cancers. The hypercoagulability attributes to increase platelet aggregation and reduce endothelial PGL_2 release. Antiphospholipid antibody syndrome has protean manifestations, including recurrent thrombosis repeated miscarriages, cardiac valve vegetations, and thrombocytopenia; it is associated with autoantibodies directly against anionic phospholipids.

3.3.3   Morphology of Thrombi

Thrombi may develop anywhere in the cardiovascular system. Their size and shape depend on the site of origin and the circumstances leading to their development. Arterial or cardiac thrombi usually begin at a site of endothelial injury or turbulence; venous thrombi characteristically occur in sites of stasis. Arterial thrombi tend to grow in a retrograde direction from the point of attachment, whereas venous thrombi extend in the direction of blood flow. The propagating tail may not be well attached and is prone to fragment to create an embolus.

3.3.3.1   Pale Thrombi

Thrombi may have grossly apparent pale or brown white. The surface of pale thrombi is rough and attaches closely to vessel wall. Microscopically, the platelets produced admixed with some fibrin and called platelets thrombi.

3.3.3.2   Mixed Thrombus

Cardiac or aortic thrombi may have grossly apparent laminations called lines of Zahn. The thrombi is firmly adherent to the injured arterial wall and are produced by alternating pale layers of platelets admixed with some fibrin and darker layers containing more erythrocytes(Figure 3-4). Lines of Zahn are significant only in that they imply thrombosis at a site of blood flow. Thrombi formed in the sluggish flow of venous blood usually resemble statically coagulated blood. Nevertheless, careful evaluation generally reveals irregular, somewhat ill-defined laminations.

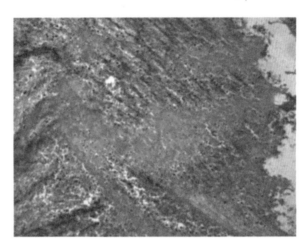

Figure 3-4　Mixed thrombus, the thrombi alternating lamination with fibrin and erythrocytes

Thrombi arising in heart chambers or in the aortic lumen are termed mural thrombi. Abnormal myocardial contraction (arrhythmias, dilated cardiomyopathy, or myocardial infarction) leads to cardiac mural thrombi, while ulcerated atherosclerotic plaque and aneurysmal dilation are the precursors of aortic thrombus formation. Arterial thrombi are usually occlusive and the most common sites are coronary, cerebral and femoral arteries. Although the thrombus is usually superimposed on an atherosclerotic plaque, the other vascular injury may be involved.

3.3.3.3　Red Thrombi

Because these thrombi forms in a relatively static environment, they tend to contain more enmeshed erythrocytes and are called red, or stasis, thrombi. Venous thrombosis(phlebothrombosis), is almost invariably occlusive, and the thrombus often creates a long cast of the vein lumen. Phlebothrombosis most commonly(90% of cases) affects the veins of the lower extremities. Less commonly, venous thrombi may occur in the upper extremities, periprostatic plexus, or the ovarian and periuterine veins; under special circumstances they might be found in the dural sinuses, portal vein, or hepatic vein.

Postmortem clots may be mistaken at autopsy for venous thrombi. Postmortem clots are gelatinous with a dark red dependent portion where erythrocytes have settled by gravity, and a yellow chicken fat supernatant, and they are commonly not attached to the underlying wall. In contrast, red thrombi are firmer and are focally attached to vessel walls, and sectioning reveals strands of gray fibrin.

Thrombi on heart valves are termed vegetations. Bacterial or fungal blood-borne infections may lead to valve damage and the development of large thrombotic masses. Sterile vegetations can also develop on non-infected valves in patients with hypercoagulable states, so-called nonbacterial thrombotic endocarditis. Less commonly, noninfective, verrucous endocarditis may occur in patients with systemic lupus erythematosus.

3.3.4　Fate of the Thrombus

If a patient survives an initial thrombotic event, thrombi undergo some combination of the following four events in the following days to weeks:

(1) Propagation

The thrombus may accumulate more platelets and fibrin, increasing vascular occlusion.

(2) Embolization

Thrombi dislodge and transport elsewhere in the vasculature.

(3) Dissolution

Activation of fibrinolytic pathways can cause rapid shrinkage and total lysis of recent thrombi. With older thrombi, extensive fibrin polymerization renders the thrombus substantially more resistant to proteolysis, and lysis is ineffectual. It is important that therapeutic infusions of fibrinolytic agents such as t-PA are effective for a short time after thrombi form.

(4) Organization and Recanalization

Thrombi can induce inflammation and fibrosis(organization), and may eventually become recanalized. Older thrombi commonly become organized. The recanalization means to re-establish vascular flow or be incorporated into a thickened vascular wall. Although the channels may not successfully restore significant flow to many obstructed vessels, recanalization can convert the thrombus into a vascularized mass of connective tissue. With time and contraction of the mesenchymal cells, the connective tissue may be incorporated into the vessel wall.

3.3.5   Clinical Correlations

Thrombi can cause obstruction of arteries and veins, and are possible sources of embolus. The significance of thrombi depends on where the thrombus occurs. Although venous thrombi may cause congestion and edema in vascular beds distal, a graver consequence is that the thrombi may embolize to the lungs and cause death. Conversely, arterial thrombi can embolize and cause tissue infarction.

3.3.5.1   Venous Thrombosis(Phlebothrombosis)

Most venous thrombi occur in the superficial or the deep veins of the leg. Superficial venous thrombi usually occur in the saphenous system. Such thrombi may cause local congestion, edema, and pain, but rarely embolize. Deep thrombi in the larger leg veins at or above the knee joint are more serious because they may embolize. Although these venous thrombi may cause local pain and distal edema, the venous obstruction may be rapidly offset by collateral channels. Therefore, deep vein thromboses are entirely asymptomatic in approximately 50% of affected patients and are recognized only in retrospect after they have embolized.

3.3.5.2   Arterial and Cardiac Thrombosis

Atherosclerosis is a major initiator of thromboses, related to the abnormal vascular flow and the loss of endothelial integrity. Cardiac mural thrombi can arise in the setting of myocardial infarction related to dyskinetic contraction of the myocardium and damage to the adjacent endocardium. Rheumatic heart disease may cause atrial mural thrombi due to mitral valve stenosis. Both cardiac and aortic mural thrombi can also embolize peripherally. Virtually any tissue may be affected, but the brain, kidneys, and spleen are prime targets because of their large flow volume.

3.3.5.3   Disseminated Intravascular Coagulation(DIC)

DIC, the insidious or sudden onset of widespread fibrin thrombi in the microcirculation, complicate a variety of disorders ranging from obstetric complications to advanced malignancy. Although these thrombi are not visible on gross inspection, they are readily apparent microscopically and may cause diffuse circulatory insufficiency, particularly in the brain, lungs, heart, and kidneys. With the development of the multiple thrombi, there is a rapid consumption of platelets and coagulation proteins. On the other hand, fibrinolytic mechanisms are activated, and an initially thrombotic disorder can evolve into a serious bleeding disorder. It is important that DIC is a potential complication of any condition associated with widespread activation of thrombin.

3.4　Embolism

Embolism is known as the process in which an abnormal substance appears intravascularly and obstructs vascular system by following blood flow, so the abnormal substance is called the embolus.

3.4.1　The Kinds of Embolus

An embolus is a detached intravascular solid, liquid, or gaseous mass that is carried by the blood to a site distant from its origin point. The embolus consequences usually cause the downstream tissues dysfunction or infarction. Thromboembolism means the vast majority of emboli derived some part of a dislodged thrombus. Rare forms of emboli are composed of fat droplets, air or nitrogen bubbles, atherosclerotic debris, tumor fragments, amniotic fluid, or foreign bodies such as bullets. Usually, an embolism should be thought to be thrombotic in origin. Depending on the original site, emboli can lodge anywhere in the vascular tree. So the clinical outcomes are best understood from the standpoint of whether emboli lodge; in the pulmonary or systemic circulation.

3.4.2　Pulmonary Thromboembolism

Pulmonary emboli are the most common form of the thromboembolic disease. The incidence of pulmonary embolism was 2–4 per 1,000 hospitalized patients. Almost all venous emboli originate from thrombi with deep leg vein above the knee level. Fragmented thrombi are carried through larger veins and pass through the right side of the heart. Depending on the size, the embolus may occlude the main pulmonary artery, impact across the bifurcation(saddle embolus), or pass out into the smaller branching arterioles. Frequently there are multiple emboli as a shower of smaller emboli from a single large thrombus. A patient having one pulmonary embolus is at high risk of having more.

The pathophysiological outcomes of pulmonary embolism depend on the size of embolus and on the cardiopulmonary status of patient. There are two important consequences of pulmonary arterial occlusion: ①an increase in pulmonary artery pressure from flow blockage and vasospasm caused by neurogenic mechanisms and/or release of mediators; ②ischemia of the downstream pulmonary parenchyma. Therefore, occlusion of a major vessel causes an abrupt increase in pulmonary artery pressure, diminished cardiac output, right-sided heart failure, and sometimes sudden death.

Most pulmonary emboli are small and silent in clinical findings. They eventually undergo organized and become incorporated into the vascular wall. Sudden death, right ventricular failure, or cardiovascular collapse occurs when a major pulmonary circulation is blocked by emboli. Embolic obstruction of medium-sized arteries may result in pulmonary hemorrhage. However, a similar embolus in the setting of left-side cardiac failure may result in a large infarct. Embolic obstruction of small end-arteriolar pulmonary branches usually results in infarction. Multiple emboli occurring over a period may cause pulmonary hypertension with right ventricular failure.

3.4.3   Systemic Thromboembolism

Systemic thromboembolism refers to emboli found in the arteries of the systemic circulation. Most systemic emboli originate are from intracardiac mural thrombi, which are associated with left ventricular infarcts and left atrial dilation. The remainder originates from aortic aneurysms, ulcerated atherosclerotic plaques, thrombi, or fragmented valvular vegetations. About 10% systemic emboli are of unknown origin.

In contrast to venous emboli, arterial emboli can travel to a wide variety of sites; the arrest point depends on the embolus origin and the relative blood flow through the downstream tissues. The major sites for arteriolar embolization include the lower extremities and the brain. The outcomes of embolization depend on the vulnerability to anoxia, the caliber of the occluded vessel and the collateral blood supply. In general, arterial emboli cause infarction.

3.4.4   Fat Embolism

Fat enters the circulation by rupture of the marrow vascular sinusoids or small venules in injured tissues. Microscopic fat globules can be found in the pulmonary vasculature after fractures of long bones or after soft-tissue crush injury. Although fat and marrow embolism occur in most individuals with severe skeletal injuries, fewer than patients show any clinical findings. Fat embolism syndrome is characterized by pulmonary insufficiency, neurologic symptoms, anemia, and thrombocytopenia, and is fatal in 10% of cases. The typical symptoms appear 1–3 days after injury as the sudden onset of tachypnea, dyspnea, and tachycardia.

The pathogenesis of fat emboli syndrome involves mechanical obstruction and biochemical injury. Fat microemboli occlude pulmonary and cerebral microvasculature, which is aggravated by platelet aggregation. This effect is further exacerbated by fatty acid release from lipid globules, causing local toxic endothelial injury. The microscopic demonstration of fat microglobules typically requires specialized techniques (frozen sections and fat stains).

3.4.5   Air Embolism

Gas bubbles within the circulation can coalesce and obstruct vascular flow, and cause distal ischemic injury. Air may enter the pulmonary circulation during obstetric or laparoscopic procedures, or as a consequence of chest wall injury. Usually, more than 100 mL of air produce a clinical effect; bubbles can coalesce to form frothy masses sufficiently large to occlude major vessels.

Decompression sickness, a particular form of gas embolism, is caused by sudden changes in atmospheric pressure. Scuba divers, underwater construction workers, and individuals in unpressurized aircraft are all at risk. When air is breathed at high pressure, increased amounts of gas become dissolved in the blood and tissues. If the diver ascends too rapidly, the nitrogen comes out of the solution in the tissues and the blood to form gas emboli, which cause tissue ischemia. Rapid formation of gas bubbles within skeletal muscles and supporting tissues in and about joints is responsible for the painful condition called the bends. Gas bubbles in the lungs vasculature cause edema, hemorrhages, and focal atelectasis or emphysema, resulting in respiratory distress called the chokes. A more chronic form of decompression sickness is called caisson disease, where the persistence of gas emboli in the bones causes multiple-focal ischemic necrosis. The heads of femurs, tibiae and humeri are most commonly affected.

Treating acute decompression sickness requires placing affected individuals in a high-pressure chamber to force the gas back into solution. Subsequent slow decompression permits gradual resorption and exhalation so that the obstructive bubbles do not reform.

3.4.6 Amniotic Fluid Embolism

An amniotic fluid embolism is a grave,uncommon complication of labor and the immediate postpartum period. The onset is characterized by sudden severe dyspnea,hypertensive shock,and cyanosis,followed by seizures and coma. If the patient survives the initial crisis,pulmonary edema typically develops,along with disseminated intravascular coagulation,due to the release of thrombogenic substances.

The underlying cause is the infusion of amniotic fluid into the maternal circulation via tears in the placental membranes and rupture of uterine veins. In the pulmonary microcirculation,histology shows squamous cells shed from fetal skin,lanugo hair,fat from vernix caseosa,and mucin derived from the fetal respiratory or gastrointestinal tracts.

3.5 Infarction

An infarct is an area of ischemic necrosis caused by occlusion of the vascular supply to the affected tissue. Infarction affecting the heart and the brain is the common and important cause of clinical illness. More than half of all deaths are an outcome of cardiovascular disease and originated from myocardial or cerebral infarction. Pulmonary infarction is a common clinical complication,bowel infarction is frequently fatal,and ischemic necrosis of the extremities is a serious problem in the diabetic population.

The vast majority of infarctions result from arterial thrombotic or arterial embolism. Uncommon causes include vessel torsion,vascular compression,or traumatic vessel rupture. Venous thrombosis can cause obstruction and congestion. Infarcts caused by venous thrombosis occur likely in organs with a single venous outflow channel.

3.5.1 Morphology

Infarctions are classified on the basis of the color(reflecting the hemorrhage amount)and the presence or absence of microbial infection. Thus,infarcts may be either anemic(white)or hemorrhagic(red)and may be either bland or septic.

3.5.1.1 Anemic Infarcts

Anemic infarcts occur with arterial occlusions in solid organs with end-arterial circulation(e. g. ,heart,spleen,and kidney),where the solidity limits the hemorrhage amount to seep into the ischemic area from adjoining capillary beds(Figure 3-5). All infarcts tend to be wedge-shaped,with the occluded vessel at the apex and the periphery of the organ forming the base. When the base is a serosal surface,there can be an overlying fibrinous exudate. The margins of infarctions are defined and slightly hemorrhagic by the narrow rim of congestion due to inflammation.

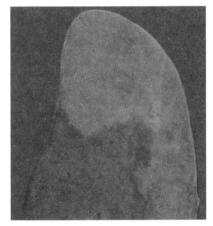

Figure 3-5 Anemic infarct,the pale infract appears at the apex of the spleen and the margin of infract shows the hemorrhage

3.5.1.2 Hemorrhagic Infarcts

Hemorrhagic infarcts(Figure 3-6)occur ①with venous occlusions(such as in ovarian torsion);②in loose tissues(e. g. ,lung)where blood can collect in infarcted zones;③in dual circulations tissues (e. g. , small intestine) , permitting flow of blood from a parallel supply into a necrotic area; ④in previously congested tissues; ⑤when flow is reestablished to a site of previous arterial occlusion.

In solid organs, the few extravasated red cells are lysed and the released hemoglobin remains in the form of hemosiderin. Thus, infarcts resulting from arterial occlusions typically become progressively paler and more sharply defined with time. In comparison, the hemorrhagic infarcts are too extensive to permit the lesion ever to become pale. After a few days, extensive hemorrhages become firmer and browner, reflecting the accumulation of hemosiderin pigment.

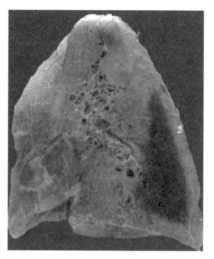

Figure 3 – 6   Hemorrhagic infarct, the infracted pulmonary appears congested and purple-red

The main histologic characteristic of infarction is ischemic coagulative necrosis. Acute inflammatory begins to develop along the margins of infarcts within a few hours and is well defined within 1−2 days. Eventually the inflammatory response is followed by a reparative response in the preserved margins. In some tissues, parenchymal regeneration can occur at the periphery. However, most infarcts are ultimately replaced by scar. In the central nervous system, ischemic injury results in liquefactive necrosis.

3.5.1.3   Septic Infarcts

occur when infected heart valve embolize or when microbes seed an area of necrotic tissue. In these cases the infarct is converted into an abscess, with a correspondingly inflammatory response and organization.

3.5.2   Factors that Influence the Development of an Infarct

Vascular occlusion can range from minimal effect to tissue necrosis, even result in organ dysfunction and sometimes death. The outcome is influenced by the following key determinants:

3.5.2.1   Anatomy of the Vascular Supply

The availability of an alternative blood supply is the most important factor of whether occlusion of an individual vessel causes damage. For example, the dual blood supply of lung by the pulmonary and bronchial artery indicates that the obstruction of pulmonary arterioles does not cause infarction until the bronchial circulation is compromised. Similarly, the liver with its hepatic artery and portal vein, and the hand and forearm with their parallel radial and ulnar arterial supply, are resistant to infarction. By contrast, the kidney and the spleen are end-arterial circulations, and vascular obstruction generally causes infarction.

3.5.2.2 Development Rate of Occlusion

Slowly developing occlusions is less to cause infarction because they allow time for the development of alternativeblood supplies. For example, small inter arteriolar anastomoses-with minimal functional flow-interconnect the three major coronary arteries in the heart. If one of the coronary arteries is slowly occluded, flow within this collateral circulation may increase sufficiently to prevent infarction, even though the major artery is completely occluded.

3.5.2.3 Tissue Vulnerability to Hypoxia

The susceptibility of a tissue to hypoxia influences the likelihood of infarction. Neurons undergo irreversible damage when deprived of their blood supply for only 3–4 minutes. Myocardial cells die after only 20–30 minutes of ischemia. By contrast, fibroblasts within myocardium remain viable after many hours of ischemia.

3.5.2.4 Oxygen Content of Blood

The partial pressure of oxygen in blood determines theconsequence of vascular occlusion. Partial flow obstruction of a small vessel in an anemic patient could cause tissue infarction, whereas it would be without effect under conditions of normal oxygen tension. With compromised flow and ventilation, congestive heart failure could lead to infarction in the setting of an otherwise inconsequential obstruction.

3.6　Edema

Edema is characterized by the accumulation of interstitial fluid within tissues. Collections of fluid are variously designated hydrothorax, hydropericardium, or hydroperitoneum in different body cavities. Anasarca is a severe and generalized edema marked by profound swelling of subcutaneous tissues and accumulation of fluid in body cavities.

3.6.1　Pathogenesis

Normally, the fluid outflow at the arteriolar end of the microcirculation is balanced by inflow at the venular end; a small net outflow of fluid is drained by the lymphatics. Either increased hydrostatic pressure or diminished colloid osmotic pressure result in the increased interstitial fluid. The increased hydrostatic and plasma osmotic pressures achieve a new equilibrium. Excess edema fluid is removed by lymphatic drainage. Clearly, lymphatic obstruction attenuates fluid drainage and cause edema. Finally, sodium retention in renal disease can also cause edema.

The edema fluid is a protein-poor transudate, with a specific gravity less than 1.012. Conversely, inflammatory edema is usually a protein-rich exudate with a specific gravity s greater than 1.020.

3.6.1.1 Increased Hydrostatic Pressure

Localized increases in hydrostatic pressure can result from an impaired venous return. For example, lower extremity deep venous thrombosis might cause edema restricted to the affected leg. With resultant systemic edema, generalized increases in venous pressure occur commonly in congestive heart failure. In congestive heart failure, the reduced cardiac output increases the capillary hydrostatic pressure, and causes reduced renal perfusion.

3.6.1.2 Reduced Plasma Osmotic Pressure

Albumin is responsible for maintaining intravascular colloid osmotic pressure. When albumin is either lost or inadequately synthesized, the decreased osmotic pressure occurs. An important cause of albumin loss is the nephrotic syndrome, in which glomerular capillary walls become leaky to lose albumin in the urine. Reduced albumin synthesis occurs in the setting of diffuses liver diseases and protein malnutrition. Regardless of the case, reduced plasma osmotic pressure leads to a net movement of fluid into the interstitial tissues.

3.6.1.3   Lymphatic Obstruction

Lymphedema of impaired lymphatic drainage is usually localized; and can result from neoplastic or inflammatory obstruction. For example, the parasitic infection filariasis can cause lymphatic and lymph node fibrosis. Women with breast cancer might be treated by resection and/or irradiation of the associated axillary lymph nodes, the loss of lymphatic drainage can cause upper extremity edema. In breast carcinoma infiltration and obstruction of lymphatics can cause edema of the overlying skin, the so-called peaud'orange (orange peel) appearance.

3.6.1.4   Sodium and Water Retention

Increased salt retention causes the increased hydrostatic pressure and the reduced vascular osmotic pressure. Excessive salt and water retention can occur with any compromise of renal function, including post-streptococcal glomerulonephritis and acute renal failure.

3.6.2   Morphology

Edema is easily recognized grossly; microscopically, edema fluid is reflected as a clearing and separation of the extracellular matrix elements with subtle cell swelling. Although any tissue in the body may be involved, edema is commonly encountered in subcutaneous tissues, lungs, and brain.

3.6.2.1   Subcutaneous Edema

Subcutaneous edema can be diffuse in regions with high hydrostatic pressures. Diffuse edema is more prominent in certain body areas because of the gravity effects, termed dependent edema. Dependent edema is a prominent feature of cardiac failure, particularly of the right ventricle. Edema due to renal dysfunction or nephrotic syndrome often manifests first in loose connective tissues. Finger pressure over edematous subcutaneous tissue displaces the interstitial fluid and leaves a finger-shaped depression, so-called pitting edema.

3.6.2.2   Pulmonary Edema

Pulmonary edema is a clinical problem frequently seen in the left ventricular failure. The lungs typically are two to three times their normal weight, and sectioning reveals frothy, blood-tinged fluid consisting of a mixture of air, edema fluid, and extravasated red cells.

3.6.2.3   Edema of the Brain

Brain Edema may be localized (e. g. , abscesses or neoplasms) or generalized, depending on the nature and extent of the pathologic process or injury. With generalized edema, the sulci are narrowed as the gyri showing signs of flattening against the skull.

3.6.3   *Clinical Correlation*

The edema effects may range from merely annoying to rapidly fatal. Subcutaneous edema is important to recognize primarily because it indicates underlying cardiac or renal disease; however, when significant it can also impair wound healing or the clearance of infection. Pulmonary edema can cause death by interfering with the normal ventilatory function and creates a favorable environment for bacterial infection. Brain edema can be serious to rapidly fatal or is severe and can cause the herniation as the increased intracranial pressure.

Chapter 4

Inflammation

Introduction

Inflammation is a very common and important basic pathological process. It occurs to the body surface where trauma, infection exist and it is also the most which are named as different disorders frequently-occurring disease of internal organs, such as furuncle, carbuncle, pneumonia, gastritis, hepatitis, nephritis, etc. The modern pathological and immunological research have shown that inflammation is not only an adaptive response by the body, but also a protective process of the body. It has the effect of reducing damage to the body, preventing the damaging agents from spreading in the body and repairing the damaged tissue. But under some circumstances, the effect of inflammatory response to the body also leads to a different degree of harm, such as severe allergic reaction caused by drugs, toxicant and fibrinous pericarditis caused by cardiac fibrous adhesion. Therefore, dialectical analysis of the two sides of inflammation is of great importance in understanding the nature of inflammation and guiding clinical practice.

4.1 Overview

4.1.1 Conception of Inflammation

Inflammation is a defensive response to injury by living tissue with a vascular system. Although invertebrates(including single-celled animals and other non-vascular multicellular animals) can also respond to injury factors, for example, phagocytosis or scavenging of harmful factors, none of these are inflammation. Only the species with blood vessels can be characterized by vascular response, preserving complex and perfect inflammatory reaction of phagocytic scavenging process. Therefore, the vascular response is the central part of the inflammatory process. The vascular reaction causes plasma and leukocytes exudation and infiltrating of leucocytes is activated. It plays the role of diluting limiting and killing damage factors in injury, as well as eliminating, absorbing the necrotic tissue. At the same time, the parenchymal cells and stromal cells regenerate and repair damaged tissue. Inflammation is essentially a complex icated pathological process that begins at the injury site, ends when the wound heals or recurrence. The damage and anti-damage are consistent throughout the inflammatory response.

4.1.2   Causes of Inflammation

Inflammatory factors are the causes of tissue damage during inflammation. There are many types of inflammatory factors, which can be summarized as the following categories.

4.1.2.1   Biological Pathogens

Biological factors are the most common and important sources of inflammation, including bacteria, viruses, rickettsia, fungi, spirochetes, and parasites, et al. Inflammation caused by biological pathogens is also called infection. Bacteria and their endotoxins or exotoxins can directly damage cells and tissues; viral replication in infected cells leads to cell necrosis; some antigens can induce tissue damage through immune responses such as parasite infections and tuberculosis.

4.1.2.2   Physical Agents

Physical agents include high temperature (burns), low temperature (frost), electric shock, ultraviolet radiation, radiation damage and mechanical trauma (cutting, crushing injury).

4.1.2.3   Chemical Agents

Chemical factors include exogenous and endogenous chemicals. Exogenous chemicals include acids, bases, oxidants, mustard gas, and certain heavy metals (mercury). Endogenous chemicals are the break down products of tissue necrosis that accumulate in the body's metabolites, such as urea and uric acid.

4.1.2.4   Allergic Reaction

When the body's immune response is abnormal, it can cause inappropriate or excessive immune reactions, causing tissue and cell damage to induce inflammation. The allergic inflammation include allergic rhinitis, urticaria, glomerulonephritis, and diseases caused by abnormal autoimmune reaction, such as rheumatoid arthritis and systemic lupus erythematosus.

4.1.2.5   Tissue Necrosis

Ischemia, hypoxia or other reasons can cause tissue necrosis. Necrotic tissue is a potentially inflammatory factor.

4.1.2.6   Foreign Bodies

The foreign bodies that enter the body through various channels, such as various kinds of metallic or wood debris, particles and surgical sutures, can cause inflammatory response due to their different antigenicity.

4.1.3   The Basic Pathological Changes of Inflammation

The basic pathological changes of inflammation are alteration, exudation, and proliferation. In general, alteration is a damaging process. Exudation and proliferation are the processes of anti-injury and repair, and exudation is the most characteristic lesion of inflammation.

4.1.3.1   Alteration

Alteration is referred to as degeneration or necrosis of local tissues or cells. Alteration can occur in both parenchymal cells and interstitial cells. Parenchymal cell alteration is characterized by cell edema, fatty degeneration, or necrosis. Mucous degeneration or fibrinous necrosis can occur in interstitial connective tissue. Alteration can be caused by direct effect of inflammatory agents, and can be mediated by blood circulation disorders or immune mechanisms. It can also be caused by indirect effects of inflammatory products. Therefore, the degree of deterioration depends on the inflammatory agents and the reaction state of the body.

4.1.3.2 Exudation

Exudation is the process of inflammation in which the fluid or cell components of the local blood vessels are emitted through the vessel wall into the tissue interstitial, body surface, mucosal surface or serous cavity. The fluid and cells is known collectively as diffusate or exudate. The exudate accumulates in the tissue gap, known as inflammatory edema. When the exudate concentrates in serous cavity, it is called inflammatory effusion(such as peritoneal effusion, pleural effusion, etc.). The inflammatory exudate and non-inflammatory transudate are different in mechanism and composition(Table 4−1), and it is of great significance to distinguish the exudate and transudate in the differential diagnosis of disease.

Table 4−1　The comparison of exudate and transudate

Difference	Exudate	Leakage
Cause	Inflammation	Non-inflammation
Protein amount	>30 g/L	<30 g/L
The proportion	>1.018	<1.018
Nucleocyte number	>1,000×10^6/L	<300×10^6/L
Rivalta test ＊	Positive	Negative
Coagulability	Self-coagulation	Non self-coagulation
Appearance	Cloudy	Tran

Note: The Rivalta test ＊ was a qualitative experiment of mucin.

4.1.3.3 Proliferation

Proliferation is a regeneration process of local tissue under the stimulation of inflammatory cytokines, disintegrating products or some physicochemical factors. In general, the proliferation of mesenchymal cells, such as endothelial cells, macrophages, and fibroblasts, can produce a large number of collagen fibers, forming inflammatory fibrosis. In some cases, the epithelial or parenchymal cells may also proliferate, such as the proliferation of epithelial cells and glands in chronic inflammation of the nasal mucosa.

The above basic lesions are consistent and interrelated throughout the process of inflammation(Figure 4−1). In different types or periods of inflammation, the extent of the three lesions were

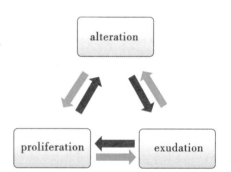

Figure 4 − 1　Schematic diagram of basic pathological changes and interrelationship in inflammation

different. In general, acute or early inflammation is dominated by alteration and exudation; chronic or later inflammation appears mainly proliferation. Although pathological changes of inflammatory response are diverse and complex, the basic lesion is the response of vascular nerve and body fluid.

4.1.4　The Local Manifestations and Systemic Responses of Inflammation

4.1.4.1　The Local Manifestations of Inflammation

Local manifestations of inflammation include redness, swelling, heat, pain and dysfunction. Redness and fever in the inflammatory region are caused by increased blood flow in local vessels, increased metabolism and enhanced heat production. A local swelling of the inflammatory area is associated with local congestion and exudation. The effect of the exudation and the accumulation of hydrogen ions in local lesions can cause pain by stimulating nerve ends. The severity of the inflammation depends on the nature of the site and the intensity of the response. For example, the infection of upper respiratory tract causes nasal mucosal swelling to nasal congestion; and the acute arthritis can cause swelling or timitation of joint movement; while liver inflammation cause liver cell metabolic disorder and liver dysfunction.

4.1.4.2　The Systemic Responses of Inflammation

The inflammatory agents can cause systemic responses of the body. The systemic acute reaction of inflammation mainly includes the number change of leukocytes and fever, which are important indications for clinical diagnosis of inflammatory or infectious diseases.

Fever is the result of endogenous and exogenous thermal stimulation of hypothalamus. Interleukin-1 (IL-1), IL-6 and tumor necrosis factor(TNF) are the most important cytokines mediating acute inflammation. IL-1 and TNF act on the thermoregulatory center of the hypothalamus, causing fever by locally producing prostaglandin E(PGE). Fever can promote the formation of antibodies, the proliferation and phagocytosis of mononuclear phagocyte system, which enhancedes the body's defensive function. However, excessive or long-term fever can affect the body's normal metabolic process, leading to dysfunction of various systems, especially nervous system.

Peripheral blood leucocytosis is of defensive significance. It is mainly related to the accelerated release of leukocytes from bone marrow depots due to IL-1 and TNF, and it often reflects the body resistance and the infection. Most of the bacterial infections lead to neutrophil increase. Certain allergies lead to eosinophils increase, and some viral infections(such as infectious mononucleosis, mumps and rubella)selectively results in lymphocytes increase. However, the peripheral blood leukocytes decrease under infection with certain viruses, rickettsia, parasites, and bacteria(such as Salmonella typhi).

Some inflammation(such as typhoid, etc.) can stimulate the proliferation of mononuclear macrophage because bacteria or toxins enter the blood and induce mononuclear macrophage to disseminate to liver, spleen and lymph nodes.

4.1.5　The Clinical Type of Inflammation

Inflammation is generally categorized into four types: peracute, acute, subacute and chronic inflammation.

4.1.5.1　Peracute Inflammation

The course of the disease lasts only a few hours to a few days. The inflammatory response is intense and can cause severe damage of tissue/organs, even leading to death. This type of inflammation is usually caused by allergic reactions, such as penicillin.

4.1.5.2　Acute Inflammation

The acute inflammation is a rapid response to injury, and the symptoms are obvious. In addition, the course of acute inflammation is short and usually lasts several days, generally no more than 1 month. Local lesions are usually dominated by exudative changes, and the majority of the cells of exudation are neutrophils. Sometimes acute inflammation can be characterized by alteration(such as acute viral hepatitis) or proliferation(such as acute glomerulonephritis).

4.1.5.3　Subacute Inflammation

The course of subacute inflammation is between acute and chronic inflammation, and it lasts about a month to several months. Most subacute inflammations are developed from acute inflammation, such as subacute severe hepatitis.

4.1.5.4　Chronic Inflammation

Chronic inflammation is characterized by slow onset, mild symptoms and long duration. It can last for months to years. Chronic inflammation can be developed from acute inflammation, or it can be chronic at the beginning. Proliferation is the main pathological morphology, but alteration and exudation are less. The infiltrated inflammatory cells are mainly lymphocytes, plasma cells and macrophages.

4.2　Acute Inflammation

Acute inflammation is an early, rapid response to the body's stimulation of proinflammatory cytokines. In acute inflammatory reactions, there are three characteristic responses: hemodynamic changes, increased vascular permeability and leukocyte exudation.

4.2.1　Changes in Vascular Reactivity and Fluid Exudation

Inflammatory vascular response is the earliest changes in inflammation, and this includes changes in hemodynamics and increased vascular permeability. Increased blood flow causes hemodynamics. Increased vascular permeability leads to leakage of plasma proteins and leukocytes to extravascular tissue.

4.2.1.1　Hemodynamic Changes

Hemodynamic changes are the basis for exudation. After tissue injury occurs during acute inflammation, hemodynamic changes occur rapidly, which include changes in vascular caliber and flow.

(1) Arteriole Spasms Shortly

Immediate vascular response is of transient vasoconstriction of arterioles. Inflammatory cytokines act on the local blood vessels of the body through the nerve reflex or inflammatory mediators, which cause transient arteriole spasm, transient ischemia of tissue. This phase lasts only a few seconds in generally.

(2) Vasodilation and Blood Flow Acceleration

Vasodilatation results in increased blood volume in microvascular bed of the area, which is responsible for local redness and fever, in the inflammatory tissue. The mechanism of inflammatory hyperemia is related to neurological and humoral factors. Duration of vasodilation depends on the length of time that pro-inflammatory agent exists, and the type as well as severity of the lesion.

(3) Slower Blood Flow

Slower blood flow result in increased vascular permeability. Extravasation of protein-rich fluids out of the blood vessels leads to a increased concentration of intravascular red blood cells, higher blood viscosity, and blocked or even stasis of blood flow, which creates conditions for leukocyte adhesion.

4.2.1.2　Increased Vascular Permeability

Increased vascular permeability is the most important cause of exudative fluid. The maintenance of normal permeability of the microcirculation vascular mainly depends on the integrity of vascular endothelial cells, and increased vascular permeability is mainly related to the following changes of vascular endothelial cells during inflammation (Figure 4-2):

(1) Endothelial Contraction

This is the most common mechanism of increased vascular permeability and is mainly associated with immediate transient response and structural reorganization of cytoskeleton.

Endothelial cells contract rapidly, this is induced by histamine, bradykinin and other inflammatory mediators, this leads to the appearing of micropores around 0.5−1.0 μm on the endothelial cells. The phase can also be called epicardial transient response because of the short half-life of these inflammatory mediators, which lasts only for 15−30 minutes. Endothelial cytoskeletal remodeling is mainly induced by cytokines (such as IL-1, TNF, IFN-γ), hypoxia and other factors.

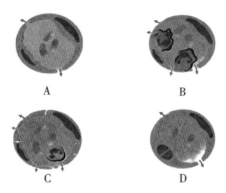

Figure 4-2　The main mechanism of vascular permeability increases

(A: The endothelial cells contract. B: Leukocyte mediate endothelial cells injury.

C: Endothelial cell penetration enhanced. D: Neonatal capillary permeability increased.)

(2) Increased Endothelial Cell Penetration

There are vesicles composed of interconnected vesicles that form the transcytoplasmic channel in the cytoplasm near the junction of endothelial cells. The process by which protein-rich liquid traverses endothelial cells through the cell channel is called transcytosis. Vascular endothelial growth factor (VEGF) and histamine, bradykinin and other inflammatory mediators can increase vascular permeability by increasing the number of pericytes and expanding the caliber.

(3) Endothelial Cell Damage

①Direct endothelial injury: It is usually caused by severe injuries, such as sever burns, pyogenic bacteria infection, which leads to endothelial necrosis and rapid increase of vascular permeability; ②Leukocyte-mediated endothelial cell injury: Toxic oxygen metabolites and proteolytic enzymes are released by leukocytes that adhere to the vascular endothelium, which leads to endothelial cell injury and detachment.

(4) Leakage of Newly Formed Capillaries

In the inflammatory repairing phase, endothelial cell connection of newly formed capillaries is not perfect. The vessel structure makes vascular permeability increase.

4.2.1.3　Liquid Leakage

It is also known as liquid exudation. Because of increased vascular wall permeability, blood components exude from blood vessel wall. Fluid exudation in acute inflammation is induced by vasodilatation and accelerated blood flow. Thus, the exosmosis of a large quantity of proteins from the blood reduced plasma colloid osmotic pressure and increased osmotic pressure of the tissue.

Exudation is an important feature of acute inflammation and plays an important defensive role in the following ways: ①Protein-rich exudates dilute the harmful substances locally; ②The antibodies, complement and lysozyme contained in the exudate are beneficial to the killing of pathogens; ③The fibrin in the exudates get into a network to facilitate the confining of inflammatory lesions and can be a scaffold for repair. In addition, fibrin in exudates is beneficial to fibroblasts to produce collagen fibers in the later stage of inflammation; ④The pathogens and toxins in the exudates are brought to the lymph nodes with lymph flow, which helps to activate the body's cellular and humoral immune responses.

However, if there is too much exudates, it would increase the pressure and block the organ, for example, pericardial effusion can result in pericardial packing, and acute inflammatory edema of the larynx which can cause suffocation; If the fibrin in the exudates cannot be dissolved and absorbed, it will form abnormal structure and result in dysfunction of local tissues and organs, such as pericardial adhesion or pericardial occlusion.

4.2.2　Leukocyte Extravasation and Phagocytosis

Leukocyte extravasation is the movement of leukocytes out of the circulatory system and towards the site of tissue damage or infection. Inflammatory cells extravasating into the tissue space is also called inflammatory cellular infiltration, which is the most important inflammatory morphological features.

Leukocyte extravasation is a very complex and continuously active process and plays an important role in the local defense. It is devided into four stages: ①margination and rolling; ②adhesion and transmigration; ③chemotaxis and activation; ④phagocytosis and degradation(Figure 4–3). The extravasated leukocyte plays an important role in local phagocytosis and immunity.

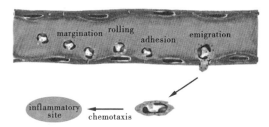

Figure 4–3　A schematic diagram of neutrophilic infiltration process

4.2.2.1　Margination and Rolling of Leukocytes

Normally leukocytes are predominantly located in the bloodstream. Because of the increased vascular dilatation and permeability as well as slower blood flow, leukocytes in capillaries go to the side flow from the axial flow in the early stage of inflammation, which is known as leukocytic margination. Then leukocytes roll on the surface of endothelial cells and does not attach to endothelial cells, known as the leukocytic pavement (Figure 4–4).

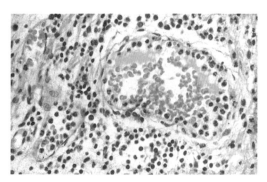

Figure 4 – 4　Neutrophilic margination and pavement

4.2.2.2   Leukocytes Adhesion and Transmigration

Peripherally marginated and pavemented neutrophils slowly roll over the endothelial cells lining the vessel wall(rolling phase). Then the such as selectins, immunoglobulins, integrins and mucin-like glycoproteins transient bond between the leucocytes and endothelial cells become firmer(adhesion phase). Adhesion molecules play an extremely important role in leukocyte adhesion. Leukocyte adhesion molecules are mostly integrins or selectins.

Leukocytes travel mainly in the lesion site of the small veins. Part cytoplasmic protrusions of the adherent leukocytes formed pseudopods, and insert into the endothelial cell gap. The whole leukocyte moves through the endothelium in the way of the amoeba, then stops for a moment and secretes the collagen enzyme that breaks down the basement membrane and finally enters the surrounding tissue. The process that leukocytes penetrate the vascular wall and get into the extravascular space is called transmigration.

4.2.2.3   Chemotaxis and Activation

A key function of leukocytes in inflammatory responses is the tropism of leukocytes to the site of injury. The aggregation of white blood cells into the inflammatory lesion is affected by their chemotactic action, and chemokines play a role in the whole process of leukocyte aggregation, which is of special significance in inflammatory response.

Chemotaxis refers to the direct movement of white blood cells along the chemical stimulus concentration gradient in the inflammatory region. Chemical stimulants that attract white blood cells are called chemotactic agents. Chemokines are divided into two categories: exogenous and endogenous chemokines. Exogenous chemokines include bacteria and usually their metabolites, and endogenous chemokines include complement components and cytokines.

4.2.2.4   Phagocytosis and Degradation

On one hand, the white blood cells that congregate in the area of the inflammation are largely consumed and have immune activity in defensive response, and on the other hand the white blood cells can cause damage and destruction to local tissue.

(1) Phagocytosis

Phagocytosis refers to the process in which white blood cells engulf and degrade pathogens, tissue fragments and foreign bodies, and this process is extremely important in the inflammatory defense response. Phagocytosis is another way for white blood cells to kill pathogens other than lysosomal enzymes.

There are mainly two kinds of phagocytes in human body: ①Neutrophils, also known as " small phagocytes", usually appear in the early stages of inflammation, acute inflammation and suppurative inflammation. Its cytoplasm contains rich neutral particles(the equivalent of lysosomal granules under the electron microscope), which contains a variety of enzymes(such as lysozyme, acid hydrolase, etc.), and it can dissolve the bacteria on the surface of the glycoprotein. ②Macrophages, also known as " large phagocyte", usually participates in specific immune response in the late inflammation, chronic inflammation and non-suppurative inflammation(tuberculosis, typhoid, etc.); the macrophages in the inflammatory region are mostly monocytes which extradavated from the blood, and differentiated into macrophages(histiocytes) in local tissues; macrophages contain many vacuoles and lysosomes, which are rich in lysozyme, acid phosphatase and peroxidase.

Phagocytosis of the microbe by macrophages involves the following 3 steps(Figure 4-5). ①Recognition and attachment: Phagocytes first identify and adhere to a pathogen by the opsonin which is a type of protein found in serum that enhances the phagocytic activity of phagocytes, mainly Fc fragment of immunoglobulin IgG and complement C3b. Phagocytes recognize bacteria that are coated with antibodies or complement then bind to the corresponding receptors via antibodies or compliment by virtue of their surface Fc receptors(FcRs) and C3b receptors. ②Engulfment: The opsonised particle or microbe bound to the surface of phagocyte is ready to be engulfed. This is accomplished by formation of cytoplasmic pseudopods around the particle due to activation of actin filaments beneath cell wall, enveloping it in a phagocytic vacuole, which are called phagosome. Phagosomes gradually break away from the cell membrane and fuse with the primary lysosomes to form a phagolysosome. Lysosomal contents play the role of killing and degradation of pathogens by the process of degranulation. ③Killing and degradation: bacteria that enter the phagocytes are mainly killed by the active oxidative metabolites. The phagocytic process causes white blood cells to produce the intermediate metabolites of oxygen during aerobic metabolism, namely, superoxide anions (O_2^-). Most of the superoxide anions are converted to H_2O_2 by spontaneous disproportionation. MPO exists in the eosinophilic granules of neutrophils, and in the presence of chlorides, the enzyme can reduce H_2O_2 to form hypochloric acid($HOCl^-$); $HOCl^-$ is also a strong oxidizer and sterilization factor that can damage the normal physiological condition of bacterial cell membrane by halide or protein/lipid oxidation, or make bacteria finally killed by enzymes activated.

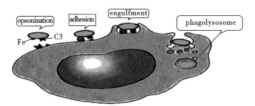

Figure 4 – 5   The process of neutrophil phagocytosis

(2)Immunity

There are two types of immunity: specific and non-specific immunity. Cells involved in the immune process are mainly lymphocytes, plasma cells and macrophages. Lymphocytes are often seen in chronic inflammation or viral infections, and they are mainly from the blood or local lymphatic tissue. Macrophages uptake antigens and deliver antigenic information to T or B lymphocytes, then sensitized T lymphocytes can produce and release lymphokines, which lead to cellular immunity; and B lymphocyte can transform into plasma cell and produce antibodies that causes the humoral immune response.

Natural killer(NK) cell is an important immune cell, it does not have T-cell receptor or produce antibodies, but it has natural killing activity. NK cells are not only associated with anti-tumor, anti-viral infection and immune regulation, but also play roles in hypersensitivity and autoimmune diseases.

(3)The Role of Tissue Damage

In the process of phagocytosis, chemokines, lysosomal enzymes, reactive oxygen radicals, prostatin and leukotrienes can be released, which can strongly induce endothelial cell and tissue damage.

4.2.3   The Inflammatory Mediators

Inflammatory mediators, also known as chemical mediators, are chemical activated factors that participate in and mediate inflammatory response, and they have the ability to cause vascular dilation, permeability, and white blood cells extravasation, which are important in the development of inflammation (Table 4-2). There are two sources for inflammatory mediators: cell-derived and plasma-derived ones. The former are usually present in intracellular granules in inflammation to stimulate the secretion or synthesis of the body; The latter are activated after a series of hydrolysis catalyzed by proteolytic enzymes which are usually present in the body. Most of the inflammatory mediators conduct their biological activity by binding to specific receptors on the surface of target cells; and one mediator can act on a variety of target cells and produce different biological effects on different cells and tissues. Most of the inflammatory mediators have a short half-life and will degrade rapidly. They will be inactivated or eliminated once they are activated or released. So the existence of mediators is in a dynamic equilibrium through the regulatory system or self-stability mechanism in our bodies. Most inflammatory mediators have the potentially damaging effects.

Table 4-2   The main medium and its role in inflammation

For use	Major inflammatory mediators
Vasodilation	Histamine, bradykinin, prostaglandin(PGI2, PGE2, PGD2, PGF2), NO
Increase the permeability of blood vessel walls	Histamine, slow excitation peptide, C3a and C5a, LTC4, LTD4, LTE4, PAF, substance P
Chemotaxis	LTB4, C5a, bacterial products, cationic proteins, chemical factors
Fever	IL-1, IL-2, TNFα, PGE$_2$
The pain	PGE$_2$, bradykinin
Tissue damage	Oxygen free radicals, lysosomal enzymes, NO

4.2.3.1   Inflammatory Mediators Released by Cells

(1) Vasoactive Amines

Vasoactive amines include histamine and serotonin, and they are present as prostatin and are released rapidly, and exert their effect once stimulated. They are often the "protagonists" of the early inflammatory response, so they are also called Fast Media. ①Histamine: It's mainly found in the mast cells in the connective tissue around the blood vessels, and in the granules of basophils and platelets in the blood. When stimulated, it is released in the form of degranulation. Factors that cause histamine release include complement fragments(such as C3a and C5a), cytokines(such as IL-1 and IL-8) and neuropeptides etc. Histamine receptors(H1, H2, H3) are present in the cell membrane, and the receptor plays a biological role in combination with histamine. The activation of H1 receptor results in the contraction of bronchial and vascular smooth muscle, and leads to vascular endothelial contraction and increased vascular permeability. Histamine also has a chemotactic effect on eosinophils. ②5-hydroxytryptamine(5-HT): It is also known as serotonin exists, mainly in platelets and enterochromaffin cells. Collagen, thrombin, ADP, platelet activating factor (PAF) and immune complexes stimulate platelet aggregation to release 5-HT. 5-HT and histamine play a similar role, they mainly function in increasing vascular permeability.

(2) Arachidonic Acid(AA) and its Metabolites

AA is an unsaturated fatty acid and present mainly in the phospholipids of various organs, for example, the prostate, brain, lung and intestine. Phospholipase A$_2$(PLA$_2$) is activated and released from the membrane phospholipid under stimulation of inflammation factors. AA itself is not inflammatory mediators, but when released, it produces prostaglandins and leukotrienes via cyclooxygenase and lipoxygenase pathways, respectively. It can also generate metabolites such as lipoxin through other pathways to play an inflammatory mediator role. ①PG: PG are the metabolites of AA by cyclo-oxygenase(COX) pathway. The important products associated with the inflammatory process are PGE$_2$, PGD$_2$, PGF$_2$ and PGI$_2$, which are synthesized by specific enzymes. Platelets, for example, contain thrombin synthase, so TXA$_2$ is mainly produced by platelets, which can cause platelet aggregation and vasoconstriction to initiate the clotting process. PGE_2 is a hypersensitive substance that causes pain in the inflammatory process by increasing the sensitivity of the skin. PGE2 is also a strong heating agent, which is used in medicine. ②Leukotriene(LT): LT is a metabolic product of AA produced by the lipoxygenase(LOX) pathway, of which the main inflammation related products are LTA_4, LTB_4, LTC_4, LTD_4 and LTE_4. LTB_4 is the activating factor of neutrophils and white blood cells, which is attached to the endothelial cells, producing oxygen free radicals and releasing lysosomes; LTC_4, LTD_4 and LTE_4 can cause strong vasoconstriction, bronchospasm and increased vascular permeability. ③Lipoxin(LX): It's also the metabolic product produced by AA through the pathway of fat and oxygenase, which has the dual function of promoting and inhibiting the inflammatory response, and its inflammatory response is mainly related to LXA_4 and LXB_4. LX may be the negative regulator of LT activity in vivo as it inhibits chemotactic reaction of neutrophils.

(3) Leukocyte Products

It mainly includes oxygen free radicals and lysosomal enzymes released by neutrophils and monocytes. ①Oxygen free radicals(OFR): This mediator mainly include superoxide anions(O_2^-), hydrogen peroxide (H_2O_2) and hydroxyl radicals(-OH), which can combine with NO in cells to form active nitrogen intermediate. When these media are released in small amounts, they can increase the expression of IL-8, certain cytokines, endothelial cell and leukocyte adhesion molecules, causing inflammation cascade and amplifying the effect. The release of these active substances will cause serious damage to the tissue. Of course, human serum, tissue fluid and host cells themselves have antioxidant mechanisms that protect the body against potential oxygen free radicals. Therefore, whether the OFR cause damage in the inflammatory response also depends on the balance between OFR and antioxidants. ②Lysosomal enzymes: Both the death of phagocytes and the exhalation of enzymes in the phagocytic process can lead to enzyme release in the lysosome. Lysosomal enzymes, such as neutral protease(elastase, collagenase, cathepsin, etc.) play an important role in destroying purulent inflammation tissue, including collagen fibers, fibrin, basement membrane, elastin and cartilage, etc; the neutral protease also cleans C3 and C5 directly, releasing anaphylaxis and kinin. On the other hand, the antiprotease system is present in human serum and tissue fluid, such as alpha 1 – antitrypsin (AAT), which is the key factor in inhibiting elastic protease in the neutrophils. If AAT is absent in lung tissues, neutral protease can not be inhibited, which will lead to emphysema throughout the whole lung.

(4) Cytokine

Cytokines are small molecules of polypeptide or glycoprotein which is produced by the immune cells (lymphocytes, monocytes), and certain non-immune cells(endothelial cells, epithelial cells, fibroblasts). Cytokines include colony-stimulating factor(CSF), IL, IFN, TNF, TGF-β, chemokine family and other cytokines(PDGF, FGF, EGF, VEGF, IGF, NGF, HGF, TGF-α, etc.), which play important roles in cellular physiology and various biological effects like the immune response and inflammation.

(5) PAF

PAF is a potent bioactive phospholipid derived from platelets, basophils, mast cells, neutrophils, monocytes and endothelial cells. By binding to the PAF receptor on the target cell membrane, PAF cause platelet aggregation and neutrophilic aggregation, adhesion and release. It also can directly act on target cells or stimulate white blood cells to synthesize other inflammatory mediators(such as reactive oxygen, LT, etc.). Clinically, PAF receptor blockers are used to prevent the binding of PAF to receptors and are therefore of therapeutic interest in diseases associated with PAF overproduction such as asthma and septic shock.

(6) NO

NO is formed by the action of L-arginine, molecular oxygen, NADPH and other auxiliary factors in different types of nitric oxide synthase(NOS), and NO is derived from endothelial cells, macrophages and specific nerve cells in the brain. There are three types of NOS isozymes in the body, including the inducible nitric oxide synthase(iNOS), endothelial cell nitric oxide synthase(eNOS) and nerve cell nitric oxide synthase(nNOS). iNOS are mainly found in macrophages and lung endothelial cells, which catalyze the production of excessive NO and participate in the inflammatory reaction. However, eNOS and nNOS participate in the production of NO in physiological state and maintain normal physiological function of the body. The main function of NO as an inflammatory medium is to relax the vascular smooth muscle and expand the blood vessels. In addition, it can reduce the aggregation and adhesion of platelets and inhibit the inflammatory response induced by mast cells.

(7)Neuropeptide

Neuropeptide is a kind of special information substance that is broadly referred to as an endogenous active substance in nerve tissue. It is characterized by low level, high activity, extensive and sophisticated function. It regulates a variety of physiological functions in the body, like pain, sleep, emotion, learning, memory and the development of the nervous system itself. For example, the presence of substance P in the lung and the nerve fiber of the gastrointestinal tract, not only participates in regulating pain signal, blood pressure and the activation of immune cells as well as endocrine cells, but also has the effect on increasing vessel wall permeability at the initial stage of inflammation. The G protein is a p-specific receptor, and a mouse without the receptor can not respond to the stimulation which is sufficient to increase the permeability of the pulmonary capillaries.

4.2.3.2   The Inflammatory Mediators of Humoral Origin

(1)Kinin System

There is a wide range of biological activity for the kininogen-kinin system. Kinin system is closely related to coagulation system, complement system, renin-angiotensin system and other cytokine system as well as various vascular activity factors, to jointly maintain normal physiological functions. The final product of the system, bradykinin, is an important inflammatory medium under kininogenase activation. Its main function is to expand the arterial artery, increase blood vessels permeability, and reduce smooth muscle contraction (such as bronchial smooth muscle). Kininases are categonrized into plasma and tissue types, and the molecular weight, physiological function, physical and chemical properties as well as immunological properties are all different for these two types of kininase. Plasma type of kininase usually activate peptide enzyme, in the form of the activated peptide enzyme(prekininogenase) then it enters the circulating bloodstream, and the activation center link is XII factor(Hageman factor) activation. First, XII factor produces a fragment(prekininogenase) under the activation by collagen and basement membrane, which changes the prekininogenase into activated kininase XII factor, and Kininogen will eventually be cracked into bioactive bradykinin under the action of kininogen. Tissue kinase is present in various secretions(saliva, pancreatic juice, tear), urine and feces. It can hydrolyze the peptides, which are converted to bradykinin by aminopeptidase.

(2)Complement System

The complement system is composed of a series of enzymes active in the serum and tissue fluid, and has the effect of increasing the permeability of blood vessels, chemotaxis and modularization. Complement is mainly synthesized by hepatocyte in plasma while it is mainly released from macrophages in the inflammatory tissue. The complement in plasma exists in an inactivated form, and can be activated by classical pathway (antigen-antibody complex), alternative pathway(pathogenic microorganism surface molecule, such as endotoxin or lipopolysaccharide) and agglutinin pathway. The activation of C3 and C5 in the complement system is the most important process. The cleavage fragments C3a, C5a and C3b are important mediators in the inflammatory process. They mainly function in three aspects: ①Anaphylaxis: The membranes of mast cells and basophils can release histamine, LT and PG, the act as mediators, causing vasodilation and increased vascular permeability; C3a and C5a cause similar pathological changes in allergic reactions, which is the so-called C5a and C3a allergy toxin(anaphylatoxin). ②Chemokines and adhesion: C5a, C3a and C4a are the potent chemokines of neutrophils, eosinophils, basophils and monocytes, and can activate white blood cells and increase the affinity of protein molecules on the surface of white blood cells to promote their adhesion to endothelial cells. ③Phagocytosis: C3b has the effect of modulating the cell wall of bacteria, which can enhance the phagocytosis of neutrophils and monocytes because there are C3b receptors on the surface of these phagocytes.

(3)Clotting System and Fibrinolytic System

Factor Ⅻ can not only activate the kinase system, but also activate blood coagulation and fibrinolysis. The blood coagulation system is activated to produce thrombin, fibrin polypeptide and factor Xa with activity of inflammatory mediators. Thrombin can promote leukocyte adhesion and fibroblast proliferation by combining to the protease-activated receptors(PAR) of platelets, vascular endothelial cells and smooth muscle cells. Thrombin also functions in the release of cytokines and inflammatory mediators, microvascular exudation, neutrophil chemotaxis and other pathological processes. Fibrin polypeptide can increase vascular permeability and it is also a chemotactic factor of leukocyte. Thrombin Xa binds to effector cell by protease receptor-1(ECPR-1), an agent that mediates acute inflammation, resulting in increased vascular permeability and enhanced leukocyte exocytosis. Activated fibrinolytic system degrades C3 and produce C3a, increasing vasodilatation and vascular permeability; fibrin degradation product(FDP) produced by fibrinolytic process has the effect of increasing vascular permeability, and fibrinolytic enzyme activate blood coagulation system by activating factors Ⅻ.

4.2.4　Morphologic Patterns of Acute Inflammation

Inflammations include three basic pathological changes: alteration, exudation and proliferation. According to the characteristics of inflammation lesions, acute inflammation may be generally divided into three types: alterative inflammation, exudative inflammation and proliferative inflammation.

4.2.4.1　Alterative Inflammation

Alterative inflammation is characterized by degeneration or necrosis of cells or tissues at the main lesion. Slight exudation and proliferation are common in severe infections, poisonings occurred in the liver, kidney, heart, brain and other parenchymal organs. The organ often exhibits the obvious dysfunction caused by the cellular degeneration or necrosis. For example, the epidemic encephalitis cause serious dysfunction of the central nervous system; in the case of toxic myocarditis caused by diphtheria exotoxin, cardiomyocyte degeneration and necrosis cause severe heart dysfunction; extensive necrosis of liver cells leads to serious liver dysfunction in acute severe viral hepatitis.

4.2.4.2　Exudative Inflammation

Exudative inflammation is the most common inflammation. A large amount of exudates are the main feature in inflammatory lesions. The exudation is different from the variance of the inflammatory factors and the reaction of the body. According to the main components of exudation, the exudative inflammation is generally classified as serous inflammation, fibrinous inflammation, suppurative inflammation, hemorrhagic inflammation and other types of inflammation.

(1)Serous Inflammation

Serous inflammation is a major inflammation with the exudation of serous fluid. Exudation is mainly composed of serum, a high concentration of albumin(3% to 5%), and a low globulin content. The electrolyte amount is the same with blood, mixed with a small number of neutrophils, fibrin and epithelial cells. Physical factors(such as high temperature), chemical factors(such as acid, alkali), biological factors(such as bacterial toxins) and snake venom can cause serous inflammation, and it can also exist in the early stages of acute inflammation. Serous inflammation often occurs in the serosa(pleura, peritoneum, pericardium), mucosa, synovium, loose connective tissue and skin. For example, after poisonous snake bites or bee stings, plasma leakage gathered in the connective tissue to form local inflammatory edema; for tuberculosis, rheumatic disease involving the serosa or synovium, a large amount of serous exudation can cause effusion of the chest, peritoneal, pericardial or joint; for the second-degree skin blisters, the serous exudation accumulates in the epidermis. The serous inflammation of mucosa, also known as serous catarrhal inflammation, is characterized by a large amount of serous discharge. For example, a large amount of serous discharge from the nasal mucosa during early stage of a cold. The term catarrh originates from Greek and means the downward drip of the serous, which is used to describe exudation that exudes outward along the mucosal surface. So catarrhal inflammation is an exudative inflammation of mucosal tissue.

The prognosis of serous inflammation is well. The effusion of the serous lymphatic vessels and blood vessels can be absorbed, and the local minor damage of epithelial tissue is easy to repair. Excessive oozing of the plasma can have adverse effects and may cause serious consequences. For example, laryngeal seroma can cause asphyxia in severe cases; pleural or pericardial effusion can result in dysfunction of lung and heart.

(2) Fibrinous Inflammation

Fibrinous inflammation is characterized by accumulation of fibrin in the exudation. Fibrinous inflammation is caused by bacterial toxins such as diphtheria, dysentery and *Streptococcus pneumonia*, or various endogenous, exogenous toxins, such as urea and mercury poisoning in uremia. The toxins lead to a large amount of fibrinogen leakage from the blood vessels, which is converted into fibrin in the necrotic tissue. With HE staining, the fibrin is red and stained with a granular, sort-like an interwoven network, accompanied with neutrophils or necrotic tissue.

Fibrinous inflammation often occurs in the mucosa(pharynx, larynx, trachea, intestine), serosa (pleura, peritoneum and peritoneum) or lung(Figure 4-6). When the fibrinous inflammation occurs in the mucosa(such as diphtheria and bacterial dysentery), the exudation of fibrin, white blood cells, necrotic mucosal tissue and pathogenic bacteria can form a layer of gray and white film(pseudomembrane) covering the mucous surface. Therefore, it is also called pseudomembranous inflammation. In diphtheria, the membrane of the pharynx and trachea is white. Because of the firm attachment of pharyngeal and diphtheria pseudomembrane with deep tissue, so the pseudomembrane is not easy to fall off(solid membranous inflammation) (Figure 4-7A/B). However, there is a loose connection between diphtheria and mucosal exudations of the trachea, and the membranous is easy to fall off(floating membranous inflammation), which may obstruct the bronchial tube and cause suffocation. Serofibrinous inflammation is common in pleural and pericardial membranes, such as tuberculous fibrous pleurisy and rheumatic pericarditis. A large amount of fibrin exudates from the heart, forms numerous villi and covers the pericardium surface, which is called a shaggy heart. Fibrous inflammation occurs in red and gray hepatic changes stage of lobular pneumonia with a large amount of fibrin exudate in the alveolar cavity. The small amount of fibrin can be dissolved by proteolytic enzyme released by neutrophils. With fewer neutrophils or increased antitrypsin activity, the excessive fibrin can cause malabsorption and result in adhesion or transformation of lobular pneumonia.

（3）Purulent Inflammation

Suppurative inflammation is characterized by a large number of neutrophils exudation, varying degrees of tissue necrosis and pus formation. It is usually caused by the infection of the septic bacteria, such as staphylococcus, streptococcus, meningococcus, and e. Coli. It also can be induced by certain chemicals, such as turpentine, ba-bean, and the necrotic tissue, which is called aseptic inflammation. Pyogenesis is the process of dissolving the necrotic tissue by a lysosomal enzyme released by neutrophils. Pus mainly contains a large number of neutrophils, pus cells（denaturation, necrotic neutrophils）, a small amount of serous, liquefactive necrotic tissue and bacteria. There are three types of suppurative inflammation：

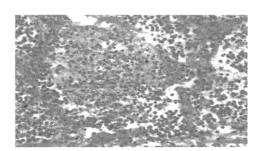

Figure 4-6   **Lobar pneumonia**

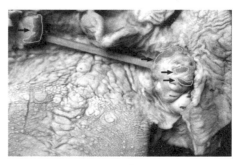

Figure 4 – 7A   **Diphtheria pseudomembrane in tonsillitis（Gross appearance）**

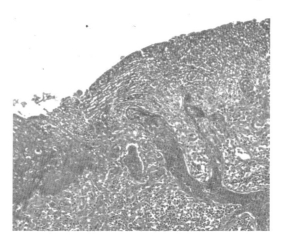

Figure 4 – 7B   **Diphtheria pseudomembrane in tonsillitis（Microscopic appearance）**

1）Abscess   An abscess is a local suppurative inflammation of the organ or tissue. An abscess is characterized by the formation of liquefactive necrosis and the cavity（pus cavity）. The abscess occurs mainly in the skin and internal organs（such as lung, liver, kidney, brain, etc. ）（Figure 4–8A/B）. Staphylococcus aureus is the common pyogenic bacteria which can produce plasma coagulase and convert the fibrinogen into fibrin to prevent bacteria spread. Staphylococcus aureus also produces the adhesion protein receptors, which may cause the spread of abscesses into the distance through the blood vessels. At the early stage of abscess, it is a focal accumulation of neutrophils and necrotice tissues. Then it becomes surrounded by vascular and fibroblastic. to form a so-called abscess membrane, which may absorb pus and limit the spread of inflammation. If the pathogen is exterminated, the pus will be absorbed and the abscess will be replaced by the granulation tissue. If the abscess does not heal, a large amount of fibrous tissue forms a thick wall of chronic abscess, which often requires an incision of pus.

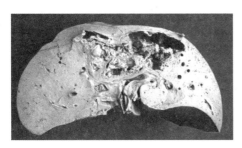

Figure 4 –8A   Hepatic abscess (Gross appearance)

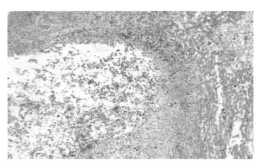

Figure 4 –8B   Hepatic abscess (Microscopic appearance)

It may lead to complications: ①ulcers; skin, mucous membrane, or synovial joints of suppurative inflammation may form deep ulcers, because of the local tissue necrosis or the limitation of collapse loss. ②sinusitis; a deep tissue abscess would break into a form or a natural tube to form a sinus. ③fistulas; the perianal abscess puncture to the skin to form the anal purulent sinus. When the abscess penetrates the inner wall of the intestine, the bowel can communicate with the skin of the body surface and form a purulent fistula(Figure 4–9).

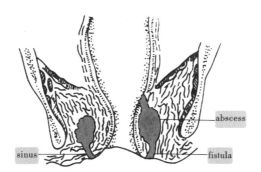

Figure 4–9   The abscess around the anus is a pattern of sinus and fistula

Some of the common examples of abscess formation are as under: ①Furuncle is an abscess occurring in a single hair follicle and its associated sebaceous glands. Furuncle appears in the areas of the rich hair follicles and sebaceous glands(such as the neck, head, face and back). ②Carbuncle is the fusion of multiple abscesses in the subcutaneous fat, fascia formation of multiple communication abscesses. Carbuncle commonly appears on the neck, back, waist, hip and other thick and tough skin. and carbuncle often requires multiple drainages.

2)Phlegmonous inflammation   Cellulitis is the diffuse inflammation of soft tissues(such as subcutaneous, mucous membrane, muscle and appendix)resulting from spreading effects of hemolytic streptococcus. It can secrete hyaluronidase to decompose hyaluronic acid and disintegrate matrix in connective tissue. It also can secrete streptokinase to dissolve fibrin. Thus, hemolytic streptococcus is easy to spread to the surrounding tissue through the interstitial and lymphatic tissue. Phlegmonous inflammation is characterized by severe tissue edema, diffuse infiltration of neutrophils(Figure 4–10), and unclear surrounding tissues. No obvious necrosis and dissolution in happens the local tissue. Light cellulitis can be absorbed without traces, but severe cellulitis can spread rapidly and cause systemic toxicity.

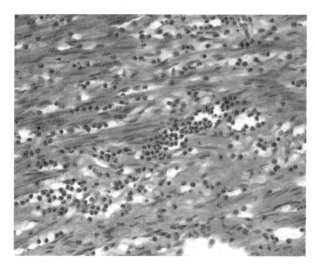

Figure 4-10   Acute phlegmonous appendicitis

3) The surface of the pus and empyema   Superficial suppuration refers to the purulent inflammation which is characterized by infiltration of neutrophils on the surface of mucosa or serous membrane, but inflammatory cells in deep tissue are not obvious. The suppurative inflammation of mucosa is also called purulent catarrhs, the pus exudation, such as suppurative urethritis, suppurative bronchitis. When the pus occurs in the membrane, the gallbladder, the fallopian tube, or the appendix, pus is accumulated in the cavity, called empyema.

(4) Hemorrhagic Inflammation

Some infections(such as anthrax, bubonic plague, leptospirosis, and epidemic hemorrhagic fever) induce vascular damage followed by hemorrhage.

The above inflammation can occur alone or can be combined, such in as serous fibrosis, hemorrhagic hemorrhage of serous and fibrinolysis. During the progress inflammation, one type inflammation may turn into another kind of inflammation. For example, serous inflammation may become fibrinous or suppurative inflammation.

4.2.4.3 Proliferative Inflammation

Although most of the acute inflammation is alteration and exudation, some acute inflammation are also characterized by cell proliferation, known as proliferative inflammation. Lesions are mainly manifested as proliferation of vascular endothelial cells, tissue cells and fibroblasts. For example, Streptococcal acute glomerulonephritis shows glomerular vascular endothelial cells and mesangial cells proliferation; mononuclear macrophage hyperplasia occurs in typhoid fever.

4.2.5 Outcome of Acute Inflammation

The variation in inflammatory response depends upon factors pertaining to the organisms(type, virulence, dose, route of entry) or host factors(systemic diseases, immune status, defect in neutrophil function, type of tissue). Acute inflammation may have variety of outcomes:

4.2.5.1 Resolution and Healing

Resolution means completely return to normal tissue after acute inflammation. This occurs when tissue changes are slight and the cellular changes are reversible and the structure and function of the original tissue are fully restored through the regenerative repair. However, when the tissue destruction is extensive, then fibrotic healing occurs.

4.2.5.2　Chronic Inflammation

Under certain instances, persisting or recurrent acute inflammation may progress to chronic inflammation. When conditions exist are the followings: ①inflammatory factor continuously exists or repeatedly acts on the body; ②the body's resistance is low; ③the treatment is inadequent.

4.2.5.3　Extension and Spread

When pathogenic microorganisms are highly toxic and the body is in low resistance, pathogenic microorganisms can propagate continuously from tissue interspace or vascular system to surrounding or whole body.

(1) Local Extension

The pathogenic microorganism of local inflammation can spread to surrounding tissues and organs through the natural channels of tissue interspace or organs. For example, Mycobacterium tuberculosis can spread to the surrounding tissue along the interstitial space. It can also spread along the bronchus to form new tuberculosis in other parts of the lung.

(2) Lymphatic Spread

Pathogenic microorganisms can invade lymphatic vessels through the interstitial space and spread into local lymph nodes, causing local lymphadenitis. For example, foot suppurative inflammation can cause inguinal lymphadenitis, tuberculosis disseminated hilar lymph node tuberculosis.

(3) Hematogenous Spread

The pathogenic microorganisms may invade the blood circulation or toxins are absorbed into the blood, causing bacteremia, toxemia, septicemia or sepsis. ①Bacteremia is defined as presence of small number of bacteria in the blood which do not multiply significantly. The patient may have no symptoms of systemic toxication. Some inflammatory diseases in the early stages are bacteremias, such as typhoid, epidemic cerebrospinal meningitis and lobular pneumonia. ②Toxemia means presence of bacterial toxins and metabolites in the blood. It can cause high fever and other systemic toxic symptoms, but the blood culture cannot find bacteria. The toxemia is often accompanied by the degeneration or necrosis of the heart, liver, kidney and other parenchymal cells. ③Septicemia means presence of rapidly multiplying, highly pathogenic bacteria in the blood, resulting in systemic toxic symptoms. The pathogenic bacteria can be found in blood culture. Clinically, patients often have chills, high fever, skin and mucous bleeding spots, swollen spleen, swollen lymph nodes, or even shock. ④Pyemia is the dissemination of small septic thrombi in the blood which cause their effects at the site where they are lodged. This can result in pyaemic abscesses or septic infarcts, which is often found in the lungs, liver, kidney, brain and skin, etc. These abscesses are small-sized, distributed more evenly. Bacterial colonies can be observed in the central and small blood vessels. This abscess is also known as an embolic abscess.

4.3　Chronic Inflammation

Chronic inflammation is defined as a prolonged process(months or even years) in which tissue destruction and inflammation occur at the same time. Most chronic inflammations originate from acute inflammation; partly due to the mild and persistent stimulation of the pro-inflammatory cytokines, such as certain virulent pathogenic microorganisms(M. tuberculosis, Treponema pallidum and Fungi, etc.) or autoimmune diseases(such as rheumatoid arthritis, systemic lupus erythematosus). Some chronic inflammations are due to long-term exposure to potentially toxic substances, for example, silicosis is due to long-term inhalation of silica(SiO_2). Recurrent and continuous progress is an important clinical feature of chronic inflammation, and its acute phase is similar to acute inflammation. Chronic inflammation is characterized by celluar proliferation(Figure 4-11). Based on the morphological characteristics, chronic inflammation can be divided into two categories: non-specific chronic inflammation and granulomatous inflammation.

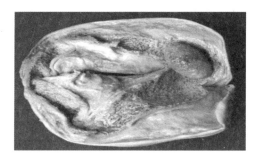

Figure 4-11　Chronic cholecystitis, with gallstone

4.3.1　Chronic non-Specific Inflammation

It is also called general chronic inflammation and is common in clinical. The proliferative cells are fibroblasts, vascular endothelial cells and parenchymal cells, accompanied by infiltrative cells, such as lymphocytes, plasma cells and macrophages(Figure 4-12). Local epithelial cells and glandular epithelium can also proliferate. Some repairing changes may occur. Granulation tissue hyperplasia, fibrosis development and scar formation play an important role in the absorbing and healing of chronic abscess, sinus, fistula and chronic mucosal ulcers. However, this repairing process might cause tissue or organ adhesion or sclerosis. For example, chronic Crohn's disease may cause intestinal stenosis and intestinal obstruction.

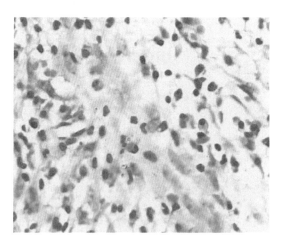

Figure 4-12　Chronic non-specific inflammation in the mucosa

There are 2 speical types of chronic non-specific inflammation:①Inflammatory polyp, a pedicled mass formed by the hyperplasia of local mucosal epithelium, glandular and granulation tissue under the long-term effect of inflammatory factors. It occurs in the cavity of organs, such as the cervix and gastrointestinal mucosa. Inflammatory polyps are generally small with a diameter of no more than 2 cm; under the microscope, the hyperplasia of mucosal epithelium, glandular and granulation tissue are obvious, and interstitial edema accompanied by chronic inflammatory cell infiltration might be observed. ② inflammatory pseudotumor, a tumor-like mass formed by the chronic inflammatory hyperplasia of tissue, often in the lung and eye socket. Under imaging examination, the morphological characteristics are similar to the tumor, known as an inflammatory pseudotumor. Under microscopy, inflammatory pseudotumor is composed of granulation tissue, fibrous tissue, inflammatory cells and hyperplasia parenchyma. The inflammatory pseudotumor of the lung is relatively complex with the chronic inflammatory cell infiltration, the significant hyperplasia of alveolar epithelial and fibrous tissue, as well as the different degree of fibrosis. It is not easy to distinguish inflammatory pseudotumor from lung tumor. Sometimes, it can only be diagnosed by pathological examination.

4.3.2   Granulomatous Inflammation

It is a chronic proliferative inflammation characterized by formation of granuloma, which is a nodular lesion characterized by the limited infiltration and hyperplasia of macrophages. The essence of granuloma is inflammation caused by delayed hypersensitivity, and the involved cells are macrophages and epithelioid cells released by the immune response. Therefore, granuloma can be defined as the aggregation of macrophages and their derived cells(such as epithelioid cells, multinucleated giant cells, etc.), with or without the presence of other inflammatory cells. The special morphological manifestations of various granulomas have important pathological diagnostic value.

4.3.2.1   The Causes of Granulomatous Inflammation

(1) Bacterial infections include tuberculosis and leprosy.

(2) Spirochetes infections include treponema pallidum and syphilis.

(3) Fungal infections include candidiasis, hairy mycosis, cryptococcosis, actinomycosis, and histoplasmosis.

(4) Parasitic infections include schistosomiasis, filariasis and ascariasis.

(5) Endogenous and exogenous foreign bodies: The former are the endogenous foreign bodies such as urate in the nodules of gout; The latter includes various metals or non-metallic substances that enter the body from the outside, such as beryllium, zirconium, surgical sutures, talcum powder, wood spines, iron chips, dust, asbestos, silica gel and mineral oil.

(6) The cause is unknown for sarcoidosis.

4.3.2.2   The Types of Granuloma

(1) Infective Granuloma

It is caused by pathogen infection such as treponema pallidum, fungi and parasites Granuloma is of diagnostic significance. For example, tuberculosis is the granulomatous inflammation caused by Mycobacterium tuberculosis, which is characterized by the formation of a typical tuberculous granuloma(tubercle). Tubercle consists of central caseous necrosis, surrounded by proliferative epithelioid cells, Langhans multinucleate giant cell, lymphocytes, and fibroblasts(Figure 4−13).

(2) Foreign Body Granuloma

It is caused by foreign bodies, e. g. , surgical suture, dust, talcum powder, wood spines, Foreign bodies are in the lesion center, surrounded by numerous macrophages, foreign body giant cells, fibroblasts and lymphocytes(Figure 4−14).

(3) Sarcoidosis Granuloma

It is a non-necrotic epithelioid granuloma that occurs during sarcoidosis. Sarcoidosis is a kind of systemic diseases with unknown etiology. Sarcoidosis can be observed in multiple systems and organs such as lymph nodes, skin, upper respiratory tract, lungs, liver, eyes, heart, nervous system, salivary glands, muscles and bones. The granuloma is mainly composed of epithelioid cells, multinucleated giant cells and lympho-cytes, without caseous necrosis.

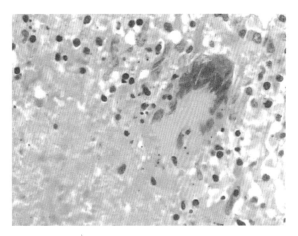

Figure 4–13   **Tubercle**

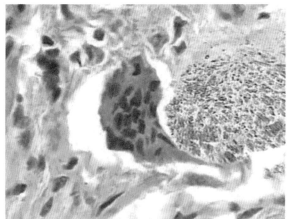

Figure 4–14   **Tophus**

4.3.2.3   The Histogeny of Granuloma? (Pathogenesis of Granuloma)

Formation of granuloma is a type Ⅳ granulomatous hypersensitivity reaction. It is a protective defense reaction by the host but eventually causes tissue destruction because of persistence of the poorly digestible antigen e. g. Mycobacterium tuberculosis, leprosy bacilli, etc.), materials that is or difficult to be degraded, e. g. suture, dust and other foreign bodies. Macrophages play an important role in secreting chemokines and aggregateing inflammatory lesions. Macrophages, being antigen-presenting cells, can present antigen to CD_4^+T lymphocytes. These lymphocytes get activated and elaborate lymphokines, which also can activate macropha-ges to improve their phagocytosis and bactericidal activity. The morphology of macrophage is modified to be epithelial cell-like appearance(Epithelioid cells). Epithelioid cells are weakly phagocytic. Fusion of adja-cent epithelioid cells can form multinucleated giant cell. Like epithelioid cells, these giant cells are weakly phagocytic but produce secretory products which help removing the invading agents.

4.3.2.4   The Components of Granuloma

(1) The Epithelioid Cells

They are modified macrophages/histiocytes which are somewhat elongated cells having slipper-shaped nucleus with 1−2 small nucleoli. The nuclear chromatin of these cells is vesicular and lightly-staining, while the cytoplasm is abundant, pale-staining with hazy outlines so that the cell membrane of adjacent epithelioid cells is closely apposed. Mitochondria, endoplasmic reticulum, ribosomes, Golgi complex and lysosomes are abundant in the cytoplasm. Although epithelioid cells are weakly phagocytic because of the absence of FC and C3b receptors on cell membrane, they also can secrete degradation enzyme and cytokines(TNF, IL-1, etc.).

(2) Multiple Nuclear Giant Cells

Multiple nuclear giant cells are fused by epithelioid cells, and their size is large(40−50 mm), with a-bundant cytoplasm and eosinophilic acid, with nuclei ranging from tens to hundreds. These nuclei may be arranged at the periphery like the horseshoe or as a flower ring, or may be clustered at the two poles (Langhans' giant cells), or they may be present centrally(foreign body giant cells). The former are com-monly seen in tuberculosis while the latter are common in foreign body tissue reactions.

Chapter 5

Neoplasm

> **Introduction**

A neoplasm or tumor is a group of cells that have undergone unregulated growth and will often form a mass or lump, and may be distributed diffusely. They have different biological behaviors and clinical manifestations. The so-called cancer usually refers to these malignant tumors which are seriously harmful to human health.

Recent evidence shows that neoplasm is the first leading cause of death in urban residents in China. In 2015, about 90.5 million people suffered from cancer. About 14.1 million new cases occur per year(not including skin cancer other than melanoma). It causes about 8.8 million deaths(15.7% of deaths)worldwide every year. The most common types of cancer are lung cancer, prostate cancer, colorectal cancer and stomach cancer in males and breast cancer, colorectal cancer, lung cancer and cervical cancer in females. In children, acute lymphoblastic leukemia and brain tumors are most common, except in Africa where non-Hodgkin lymphoma occurs more often.

This chapter describes the basic pathologic properties of neoplasia, including the nature of benign and malignant neoplasms and the molecular basis of neoplastic transformation. We also discuss the host response to neoplasms and the clinical features of neoplasia.

5.1 Definition and General Morphology of Neoplasm

Neoplasm is an abnormal growth of tissue which usually(but not always)forms a local mass. When it forms a mass, neoplasm is commonly referred to as a tumor. *Tumor*, Latin for *swelling*, originally meant any form of swelling, neoplastic or not. The word "*Neoplasm*" is from ancient Greek *neo*-"new" and *plasm*-"formation". Some neoplasms do not form a tumor, such as leukemia and most forms of carcinoma in situ.

The process of the neoplasm formation is called neoplasia, which is the result of severe disorders of cell growth regulation with kinds of tumorigenic factors. Neoplasia literally means "new growth", which is caused by an abnormal proliferation of cells, usually named as neoplastic proliferation. The characteristics of neoplastic proliferation are ①uncoordinated, uncontrolled and harmful growth of cells; ②clonal proliferation of cells; ③varying degrees of dedifferentiation; ④a certain degree of autonomy.

The concept contrary to the neoplastic proliferation is non-neoplastic proliferation. It is usually a controlled and limited process which is coordinated with the needs of the body and occurs in the conditions of normal cell renewing, defense response caused by injury and reparation. For example, the proliferation of endothelium and fibroblast in the inflammatory granulation tissues is non-neoplastic. It generally will not continue after the cessation of the stimuli which evokes the changes. Cells or tissues of non-neoplastic proliferation are polyclonal and capable of differentiation and maturation.

Various factors that cause tumor formation are called tumorigenic agents. Substances that cause the formation of a malignant tumor are called carcinogens. Research over the past few decades has shown that neoplasia is a complicated process resulting from the accumulation of multiple genetic mutations.

The nature of a neoplasm is mainly determined by pathological observations (including gross and microscopic morphological examinations) of specimens from biopsy and surgical excision.

5.1.1   Gross Appearance of Neoplasm

Attention should be paid to the number, size, shape, color and texture of tumor in gross observation because the above information is helpful for determining the type and benign and malignant tumor.

5.1.1.1   Number

The tumor can be single or multiple. Some tumors, such as carcinoma of digestive tract are usually single; other types of tumor often show as multiple masses, for example the patients with neurofibromatosis can have dozens or even hundreds of masses. When physical examination is performed for tumor patients or surgical specimens are examined, it should be avoided noticing obvious tumor and neglecting the possibility of multiple tumors.

5.1.1.2   Volume

The volume of the tumor can be very different. Tiny tumors, such as thyroid microcarcinoma, are difficult to observe by naked eyes. They need to be observed under microscope. A large tumor can weigh up to several kilograms or even tens of kilograms, such as cystadenoma occurring in the ovary. The volume of a tumor is related to many factors such as the nature(benign or malignant), location, growth rate and so on. Tumor that occurs on the body surface or in large body cavity has plenty of space and large volume. On the contrary, tumor that occurs in a narrow space and closed cavity like cranial cavity and spinal canal is usually small because of growth restriction.

Generally speaking, the larger the malignant tumor, the easier it is to metastasize. Therefore, the volume of malignant tumor is an important index of tumor stage. In some tumor types (gastrointestinal stromal tumor), volume is also an important index to predict tumor biological behavior.

5.1.1.3   Shape

The shape of tumor can be different because of its different histological type, location, growth mode, its good and evil nature. In medicine, we use some typical terms to describe the shape of a tumor, such as papillary, villous, polypoid, nodular, lobular, infiltrative, ulcerative, cystic. Common shapes of tumors are shown in Figure 5-1.

5.1.1.4   Color

The color of the tumor is determined by the color of tumor tissues, cells and products. The cut surface of fibrous tumor is mostly gray-white. The lipoma is yellow and the hemangioma is often red. Some secondary changes occur in tumor, such as degeneration, necrosis and bleeding, which can change the original color of the tumor. Melanoma cells produce melanin, which makes the tumors dark brown.

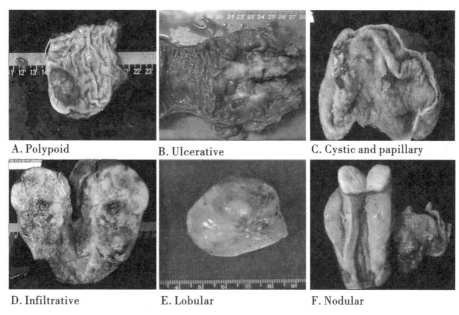

A. Polypoid   B. Ulcerative   C. Cystic and papillary

D. Infiltrative   E. Lobular   F. Nodular

Figure 5-1   Common shapes of neoplasms

5.1.1.5   Texture

Types and the proportion of tumor cells to interstitial tissue determine the texture of the tumor. Lipoma is soft. Less interstitial tumors, such as colorectal adenoma, are soft. Invasive carcinoma with fibrous tissue reaction is hard.

5.1.2   Microscopic Morphology of Neoplasm

The tissue morphology of the tumor is ever-changing and the basis of histopathological diagnosis of tumor. All tumors have two basic components: the parenchyma and the host-derived stroma. Neoplastic cells constitute the parenchyma and their morphology, composition and products are the main basis for judging the differentiation and histological classification of tumors. Tumor stroma is usually made up of connective tissue and blood vessels, which supports and nourishes the parenchyma of the tumor. Neoplastic cells stimulate angiogenesis which is the key factor for tumor to continue to grow. Infiltration of lymphocytes is also seen in tumor stroma, which may be related to the body's immune response to tumor tissue.

5.2   Differentiation and Atypia of Neoplasm

Tumor differentiation refers to the similarity between tumor tissue and some normal tissue in morphology and function. The degree of similarity is called tumor differentiation. For example, tumors similar to adipose tissue suggest that they differentiate into adipose tissue. The more the neoplastic cells resemble their normal forebears in morphology and function, the better the differentiation of the neoplasm, which is termed as well-differentiated. On the contrary, the smaller the similarity with normal tissue, the less differentiated or poorly differentiated. A poorly differentiated tumor, which is unable to determine the direction of its differentiation, is called undifferentiated tumor.

Tumor atypia refers to the difference between the neoplastic parenchyma and the corresponding normal tissues in tissue structure and cell morphology (Figure 5-2). Architectural atypia of the neoplasms is the difference in tissue structure and spatial arrangement between neoplastic cells and the corresponding normal tissues. For example, in squamous cell carcinoma or carcinoma in situ of esophagus, there is an obvious disorder of squamous epithelium. In gastric adenocarcinoma, glandular epithelium is formed with irregular glands or glandular structure. In endometrial adenocarcinoma, normal endometrial stroma disappears between glands.

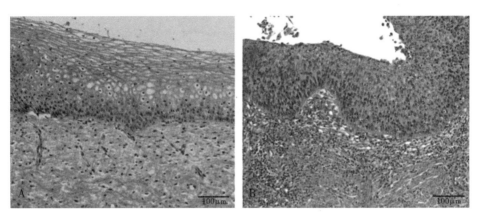

Figure 5-2   Normal stratified squamous epithelium(A); Architectural atypia(B) (H&E,200×)

Cellular atypia of the neoplasms has many manifestations, including ①Cell volume abnormality. Some of neoplastic cells are characterized by increased cell volume, some of which are primitive small cells. ②Pleomorphism. The size and shape of tumor cells are very different. Sometimes, tumor giant cells appear in tumor tissue. ③The increase of nuclear-to-cytoplasm ratio. It is the prominent hallmark of neoplasm, especially of malignant neoplasm, that the nuclei are large disproportionately for the cells with the nuclear-to-cytoplasm ratio that increases from the normal 1 : 4 or 1 : 6 to approach 1 : 1. ④Nuclear pleomorphism. The nuclear shape is variable and often irregular with the appearance of giant nuclei, double nuclei, multiple nuclei and weird or bizarre nuclei. The chromatin is often coarsely clumped and unevenly distributed under the nuclear membrane(hyperchromatic), which results from the increase of DNA in nuclei. ⑤Distinctive and large nucleolus. The number of nucleoclus is increased. ⑥Increase in nuclear mitosis. Abnormal mitoses (pathological mitotic figures) can be observed sometimes, such as asymmetrical or multipolar mitoses (Figure 5-3).

Atypia is a manifestation of disturbance of maturation and differentiation in neoplastic tissues and cells; and also an important indicator to distinguish between benign and malignant neoplasms. Benign neoplasms usually show light inconspicuous cellular atypia, but still have different degrees of architectural atypia. For malignant neoplasms, both cellular atypia and architectural atypia are obvious. The greater the atypia, the lower the maturity and differentiation, the greater the difference between the neoplasms and the corresponding normal tissues. The obvious atypia is called anaplasia. Most of the anaplastic neoplasms are highly malignant which show the characteristics of anaplasia.

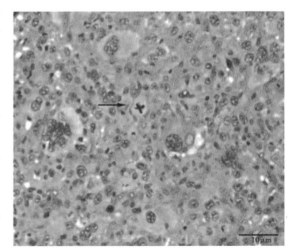

Figure 5-3   Nuclear pleomorphism. The tumor cells present marked pleomorphism in size and shape, with multiple or bizarre nuclei and multipolar mitoses (arrow) (H&E,400×)

5.3   Nomenclature and Classification of Neoplasm

The nomenclature and classification of neoplasm are important parts of pathological diagnosis of neoplasm, and also important for clinical practice. Medical staff should understand the meaning of these names in tumor pathological diagnosis and use them properly.

5.3.1   The Principle of Nomenclature

There are a wide variety of human neoplasm and complex naming. Neoplasm is usually named according to its tissue or cell type and biological behavior.

5.3.1.1   General Principles of Tumor Nomenclature

The nomenclature of benign neoplasm

In general, benign neoplasms are designated by attaching the suffix-oma to the tissue or cell type from which the neoplasm arises. For example, a benign tumor arising from glandular epithelium is called an adenoma; a benign tumor of smooth muscle is leiomyoma.

The nomenclature of malignant neoplasm

Malignant neoplasm of the epithelial tissue is called carcinoma. Carcinomas show some features of epithelial differentiation, designated by adding the "carcinoma" after the name of the epithelium. For example, the malignant neoplasm of the squamous epithelium is termed as squamous cell carcinoma; the malignant neoplasm of the glandular epithelium is named adenocarcinoma. Some carcinomas have more than one kind of epithelial differentiation, for example adenosquamous carcinoma of lung has both squamous cell carcinoma and adenocarcinoma component. Undifferentiated carcinoma refers to a cancer which can be identified as carcinoma with morphology or immunophenotype, but lacking specific epithelial differentiation characteristics.

Malignant neoplasm of the mesenchymal tissues is called sarcoma. Mesenchymal tissues include fibrous tissue, adipose tissue, muscle, blood vessel, lymph vessel, bone and cartilage. Sarcomas show the characteristics of differentiation to some kinds of mesenchymal tissues, designated by adding the "sarcoma" after the name of the mesenchymal tissue, such as fibrosarcoma, liposarcoma, leiomyosarcoma, osteogenic sarcoma. Undifferentiated sarcoma refers to a sarcoma which can be identified with morphology or immunophenotype, but lacking specific mesenchymal differentiation characteristics. Carcinosarcoma is a malignant neoplasm containing two components of carcinoma and sarcoma. It should be emphasized that in pathology, carcinoma is a malignant neoplasm of epithelial tissue. Cancer refers to all malignant neoplasms, including carcinoma and sarcoma.

5.3.1.2   Exceptional Conditions of Tumor Nomenclature

In addition to the general rules mentioned above, neoplasm is sometimes named in combination with the morphological characteristics. For example, adenoma that forms papillary and cystic structures is called papillary cystadenoma; adenocarcinoma with papillary and cystic structures is named papillary cystadenocarcinoma.

Due to historical reasons, the names of a few tumors have been established by usage, not completely following the above principles. ①The morphology of some tumors is similar to that of some immature cells or tissues during development. They are called blastoma. Benign blastoma includes osteoblastoma; malignant blastoma, such as neuroblastoma, medulloblastoma and nephroblastoma. ②Leukemia, lymphoma and seminoma are malignant neoplasms actually, despite of the end of oma and mia in name. ③Some malignant tumors are neither carcinoma nor sarcoma, but are directly called malignant oma, such as malignant melanoma, anaplastic(malignant)meningioma, malignant teratoma and malignant schwannoma. ④Some tumors are named after the scholars who initially described or studied the tumor, such as Ewing sarcoma, Hodgkin lymphoma. ⑤Several neoplasms are named in the form of neoplastic cells, for example clear cell sarcoma. ⑥"-omatosis" in the names of neurofibromatosis, lipomatosis, angiomatosis, etc, mainly refers to the state of multiple tumors. ⑦Teratoma is an omnipotent tumor occurring in the gonadal or embryonic remaining parts, often occurring in the gonadal gland, usually containing a variety of components of more than two germ layers. It is divided into two types of benign and malignant teratoma.

5.3.2   Classification

The classification of neoplasm is mainly based on the tissue type, cellular type and biological behavior, including clinicopathological characteristics and prognosis of various neoplasms. The classification of common tumors is shown in Table 5-1. There are more detailed classifications of tumors in each organ system.

Different types of neoplasms have different clinicopathological features, therapeutic response and prognosis. The correct classification of neoplasms is an important basis for the formulation of treatment plans and the prognosis of patients. Classification is also the basis of the diagnosis and research of neoplasms. Proper classification helps to define diagnostic criteria and unify diagnostic terminology, which is the premise of clinical pathological diagnosis. Unified diagnostic criteria and terms are also the basic requirements for disease statistics, epidemiological investigation, etiological and pathogenetic study and comparative analysis of the results of different institutions.

Table 5-1   Nomenclature of neoplasms

Tissue of origin	Benign	Malignant
Tumors of epithelial origin		
Stratified squamous cell	Squamous cell papilloma	Squamous cell carcinoma
Basal cells		Basal cell carcinoma
Glandular epithelial cell	Adenoma	Adenocarcinoma
Urinary tract epithelium	Urothelial papilloma	Urothelial carcinoma
Tumors of mesenchymal origin		
Fibrous tissue	Fibroma	Fibrosarcoma
Adipose tissue	Lipoma	Liposarcoma
Smooth muscle	Leiomyoma	Leiomyosarcoma
Striated muscle	Rhabdomyoma	Rhabdomyosarcoma
Blood vessels	Hemangioma	Angiosarcoma
Lymph vessels	Lymphangioma	Lymphangiosarcoma
Bone, cartilage	Osteoma, chondroma	Osteogenicsarcoma, chondrosarcoma
Lymphoid hematopoietic issue		
Lymphatic cells		Lymphomas
Hematopoietic cells		Leukemias
Nervous tissue, meninges		

Continue to Table 5-1

Tissue of origin	Benign	Malignant
Gliocyte		Diffuse astrocytomas
Neuron	Gangliocytoma	Neuroblastoma, medulloblastoma
Meninges	Meningioma	Anaplastic meningioma
Schwann cells	Schwannoma	Malignant schwannoma
Other neoplasms		
Melanocytes	Nevus	Malignant melanoma
Placental trophoblast cells	Hydatidiform mole	Choriocarcinoma
Germ cells		Seminoma, embryonal carcinoma
Totipotential cells in gonads or in embryonic rests	Mature teratoma	Immature teratoma, teratocarcinoma

WHO (World Health Organization) invites experts worldwide to classify neoplasms in different systems, constantly revises it according to the progress of clinic and basic research. Now the WHO tumor classification is widely used in the world.

Pathological diagnosis of neoplasm not only relies on the clinical manifestation of patients, medical imaging and morphologic features but also the expressions of specific molecules in tumor cells. For example, the expressions of desmin in myogenic tumor, cluster of differentiation (CD) antigen on the surface of lymphatic cells, various cytokeratins (CK) in epithelium, human melanoma black 45 (HMB45) in malignant melanoma cells can be detected by immunohistochemical (IHC) method (Figure 5-4). Ki67 and other markers can be used to detect the proliferative activity of tumor cells, which helps to assess their biological behavior and prognosis (Figure 5-5). These markers are important tools for modern pathological diagnosis. Immunological markers play an increasingly important role in tumor diagnosis.

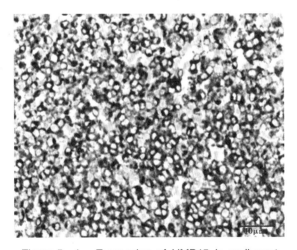

Figure 5-4　Expression of HMB45 in malignant melanoma (IHC, 200×)

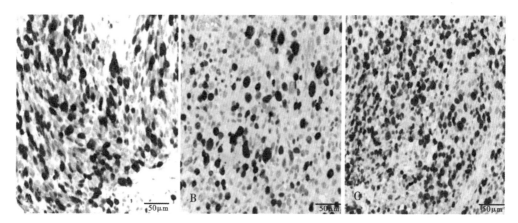

Figure 5-5   Strong nuclear positivity of Ki67 in poorly-differentiated carcinoma (A), sarcoma (B) and lymphoma (C) (IHC, 200×)

Table 5-2 lists common immunological markers and cell or tissue type that usually expresses these markers in tumor diagnosis. It must be noted that most of the immunological markers do not have absolute specificity. It is usually necessary to use a set of markers, good positive and negative controls at the same time, to help to contirm the histopathologic diagnosis of histology. Otherwise it can easily lead to inappropriate conclusions.

An increasingly in-depth study of the molecular mechanism of tumorigenesis provides a new direction for the classification, diagnosis and treatment of neoplasms. In addition to the morphological and biological behavior of various tumors, the latest version of WHO's organ system tumor classification also takes into consideration the characteristic cytogenetics and molecular genetic changes. In recent years, the DNA chip technology has been used to detect the gene expression profiles of tumor cells in a large scale, and the characteristic expression profiles associated with biological behavior or treatment response and prognosis are also shown in some tumors. Molecular diagnosis has been one of the important means of tumor pathological diagnosis. Table 5-3 lists cytogenetic changes of some neoplasms.

Table 5-2   Common immunohistochemical markers of neoplasm

marker	common positive cells or tumor types
Alpha fetal protein, AFP	Fetal liver, yolk sac, hepatic carcinoma, yolk sac tumor
CD3	T lymphatic cell, T cell lymphoma
CD15	Granulocyte, R-S cell (Hodgkin lymphoma), some adenocarcinoma
CD20	B lymphatic cell, B cell lymphoma
CD30	R-S cell (Hodgkin lymphoma), large cell anaplastic lymphoma, embryonal carcinoma
CD31	Endothelium, neoplasm of blood vessel
CD34	Endothelium, neoplasm of blood vessel, gastrointestinal stromal tumors, solitary fibrous tumor
CD45	Leukocyte, neoplasm of ymphoid hematopoietic tissue
CD45RO	T lymphatic cell, T cell lymphoma
CD68	Macrophage

Continue to Table 5-2

marker	common positive cells or tumor types
CD79a	B lymphatic cell, B cell lymphoma
calcitonin	thyroid parafollicular cells, thyroid medullary carcinoma
chromogranin A, CgA	Neuroendocrine cell, neuroendocrine neoplasm, pituitary adenoma
Cytokeratin, CK	Epithelium, mesothelial cell, carcinoma, mesothelioma
desmin	Muscle cell, leiomyoma, leiomyosarcoma, rhabdomyosarcoma
Epithelial membrane antigen, EMA	Epithelium, carcinoma, Meningioma
Glial fibrillary acidic protein, GFAP	Gliocyte, astrocytoma
HMB45	Melanoma, angioleiomyolipoma, PEComa
Ki67	Proliferative cell
Placental alkaline phosphatase, PLAP	Germ cell tumor
Prostate specific antigen, PSA	Prostate epithelium, prostate carcinoma
S-100	Nervous tissue, adipose tissue, Langerhans histocyte, schwannoma, adipose tissue tumor, melanoma
Smooth muscle actin, SMA	Smooth muscle cell, myofibroblast, leiomyoma, myofibroblast tumor
Synaptophysin, Syn	Neuron, neuroendocrine cell, neuron tumor, neuroendocrine neoplasm

Table 5-3　Cytogenetic changes of some neoplasm

Type of tumor	cytogenetic changes
Carcinoma of the lung	del(3)(p14-23)
Renal carcinoma	del(3)(p14-23), t(3;5)(p13;q12)
Nephroblastoma(Wilm's tumor)	del(11)(p13)
Dermatofibrosarcoma protuberant	t(17;22)(q22;q13)
Myxoidliposarcoma	t(12;16)(q13;p11), t(12;22)(q13;q11-12)
Synovial sarcoma	t(x;18)(p11;q11)
Rhabdomyosarcoma	t(2;13)(q35-37), t(1;13)(q36;q14)
Myxoid chondrosarcoma	t(9;22)(q22;q12)
Astrocytoma	del(9)(p13-24)
Neuroblastoma	del(19)(p32-26)
Retinoblastoma	del(13)(q14)
Primitive neuroectodermal tumors(PNET)	t(11;12)(q24;q12), t(21;22)(q22;q12), t(7;22)(p22;q12), t(17;22)(q12;q12), t(2;2 2)(q33;q12)

5.4 Growth and Spread of Neoplasm

In addition to continuous growth, malignant tumor also has local invasion, and even spreads to other parts through metastasis.

5.4.1 The Growth of Neoplasm

5.4.1.1 The Growth Pattern of Neoplasm

There are three main growth patterns of neoplasm: expansile, exophytic and invasive growth patterns.

Benign tumors in solid organ are mostly expansile. The growth rate of benign tumor is slower. As the volume increases, the tumor pushes but not invades surrounding tissues. The benign tumor is well circumscribed and can form a complete fibrous capsule around the tumor. Encapsulated tumor can often be pushed and easily removed without recurrence. The effect of expansile growth pattern on local organ and tissue is mainly squeezing.

Exophytic growth refers to the growth of a neoplastic protrusion on the surface of body or organ(such as the digestive tract)and in the cavity(such as thoracic cavity, peritoneal cavity). The neoplastic protrusion can be papillary, polypoid, fungating or cauliflower. Both benign and malignant neoplasms can grow exogenously, but malignant neoplasms often infiltrate at the base of neoplastic protrusion. Due to the rapid growth of malignant tumor, the blood supply of the central part of the tumor is relatively inadequate. So tumor cells are prone to necrosis, and the necrotic tissues fall off to form an ulcer with an uneven bottom and a marginal bulge.

Invasive growth usually is a hallmark of malignancy. Invasion refers to the phenomenon that neoplastic cells grow into and destroy the surrounding tissue including tissue space, lymph and blood vessels. Invasive tumor has no capsule and no clear borderline with the adjacent normal tissue. It isn't easily moved with palpation. During the operation, a larger area of the surrounding tissues should be removed. If the resection is not complete, it tends to recur after surgery. In surgery, it is helpful for the surgeon to determine if it needs to be expanded through rapid frozen section examination of the marginal tissues by pathologist.

5.4.1.2 The Growth Characteristics of Neoplasm

The growth rate of different tumors is very different. Benign tumors usually grow slowly, for years or even decades. Malignant tumors grow faster, especially those with poor differentiation. They can form an obvious mass in short time. There are many factors that affect the growth rate of tumor, such as the doubling time of tumor cells, growth fraction, the proportion of tumor cell formation and death.

The doubling time of tumor cells refers to the time required for cell division to propagate into two progeny cells. The doubling time of most malignant tumor cells is not faster than that of normal cells, so the rapid growth of malignant tumor may not be caused by the shortened time of tumor cell doubling. Growth fraction refers to the proportion of cells that proliferate in the tumor cell population. The cells that proliferate are constantly dividing and proliferating. This process of division and proliferation is called a cell cycle, including G1, S, G2 and M stages. In the early stage of malignant tumor, cell division and proliferation are active, and the growth fraction is high. With the growth of tumor, some tumor cells enter quiescent stage(G0 stage)and stop dividing and proliferating. Many anti-tumor chemotherapeutic agents play a role in interfering with cell proliferation. Therefore, tumors with high growth fraction are sensitive to chemotherapy. If a tumor has large number of non proliferative cells, it may be less sensitive to chemotherapeutic drugs. Radiation therapy or surgery can be performed to reduce or remove most of the tumor. At this time, the residual G0 tumor cells can enter the proliferation period and increase the sensitivity of the tumor to chemotherapy. To promote tumor cell death and inhibit tumor cell proliferation are two important ways of tumor therapy.

5.4.1.3   The Angiogenesis of Neoplasm

Neoplasm cannot continue to grow beyond the size of 1–2 mm in diameter unless it has the ability to induce neoangiogenesis. Neoplastic cells themselves and inflammatory cells(mainly macrophages)can produce angiogenesis factors such as vascular endothelial growth factor(VEGF)to induce neovascularization. The combination of angiogenic factors and their receptors which are located on the surface of vascular endothelial cells and fibroblasts, can stimulate the division of endothelial cells and capillary sprouting growth. Recent evidence shows that neoplastic cells themselves can form a vascular-like tubular structure with the basement membrane, which can communicate with the blood vessels as a microenvironment or microenvironmental component that does not depend on angiogenesis. It is called vasculogenic mimicry. Inhibition of tumor angiogenesis or "vasculogenic mimicry" is an important topic of anti-tumor research.

5.4.1.4   The Progression and Heterogeneity of Neoplasm

The increasing invasion of malignant tumors during growth is called the progression of tumors, showing as the speed of growth increases, the infiltration of the surrounding tissue and the occurrence of distant metastasis. Tumor progression is related to its increasing heterogeneity. Although neoplasms are derived from monoclonal proliferation of a single malignant transformation cell, progeny cells may have the different changes in genes or other large molecules, variations in the growth rate, invasive ability, the response to growth signal and the sensitivity to anticancer drugs in the process of growth. At this time, the tumor cell population is no longer made up of exactly the same tumor cells but heterogeneous subclones with their respective characteristics. In the process of tumor progression which acquires heterogeneity, cells with growth advantages and strong invasiveness overwhelm cells with no growth advantages and weak invasiveness.

In recent years, the study of leukemia, breast cancer, glioma and other tumors shows that although a tumor is made up of a large number of tumor cells, there are a few cells that have the ability to start and maintain tumor growth and self-renewal, which are called cancer stem cells(CSC), tumor stem cells(TSC), or tumor initiating cells(TIC). CSCs were first described in tumors of hematopoietic origin and have now been identified in several types of solid tumors, such as cancers arising in the breast, lung, prostate, colon, brain, head and neck, pancreas and skin. Long-term self-renewal potential, quiescence and resistance to chemotherapy and radiotherapy are proprieties associated with CSCs. Further research on CSCs will help to understand the tumorigenesis, growth and response to treatment, and explore the new therapeutic treatment.

5.4.2   The Spread of Neoplasm

Malignant tumors not only infiltrate in the primary site, adjacent organs or tissues but also spread to other sites of body by various ways. Local invasion and metastasis are the most important biological characteristics of malignant tumors.

5.4.2.1   Local Invasion and Direct Spreading

Direct spreading denotes the phenomenon that as malignant tumors continue to grow, tumor cells often infiltrate along tissue gaps or nerve bundle to damage adjacent organs or tissues. For example, advanced cervical cancer directly spreads to rectum and bladder.

The mechanisms of local invasion and direct spreading are quite complicated. Taking cancer as an example, it can be roughly summed up in four steps(Figure 5–6). ①The reduction of adhesion molecules on the surface of cancer cells. On the surface of normal epithelium, there are a variety of cell adhesion molecules(CAMs). The interaction between them helps to bind cells together and prevent cell migration. The reduction of adhesion molecules on the surface of cancer cells causes cells to separate from each other. ②The increased attachment of cancer cells to the basement membrane. The attachment of normal epithelium to the basement membrane is mediated by some molecules at the basal surface of the epithelium such as laminin (LN) receptor. Cancer cells express more LN receptors, increasing the attachment of cancer cells to the basement membrane. ③The degradation of extracellular matrix (ECM). Cancer cells produce proteinase such as type IV collagenase to dissolve the extracellular matrix components, cause partial defect in the basement membrane and subsequently help cancer cells to pass through. ④The migration of cancer cells. Cancer cells move through the basement membrane defect by amoeboid movement. After that, cancer cells further dissolve interstitial connective tissue and move in the interstitium. When cancer cells reachthe wall of the vessel, they pass through the basement membrane of blood vessels in a similar way into the blood vessels.

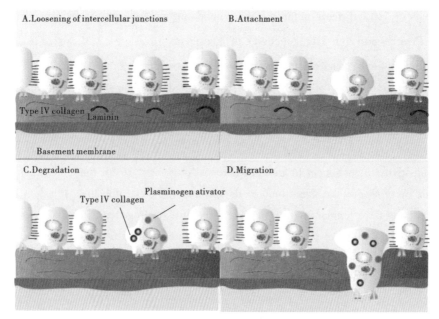

Figure 5-6　The mechanisms of local invasion and direct spreading of neoplasm

Metastasis: The term metastasis denotes the process that malignant tumor cells migrate to other site and continue to grow to form the same type of tumor by invading lymph vessels, blood vessels or body cavity from the original site. Tumor formed by metastasis is called metastatic tumor or secondary tumor. Metastasis is an important feature of malignant tumors, however not all malignant tumors can metastasize. For example, basal cell carcinoma of the skin can cause damage to local tissues, but rarely metastasize.

5.4.2.2　Malignant Tumors Metastasize Through the Following Ways

(1)Lymphatic Metastasis

Neoplastic cells invade the lymph vessels(Figure 5-7) and reach the local lymph nodes(regional lymph nodes) by lymphatic flow. For example, the carcinomas of the upper outel quadrant of the breast usually metastasize to the ipsilateral axillary lymph nodes to form metastatic breast cancer of the lymph nodes. Tumor cells first gather at marginal sinus and then involve the whole lymph node, leading to the enlargement of lymph nodes and the hardening of the texture. The tumor invades the capsule and allows the neighboring lymph nodes to merge into clusters. The metastasis of local lymph nodes can continue to transfer to other lymph nodes at the next stop of the lymphatic circulation and finally enter the blood flow through the thoracic duct.

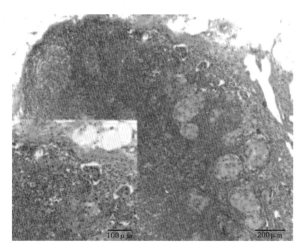

Figure 5-7   Lymphatic metastasis of papillary thyroidcarcinoma(H&E,100×)

(2)Hematogenous Metastasis(Figure 5-8)

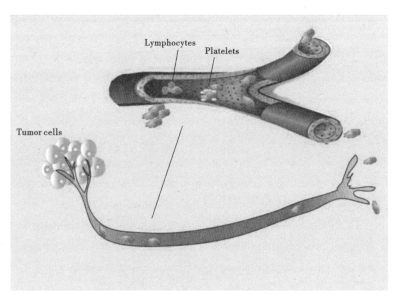

Figure 5-8   The mechanism of hematogenous metastasis of malignant tumors

After cancer cells invade the blood vessels,they can reach distant organs with blood flow,continue to grow and form metastases. Because the venous wall is thinner and the pressure in the tube is relatively low, tumor cells often pass through the vein into the blood and a few can also be connected to the lymphatic vessels. The tumor cells that invade the systemic circulatory vein reach the lung through the right heart and form a metastatic tumor in the lung,such as lung metastases from osteosarcoma. The tumor cells that invade the portal venous system first form hepatic metastasis,such as hepatic metastasis of gastrointestinal carcinoma. Tumor cells of primary lung tumor or intrapulmonary metastatic tumor can invade the pulmonary vein directly or enter the pulmonary vein through the pulmonary capillary. Then they metastasize to all organs through the left heart with the blood flow of the aorta,such as brain,bone,kidney and renal adrenal gland.

Thus, the metastatic tumors of these organs usually occur after lung metastasis. Additionally, tumor cells that invade the chest, waist and pelvic vein can enter the vertebral venous plexus through anastomotic branches, for example, prostate cancer can metastasize to the spine through this pathway, and then to the brain without lung metastasis.

Malignant tumors can involve many organs through hematogenous metastasis, but the most frequently involved organs are lung and liver. So clinically it is necessary to carry out imaging examination of lung and liver for judging whether there is a hematogenous metastasis or not and determining the patient's clinical staging and treatment plan. The morphologic features of metastatic tumor are clearly demarcated, often multiple, scattered, much closer to the surface of the organ. Metastatic tumors located at the surface of the organ form cancer umbilicus due to the central hemorrhage, necrosis and subsidence of cancer nodules.

Malignant tumor cells that enter the blood vessels do not always migrate to other organs to form metastases. Mostly single cancercell is destroyed by natural killer cells, but the tumor cells agglutinated with platelets form an uneasily eliminated tumor cell plug, which can adhere to the vascular endothelial cells and then pass through the vascular endothelium and the basement membrane to form a new metastatic tumor. In the course of tumor progression, there are subclones with different invasiveness. Highly invasive subcellular clones are easy to form widespread hematogenous dissemination.

The location of tumor metastasis is affected by the location of primary tumor and blood circulation. However, some tumors show affinity for some organs. For example, lung cancer easily metastasizes to the adrenal and brain; thyroid carcinoma, renal carcinoma and prostate cancer preferentidally metastasize to the bone; breast cancer often metastasizes to lung, liver, bone, ovary and so on. These phenomena may be related to the following factors: ①The ligands on the endothelial cells of these organs can specifically identify and bind the adhesion molecules on the surface of some cancer cells. ②These organs release the chemotactic factors that attract some cancer cells. ③This is the result of negative selection, that is, the environment of some tissues or organs is not suitable for tumor growth, for example, enzyme inhibitors in tissues are not conducive to the formation of metastases.

(3) Seeding Metastasis

When a malignant tumor occurring in the thoracic or abdominal cavity penetrates to the organ surface, the tumor cells can fall off and grow on the surface of the other organs of the body like sowing, forming multiple metastatic tumors. This dissemination is called seeding metastasis. It is common in malignant tumor of abdominal organ. For example, mucinous carcinoma of the gastrointestinal tract invades the serosa and can be implanted into the greater omentum, peritoneum, pelvic organs, such as the ovary. In the ovary, there is a bilateral ovarian growth, and a diffuse infiltration of carcinoma of the signet ring cells with mucus. This special type of ovarian metastatic tumor is called Krukenberg tumor. It should be noted that Krukenberg tumors are not necessarily seeding metastases, but metastases through lymphatic and blood channels.

The implant metastasis of the serous cavity is often accompanied by serous effusion, caused by the block of subserous lymphatics or capillaries by tumor embolus, the increase of capillary permeability, the blood leakage, and the bleeding induced by tumor cells destroying blood vessels. The effusion of the body cavity may contain unequal tumor cells. It is one of the important ways for the diagnosis of malignant tumor to extract the effusion of the body cavity for cytological examination in order to find the malignant tumor cells.

5.5   Grading and Staging of Neoplasm

Grading of malignancies is an indicator of malignancy. The malignancies are graded on the basis of the degree of differentiation, atypia and the number of mitoses. Three categories of grading are used mostly. Grade Ⅰ is well differentiated with low malignancy. Ⅱ grade is moderately differentiated. Ⅲ grade is poorly differentiated. Some tumors use two categories (low grade and high grade). It should be noted that Ⅰ, Ⅱ, Ⅲ grade are not equivalent to biological behavior codes in the international classification of diseases ICD-O.

Tumor staging refers to the growth and spread of malignant tumors. The larger the tumor size, the wider the growth and dissemination, the worse the prognosis. The following factors should be considered in tumor staging: the size of the primary tumor, the depth of in filtration, the scope of infiltration, the involvement of adjacent organs, the local and distant lymph node metastasis, the distant metastasis, and so on.

The staging system widely used in the world is TNM classification system. T refers to the primary tumor. N refers to regional lymph node involvement, and M refers to metastasis. TNM staging varies for specific forms of cancer, but there are general principles. The primary lesion is characterized as T1 to T4 with the increase of tumor volume and the extent of adjacent tissue involvement. T0 is used to indicate an in situ lesion. N0 means no nodal involvement, whereas N1 to N3 represents the increase of the degree and range of lymph node involvement. M0 means no distant metastasis, whereas M1 indicates the presence of metastasis.

5.6   Effects of Neoplasms on the Host

Benign tumors are composed of well-differentiated tumor cells. They grow slowly in local sites and usually do not infiltrate and metastases. Therefore, benign tumors generally have relatively little influence on the body, mainly manifested by local compression and obstructive symptoms. The occurrence or severity of these symptoms is mainly related to the location and secondary changes of the tumor. For example, benign tumors on the body surface do not have significant effect on the body except for a few local symptoms. However, if they occur in the cavity or an important organ, they may cause more serious consequences. For example, a leiomyoma that protrudes into the intestinal cavity can cause severe intestinal obstruction or intussusception. Intracranial benign tumors may lead to increased intracranial pressure and the corresponding neurological symptoms due to oppression of the brain tissue and obstruction of the ventricular system. Sometimes benign tumors have secondary changes and also affect the body to varying degrees. For example, uterine submucosal leiomyomas are often accompanied by superficial erosion or ulceration of the endometrium, which may lead to bleeding and infection. Benign tumors of the endocrine gland can secrete too many hormones and cause symptoms. For example, pituitary growth adenomas secreting excessive growth hormone can cause gigantism or acromegaly.

Malignant tumors are poorly-differentiated, rapidly growing, infiltrating, and destroying the structure and function of organs. They also metastasize. The effects of malignant tumors on the host are serious, and the therapeutic effect is not satisfactory. The patient's mortality is high and the survival rate is low. In addition to the symptoms of local compression and obstruction, malignant tumors are also prone to ulcers, bleeding, and perforation. Tumors involving local nerves can cause stubborn pain. Tumor products or combined infection can cause fever. Malignant tumors of the endocrine system, including those of the diffuse neuroendocrine system(DNES) such as carcinoids and neuroendocrine carcinomas, produce biogenic amines or polypeptide hormones and cause endocrine disorders. Patients with advanced malignant tumors often develop cancer cachexia, which is characterized by severe body weight loss, anemia, anorexia, and general weakness. The occurrence of cancer cachexia may be mainly the result of tumor tissue itself or cytokines produced by body reactions.

Some non-endocrine tumors may also produce and secrete hormones or hormone-like substances, such as adrenocorticotropic hormone(ACTH), calcitonin, growth hormone(GH), parathyroid hormone(PTH), resulting in endocrine symptoms, which is called ectopic endocrine syndrome. This type of tumors are mostly malignant, with a majority of carcinomas, such as lung carcinoma, stomach carcinoma, and liver carcinoma. The production of heterotopic hormones may be related to abnormal gene expression in tumor cells.

Ectopic endocrine syndrome belongs to paraneoplastic syndrome. The generalized paraneoplastic syndrome refers to some lesions and clinical manifestations that cannot be explained by the direct spread or distant metastasis of the tumor, and are caused by tumor products(such as ectopic hormones) or abnormal immune responses(such as cross-immunity). Patients exhibit abnormalities of many systems, including endocrine, neural, digestive, hematopoietic, bone, joint, kidney and skin. It should be noted that endocrine tumors (such as pituitary adenomas) produce lesions or clinical manifestations that are caused by endocrine-inherent hormones(such as growth hormone), which do not belong to paraneoplastic syndromes.

Some tumor patients show paraneoplastic syndrome before finding tumors. The tumors will be found in time if the paraneoplastic syndrome is considered carefully and further looked for its causes by medical staff. In addition, when tumor patients have such symptoms, the possibility of paraneoplastic syndrome should be taken into account and it should not be mistaken as metastasis.

5.7 Identification Between Benign and Malignant Neoplasms

The biological behaviors of tumors and their influences on hosts vary greatly. Most tumors are divided into benign or malignant. Benign tumors are generally easy to betreated and with a good therapeutic reaction. Malignant tumors are harmful, treatment measures are complex, and the results are not satisfactory. If a malignancy is misdiagnosed as a benign tumor, the treatment may be delayed or incomplete. Conversely, misdiagnosing of a benign tumor as a malignancy can lead to overtreatment. Therefore, it is of great significance to distinguish benign and malignant tumors. The main differences between benign and malignant tumors are listed in Table 5-4.

Table 5-4　Differences between benign and malignant neoplasms

	Benign neoplasm	Malignant neoplasm
Differentiation	Well differentiated, minor atypia	Poorly differentiated, obvious atypia
Mitosis	No or less, without pathological mitotic figures	Many, with pathological mitotic figures
Growth rate	Slow	Fast
Growth pattern	Expansive or exogenous growth	Invasive or exogenous growth
Secondary changes	Uncommon	Common, such as bleeding, necrosis, ulceration, etc

Continue to Table 5-4

	Benignneoplasm	Malignantneoplasm
Metastasis	No	Yes
Recurrence	No or less	Often
Impact on hosts	Less, local oppression or obstruction	More, destroy the tissue of the original site and metastatic sites, Necrosis, hemorrhage, and infection; cachexia

Some tumors cannot be classified as benign or malignant directly. They need to be evaluated for the risks of recurrence and metastasis(low, medium, and high)based on their morphological characteristics. In some types of tumors(such as ovarian serous tumors), in addition to typical benign tumors(such as ovarian serous papillary cystadenoma)and typical malignant tumors(such as ovarian serous papillary cystadenocarcinoma), there are also borderline tumors with the tissue morphology and biological behavior between benign and malignant, such as ovarian borderline serous papillary cystadenoma. Some borderline tumors have a tendency to develop malignant; the malignant potential of some borderline tumors is difficult to determine at present. Further studies are needed to further understand its biological behavior.

Tumor-like lesions or pseudoneoplastic lesions are not true tumors. However their clinical manifestations or histological morphology are similar to those of tumors. Some tumor-like lesions may be mistaken for malignant tumors. Therefore, it is important to recognize these lesions and have full consideration in differential diagnosis.

It must be emphasized that benign or malignant tumors refer to their benign or malignant biological behaviors. Pathologically, in most cases it is feasible to judge benign or malignant tumors by their morphological changes and subsequently estimate their biological behavior and prognosis. At present, pathologic diagnosis is the most important in all tumor detection methods. However, it must be recognized that there are many complex factors that affect the biological behavior of a tumor. Though pathologists observe some of their characteristics(tumor morphology, immunophenotype, etc.), many factors(especially changes at molecular level)are less known. In addition, the histological diagnosis will inevitably encounter technical problems such as whether the tissue sample is representative. Therefore, this prognosis assessment is not very accurate. When performing pathological diagnosis, pathologists not only need to rely on the diagnostic criteria generally accepted in the field at that time and their own experience and judgment, but also pay attention to clinicopathological correlation, which means taking full account of the patient's clinical condition, imaging data, and other test results. In medical practice, the role of the pathologist is a consultant, who provides diagnosis by considering clinical and pathological information comprehensively. When formulating treatment plans, each physician has the responsibility to fully consider the clinical and pathological links and make reasonable judgments and decisions. Patients and their families often lack understanding of the complexity of the diagnosis and treatment of diseases(including tumors), and often expect simple and definitive answers to all questions(benign or malignant, treatment response, survival, etc.). All physician(including pathologists)have the responsibility to use various opportunities to educate the public and make them fully aware of the complexities of the diagnosis and treatment of these diseases.

5.8   Brief Introduction of Common Neoplasms

This section describes the general clinical and pathological features of some common tumors. In the chapters of systemic diseases in this book, a more detailed introduction to common tumors in various organ systems is provided.

5.8.1 Epithelial Tumors

Epithelial tissues include covering and glandular epithelia. Epithelial tumors are very common. Most malignant tumors of the human body are malignant epithelial tumors (carcinomas), which are extremely harmful to human beings.

5.8.1.1 Benign Epithelial Tumors

(1) Papilloma

Papilloma occurs in the areas covered by squamous epithelium, urinary tract epithelium and so on, known as squamous cell papilloma (Figure 5-9), urothelial papilloma, etc. It grows exogenously to the surface of the body or cavity, forming finger or papillary protrusion and may also be cauliflower or villous. The root of the tumor may have pedicles connected to normal tissue. Microscopically, the axis of the papilla consists of interstitial components, such as blood vessels and connective tissue, and the surface is covered with epithelium.

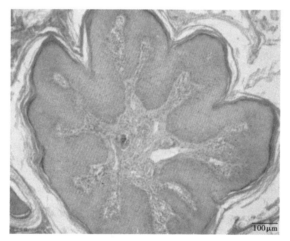

Figure 5 – 9   Squamous cell papilloma of skin
(H&E, 100×)

(2) Adenoma

Adenoma is a benign tumor of the glandular epithelium and commonly occurs in intestine, breast, and thyroid, etc. Mucosal adenomas are mostly polypoid; adenomas in the glandular organs are mostly nodular with clear boundaries to the surrounding normal tissue. The glands of adenomas are similar to those of the corresponding normal tissues and may have secretory functions.

According to the composition or morphological characteristics of adenomas, they are divided into tubular adenoma, villous adenoma, cystadenoma, fibroadenoma, pleomorphic adenoma, etc.

(3) Tubular Adenoma and Villous Adenoma

Tubular adenoma and villous adenoma are common in colon and rectal mucosa, often polypoid, and may have pedicle connected to the mucosa. However, some adenomas are sessile or flat. Microscopically, the glandular epithelium of tumor forms well differentiated tubules or villous structure or mixed structures (called tubulovillous adenomas). Villous adenomas have a higher risk of developing carcinoma, especially those with larger volumes. In familial adenomatous polyposis (FAP), the risk of adenoma developing carcinoma is extremely high, and patients with carcinoma are younger.

（4）Cystadenoma

Cystadenoma results from the accumulation of glandular secretions in the adenoma and enlargement of the lumen. Grossly, the cysts with different sizes can be seen, often occurring in the ovary and so on. There are two main types of ovarian cystadenoma: serous papillary and mucinous cystadenomas. In serous papillary cystadenoma, the glandular epithelium shows papillary growth inside the cyst and secretes serous fluid. In mucinous cystadenoma, the glandular epithelium secretes mucus with a multilocular and smooth wall, and less papillae.

5.8.1.2　Malignant Epithelial Tumors

Carcinoma is the most common human malignancy. The incidence of carcinoma increases significantly among people over the age of 40.

Carcinomas that occur on the surface of the skin and mucosaare polypoid, umbellate-like or cauliflower-like, often with necrosis and ulcers on the surface. Carcinomas in the organ often show irregular nodule, infiltrating the surrounding tissues like tree roots or crab feet. The texture is hard and the cut surface is often grayish white. Microscopically, cancer cells are arranged in nests, acini, ducts or cords with a clear boundary to the surrounding interstitium. Sometimes cancer cells diffusely infiltrate in the interstitium. Metastasis of carcinoma usually occurs in the early stage of lymphatic metastasis and late stage of hematogenous metastasis.

（1）Squamous Cell Carcinoma

Squamous cell carcinoma often occurs in the areas covered by squamous epithelium, such as skin, mouth, lips, esophagus, larynx, cervix, vagina and penis. Some regions, such as bronchus and bladder, are not covered by squamous epithelium normally, but they can develop squamous cell carcinoma on the basis of squamous metaplasia. Grossly, squamous cell carcinoma is generally cauliflower-like or ulcerative. Microscopically, in well-differentiated squamous cell carcinomas, lamellar keratins(called keratin pearls or cancer pearls)appear in the center of cancer nests(Figure 5−10). Intercellular bridges can also be seen between cells. In poorly-differentiated squamous cell carcinomas, there is no keratinization and less or no intercellular bridges.

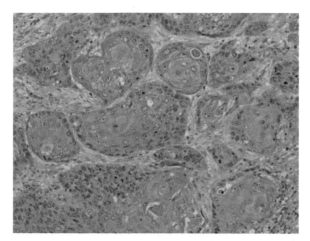

Figure 5−10　Well-differentiated squamous cell carcinoma. Keratin pearls present in the center of cancer nests(H&E,200×)

（2）Adenocarcinoma

Adenocarcinoma is a malignant tumor of glandular epithelium, which is commonly seen in the gastrointestinal tract, lung, breast, and female reproductive system. The cancer cells form glands or adenoids with different sizes, irregular shapes and arrangement. Cells are often arranged in multiple layers, with different sizes of nuclei and many mitotic figures (Figure 5–11). Papillary structure predominant adenocarcinoma is called papillary adenocarcinoma. Adenocarcinoma with highly dilated cystic cavity is called cystadenocarcinoma. Cystic adenocarcinoma with papillary growth is called papillary cystadenocarcinoma.

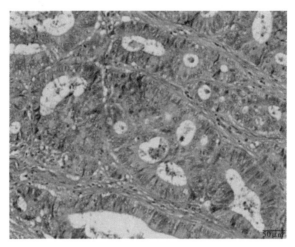

Figure 5–11　Adenocarcinoma. The tumor cells are arranged in glandular and cribriform structure (H&E, 200×)

Adenocarcinoma that secretes large amounts of mucus is called mucinous carcinomas or colloid carcinomas, commonly seen in the stomach and large intestine. Grossly, the tumor tissue is grayish white, moist and translucent like jellies. Microscopically, the dilated glandular cavities contain a large amount of mucus. Mucus pools can be formed due to disintegration of the glands, and cancerous cells float in the mucus. Sometimes the mucus accumulates in cancer cells and pushes the nucleus to one side, making the appearances of signet rings, known as signet-ring cells. Carcinomas with predominant signet ring cells are called signet-ring cell carcinomas.

(3) Basal Cell Carcinoma

Basal cell carcinoma often occurs in the head and face of the elderly. Microscopically, cancerous nests consist of deeply stained basal cell-like cancerous cells (Figure 5–12). There are superficial and nodular subtypes. The carcinoma grows slowly, often forms ulcers on the surface and infiltrates deep tissues. It rarely metastasizes. Clinically, it shows low grade malignancy and is sensitive to radiation therapy.

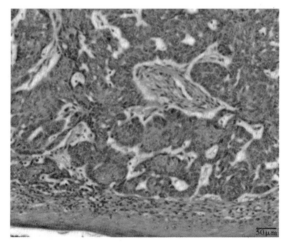

Figure 5–12　Basal cell carcinoma of skin (H&E, 200×)

（4）Urothelial Carcinoma

Urothelial carcinoma occurs in the bladder, ureter or renal pelvis. It can be papillary or non-papillary. It is divided into low-grade and high-grade urothelial carcinoma. The higher tumor grade they have, the more prone to relapse and deep infiltration. Those with lower grade also have a tendency to relapse. In some cases, the tumor grade increases after recurrence.

5.8.2　Mesenchymal Tumors

There are many types of mesenchymal tumors, including those from adipose tissue, blood vessels, lymphatic vessels, smooth muscle, striated muscle, fibrous tissue and bone tissue. It is customary to classify peripheral nerve tissue tumors into mesenchymal tumors. The tumors of mesenchymal tissue except bone tumors are also known as soft tissue tumors.

Benign tumors are common in mesenchymal tissue tumors, and malignant tumors(sarcomas) are less common. In addition, there are a lot of tumor-like lesions in the mesenchymal tissue, forming clinically visible "masses", but not true tumors. Some tumor-like lesions mimic sarcomas, making them difficult to be diagnosed.

5.8.2.1　Benign Mesenchymal Tumors

（1）Lipoma

Lipoma occurs mainly in adults and is the most common benign soft tissue tumor. It often occurs in the subcutaneous tissues of the back, shoulders, neck and extremities. Grossly, a lipoma is usually lobulated with capsule. It is soft with yellow cut surface, just like adipose tissue(Figure 5-13). The diameter varies from a few centimeters to several tens of centimeters. It is single or multiple. Microscopically, it looks like normal adipose tissue with irregular lobules and fibrous septa. It is easy to be removed by surgery.

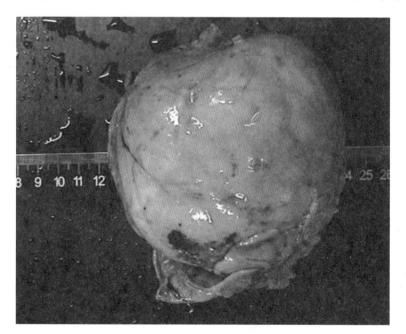

Figure 5-13　Lipoma. Usually lobulated, with intact capsule

（2）Hemangioma

Hemangioma is common and occurs in many sites, such as skin, muscle(muscle hemangioma), and visceral organs, etc. It is divided into capillary hemangioma, cavernous hemangiomas(Figure 5-14), venous hemangioma and etc. Hemangioma often has no capsule and is not clearly defined. Skin or mucosal hemangioma usually protrudes as bright red or dark red masses or purple spots above the surface. Visceral hemangioma is mostly nodular. Diffuse cavernous hemangiomas occurring in limb soft tissues may cause limb enlargement. Hemangioma is more common in children and may be congenital. It may grow up with the development of the body, cease to develop in adults or even regress spontaneously.

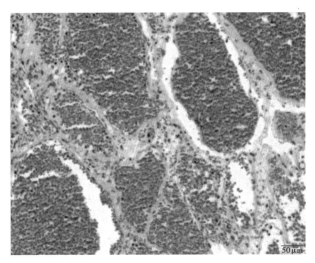

Figure 5 – 14   Cavernous hemangiomas. The tumoriscomposed of thinvessels of different sizes(H&E, 200×)

(3) Lymphangioma

Lymphangioma is composed of hyperplastic lymphatic vessels containing lymphatic fluid. Lymphatic vessels exhibit dilated and fused cysts and contain a large amount of lymphatic fluid, also called cystic hygroma. It is common in children.

(4) Leiomyoma

Leiomyoma is common in the uterus. The tumor is composed of relatively uniform spindle cells, resembling normal smooth muscle cells. The nucleus is long-barreled and blunt at both ends. Tumor cells are arranged in bundles and woven. The mitotic figure is rare.

(5) Chondroma

Chondroma originated from periosteum is called periosteal chondroma. Chondroma originated from the bone marrow cavity of the hand, foot and long bones of the extremities is called enchondroma, which may cause expanding of the bone with thin bone shells outside. The cut surface is light blue or silver white, translucent with calcification or cystic degeneration. Microscopically, the tumor is composed of mature hyaline cartilage and shows irregular lobules, which are surrounded by loose fibrovascular stroma. Chondromas occurring in the pelvis, sternum, ribs, long bones or vertebrae are prone to malignancy; and those occurring in the finger(toe)bone are rarely malignant. Pathological diagnosis and differential diagnosis of chondroma are dependent on comprehensive analyses of site, imaging and tissue morphology.

5.8.2.2   Malignant Mesenchymal Tumors

Malignant mesenchymal tumors are collectively referred to sarcomas and less than carcinomas. Some types of sarcomas often occur in children or adolescents. For example, embryonal rhabdomyosarcoma is common in children, and 60% of patients with osteosarcoma are under 25 years of age. Some sarcomas occur mainly in middle-aged and elderly people, such as liposarcoma. Sarcomas are usually large and fish flesh-like in appearance in the cut surface, prone to have secondary changes including hemorrhage, necrosis, and cystic degeneration. Microscopically, most sarcoma cells do not form nests. They proliferate diffusely and are poorly demarcated with the interstitium. There are less interstitial connective tissues but more abundant blood vessels in sarcomas. Thus sarcomas usually metastasize via blood vessels.

The difference between carcinoma and sarcoma is listed in Table 5-5.

Table 5-5   Difference betweens carcinoma and sarcoma

	Carcinoma	Sarcoma
Tissue differentiation	Epithelial tissue	Mesenchymal tissue
Incidence	Higher. It is 9 times more than the sarcoma. More common in adults over 40 years old	Lower. Some types mainly occur in young people or children; some types are mainly seen in middle-aged people
Gross features	Hard texture, grayish-white	Soft, grayish-red, fish-flesh appearance
Microscopic features	More cancer nests; a clear boundary between parenchyma and mesenchyma. Hyperplasia of the fibrous tissue in the stroma	Diffuse distribution of tumor cells. Unclear boundary between the parenchyma and the mesenchyma. Abundant blood vessels and less fibrous tissue in the stroma
Reticular fiber	Seen around the cancer nests. There are no reticular fibers around each cancer cells	There are many reticular fibers around each sarcoma cells
Metastasis	Mostly via lymphatic pathway	Mostly via blood pathway

（1）Liposarcoma

Liposarcoma is one of the most common sarcomas in adults. It often occurs in deep soft tissues, retroperitoneal region, etc. It is commonly seen in adults, rare in youngsters. Grossly, most are nodular or lobular, mimicking lipoma. Some may be mucous or fish flesh-like. Tumor cells show a variety of morphology and are characterized by the appearance of lipoblasts. There are lots of lipid vesicles of varying sizes in the cytoplasm, which extrude the nucleus and form a pressure trace(Figure 5-15). It can be divided into several subtypes: well-differentiated liposarcoma, myxoid/round cell liposarcoma, pleomorphic liposarcoma, and dedifferentiated liposarcoma.

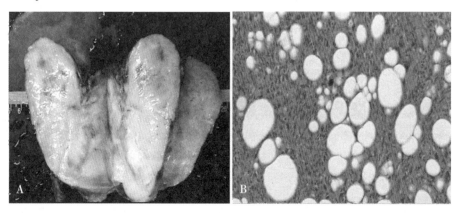

Figure 5-15   Liposarcoma. Fish flesh-like macroscopically(A) ; Microscopically lipid vesicles of varying sizes in background of sarcoma(B, H&E, 200×)

(2) Rhabdomyosarcoma

Rhabdomyosarcoma is common in infants and younger children under 10 years, and rare in adults. It occurs frequently in the head and neck, genitourinary tract etc., occasionally in the limbs. The tumor is composed of rhabdoblasts from different stages of differentiation(Figure 5–16). The cytoplasm of well-differentiated rhabdomyoblast is red. Sometimes the longitudinal or transverse lines are visible. Histologically, there are subtypes such as embryonal rhabdomyosarcoma (including sarcoma botryoides) , alveolar rhabdomyosarcoma, and pleomorphic rhabdomyosarcoma. Rhabdomyosarcoma is highly malignant, grow rapidly, and is easy to metastasize early with poor prognosis.

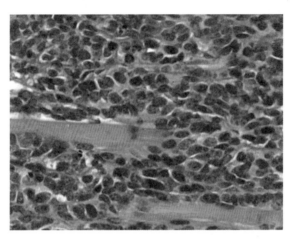

Figure 5–16 Embryonal rhabdomyosarcoma. Various differentiated rhabdomyoblast with eosinophilic cytoplasm and residual normal skeletal-muscle (H&E,200×)

(3) Leiomyosarcoma

Leiomyosarcoma occurs in the uterus, soft tissue, retroperitoneum, mesentery, omentum and skin, mostly seen in middle-aged and elderly. The presence of coagulative necrosis and number of mitotic figures are very important for the diagnosis of leiomyosarcoma and evaluation of its malignancy.

(4) Angiosarcoma

Angiosarcoma occurs in skin, breast, liver, spleen, bone and soft tissue. Cutaneous angiosarcoma is more common, especially in the skin of the head and face. The tumors bulge from the surface of the skin, appearing as dark red or grayish white papule or nodular. They are prone to necrosis and hemorrhage. Microscopically, tumor cells show different degrees of atypia, forming vascular cavity-like structures with various sizes and irregular shapes, and vascular cavities are often anastomosed to each other(Figure 5–17). In poorly differentiated angiosarcoma, tumor cells proliferate in solid. The formation of the vascular cavity is not obvious or only fissured, which contains red blood cells.

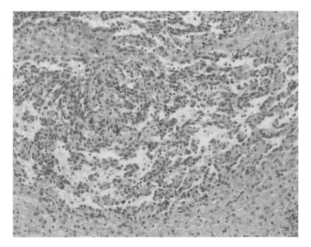

Figure 5–17 Angiosarcoma of scalp. The lesions show obvious vasoformative growth, with anastomosing channels(H&E,200×)

(5) Fibrosarcoma

Fibrosarcoma often occurs in the subcutaneous tissue of the extremities. The tumor is infiltrative, grayish-white and fish flesh-like at the cut surface, often accompanied by hemorrhage and necrosis. The typical microscopic morphology is that atypical spindle cells arrange in the "herringbone" pattern. The infantile fibrosarcoma, which occurs in infants and young children, has a better prognosis than adult one.

In the past, fibrosarcoma was considered to be a common sarcoma of soft tissue. Later studies showed that many of them were not fibrosarcomas, but other sarcomas or sarcoma-like lesions. Most of the "fibrosarcomas" described in the earlier literature have now been classified into other types of tumor. The concept and classification of fibrous tissue and fibroblast neoplasms have undergone great changes and development in recent years.

(6) Osteosarcoma

Osteosarcoma is the most common bone malignancy and often seen in young people. It occurs in the metaphysis of long bones, especially the lower end of the femur and the upper end of the tibia. At the cut surface, it is grayish white and fish flesh-like, commonly accompanied with hemorrhage and necrosis. The tumor destroys the bone cortex and raises the outer membrane of its surface (Figure 5-18). Triangular bulge is formed between the bone cortex of the upper and lower ends of the tumor and the periosteum, due to the formation of new bone created by the periosteum, thus constitutes the Codman triangle observed by X-ray examination. Since the periosteum is lifted, radial reactive new trabecular bones are formed between the periosteum and cortical bone. The trabecular bones are vertical to the bone surface, showing daylight radiate shadow on the X-ray. These imaging features are characteristics of osteosarcoma. Microscopically, the tumor cells are obviously atypical, spindle-shaped or polygonal, and directly form neoplastic bone tissue or bone tissue, which is the most pivotal histological evidence for the diagnosis of osteosarcoma (Figure 5 – 18). Chondrosarcoma and fibrosarcoma-like components can also be found in osteosarcoma. Osteosarcoma is highly malignant and grows rapidly. Most of them are found to metastasize via bloodstreams before diagnosis.

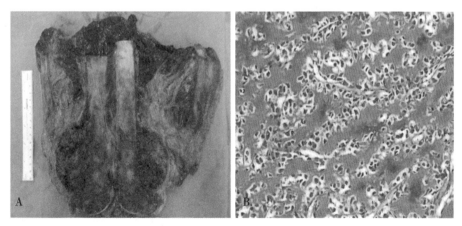

Figure 5-18   Osteosarcoma. The tumor infiltrates medullary cavity and destroys the cortex(A) ; Microscopically trabecalue of neoplastic woven bone tissue is lined by spindle-shaped or polygonal tumor cells(H&E,200×)

(7) Chondrosarcoma

The age of onset is mostly from 40 to 70 years old. Chondrosarcoma occurs commonly in the pelvis, and less in the femur, tibia and scapula, etc. Grossly, the tumor is located in the marrow cavity, showing a pale, translucent lobular mass. Microscopically, there are abnormal chondrocytes in the cartilage matrix, with large and dark stained nuclei, prominent nucleoli, and much mitosis (Figure 5–19). Many diploid, megakaryocytic and multinuclear tumor giant cells appear. Chondrosarcoma usually grows slower than osteosarcoma and metastasizes later.

Figure 5 – 19   Chondrosarcoma. Abnormal chondrocytes with large and dark nuclei form cartilage lobule of different size (H&E, 200×)

5.8.3 Neuroectodermal Tumor

Some parts of early embryonic ectoderm develop into the nervous system called neuroectoderm, including the neural tube and neural crest. The neural tube develops into the cerebrum, spinal cord, retinal epithelium, etc. Nerve ganglia, Schwann cells, melanocytes, and adrenal medulla chromaffin cells originate from the neural crest. There are many types of tumors originating from neuroectodermal blasts.

About 40% of the primary tumors of the central nervous system are gliomas. In children with malignant tumors, the incidence of intracranial malignancies is next only to leukemia. The common tumors in the peripheral nervous system are neuromyeloma and neurofibroma.

Retinoblastoma arises from the retinal embryonic basal, and tumor cells are naive small round cells with a morphology similar to that of undifferentiated retinoblasts, showing a characteristic Flexener-Wintersteiner rosette. Most of the tumors are seen in infants under 3 years old and with a poor prognosis.

Malignant melanoma (Figure 5–20) is more common in the skin and mucous membranes, occasionally in visceral organs. Malignant melanoma of the skin can develop from melanocytic nevus. The tumor cells can be pigmented or not. Tumor staging is closely related to its prognosis.

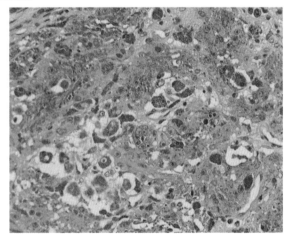

Figure 5–20   Malignant melanoma of skin. The tumor cells showing obvious eosinophilic nucleoli, with pigment in the cytoplasm (H&E, 200×)

5.9 Precancerous Diseases(or Lesions), Atypical Hyperplasia, and Carcinoma in Situ

Although some diseases(or lesions) are not malignant tumors, they have the potential to develop into malignant tumors, thus the patients have an increased risk of developing the corresponding malignancy. These diseases or lesions are called precancerous diseases or precancerous lesions. It should be noted that precancerous diseases(or lesions) will not certainly develop into malignant tumors.

It will take a long time to develop from precancerous lesions to cancer. In epithelial tissues, sometimes atypical hyperplasia or dysplasia is firstly observed, then it develops into carcinoma in situ(CIS), and subsequently invasive carcinoma.

5.9.1 Precancerous Diseases(or Lesions)

Precancerous diseases(or lesions) may be acquired or inherited. People with inherited cancer syndromes have some chromosomal and genetic abnormalities that increase their chances of developing certain tumors. Acquired precancerous diseases(or lesions) may be associated with certain lifestyle habits, infections, or some chronic inflammatory diseases.

5.9.1.1 Adenomas of Large Intestines

It is common. The lesion may be single or multiple. There are two common subtypes: villous adenoma and tubular adenoma. Villous adenomas are more likely to develop into carcinoma. Familial adenomatous polyposis(FAP) almost always develops into carcinoma.

5.9.1.2 Mammary Fibrocystic Disease

There is an increased risk of carcinogenesis in mammary fibrocystic disease with atypical hyperplasia of ductal epithelium. The breast fibrocystic disease is common in women around the age of 40, mainly characterized by cystic dilatation of the breast duct, and proliferation of lobular and ductal epithelial cells.

5.9.1.3 Chronic Gastritis and Intestinal Metaplasia

There is a certain relationship between gastric intestinal metaplasia and gastric carcinogenesis. Chronic gastritis with H. pylori infection is associated with gastric mucosa-associated lymphoid tissue(MALT) lymphoma and gastric adenocarcinoma.

5.9.1.4 Ulcerative Colitis

Ulcerative colitis a kind of inflammatory bowel disease. Colon adenocarcinoma may occur on the basis of recurrent ulcers and mucosal hyperplasia.

5.9.1.5 Chronic Ulcer

Squamous epithelial hyperplasia and atypical hyperplasia may further develop into cancer due to long-term chronic irritation.

5.9.1.6 Leukoplakia

Leukoplakia often occurs in the oral cavity, vulva, etc. It exhibits hyperplasia, hyperkeratosis and atypia of squamous epithelium. Grossly, white patches appear. It may develop into squamous cell carcinoma if untreated for a long time.

5.9.2 Dysplasia and Carcinoma in Situ

In the past years, the term atypical hyperplasia was often used to describe cell proliferation with atypia. It is mostly used in epithelial lesions, including covered epithelium (such as squamous epithelium and urothelium) and glandular epithelium (such as breast duct epithelium, endometrial glandular epithelium). Since atypical hyperplasia is found not only in neoplastic lesions, but also in repair, inflammation, etc. (so-called reactive atypical hyperplasia), in recent years, the academic community tends to use the term dysplasia to describe atypical hyperplasia associated with tumorigenesis.

Dysplasia is divided into mild, moderate and severe grades. In the case of covered epithelium, mild dysplasia means less pleomorphic, involving the lower 1/3 layer of the epithelium; Moderate dysplasia involves the lower 2/3 layer of the epithelium; severe dysplasia shows most pleomorphic, involving more than 2/3 layer of the epithelium. Mild dysplasia can return to normal, while moderate to severe dysplasia is difficult to reverse.

The term of carcinoma in situ is usually used for epithelial lesions. It refers to dysplastic cells that are the same with cancer cells in the aspects of morphological and biological characteristics, involves the entire layer of epithelium, but not penetrates the basement membrane. Therefore, sometimes it is also called intra-epithelial carcinoma. In situ carcinoma is commonly seen in squamous epithelium or urinary tract epithelium, such as the cervix, esophagus, skin, bladder, etc. It is also found in the squamous metaplasia of mucosal surface, such as the squamous metaplasia of the bronchial mucosa. If the ductal epithelium of the breast is cancerous but does not invade the basement membrane and infiltrate into the interstitium, it is called ductal carcinoma in situ. Detection and treatment of a carcinoma in situ in time will prevent it from developing into invasive carcinoma. An important task for cancer prevention and control is to establish a technical method for early detection of carcinoma in situ.

At present, the concept of intraepithelial neoplasia is often used to describe the continuous process of epithelial dysplasia to carcinoma in situ. Mild dysplasia is called intraepithelial neoplasia grade I, moderate dysplasia called intraepithelial neoplasia grade II, and severe dysplasia and carcinoma in situ is called intraepithelial neoplasia grade III. Severe dysplasia and carcinoma in situ are collectively called grade III, mainly due to the difficulties of distinguishing them completely, and the principles of the treatment are basically the same.

5.10 Molecular Detection of Neoplasm

The molecular targeted therapy has achieved great success with the characteristics of specificity and effectiveness. It aims at reversing the malignant biological behavior of tumor cells at molecular levels, such as cell signal transduction pathways, oncogenes and tumor suppressor genes, cytokines and receptors, anti-angiogenesis and suicide genes. As a new mode of biological treatment, the molecular targeted therapy only fights tumor cells and has little effect on normal cells.

The current detection methods include polymerase chain reaction (PCR) and sequencing, immunohistochemistry (IHC) assay, fluorescence in situ hybridization (FISH) or chromogenic in situ hybridization (CISH), etc. The proteomics and genomics approaches are used to detect more precise targets for continuous advancement of molecular targeted therapies.

Currently, there are more than 10 kinds of molecular targets. Here we list some common targets.

5.10.1 HER-2

As a member of the EGFR family and a protein with receptor tyrosine kinase activity, the HER-2 protein plays a pivotal role in controlling the activation of cell conduction pathways, such as epithelial cell growth, differentiation, adhesion, and activation. HER-2 is over-expressed in about 20% of breast cancer patients, which indicates a poor prognosis. In addition, HER-2 over-expression is observed in lung carcinoma, pancreatic carcinoma, gastric carcinoma, and ovarian carcinoma.

The targeted therapeutic drug trastuzumab (Herceptin), antagonizes the growth-promoting effect of HER-2 family by down-regulating HER-2 gene expression and mediates antibody-dependent cell-mediated cytotoxicity(ADCC). It has no effect on HER-2 negative tumor cells or normal cells. Therefore, the expression of HER-2 in tumor tissues must be detected before the use of trastuzumab treatment.

In recent years, the study of trastuzumab in the treatment of gastric carcinoma has become a hot topic. HER-2 is over-expressed in 10% to 55% of gastric carcinoma. About 20% of gastric cancer patients with HER-2 over-expression have poor prognosis. Recently, trastuzumab combined with chemotherapy is used for HER-2 positive gastric and gastroesophageal junctional tumors, which shows survival advantage without increasing the toxicity of chemotherapeutic drugs. Thus, it can be an option for HER-2 positive advanced gastric carcinoma patients.

5.10.2 EGFR Gene Mutation

EGFR is over-expressed and/or mutated in multiple tumors. The mutated EGFR selectively activates Akt signaling proteins and transcriptional activators. Then the activation of STAT signaling pathway prolongs cell survival, leading to uncontrolled tumor cell growth and increased malignancy. In recent years, molecular targeted drugs targeting EGFR have attracted more and more attention. Among them, EGFR-tyrosine kinase inhibitors(TKI), gefitinib and erlotinib, have been used clinically for the treatment of advanced non-small cell lung cancer(NSCLC). Gefitinib is especially effective in Asian women, non-smoking, and adenocarcinoma subgroup. It is also effective for the treatment of head and neck tumors, prostate cancer and breast cancer. Erlotinib is used primarily for the patients with advanced and metastatic NSCLC.

Evidences hows that the EGFR gene status is the most critical predictor of EGFR-TKI efficacy. EGFR gene mutations occur frequently in women, non-smokers, adenocarcinomas, and Asian populations. The detection of EGFR gene mutation status can be performed by PCR and sequencing.

5.10.3 K-ras, BRAF Gene Mutations and EGFR Monoclonal Antibody

Proto-oncogene K-ras plays a key role in the development of multiple tumors. The RAS protein, also known as P21 protein, is a membrane GTP/GDP binding protein. When the K-ras gene is mutated, it is not affected by the status of the upstream EGFR gene and always in an activated state, which continuously stimulates cell growth and leads to tumorigenesis. K-ras mutations are observedin a variety of tumors, including pancreatic and colorectal cancers(30% to 50%), etc. The point mutations of the K-ras gene are mainly concentrated in codon 12 and codon 13, which account for more than 90% of all mutations.

The BRAF gene is a member of the RAF family and encodes a serine/threonine protein kinase which is the most critical activating factor for the MEK/ERK signaling pathway. There are different proportions of BRAF mutations in a variety of human malignancies such as malignant melanoma, colorectal cancer, lung cancer, thyroid cancer, liver cancer, and pancreatic cancer. The most common mutations are V600E and V600K, which activate the BRAF protein and subsequently lead to the activation of MEK/ERK signaling pathway to promote cell growth and even tumorigenesis.

Cetuximab and Panitumumab are human murine chimeric IgG monoclonal antibodies directed against the extracellular domain of EGFR that bind to cell surface receptors to produce ADCC activity, regardless of the presence or absence of EGFR mutations in cells. Cetuximab is currently the first line of treatment for advanced metastatic colorectal cancer(mCRC). After adding cetuximab to conventional chemotherapeutics, the patient's objective response rate is significantly improved and survival is prolonged. BRAF mutations are resistant to both drugs, and the survival rate is significantly lower than other patients. The new version of the NCCN Clinical Guideline for Colorectal Cancer states that all patients with mCRC should detect mutation status of both K-ras and BRAF genes, and only patients with wild-type K-ras and BRAF should be recommended for cetuximab.

5.10.4   C-kit and PDGFR-α

The KIT protein encoded by the c-kit gene, is a transmembrane receptor tyrosine kinase. It is a receptor of stem cell factor(SCF). When combined with SCF, KIT protein activates the corresponding signaling pathway and promotes cell proliferation, division, and survival. C-kit gene mutations occur in more than 90% of patients with gastrointestinal stromal tumors(GIST). Deletions or point mutations of c-kit exons 11, 9, 13, and 17 are common. The activation of KIT protein is no longer regulated by the ligand SCF when c-kit mutated, and the sustained activation of KIT tyrosine kinase results in the inhibition of apoptosis and uncontrolled proliferation, and finally resulting in the formation of tumors. In another 10% to 15% of GIST patients, there was no c-kit mutation but PDGFR-α gene mutation. The protein PDGFR-α encoded by the PDGFR-α gene shares the same type Ⅲ tyrosine protein kinase family as c-kit. PDGFR-α is activated by binding to ligand PDGF and activates phosphorylation pathways and other changes of phosphatidylinositol, CAMP and various proteins, which may promote DNA synthesis, cell division and proliferation, and cause malignant tumor.

Imatinib(also known as Gleevec)is a tyrosine kinase inhibitor that selectively inhibits the proto-oncogenes abl, Abl-Bcr, c-kit, and PDGF receptor tyrosine kinase and inhibits kinase or substrate proteins, and inactivation of tyrosine phosphorylation blocks the signal transduction and achieves therapeutic goals. Most major KIT mutations occur in exon 11, and this mutation is favorable for imatinib therapy; however, patients with a KIT mutation in exon 9, which accounts for 10%−20% of GIST cases, were poor responders to imatinib therapy. Detection of mutations in the corresponding exons of c-kit and PDGFR-α gene is an important indicator for predicting the efficacy of imatinib. GIST patients should be tested for c-kit and PDGFR-α prior to treatment with imatinib.

5.11   Molecular Basis of Carcinogenesis

With the development of molecular biology and technical improvement in DNA sequencing methods, the etiology and molecular basis of cancer is coming to light. Carcinogenesis is a multistep process caused by the dysfunction of regulatory genes related to cell growth and proliferation. Accumulation of nonlethal DNA damages caused by environmental and genetic carcinogenic factors synergistically or sequentially is the essence of neoplasm. Four classes of gene disorders including activation of proto-oncogenes, silencing of tumor suppressor genes, mutation of genes that related to programmed cell death(apoptosis) and changes of genes involving in DNA repair lay at the heart of carcinogenesis.

5.11.1　Activation of Proto-oncogene

Proto-oncogenes are generally vital regulatory genes that encode growth factors, growth factor receptors, signal-transducing proteins and transcription factors in normal cells. The corresponding oncogenes are activated or mutated proto-oncogenes, which encode oncoproteins that serve excessive normal function similar to their normal counterparts or impart completely new functions. Oncoproteins can continuously transform normal cells to malignant cells that are self-sufficient in growth. The well characterized oncogenes and their related human cancers are listed in Table 5-6.

Table 5-6　Selected oncogenes, mode of activation and associated human tumors

Category	Proto-oncogene	Mode of activation	Associated Tumors
Growth Factors			
PDF-βchain	*SIS*	Overexpression	Astrocytoma
FGF	*HST*-1	Overexpression	Osteosarcoma, Stomach cancer,
	INT-2	Amplification	Bladder cancer, Breast cancer, Melanoma
Growth Factor Receptors			
EGF-receptor family	ERBB1 (EGFR)	Mutation	Adenocarcinoma of lung
	ERBB2 (HER)	Amplification	Breast carcinoma
FMS-like tyrosine kinase 3	FLT3	Point mutation	Leukemia
Proteins Involved in Signal Transduction			
GTP-binding (G) proteins	KRAS	Point mutation	Colon, lung, and pancreatic tumors
	HRAS	Point mutation	Bladder and kidney tumors
	NRAS	Point mutation	Melanomas, hematologic malignancies
	GNAQ	Point mutation	Uveal melanoma
	GNAS	Point mutation	Pituitary adenoma, other endocrine tumors
Non-receptor tyrosine kinase	ABL	Translocation	Chronic myelogenous leukemia
		Point mutation	Acute lymphoblastic leukemia
RAS signal transduction	BRAF	Point mutation, Translocation	Melanomas, leukemias, colon carcinoma, others
Nuclear Regulatory Proteins			
Transcriptional activators	MYC	Translocation	Burkitt lymphoma
	NMYC	Amplification	Neuroblastoma
	LMYC	Amplification	Small cell lung cancer
Cell Cycle Regulator			
Cyclins	CCND1 (Cyclin D1)	Translocation	Mantle cell lymphoma, multiple myeloma
		Amplification	Breast and esophageal cancers
Cyclin-dependent kinase	CDK4	Amplification or point mutation	Glioblastoma, melanoma, sarcoma

The transformation of proto-oncogenes to oncogenes is called activation. Commonly, this process is accomplished through the following mechanisms: ①Point mutation. The point mutation of RAS protein is an example. RAS proteins are growth-promoting, signal-transducing proteins belonging to membrane-associated small G proteins that bind guanosine nucleotides. They normally bind to guanosine diphosphate(GDP) and stay at the quiescent state. A point mutation(G->T) in coden 12 changes a glycine(Gly) to Valine(Val), and hence lose the activity of GTPase, through which target cells escape the upstream signal control and are persistently activated in proliferation. ②Gene amplification. Excessive replication of target genes will lead to the over-expression of gene products and constitutive activation of its downstream signal transduction. For example, the abnormal HER2(*eRBB*2) amplification is observed in certain breast cancers, leading to a persistent downstream tyrosine kinase activity. ③Chromosomal translocation. The proto-oncogene located chromosomal segment is translocated to another chromosome, resulting in abnormal expression, structure or functions of the proto-oncogene. In Burkitt lymphoma, cell growth regulator MYC located in chromosome 8 is translocated to chromosome 14 behind a strong promoter, leading to the excessive transcription and overexpression of the transcription factor MYC. Chromosomal translocation might also lead to the formation of fusion proteins, such as the translocation of proto-oncogene *abl* in chronic myelogenous leukemia(CML). The newly formed Bcr/Abl fusion protein is a dysfunctional oncoprotein that promotes the malignant transformation of target cells.

5.11.2 Silencing of Tumor Suppressor gene

Tumor suppressor genes, or anti-oncogenes, are also essential regulatory genes in cellular growth and proliferation. They can be transcription factors, cell cycle inhibitors, signal-transducing molecules, cellular membrane receptors or DNA damage regulators. Different from oncogenes, tumor suppressor genes exert their opposite function on cell growth and proliferation. Mutated tumor suppressor genes in both alleles will lead to the failure of growth inhibition and induce the occurrence of cell transformation. Many of our concepts of tumor suppressor genes are derived from RB and p53, two well characterized tumor suppressor genes at present. Their products are both nuclear transcription factors. The well characterized tumor suppressor genes and their associated human cancers are listed in Table 5-7.

Table 5-7   Selected tumor suppressor genes and associated familial syndromes and cancers

Gene	Protein	Function	Familial Syndrome	Sporadic Cancer
Inhibitors of Mitogenic Signaling Pathways				
APC	Adenomatous polyposiscoli protein	Inhibitor of WNT signaling	Familial colonic polyps and carcinomas	Carcinomas of stomach, colon, pancreas; melanoma
*NF*1	Neurofibromin-1	Inhibitor of RAS/MAPK signaling	Neurofibromatosis type 1 (neurofibromas and malignant peripheral nerve sheath tumors)	Neuroblastoma, juvenile myeloid leukemia
*NF*2	Merlin	Cytoskeletal stability, Hippo pathway signaling	Neurofibromatosis type 2 (acoustic schwannoma and meningioma)	Schwannoma, meningioma
Inhibitors of Cell Cycle progression				
RB	Retinoblastoma (RB) protein	Inhibitor of G1/S transition during cell cycle progression	Familial retinoblastoma syndrome (retinoblastoma, osteosarcoma, other sarcomas)	Retinoblastoma; osteosarcoma carcinomas of breast, colon, lung

Continue to Table 5-7

Gene	Protein	Function	Familial Syndrome	Sporadic Cancer
Inhibitors of "Pro-growth" Programs of Metabolism and Angiogenesis				
VHL	Von Hippel Lindau (VHL) protein	Inhibitor of hypoxiain-duced transcription fac-tors(e. g. ,HIF1α)	Von Hippel Lindau syndrome (cerebellar hemangioblastoma, retinal angioma, renal cell car-cinoma)	Renal cell carcinoma
Inhibitors of Invasion and Metastasis				
CDH1	E-cadherin	Cell adhesion, inhibition of cell motility	Familial gastric cancer	Gastric carcinoma, lobular breast carcinoma
Enablers of Genomic Stability				
TP53	p53 protein	Cell cycle arrest and ap-optosis in response to DNA damage	Li-Fraumeni syndrome (di-verse cancers)	Most human cancers
DNA Repair Factors				
BRCA1, BRCA2	Breast cancer-1 and breast cancer-2 (BRCA1 and BRCA2)	Repair of double-stran-ded breaks in DNA	Familial breast and ovarian carcinoma; carcinomas of male breast; chronic lympho-cytic leukemia(BRCA2)	Rare

5.11.2.1   Retinoblastoma Gene(*RB gene*)

RB is the first discovered tumor suppressor gene that was identified by studying a rare disease, familial retinoblastoma. Familial and sporadical retinoblastomas are two different types of retinoblastoma. Interesting-ly, most familial retinoblastoma patients are predisposed to develop tumor at the early age in both eyes and have high risk of developing other soft-tissue sarcomas. Sporadical retinoblastoma patients, however, have a relative late onset of tumor in one eye and are not at an increased risk of developing other types of cancer. This could be well explained by the "Two hit hypothesis" proposed by Knudson in 1974. The Knudson's hy-pothesis suggests that RB gene must exist and retinoblastoma develops only when two RB gene alleles are both mutated. In the familial case, children inherited a copy of defective RB allele(first hit) in the germ-line, and the other copy of RB allele is normal. Retinoblastoma develops when the normal RB allele is muta-ted(second hit), and it is relatively easy to take place. In the sporadical case, retinoblastoma occurs when two normal RB alleles undergo spontaneous somatic mutation. The possibility of this event is relatively low.

Mutation of both alleles of *RB* gene at chromosome locus 13q14, are required to produce retinoblasto-ma. In addition, transformation of normal RB gene to retinoblastoma cells can reverse their tumor pheno-type. The loss of RB gene is also found in other types of tumors including bladder cancer, lung cancer, breast cancer and osteosarcoma. The RB protein is a vital governor of proliferation through negatively regula-ting the G1/S cell cycle transition. In G1 stage, hypophosphorylated RB in complex with E2F transcription factor family inhibits the transcription of proteins that are required in S phase of the cell cycle (Figure 5-21). The activation of cdk4/6 phosphorylates RB and releases E2F, which can active the transcription of S phase proteins. The mutation of RB can result in an uncontrolled E2F activity and then cells lose their control of G1/S transition.

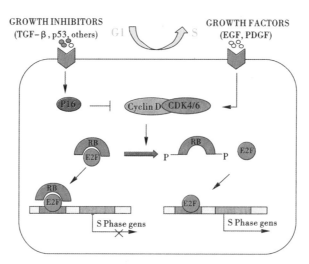

Figure 5-21 The role of RB in regulating the G1-S checkpoint of the cell cycle

5.11.2.2 P53 Tumor Suppressor Gene

P53 located in chromosome 17 is another extensively studied tumor suppressor gene in human cancers. Loss of p53 function is detected in 50% of human tumors, indicating its critical role in preventing cancer development. Increased p53 protein is detected in cells when there is cellular stress or primarily DNA damage. Once activated, P53 works as a specific transcription factor that stimulates the transcription of p21, which can stop the cell cycle at G1 stage until the damage is repaired or the cells undergo programmed cell death(apoptosis). In healthy cells, p53 is association with MDM2, an E3 ubiquitin ligase, leading to the ubiquitization and degradation of P53. As a result, p53 is virtually undetectable in normal cells. With the loss or mutation of p53 function, DNA damage goes without repair, cells undergo mitotic replication rather than apoptosis, and mutations accumulate in oncogenes and other cancer genes. As a result, cells are predisposed to malignant transformation.

5.11.2.3 Other Tumor Suppressor Genes

Mutations of adenomatous polyposis coli(APC) are associated with familial adenomatous polyposis, in which patients develop thousands of adenomatous polyps in the colon. *APC* is a tumor suppressor that involves in down-regulating WNT signaling pathway, which has a major role in controlling cell fate, adhesion and cell polarity. APC participates in the degradation of β-catenin to stop its nuclear translocation and the following activation of c-myc. Mutation or dysfunction of NF1 gene located in chromosome 17 develops neurofibromatosis type Ⅰ. Neurofibromin, the protein product of the *NF*1 gene, contains a GTPase-activating domain that keeps RAS inactive. On the contrary, loss-of-function mutation in NF1 gene leads to a persistently activated RAS and uncontrolled cell proliferation. A large amount of tumor suppressor genes have been identified during the past decades including E-Cadherin, CDKN2A, PTEN, NF2, WT1, PATCHED, VHL and so on. There is no doubt that more tumor suppressor genes remain to be discovered.

5.11.3 Dysfunction of Apoptosis Related Genes

Accumulation of malignant transformed cells may not only result from activated proto-oncogenes or silenced tumor suppressor genes, but also from mutated genes that regulate programmed cell death. Dysfunction of apoptosis-regulating genes results in less cell death and enhanced survival of the cells. It's no doubt that apoptosis of cancer cells is linked to the key points of apoptotic signaling pathways. Pro-apoptotic and anti-apoptotic members of the BCL2 family of proteins are well-known apoptotic regulatory proteins. The pro-apoptotic proteins BAX and BAK are required for apoptosis and directly promote mitochondrial permeabilization that triggers apoptosis. Over-expression of anti-apoptotic members including BCL2, BCL-XL, and MCL1 prevent cells from apoptosis. Apoptosis is also initiated when CD95/Fas is activated by its ligand, CD95L/FasL, leading to the recruitment of caspases to cleave DNA and causing cell death. Dysfunction of CD95/Fas or caspase family members prevents cells from apoptosis and leads to their malignant transformation.

5.11.4   Dysfunction of Genes Regulate Repair of Damaged DNA

Both external factors including ionizing radiation, ultraviolet radiation, and internal DNA replication mistakes can cause DNA damages. In normal cells, minor DNA damages can be repaired. Mutations tend to accumulate in cells with mutated DNA repair genes, followed by their malignant transformation. Defective in DNA repair system, Xerodermapigmentosum patients are at an increased risk of developing skin cancers, due to the accumulation of UV induced DNA damage.

5.11.5   Activated Telomerase

Telomeres are short repeated DNA sequences located at the end of chromosome that are important for chromosome replication through preventing chromosomes from fusion and degradation. Except germ cells, most somatic cells do not have the activity of telomerase that can recover the length of telomere. Normal somatic cells have limited capacity of replication also because of the telomere attrition. The length of telomere is shortened progressively as the times of DNA replication increase. The telomerase activity is reactivated in most malignant tumor cells, resulting in stable telomere length and indefinite cell proliferation.

5.11.6   Epigenetic Changes

Besides changes in Nucleotide sequence, epigenetics changes including histone modification and DNA methylation, which regulate gene expression and genetic changes. Numerous mutations involving genes that encode epigenetic regulatory proteins have been identified by cancer genomes sequencing. DNA methylation, a modification created by DNA methyltransferases, is considered as a vital regulatory mechanism of gene expression. Abnormal DNA methylation of key promoters is commonly seen in tumor cells, including both hypermethylation of tumor suppressor genes and hypomethylation of oncogenes. DNA hypermethylation leads to the decreased expression of tumor suppressor genes such as RB and VHL. Hypomethylation of CpG repeated sequences rich in noncoding areas of the genome decreases the stability of DNA molecules, and triggers the malignant phenotype. Histone modifications catalyzed by enzymes are associated with chromatin regulatory complexes. Methylation and acetylation of histones are tightly associated with DNA replication, transcription and damage repair. Dysfunction of histone modification also contributes to carcinogenesis. In recent years, non-coding RNAs have been paid more attention as generalized epigenetic factors that can regulate gene expression. The progress in the regulatory roles of non-coding RNAs contributes to the identification of the complicated mechanisms behind carcinogenesis.

5.11.7   Carcinogenesis is a Multi-step Process

Malignant tumors must develop several fundamental abnormalities resulting from the stepwise accumulation of multiple mutations to produce a fully malignant tumor. In the laboratory, normal epithelial cells bearing a series of mutations including activation of RAS, inactivation of RB, P53 and PP2A, can complete malignant transform ation. However, these mutations never occur simultaneously, but gradually accumulate during the natural development of human cancers. Development of colon carcinoma is a classic example of incremental acquisition of malignant phenotypes. Colon carcinoma involves a series of morphologically identifiable stages. Colon epithelial hyperplasia occurs first followed by the formation of adenomas, and then the ultimate malignant transformation. Molecular mechanisms at each of these stages are well illustrated(Figure 5–22). Defective of the tumor suppressor gene *APC* and the following activation of RAS occur first to induce epithelial hyperplasia and adenomas. Loss of a tumor suppressor gene on 18q and loss of *P53* contribute to the ultimately malignant transformation. Similar situation also exists in other epithelial cancers although the precise temporal sequence of mutations may be different in each organ and tumor type.

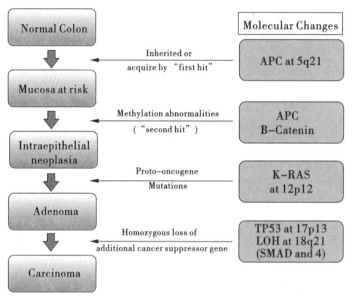

Figure 5–22   Molecular mechanism for the evolution of colorectal cancer

5.12   Etiology of Neoplasms

Environmental tumorigenic factors induce the development of tumors through multiple molecular pathways discussed above. However, the identification of tumorigenic factors is not easy as most tumors develop a while after exposure to those factors. Carcinogens are materials that can trigger carcinogenesis. Carcinogens play a vital role in the initiation and promotion of tumors.

5.12.1   Chemical Carcinogens

Hundreds of chemicals have been identified as carcinogens to both animals and humans. Most of the chemical carcinogens are mutagens that covalently bind to DNAs and induce the following DNA structure changes. They usually involves in the initiation of carcinogenesis.

5.12.1.1   Direct-acting Carcinogens

Minority of carcinogens are direct-acting carcinogens that are carcinogenic without metabolic conversion. Most of them(mainly alkylating and acylating agents) are weak carcinogens that have little impact on cancer initiation. Some of weak carcinogens are even cancer chemotherapeutic drugs, such as alkylating a-gents. Although they are carcinogens to acute myeloid leukemia, in some cases, they successfully cure, con-trol or delay the recurrence of certain types of cancer including leukemia, lymphoma and ovarian carcino-mas.

5.12.1.2   Indirect-acting Carcinogens

Indirect-acting carcinogens refer to most chemicals that require metabolic conversion to become active carcinogens. Polycyclic hydrocarbons presented in fossil fuels are the most potent indirect-acting carcino-gens. Benzo[a]pyrene, the active component of soot, is the product of tobacco combustion in cigarettes and contributes to the high incidence of lung cancer. Polycyclic hydrocarbons produced from smoked meats and fish are associated with gastric cancers. The aromatic amines and azo dyes widely used in the aniline dye and rubber industries are other class of indirect-acting carcinogens. Nitrates and nitrites used in the process-ing of meat contribute to the development of digestive tract tumors. Aflatoxin from moldy food, especially in moldy peanuts and corns, strongly triggers hepatic cancer through inactivating the tumor suppressor gene p53.

5.12.2   Radiation Carcinogenesis

UV rays of sunlight, as well as electromagnetic and particulate radiation, are all carcinogenic. UV light is one of the clearly identified causation of skin cancer through inducing the formation of pyrimidine dimers in DNA. In normal person, this DNA damage can be repaired by nucleotide excision repair pathway. The he-reditary disorder *xeroderma pigmentosum* patients, as discussed previously, tend to develop skin cancer be-cause of the loss of DNA damage repair enzymes. Electromagnetic and particulate radiations including X-rays, γ rays, α particles, β particles, protons and neutrons cause the break, translocation and mutation of chromosome, which can activate oncogenes and inactivate tumor suppressor genes to stimulate the malignant transformation of damaged cells.

5.12.3   Microbial Carcinogenesis

Most microbial carcinogens are tumor viruses including DNA and RNA tumor viruses. Recent research indicates that some bacteria are important for the development of gastritis and gastric ulcer. For example, Helicobacter pylori are tightly associated with some gastric tumors.

5.12.3.1   Oncogenic DNA Tumor Virus

In infected host cells, DNA viruses integrate their genome into host genome and ultimately trigger the malignant transformation of host cells. Various oncogenic DNA viruses that cause tumors in animals and hu-mans have been identified including human papilloma virus(HPV), Epstein-Barr virus(EBV), hepatitis B virus(HBV), Merkel cell polyoma virus, and Kaposi sarcoma herpesvirus(human herpesvirus 8). The onco-genic potential of HPV attributes to the activities of two viral genes encoding E6 and E7, which can bind to RB and P53, respectively, resulting in uncontrolled cellular growth and malignant transformation. EBV is closely associated with the pathogenesis of several human tumors including Burkitt lymphoma and nasopha-ryngeal carcinoma. EBV infected B lymphocyte undergo polyclonal proliferation, and the following mutations ultimately cause malignancies. HBV and HCV infection have been demonstrated closely related with the de-velopment of hepatocellular carcinoma, and the chances of HBV infected patients are 200 times easier to de-velop hepatocellular carcinoma. The oncogenic effects of HBV and HCV are multifactorial and the dominant one seems to be immunologically mediated chronic inflammation, hepatocyte injury and regeneration, and genomic damage.

5.12.3.2 Oncogenic RNA Tumor Virus

RNA tumor viruses are retroviruses that transform host cells directly through integrating virus oncogene to host genome, or indirectly through over-expression and activation of host oncogenes. Human T-Cell Leukemia Virus Type 1(HTLV-1) is the only human retrovirus that is firmly implicated in the pathogenesis of cancer. HTLV-1 causes adult T-cell leukemia/lymphoma(ATLL) that is mainly endemic in certain parts of Japan and the Caribbean basin. The activity of HTLV-1 is associated with the products of its Tax gene that actives the transcription of host genes including c-fos, c-sis, GM-CSF, IL-2 and its receptors, which further stimulate the proliferation of T-lymphocytes.

5.12.4 Helicobacter pylori

H. pylori are incriminated as the major cause of gastritis and peptic ulcers, and the first bacterium that is classified as a carcinogen. H. pylori infection has also been demonstrated to be closely related with the genesis of both gastric adenocarcinomas and gastric lymphomas.

5.13 Neoplasm and Genetics

Beside senvironmental tumorigenic factors, hereditary factors also account for the development of many caner types. Patients with inherited cancer syndrome are more likely to develop neoplasms because of their defective genes and abnormal chromosomes. The well-identified inherited cancer syndromes are also listed in Table 5-2:

5.13.1 Autosomal Dominant Inherited Cancer Syndrome

The predisposition to autosomal dominant inherited cancers follows an autosomal dominant pattern of inheritance and a defective copy of gene increases the chance of tumorigenesis. Patients with familial retinoblastoma, discussed previously, ware inherited a copy of defective RB allele from parental generation. Retinoblastoma develops when the normal RB allele is mutated. Some precancerous lesions including familial adenomatous polyposis and neurofibromatosis are autosomal dominant inherited. In these diseases, tumor suppressor genes, such as RB, APC and NF1, are mutated or lost.

5.13.2 Autosomal Recessive Inherited Cancer Syndrome

The predisposition to recessive inherited cancers follows an autosomal recessive pattern of inheritance that both gene alleles are mutated. One example is xerodermpigmentousum mentioned before. Exposed to UV light, xerodermapigmentosum patients with defective nucleotide excision repair are at the increased risk of developing skin cancer. Besides xerodermpigmentousum, syndromes involving defects in DNA repair system constitute a group of inherited recessive disorders, such as bloom syndrome, ataxia-telangiectasia, and Fanconi anemia.

5.13.3 Familial Cancer

Some common types of cancers, such as breast, ovary, colon and brain cancers, have been reported to occur in a familial pattern. Since multiple factors are involved in the inheritance of familial cancers, the transmission pattern of familial cancer is not easy to rule out.

5.14   Host Defense Against Neoplasm: Tumor Immunity

Cells that undergo malignant transformation can be recognized and destroyed by host immune system. Tumor antigen and antitumor effector mechanisms are the main contents of tumor immunology. Immune surveillance is the normal function of the immune system to recognize the merging malignant cells and destroy them. However, immune surveillance is imperfect, and some malignant cells successfully escape the policing through producing a number of factors that promote immune tolerance and immune suppression.

5.14.1   Tumor Antigens

Tumor antigens that elicit host immune response are broadly classified into two categories. They are, tumor specific antigen(TSA) that are present only in tumor cells, and tumor-associated antigen(TAA) that are present both in tumor cells and some normal cells. According to their molecular structure and source, tumor antigens can also be classified into the following classes: ①Products of mutated proto-oncogenes, tumor suppressor genes, and neutral "passenger" genes. These products, such as peptides derived from mutated oncoproteins of RAS, p53, and BCR-ABL, enter the traditional antigen-processing pathway and recognized by $CD4^+/CD^+8$ T Cells. ②Aberrantly expressed cellular proteins. One example of such antigen is tyrosinase, which is also expressed in normal melanocytes and melanomas involved in melanin biosynthesis. They fail to be recognized by immune system in normal cells because of their limited amount. ③Antigens produced by oncogenic viruses. Human immune system plays a surveillance role where by cytotoxic T lymphocytes(CTLs) can recognize antigens produced by HPV and EBV. ④Oncofetal antigens. Oncofetal antigens, such as carcinoembryonic antigen (CEA) and α-fetoprotein (AFP), are highly expressed in cancer cells and fetal tissues. With the development of detection techniques, small amount of them are even found in normal tissues. ⑤Altered cell surface glycolipids and glycoproteins. Abnormal expressions or forms of surface glycoproteins and glycolipids are observed in most tumors. Abnormal forms of MUC-1, expressed on both breast and ovarian carcinomas, have been used for diagnostic and therapeutic studies. ⑥Cell type-specific differentiation antigens. These antigens are specific for particular lineages or differentiation stages of various cell types.

5.14.2   Antitumor Effector Mechanisms

Although antibodies produced by cancer patients can recognize tumor antigens, cell-mediated immunity is still the dominant antitumor mechanism in vivo. The main effector cells are:

CTLs. The antitumor effect of CTL sismainly accomplished through reacting against virus-associated neoplasms, such as EBV-and HPV-induced tumors.

Natural killer(NK) cells. NK cells function as the first line against human tumors. They are lymphocytes that can destroy tumor cells without primary sensitization. With the activation of IL-2 and IL-15, NK cells increase their activities against human tumors.

Macrophages. Activated macrophages kill tumors in a manner similar to killing microbes. They can exhibit cytotoxicity even without the appearance of T cells. Interferon-γ, cytokine secreted by T cells and NK cells is the potent activators of macrophages, as a result, T cells, NK cells and macrophages may collaborate in the antitumor process.

5.14.3   Immune Surveillance and Escape

The term "Immune surveillance" was first proposed as a normal function of the immune system against emerging malignant cells. This has been supported by many observations: One strong argument is that persons with congenital immunodeficiencies are 200 times easier to develop cancers compared with the immunocompetent individuals. Another is the positive response of advanced cancer to the newly developed therapeutic agents that function through stimulating the host T-cell response. Furthermore, transplant recipients and persons with acquired immune deficiency syndrome (AIDS) also have an increased incidence of malignancies.

However, most cancers occur in immunocompetent persons indicating that tumor cells must develop mechanisms to escape extermination by immune system in the hosts. The possible escape mechanisms have been proposed: ①Selective outgrowth of antigen-negative variants. Only the weak immunogenic mutants can survive during the tumor progression. ②Loss or reduced expression of MHC molecules. Tumor cells with abnormal levels of HLA class I molecules, may escape the attack of CTLs. ③Activation of immunoregulatory pathways. Tumor cells might inhibit tumor immunity by engaging the immune regulatory pathways. ④Secretion of immunosuppressive factors by cancer cells. Host immune responses are suppressed by tumor products, such as TGF-β, a potent immunosuppressant, secreted in large quantities of tumors. ⑤Induction of regulatory T cells (Tregs). Tumors products might reach the "immune escape" through favoring the development of immunosuppressive regulatory T cells.

Chapter 6

Environmental and Nutritional Diseases

❯ Introduction

The field of environmental pathology includes all such diseases caused by environment factors, most of which is man-made. In addition, overnutrition and malnutrition are also discussed in this chapter. The WHO estimates that 80% cases of cardiovascular disease and type 2 diabetes mellitus, and 40% of all cancers are preventable by avoidance of tobacco, healthy diet and physical activity. There are many factors that have been considered to affect human health as under: ①Industrial effluents and automobile exhausts. ②Accumulation of wastes. ③Unsatisfactory disposal of radioactive and electronic waste.

6.1 Environmental Pollution

Environmental pollution refers to natural or man-made destruction, which adds harmful substances to the environment and exceeds the self-purification capacity of the environment. Any agent-chemical, physical or microbial, that alters the composition of the environment is called pollutant. On the other hand, our personal environment gets affected by smoking of tobacco, water we drink and food we eat. Therefore, in this part, we briefly discuss the health effects of smoking, environmental compounds and air pollution.

6.1.1 Air Pollution

People live in a certain environment and cannot do without air. If people are exposed to polluted air for a long time, their health will be damnified. Air pollution is a major cause of morbidity and mortality worldwide, especially for those who already have pulmonary or myocardial disease. Inhaling polluted air can cause various diseases or cause lesions in many organs and systems (Table 6 – 1). Fine particulate matter (PM 2. 5) is a well-known air pollutant threatening public health. Studies has confirmed that long-term exposure to the particles could reduce the pulmonary function, cause exacerbation of asthma and chronic obstructive pulmonary disease, and increase incidence and mortality of lung cancer. Some of the pollutants have only foud in specific locations (such as coal dust, silica, and asbestos), others are general pollutants present widespread in the ambient atmosphere (e. g. sulphur dioxide, nitrogen dioxide, and carbon monoxide).

The effects of pollutants on human health are related to the following factors:

1) exposure time;

2) total dose of exposure;

3) impaired ability of the host to clear inhaled particles; and

4) particle size of 1-5 μm capable of getting impacted in the distal airways to produce tissue injury.

Table 6-1　Examples of common air pollutants

Pollutant	Source(s)	Consequences
Sulfur dioxide(SO_2)	Coal smoke Tobacco	Mucosal irritation
Carbon monoxide(CO)	Car exhaust Gas stove	Anoxia(death)
Polychlorinated biphenyls(PCBs)	Air spray Refrigerators	Undefined
Formaldehyde	Laboratory fumes House insulation	Mucosal irritation
Carbon	Smog Mining Coal smoke	Anthracosis
Quartz(silica)	Stone cutting	Silicosis
Asbestos Fine particulate matter(PM 2.5)	Insulation Shipbuilding Industrial emission Car exhaust	Asbestosis Interstitial pneumonia, fibrosis, other diseases

6.1.1.1　Outdoor Air Pollution

Air pollution is a very critical issue worldwide, particularly in developing countries. The six most common pollutants in the air are sulfur dioxide, carbon monoxide, ozone, nitrogen dioxide, lead and particulate matter. Usually, these agents produce well-known smog(smog and smog), sometimes suffocating large cities such as Beijing, Shanghai, Houston, Cairo, New Delhi, Mexico City and Hong Kong. Although the respiratory system bears the brunt, all organs in the body are involved in. Major health effects of outdoor pollutants are summarized in Table 6-2.

1) Ozone(O_3) is produced by interaction of ultraviolet(UV) radiation and oxygen(O_2) in the stratosphere and naturally accumulates in the so-called ozone layer 10 to 30 miles above the earth's surface. The ozone layer absorbs a lot of ultraviolet radiation from the sun, thus protecting the living things on the earth. Ozone on the earth's surface is a gas formed by the reaction of nitrogen oxides and volatile organic compounds in the presence of sunlight. These chemicals are emitted by industrial emissions and motor vehicle exhaust.

Generally, ozone inhalation only causes upper respiratory tract inflammation and mild symptoms(pulmonary dysfunction and chest discomfort). However, excessive exposure or prolonged exposure can pose a risk to patients with asthma or emphysema.

Together with other toxic gases, even low-level exposure to ozone can also damage lung function. Unfortunately, air pollutants often combine to create a veritable "witches' brew" of ozone and other agents such as sulfur dioxide and particulates.

2) Sulfur dioxide is produced by power plants burning coal and oil, smelting copper, and paper mills as a byproduct. When released into the air, it can be converted to sulfur trioxide, which forms sulfuric acid when exposed to water, which can cause damages of nasopharynx and lead to difficulty in breathing and asthma attacks in susceptible individuals.

3) Particulate matter(PM) is a type of air pollution that comprises a heterogeneous mixture of different particle sizes and chemical compositions. There are various sources of fine PM(PM 2.5), and the components may also have different effects on people. In general, the coarse particles with a particle size of 2.5

microns to 10 microns mainly come from the road dust, and the fine particles under 2.5 microns(PM 2.5) are mainly from the combustion of fossil fuels(such as motor vehicle exhaust and coal burning), volatile organic compounds and so on. When the concentration of PM 2.5 increased by 10 micrograms per cubic meter, the lung function of residents in air pollution area dropped by about 26 milliliters. If the concentration of PM 2.5 exceeds 75 micrograms per cubic meter, then the risk of chronic obstructive pulmonary disease is 2.53 times than that of 35 micrograms per cubic meter. Although the particles have not been well characterized chemically or physically, fine or ultrafine particles less than 10 μm in diameter are the most harmful. They are readily inhaled into the alveoli, where they are phagocytosed by macrophages and neutrophils, which respond by releasing a number of inflammatory mediators, such as IL-1. In contrast, particles that are greater than 10 μm in diameter are of lesser consequence, because they are usually blocked by nasal hair in the nasal cavity, or are captured by airway mucous epithelium, and are excreted with sputum through cilia swing.

Table 6-2　Health damage caused by outdoor air pollution

Pollutant	Populations at Risk	Effects
Sulfur dioxide	Healthy adults	Increased respiratory symptoms
	Individuals with chronic lung disease	Increased mortality
	Asthmatics	Increased hospitalization
		Decreased lung function
Acid aerosols	Healthy adults	Altered mucociliary clearance
	Children	Increased respiratory infections
	Asthmatics	Decreased lung function
		Increased hospitalizations
Nitrogen dioxide	Healthy adults	Increased airway reactivity
	Asthmatics	Decreased lung function
	Children	Increased respiratory infections
Ozone	Healthy adults and	Decreased lung function
	children	Increased airway reactivity
		Lung inflammation
		Decreased exercise capacity
		Increased hospitalizations
Particulates	Children	Increased respiratory infections
	Individuals with chronic lung or heart disease	Decreased lung function
	Asthmatics	Excess mortality
		Increased attacks

6.1.1.2　Tobacco Smoking

Smoking is a global problem endangering health. Cigarette smoke contains over 60 known carcinogens, plus toxic metals and formaldehyde. Tobacco contains several harmful constituents including nicotine, many carcinogens, carbon monoxide and other toxins(Table 6-3). The WHO report shows that smoking is harmful to human beings in many ways, these include mainly asthma, pneumonia, lung cancer, hypertension, heart disease and reproductive dysplasia. The harm caused by smoking is related to many factors, the most important of which is dose of exposure expressed in terms of pack years. It is estimated that the life expectancy of a person who smokes 2 packs of cigarettes at the age of 30 is 8 years less than a non-smoker. After quitting smoking, the higher mortality slowly declines and the beneficial effect reaches the level of non-smokers after 20 or more of smoke-free years.

Table 6-3　Health hazards caused by the main components in tobacco smoke

Constituents	Adverse Effect
Tar Polycyclic aromatic hydrocarbons Nitrosamines Benzopyrene	Carcinogenesis
Nicotine	Ganglionic stimulation and depression, tumor promotion
Phenol	Tumor promotion; mucosal irritation
Formaldehyde Nitrogen oxide	Toxicity to cilia; mucosal irritation
Carbon monoxide	Reduced oxygen transport

(1) mechanism

The mechanisms of smoking caused by disease include the following:

1) It directly affects the respiratory tract mucosa and causes bronchitis. Cigarette smoke increases the recruitment of leukocytes to the lung, increasing local elastase production and subsequent injury to lung tissue that leads to emphysema.

2) Carcinogensis. A variety of components in the smoke can cause cancer, particularly polycyclic hydrocarbons and nitrosamines, which are potent carcinogens in animals and probably involves in the causation of lung carcinomas in humans (Table 6-3; Table 6-4). The risk of developing lung cancer is related to the intensity of exposure, frequently expressed in terms of "pack years" (e. g. , one pack daily for 20 years equals 20 pack years) or in cigarettes smoked per day. In addition to lung cancer, smoking can also cause oral, esophageal, pancreatic and bladder cancer.

Smoking increases the incidence of cancer on the premise of other carcinogens. A classic example is that smoking increases the incidence of lung cancer in asbestos workers by 10 times. The combination of tobacco (chewed or smoked) and alcohol consumption has multiplicative effects on the risks of oral, laryngeal, and esophageal cancers.

Table 6-4　Organ specific carcinogens produced by smoking

Carcinogen(s)	Organ
Polycyclic aromatic hydrocarbons 4-(Methylnitrosoamino)-1-(3-pyridyl)-1-butanone(NNK) 210Polonium	Lung, larynx
NNK, NNN, 210polonium	Oral cavity; snuff
Polycyclic aromatic hydrocarbons, NNK, NNN	Oral cavity; smoking
N'-Nitrosonornicotine(NNN)	Esophagus
NNK	Pancreas
4-Aminobiphenyl, 2-naphthylamine	Bladder

3) Atherosclerosis is considered to be associated with smoking. Coronary atherosclerosis can cause myocardial ischemia, and even myocardial infarction. The mechanism of atherosclerosis induced by smoking may be related to increased platelet aggregation. Smoking is an important modifiable risk factor for the development of cardiovascular disease such as coronary artery disease, stable angina, acute coronary syndromes, sudden death, stroke, peripheral vascular disease, congestive heart failure, erectile dysfunction and aortic aneurysms via initiation and progression of atherosclerosis, which is responsible for approximately 140,000 premature deaths from cardiovascular diseases each year. Smoking has a multiplicative effect on atherosclerosis risk when combined with hypertension and hypercholesterolemia.

4) Smoking during pregnancy increases the risk of spontaneous abortion and premature birth, causing intrauterine growth retardation; however, birth weights of infants whose mothers stopped smoking before pregnancy are normal.

5) Second hand smoke, also known as passive smoking, and environmental tobacco smoke, is a mixed smog from cigarette or other tobacco products released from the end of the combustion and tobacco smoke exhaled by smokers. It is also the most widespread and serious indoor air pollution. It is a major cause of death worldwide. Studies have shown that second-hand smoke contains tar, ammonia, nicotine, suspended particulates, PM 2.5, polonium 210 and more than 4,000 kinds of harmful chemicals and dozens of carcinogens.

Secondhand smoke is more harmful to passive smokers than active smokers, especially to young children. The survey shows that in China, the main victims of passive smoking are women and children. Although they do not smoke themselves, they often suffer from secondhand smoke in the family and public places. In addition, workplace, venue, and so on, will often become a secondhand smoke flooding place. Although they do not smoke cigarettes directly, inhalation can still cause harm to the body. It is estimated that the relative risk of lung cancer in nonsmokers exposed to environmental smoke is about 1.3 times than that in nonsmokers who are not exposed to smoke. Secondhand smoke greatly increases the risk of atherosclerosis and fatal myocardial infarction. In addition, it also increases the number of respiratory infections and asthmatic attacks in children, the risk of sudden infant death syndrome (SIDS) and middle ear infections in young children, and the number of low birth weight infants born to exposed mothers.

(2) Tobacco-Related Diseases

Tobacco contains numerous toxic chemicals having adverse effects varying from minor throat irritation to carcinogenesis. The relative risk of major diseases in tobacco smokers compared to non-smokers and accounting for higher mortality include the following (in descending order of frequency):

1) Cancer of the lung: Cigarette smoke contains more than 3,000 toxic chemicals. According to statistics, smoking 10 cigarettes a day, the incidence of lung cancer increased by 13 times, if smoking 20 cigarettes a day, the incidence of lung cancer increased by 20 times, smoking 40 a day, lung cancer incidence rate increased by 65 times.

2) Chronic obstructive pulmonary disease (COPD): Smoking is the primary risk factor for the onset of COPD. The longer the smoking time and the greater the amount of smoking, the higher the prevalence rate. The prevalence rate of smokers is a times higher than non-smokers. Twenty-five percent of the heavy smokers will eventually develop into COPD, while 90% of the COPD fatients are smokers. According to statistics, the prevalence rate of smokers who smoke more than 40 cigarettes per day is 75.3%.

3) Cerebrovascular accidents and cardiovascular diseases: Coronary heart disease: Smoking is a major risk factor for many cardiovascular and cerebrovascular diseases. The incidence of coronary heart disease, hypertension, cerebrovascular disease and peripheral vascular disease of smokers increased significantly.

Statistics show that 75% of patients with coronary heart disease and hypertension have history of smoking. The incidence of coronary heart disease is 3.5 times higher than that of non-smokers. The mortality of coronary heart disease is 6 times higher than that of the latter. The incidence of myocardial infarction is 2−6 times higher than that of the latter.

4) Somking during pregnancy is associated with high risk of lower birth weight of foetus, high perinatal mortality and intellectual deterioration of newborn.

6.1.1.3 Carbon Monoxide Posioning

Carbon monoxide(CO) is a nonirritating, colorless, tasteless, odorless gas. It is produced by the incomplete oxidation of carbonaceous materials. Carbon monoxide poisoning is caused by inhalation of carbon containing substances which was incompletely combusted. The mechanism of poisoning is that the affinity of carbon monoxide and hemoglobin is 200−300 times higher than the affinity of oxygen and hemoglobin, so carbon monoxide is easily combined with hemoglobin to form carbo-oxy hemoglobin, which causes hemoglobin to lose the capacity of oxygen carrying, causing tissue asphyxia. Hypoxia leads to central nervous system (CNS) depression, which develops so insidiously that victims often are unaware of their plight and are unable to help themselves. Systemic hypoxia appears when the hemoglobin is 20% to 30% saturated with CO, and unconsciousness and death are probable with 60% to 70% saturation.

1) Acute carbon monoxide poisoning is common in accidents and suicides. The clinical manifestations were mainly anoxia, and its severity was proportional to the saturation of HbCO. People with light poisoning have headeche, weakness, verhgo, in breathing people with have headache, weakness, vertigo, difficulty in breathing while working, when HbCO saturation is 10% to 20%. In patients with moderate poisoning, the symptoms were aggravated when the skin and mucous membranes were cherry red(Figure 6−1). The patients could have nausea, vomiting, blurred consciousness, deficiency or coma, and the saturation of HbCO reached 30% to 40%. The havily poisoned people went into a oleep coma, accompanied by hyperthermia, increased muscle tension and paroxysmal or tonic spasm, when HbCO saturation was >50%. Some patients have blisters and redness on the chest and extremities, mainly due to autonomic neurotrophic disorders. Some patients with acute CO poisoning were awakened after the coma, after 2−30 days of false recovery, they would be comatose again, and there were psychosis of dementia with dementia, tremor paralysis syndrome, sensorimotor disorder or peripheral neuropathy, also called acute carbon monoxide poisoning delayed encephalopathy. Patients often have brain edema, pulmonary edema, myocardial damage, arrhythmia and respiratory depression, which can cause death. If a cadaver is dissected, the visceral organs may appear cherry-red(Figure 6−1).

Of course, if death occurs rapidly, morphologic changes may not be present; with longer survival, the brain may be slightly edematous and exhibit punctate hemorrhages and hypoxia induced neuronal changes. These changes are not specific; they simply imply systemic hypoxia. In victims who survive CO poisoning, complete recovery is possible; however, impairments of memory, vision, hearing, and speech sometimes remain.

2) When someone has long-term exposure to low concentration of CO, chronic poisoning will happen, and the clinical manifestations are headache, dizziness, memory loss, lack of concentration and palpitation. As a result, with low-level persistent exposure to CO, carboxyhemoglobin may accumulate to a life-threatening concentration in the blood. The slowly developing hypoxia can evoke widespread ischemic changes in the brain, particularly in the basal ganglia and lenticular nuclei. With cessation of exposure to CO, the patient usually recovers, but there may be permanent neurologic damage.

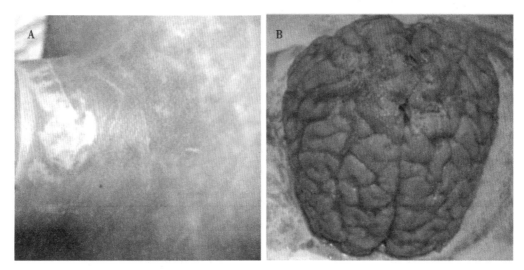

Figure 6-1   Carbon monoxide(CO) poisoning. A faulty natural gas room heater caused this fatal poisoning. The characteristic cherry-red coloration of skin and brain persists in death. CO binds irreversibly with hemoglobin to produce bright red hemoglobin, which retains its color even though no oxygen is present. (Picture A has been was originated from coroner Luo hui, Police Station of Boluo county, Guangdong Province; Picture B has been was originated from professor Zhang lushun, Chengdu Medical College)

6.1.1.4 Agricultural Exposures

In the process of agricultural production, pesticide is essential to ensure output. Pesticide refers to chemical agents used in agriculture to control plant diseases and insect pests and regulate plant growth. Many kinds of pesticides can be divided into insecticides, acaricides, rodenticides, nematides, mollusks, fungicides, herbicides, plant growth regulators and so on. According to the sources of raw materials, they can be divided into mineral source pesticides (inorganic pesticides), biological pesticides (natural organisms, microbes, antibiotics, etc.) and chemical synthesis of pesticides. According to the chemical structure, pesticides can be classified as organic chlorine, organophosphorus, organic nitrogen, organic sulfur, carbamate, pyrethroid, amide, urea, ether, phenols, phenoxy carboxylic acids, amidamides, three azoles, heterocyclics, benzoic acids, organometallic compounds, and so on.

1) Organophosphorus pesticide(OPS) is the most widely used insecticide in China. It mainly includes dichlorvos, parathion(1605), Phi phoxim(3911), internal phosphorus(1059), dimethoate, dimethoate and malathion(4049). Every year, millions of people around the world suffer from acute organophosphorus poisoning. About 300 thousand of them die, and most of them happen in developing countries. There are three ways organophosphorus pesticides can enter the body: entering throug the mouth-or taking orally (in suicides), by the skin or/and mucous membrane, and by the respiratory tract.

Acute organophosphorus pesticide poisoning(AOPP) refers to a series of injuries caused by a large amount of organophosphorus pesticides that enter the body in a short period of time. It mainly includes cholinergic excitation or crisis in acute poisoning patients, followed by intermediate syndrome(IMS) and delayed peripheral neuropathy(OPIDPN). Cholinergic crises are more common in patients taking large doses of cholinesterase inhibitors, including organophosphate poisoning. Before the crisis, the patient often showes obvious adverse reactions of cholinesterase inhibitors, such as nausea, vomiting, abdominal pain, diarrhea, sweaty, tears, wet cold skin, increased oral secretion, muscle fascicular tremor, emotional excitement, anxiety and other mental symptoms. When the cholinergic crisis occurs, the clinical manifestations include vomiting, abdominal pain, diarrhea, pupil reduction, Dohan, saliva, increased tracheal secretions, heart rate slowing, muscle tremor, spasmodic and contraction.

2) Organochlorine pesticide poisoning is commonly caused by organochlorine pesticides such as DDT, chlorid, etc. Organochlorine pesticides have been widely used. Since it is difficult to be degraded and remains in agricultural products for a long time affecting humans health, it have been gradually replaced. Poisoning is mostly caused by improper protection, food poisoning or suicide, and also for homicide. It can inhibit the metabolism of inositol, stimulate the excitement of central nervous system, and damage organs such as liver and kidney. Clinical manifestations of moderate poisoning include severe vomiting, sweating, salivating, blurred vision, muscle tremors, convulsions, palpitations, lethargy and so on. When a person is seriously poisoned, the clinical manifestations are epileptic seizures, coma, even respiratory failure or heart to fibrillation, and can cause liver and kidney damage.

3) Chronic poisoning refers to the exposure to poison in the body for a long time with small doses, causing some changes in the body's physiological, biochemical and pathological aspects, with a series of clinical signs and symptoms. Chronic human exposure to low level agricultural chemicals is implicated in cancer, chronic degenerative diseases, congenital malformations and impotence, but the exact cause-and-effect relationship is lacking.

WHO conducted a statistical analysis of 19 major agricultural countries in the world in 2013, and found that there were about 3 million cases of pesticide poisoning caused by pesticide residues in these countries, of which 500 thousand were acute poisoning. More than 75% of the mortality rate is occurring in developing countries due to veadily availability and indiscriminate use of hazardous pesticides which are otherwise banned in developed countries. Pesticide residues in food items such as in fruits, vegetables, cereals, grains, pulses etc. is of greatest concern.

6.1.1.5 Industrial Exposure

1) Volatile organic solvents. Volatile organic compounds(VOC) is the general term of volatile organic compounds with a melting point below room temperature, and whose boiling point range is between 50-260 ℃. Organic solvents are widely used in huge quantities worldwide. The harm of VOC is very obvious. When the concentration of VOC exceeds a certain concentration in the living room, people feel headache, nausea, vomiting and weakness in the extremities for a short time. VOC also can damage human liver, kidneys, brain and nervous system.

Occupational exposure of rubber workers to benzene and 1,3-butadiene increases the risk of leukemia. Benzene poisoning can be divided into acute benzene poisoning and chronic benzene poisoning. Acute benzene poisoning refers to the pathophysiological process that occurs mainly in the central nervous system as an organic solvent containing benzene or inhaling high concentration of benzene vapor. Chronic benzene poisoning refers to benzene and its metabolite phenols, which directly inhibit the nuclear division, cause gene mutation and affect the hematopoietic function of the bone marrow. The clinical manifestation was a continuous decrease in white blood cell counts, which eventually developed into aplastic anemia or leukemia.

Butadiene is a colorless gas with sweet and aromatic odor. its molecular weight is 54.1, and the freezing point is 108.9 ℃, and the boiling point is -4.4 ℃. It is soluble in organic solvents, and the solubility in water is 0.38%. It is low toxic. It has the effect of anesthesia and stimulation. Its anesthetic effect is stronger than that of propane, but it is only half of butene.

2) Metals. Heavy metal poisoning refers to poisoning caused by heavy metal elements or compounds whose atomic weight is greater than 65, such as mercury poisoning and lead poisoning. Because heavy met-

als can alter the structure of protein irreversibly and affect the function of tissue cells and affect human health.

Mercury is silver white liquid metal and evaporates at room temperature. Mercury poisoning is often a chronic poisoning. It often occurs in production activities, resulting in long-term inhalation of mercury vapor and mercury compound dust. The main symptoms were mental nerve abnormalities, gingivitis and tremor. Acute mercury poisoning is caused by inhalation of large amounts of mercury vapor or intake of mercury compounds. For those who are allergic to mercury, poisoning can occur even if they are partially coated with mercury matrix preparations.

Lead is a widespread industrial pollutant, which can affect the functions of the human nervous system, the cardiovascular system, the skeletal system, the reproductive system and the immune system, and cause the diseases of the gastrointestinal tract, the liver and kidney, and the brain. As for lead poisoning, there will be special discussion in the following chapter.

3) Bisphenol A is used in industry to synthesize polycarbonate(PC), epoxy resin and other materials. Since 1960s, bisphenol A has been used to make plastic(milk) bottles, infant cups, food and beverage(milk powder) cans inner coating. Bisphenol A is everywhere, from mineral water bottles, medical devices to food packaging. Every year, 27 million tons of plastic containing BPA are produced worldwide. BPA can lead to endocrine disorders, threaten the health of the fetus and children. Obesity caused by cancer and metabolic disorders is also thought to be related to bisphenol A. It is believed that bottles containing bisphenol A can induce precocious puberty in the European Union countries.

4) Vinyl chloride is an important monomer used in polymer chemical industry. It can be made from ethylene or acetylene. It is a colorless, liquefied gas, boiling point 13.9 ℃, critical temperature 142 ℃, critical pressure 5.22 MPa. It forms an explosive mixture with the air. The explosion limit is 4% to 22% (volume). It is more explosive under pressure. It is necessary to pay attention to the sealing and nitrogen seal of the container and the addition of a small amount of inhibitor. Vinyl chloride is a toxic substance. Exposure to vinyl chloride for a long time may lead to hepatic angiosarcoma, a rare type of liver tumor.

5) Environmental dusts. Dusts refers to solid particles suspended in the air. It is customary to have many names for dust, such as mineral dust, sand dust and powder. According to the international organization for standardization, the solid suspended solids with particle size less than 75 μm are defined as dust. Too much dust in the atmosphere will have a disastrous effect on the environment. Exposure to these agents nearly always occurs in the workplace. Inhalation of *mineral dusts* causes chronic, nonneoplastic lung diseases called pneumoconioses. The most common pneumoconioses are caused by exposures to coal dust(in mining of hard coal), silica(in sandblasting and stone cutting), asbestos(in mining, fabrication, and insulation work), and beryllium(in mining and fabrication). The increased risk of cancer as a result of asbestos exposure, however, extends to family members of asbestos workers and to other persons exposed outside the workplace. Pneumoconioses and their pathogenesis are discussed in Chapter 8.

Table 6-5   Diseases related to occupational exposure

Toxicant(s)	Effect(s)
Solvents, acrylamide, methyl chloride, mercury, lead, arsenic, DDT	Peripheral neuropathies
Chlordane, toluene, acrylamide, mercury	Ataxic gait
Alcohols, ketones, aldehydes, solvents	CNS depression
Ultraviolet radiation	Cataracts
CO, lead, solvents, cobalt, cadmium	Heart disease

Continue to Table 6-5

Toxicant(s)	Effect(s)
Isopropyl alcohol, wood dust	Nasal cancer
Radon, asbestos, silica, bis(chloromethyl)ether, nickel, arsenic, chromium, mustard gas	Lung cancer
Grain dust, coal dust, cadmium	Chronic obstructive lung disease
Beryllium, isocyanates	Hypersensitivity
Ammonia, sulfur oxides, formaldehyde	Irritation
Silica, asbestos, cobalt	Fibrosis
Vinyl chloride	Liver angiosarcoma
Mercury, lead, glycol ethers, solvents	Toxicity
Naphthylamines, 4-aminobiphenyl, benzidine, rubber products	Bladder cancer
Lead, phthalate plasticizers	Male infertility
Cadmium, lead	Female infertility
Mercury, polychlorinated biphenyls	Teratogenesis
Benzene, radon, uranium	Leukemia
Polychlorinated biphenyls, dioxins, herbicides	Folliculitis and acneiform dermatosis
Ultraviolet radiation	Cancer

6.2 Chemical and Drug Injury

Everyone is exposed to different kinds of chemicals and drugs. These chemicals and drugs are broadly divided into the following two categories: ①Therapeutic(iatrogenic) agents e. g. drugs, which when administered indiscriminately are associated with adverse effects. ②Non-therapeutic agents e. g. alcohol, lead, carbon monoxide, drug abuse.

6.2.1 Therapeutic(Iatrogenic) Drug Injury

Usually, the treatment of diseases is inseparable from the drugs. Of course, if used inappropriately, it can also cause a human injury. Though the basis of patient management is rational drug therapy, nevertheless adverse drug reactions do occur in 2% -5% of patients(Table 6-6). In general, the risk of adverse drug reactions increases with increasing number of drugs administered.

Drug-induced injury refers to abnormal reactions or diseases, such as disorders of physiological and biochemical processes, structural changes and other diseases, which are the consequences of drug adverse reactions, in the course of drug use, such as prevention, diagnosis or treatment. Drug induced injuries can be divided into two categories. The first type of injuries are due to side effects of drugs, excessive doses or injury caused by drug interactions. Such injuries can be prevented by rational use of drugs, with little harm. The second type is allergic reactions or allergy or specific reactions. This kind of injuries are difficult to prevent, and their incidence is low, but it is very harmful. It often leads to death. Drugs can cause a variety of diseases, such as arrhythmia, diffuse pneumonia, pulmonary fibrosis, violent hepatitis, chronic active hepatitis, nephrotic syndrome or renal failure, dermatitis, aplastic anemia, hemolytic anemia, mental disorder, gastrointestinal bleeding and cancer, etc.

6.2.1.1   Cause of Iatrogenic Drug Injury

Adverse effects of drugs may appear due to：①overdose；②genetic predisposition；③exaggerated pharmacologic response；④interaction with other drugs；⑤unknown factors. Some of the common forms of iatrogenic drug injuries and the offending drugs are listed in Table 6-6.

Table 6-6   Therapeutic drug injury

Adverse Effect	Offending Drug
Gastrointestinal Tract	
Gastritis, peptic ulcer	Aspirin, nonsteroidal anti-inflammatory drugs (NSAIDs)
Jejunal ulcer	Enteric-coated potassium tablets
Pancreatitis	Thiazide diuretics
Liver	
Cholestatic jaundice	Phenothiazines, tranquilisers, oral contraceptives
Hepatitis	Halothane, isoniazid
Fatty change	Tetracycline
Nervous System	Anticoagulants,
Cerebrovascular accidents	Oral contraceptives
Peripheral neuropathy 8th nerve deafness	Vincristine, antimalarials Streptomycin
SKIN	
Acne	Corticosteroids
Urticaria	Penicillin, sulfonamides
Exfoliative dermatitis,	Penicillin, sulfonamides,
Stevens-Johnson syndrome	phenyl butazone
Fixed drug eruptions	Chemotherapeutic agents
Heart	
Arrhythmias	Digitalis, propranalol
Congestive heart failure	Corticosteroids
Cardiomyopathy	Adriamycin
Blood	
Aplastic anaemia	Chloramphenicol
Agranulocytosis, thrombocytopenia	Antineoplastic drugs
Immune haemolytic anaemia	Penicillin
Megaloblastic anaemia	Methotrexate
Lungs	
Alveolitis, interstitial pulmonary fibrosis	Anti-neoplastic drugs
Asthma	Aspirin, indomethacin
Kidneys	
Acute tubular necrosis	Gentamycin, kanamycin
Nephrotic syndrome	Gold salts
Chronic interstitial nephritis, papillary necrosis	Phenacetin, salicylates
Metabolic effects	
Hypercalcaemia	Hypervitaminosis D, thiazide diuretics
Hepatic porphyria	Barbiturates
Hyperuricaemia	Anti-cancer chemotherapy

Continue to Table 6-6

Adverse Effect	Offending Drug
Female Reproductive Tract	
Cholelithiasis, thrombophlebitis, thromboembolism, benign liver cell adenomas	Long-term use of oral contraceptives
	Diethylstilbesterol by pregnant women
Vaginal adenosis, adenocarcinoma in daughters	Thalidomide in pregnancy
Foetal congenital anomalies	

6.2.2　Alcoholism

Alcoholism, commonly known as drunkenness, refers to the abnormal state of the body after drinking a large amount of alcohol(ethanol) at a time and result in the most serious injury to the nervous system and the liver.

After alcohol is absorbed, metabolism is divided into three steps: first, ethanol is converted into acetaldehyde by ethanol dehydrogenase; then acetaldehyde is oxidized into acetic acid by acetaldehyde dehydrogenase; finally the acetic acid will be decomposed into carbon dioxide and water. Acetaldehyde can cause the secretion of adrenaline and norepinephrine. At this point, the patient's characteristics are flushing and rapid heartbeat. Alcohol has direct neurotoxicity, cardiotoxicity and hepatotoxicity, so patients have a series of nervous system abnormalities, and even coma and shock after poisoning. In addition, alcohol can cause heart disease, hypoglycemia and metabolic acidosis

It is divided into two kinds of acute poisoning and chronic poisoning. The former can cause serious injuries to the patient in a short time and can even lead to death directly or indirectly. The latter causes cumulative damage to patients, such as alcohol dependence, mental disorders, alcoholic cirrhosis, and the induction of certain cancers(oral and tongue cancer, esophageal cancer, and liver cancer).

Alcohol dependence is characterized by higher tolerance. The usual dose is not sufficient to cause comfor-teffect and needs to consume more and more amounts to experience the desired effect for an alcoholic. Dependence also prompts withdrawal symptoms, such as nausea, sweating, tremors, and anxiety when the person attempts to go without alcohol.

The adverse effects—acute as well as chronic, are related to the quantity of alcohol content imbibed and duration of consumption. Generally, 10mg of ethanol is present in: ①one can of beer(or half a bottle of beer); ②120 ml of neat wine; ③30 ml of 43% liquor(small peg). A daily consumption of 40mg of ethanol (4 small pegs or 2 large pegs) is likely to be harmful; intake of 100mg or more daily is certainly dangerous.

6.2.2.1　Acute Alcoholism

After drinking, about 20% of alcohol was absorbed in the stomach, and 80% absorbed in the duodenum and small intestine. The toxic dose and lethal dose of alcohol vary from person to person. The toxic dose is generally 70-80 grams and the lethal dose is 250-500 grams. Whether the poisoning occurs after drinking is related to the following factors: ①limosis(when a person drinks on an empty stomach, the rate of alcohol is absorbed quickly); ②Fat intake(the fat foods can slow the absorption of alcohol); ③The gastrointestinal function and the ability of the human conversion agent to treat alcohol.

(1)Central Nervous System

Alcoholic brain injury refers to chronic damage of frontal lobe and limbic system related to memory and advanced mental functions caused by alcohol consumption. The clinical manifestations of alcoholism include alcohol induced amnesia syndrome and frontal lobe syndrome. The main manifestations of amnesia syndrome are short-term memory impairment, and the manifestation of frontal lobe damage syndrome include the defects of abstract thinking, concept formation, planning and complex information processing, while other cognitive functions are relatively intact and clear consciousness.

Alcohol acts as a CNS depressant; the intensity of effects of alcohol on the CNS is related to the quantity consumed and duration over which consumed, which are reflected by the blood levels of alcohol:

1) Initial effect of alcohol is on subcortical structures which is followed by disordered cortical function, motor ataxia and behavioral changes. These changes are apparent when blood alcohol level does not exceed 100 mg/dL which is the upper limit of sobriety in drinking as defined by law-enforcing agencies in most countries while dealing with cases of driving in drunken state.

2) Blood level of 100–200 mg/dL is associated with depression of cortical centres, lack of coordination, impaired judgement and drowsiness.

3) Stupor and coma supervene when blood alcohol level is about 300 mg/dL.

4) Blood level of alcohol above 400 mg/dL can cause anaesthesia, depression of medullary centre and death from respiratory arrest.

However, chronic alcoholics develop CNS tolerance and adaptation and, therefore, can withstand higher blood levels of alcohol without such serious effects.

(2) Stomach

Acute poisoning can cause gastric ulcer, gastric bleeding, and acute gastritis.

(3) Liver.

Severe alcoholism can induce extensive necrosis of liver cells and even liver failure, ie, alcoholic hepatitis. Alcoholic hepatitis is characterized by fatigue, anorexia, weight loss, hepatomegaly, and in more severe cases, fever, jaundice, and vomiting. Alcoholic hepatitis represents an acute presentation of alcoholic liver disease. Acute alcoholic injury to the liver is explained in Chapter 9.

6.2.2.2 Chronic Alcoholism

Chronic alcoholism produces widespread injury to organs and systems. Contrary to the earlier belief that chronic alcoholic injury results from nutritional deficiencies, it is now known that most of the alcohol-related injuries in different organs are due to toxic effects of alcohol and accumulation of its main toxic metabolite, acetaldehyde, in the blood. Other proposed mechanisms of tissue injuries in chronic alcoholism are free-radical mediated injuries and genetic susceptibility to alcohol-dependence and tissue damage.

Some of the more important organ effects in chronic alcoholism are as under:

(1) Nervous System

Chronic alcohol abuse can cause serious damages to the brain. The main lesion is the loss of neurons, which affects the whole brain, especially in the cerebellum. Neuronal loss in alcoholics occurs in discrete anatomical regions. In the cerebral cortex, the loss is restricted to the superior frontal cortex, but the magnitude of this loss(mean 23 percent) is too small to be reliably detected by routine non-quantitative evaluation.

Neuronal loss does not occur from the primary motor cortex or hippocampus. In subcortical regions, there is neuronal loss from the supraoptic and paraventricular nuclei of the hypothalamus, but not from the mamillary bodies, anterior and dorsomedial nuclei of the thalamus, serotonergic dorsal raphe, basal forebrain or cerebellum. Neuronal loss from the hypothalamus is related to maximum daily alcohol consumption.

In addition, there is another disease, named fetal alcohol syndrome. Fetal alcohol syndrome(FAS) results from maternal alcohol use during pregnancy, possibly complicated by genetic risk factors. The adverse effects of alcohol on the developing human fetus consist of a spectrum of structural anomalies and behavioral and neurocognitive disabilities, most accurately termed the fetal alcohol spectrum disorders(FASD). Autopsy and brain imaging studies indicate reductions and abnormalities in overall brain size and shape, specifically in structures such as the cerebellum, basal ganglia and corpus callosum.

(2)Liver

Alcoholic liver disease is a disorder of liver cell structure and/or dysfunction due to excessive consumption of alcohol. There is a wide spectrum of histology for alcoholic liver disease that includes that of steatosis, steatohepatitis, alcoholic hepatitis(without steatosis), alcoholic foamy degeneration, cholestasis, veno-occlusive disease (VOD), central hyaline sclerosis, and micronodular cirrhosis. Initially, it is usually manifested as fatty liver, which can develop into alcoholic hepatitis, alcoholic liver fibrosis and alcoholic cirrhosis(severe scarring), which is associated with liver failure, intestinal hemorrhage, and liver cancer.

(3)Pancreas

Chronic calcifying pancreatitis and acute pancreatitis are serious complications of chronic alcoholism.

(4)Gastrointestinal Tract

Alcohol abuse is associated with gastritis, gastric and esophageal ulcers, fatal intestinal bleeding, and increased risk for cancers of the mouth and esophagus. Gastritis, peptic ulcer and oesophageal varices associated with fatal massive bleeding may occur.

(5)Cardiovascular System

Alcohol abuse is associated with dilated cardiomyopathy and increased risk of cardiovascular disease. By contrast, moderate social consumption of alcohol is protective. Level of HDL(atherosclerosis-protective lipoprotein) has been shown to increase with moderate consumption of alcohol.

(6)Endocrine System

In men, testicular atrophy, feminisation, loss of libido and potency, and gynaecomastia may develop. These effects appear to be due to lowering of testosterone levels.

(7)Blood

Haematopoietic dysfunction with secondary megaloblastic anaemia and increased red blood cell volume may occur.

(8)Immune System

Alcoholics are more susceptible to various infections.

(9)Pregnancy

Even small amounts of alcohol have adverse effects on the fetus. Fetal alcohol syndrome may be the result.

(10)Cancer

A meta analysis of alcoholism and alcoholism in the National Institute showed that drinking was the strongest factor associated with the risk of oral cancer, pharynx, esophageal and larynx cancer. Drinking also significantly increases the risk of gastric cancer, rectal cancer, liver cancer, breast cancer and ovarian cancer. Excessive drinking has the highest risk of cancer, and even a small amount of alcohol consumption increases the risk of cancer.

6.2.3 Drug Abuses

Drug abuse means that drug abuse personnel who are addicted to any substance other than alcohol and nicotine that is used in excess to achieve an altered mood. This use has nothing to do with medical purposes, and the result is that abusers are dependent on the substance, forcing them to pursue their use without ending. Once they are addicted to the drug, they will not be able to extricate themselves. Drug abuse is associated with suicide, homicide, assaults, motor-vehicle injury, HIV infection, pneumonia, mental illness, hepatitis, and sudden death from cardiac disease or coma.

Addiction can be psychological, physical, or both. In physical addiction, body systems become physiologically dependent on the drug and withdrawal may produce physical effects ranging from anxiety to seizures and death. Psychological addiction is self-explanatory. Tolerance comes from chronic use of drugs. Abstinence from the drug decreases tolerance, a feature that can be dangerous.

Drug abuse in pregnancy is dangerous for the fetus. Like maternal alcohol use, maternal drug use may be associated with prematurity and birth defects. Some babies are also addicted, and these babies must be slowly placed under detoxification.

Drugs can be ingested, sniffed or inhaled, or injected. Greater effect is produced by injection or by sniffing or inhaling(including smoking)for quicker absorption into the bloodstream. Ingestion produces less of the desired effect because intestinal absorption is slow.

Illegal drugs fall into four main categories: depressants, stimulants, narcotics, and hallucinogens. Some of the commonly abused drugs and substances are as under: derivatives of opium.

Alkaloids extracted from opium and derivatives in vivo and in vitro can interact with the specific receptors of central neurons, relieve pain and produce happiness. Opioid and its semisynthetic derivatives include morphine, two ethyl morphine(heroin), hydrogenated morphine, codeine and oxycodone. The synthetic morphine substances include propiophene, fentanyl, methadone, pethidine, and agonist antagonist, tazocine. Large doses of opioids can cause stupor, coma and respiratory depression.

Repeated use of opioids will cause tolerance and neural adaptation, which is related to rebound hyperactivity after withdrawal. Opioid withdrawal syndrome includes craving, anxiety, bad mood, yawning, sweating, goose bumps, tears, runny nose, nausea or vomiting, diarrhea, pain spasm, muscle pain, fever, and insomnia.

The use of morphine, such as intravenous use, has many physical consequences, including hepatitis B, hepatitis C, HIV infection, septicemia, endocarditis, pneumonia and lung abscess, thrombotic phlebitis and rhabdomyolysis, as well as psychological and social damage.

Heroin is a semi synthetic drug derived from morphine alkaloids. It is commonly known as a number of white powder and white flour. It is the essential product of the opioid drug series. Generally, it includes heroin(two acetyl morphine), heroin salt(heroin hydrochloride, nitrate, tartrate and citrate)and the hydrate of heroin salt.

Heroin has great harm to the physical and mental health of human beings. Long term absorption and injection of heroin can cause disintegration of personality, psychopathy and reduced life expectancy, especially the most obvious injury to the nervous system. Heroin has a wide range of adverse physical effects that can be categorized etiologically according to ①the pharmacologic action of the agent; ②reactions to the cutting agents or contaminants; ③hypersensitivity reactions to the drug or its adulterants; ④diseases transmitted through the sharing of needles.

Some of the most important adverse effects of heroin are the following:

(1)Sudden Death

Sudden death means that a person who is healthy or seemingly healthy, dies in a short time due to natural illness. Heroin-induced death is usually caused by overdose. However, sudden death sometimes is due to a loss of tolerance for the drug, such as after a period of incarceration. The mechanisms of death include profound respiratory depression, arrhythmia and cardiac arrest, and pulmonary edema.

(2)Pulmonary Disease

Pulmonary complications include edema, septic embolism, pulmonary abscess, opportunistic infections, talcum and other foreign body granulomas with adulteration. Although granulomas occurs mainly in the lungs, they are sometimes found in the spleen, liver and lymph nodes to drain the upper limbs. Examination under polarized light often highlights the trapped talc crystals, sometimes wrapped in foreign body giant cells.

(3) Infections

Infection is a common complication of heroin abuse. The most common sites are skin and subcutaneous tissue, heart valves, liver and lungs. More than 10% of the patients hospitalized with heroin abuse have endocarditis, which often takes a distinctive form involving right-sided heart valves, particularly the tricuspid. Most cases are caused by *Staphylococcus aureus*, but a few cases are caused by fungi and other pathogens. Viral hepatitis is the most common infection among drug addicts and is obtained through sharing dirty needles. This has also led to a very high incidence of human immunodeficiency virus (HIV) infection among intravenous drug users.

(4) Skin Lesions

Skin damage may be the most common symptom of heroin addiction. Acute lesions include abscesses, cellulitis and ulcers caused by subcutaneous injection. Scarring at injection sites, hyperpigmentation over commonly used veins, and thrombosed veins are the usual sequelae of repeated intravenous inoculations.

(5) Renal Problems

Heroin can also cause kidney damage. The most common two forms are amyloidosis (usually secondary to skin infection) and focal glomerulosclerosis, both of which cause proteinuria and nephrotic syndrome.

6.2.4 Lead Poisoning

Lead can cause a series of physiological and biochemical changes to affect the functions of the central and peripheral nervous system, the cardiovascular system, the reproductive system and the immune system, and cause the diseases of the gastrointestinal tract, the liver and kidney, and the brain. Children and pregnant women are especially vulnerable to lead. Lead poisoning reduces children's intelligence, learning ability, perception and understanding, inattention, hyperactivity, impulsiveness, and obstacles to language learning.

6.2.4.1 The Effects of Lead Exposure Include the Following

1) The neurotoxic effects of lead are attributed to the inhibition of neurotransmitters caused by the disruption of calcium homeostasis.

2) Lead interferes with the normal remodeling of cartilage and primary bone trabeculae in the epiphyses in children. This causes increased bone density detected as radiodense lead lines.

3) Lead inhibits the healing of fractures by increasing chondrogenesis and delaying cartilage mineralization.

4) Lead affects the synthesis of hemoglobin. Porphyrin metabolism disorder is one of the important and early changes in the mechanism of lead poisoning. Porphyrin is an intermediate in the process of hemoglobin synthesis, and it is affected by a series of sulfhydryl enzymes in the process of hemoglobin synthesis. It has been proved that lead at least inhibits the delta aminolevulinic acid dehydrase (delta aminovalerate dehydrase, ALAD), fecal porphyrin oxidase and ferrous complex enzyme. ALAD is a metalloenzyme which consists of 8 identical subunits and 8 zinc ions. Zinc ions play an important role in the activity and stability of enzymes. Lead can replace the zinc ions of the active site, inhibit the activity of ALAD, and inhibit the formation of ALA, which leads to the increase of ALA in the blood. Of course, the ALA from urine is also increased. In addition, lead can also inhibit the activity of fecal porphyrin oxidase and prevent the oxidation of

fecporphyrin III to protoporphyrin IX, which results in the increase of fecal porphyrin in blood and increased excretion of fecal porphyrin in urine. Lead can also inhibit the ferrous complex enzyme, so that protoporphyrin IX cannot be combined with two valent iron to be heme. Protoporphyrin in erythrocytes can bind with abundant zinc in mitochondria of red blood cells, resulting in increased zinc protoporphyrin. Therefore, urinary ALA, faecal porphyrin and hematoporphyrin or zinc protoporphyrin are all diagnostic indicators of lead poisoning.

6.2.4.2   Morphological Changes of Lead Poisoning

The major anatomic targets of lead toxicity are the bone marrow and blood, nervous system, gastrointestinal tract, and kidneys.

1) Blood and marrow changes occur fairly rapidly and are characteristic. Lead poisoning can lead to anemia. Due to the disorder of hemoglobin synthesis, compensatory hyperplasia of erythrocytes in bone marrow is occurs. The dot cells, reticulocytes and erythrogranulocytes in the blood increased. The basophilic substances of these three red blood cells contain mitochondria and microsomal fragments and RNA. The inhibition of ferrochelatase by lead may result in the appearance of a few ring sideroblasts, red cell precursors with iron-laden mitochondria that are detected with a Prussian blue stain. In the peripheral blood the defect in hemoglobin synthesis appears as a microcytic, hypochromic anemia that is often accompanied by mild hemolysis. Even more distinctive is a punctate basophilic stippling of the red cells.

2) Brain damage is prone to occur in children. Lead can easily pass through the placenta, and lead can also easily pass through the blood-brain barrier because of the immature endothelial cells in the developing mesencephalon. It can be very subtle, producing mild dysfunction, or it can be massive and lethal. In young children, sensory, motor, intellectual, and psychologic impairments have been described, including reduced IQ, learning disabilities, retarded psychomotor development, blindness, and in more severe cases, psychoses, seizures, and coma. Lead toxicity in the mother may impair brain development in the prenatal infant. At the more severe end of the spectrum lies marked brain edema, demyelination of the cerebral and cerebellar white matter, and necrosis of cortical neurons accompanied by diffuse astrocytic proliferation. In adults the CNS is less often affected, but frequently a peripheral demyelinating neuropathy appears, typically involving the motor nerves of the most commonly used muscles. Thus, the extensor muscles of the wrist and fingers are often the first to be affected(causing wristdrop), followed by paralysis of the peroneal muscles(causing footdrop).

3) The gastrointestinal tract is also a major source of clinical manifestations. The mucous membrane of the digestive tract has the ability to secrete lead. In the process of lead XX, lead plays a direct role in the gastric mucosa, destroys the ability of gastric mucosa regeneration, and causes inflammatory changes in the gastric mucosa. Studies have shown that the detection rate of pathological damages of gastric mucosa in patients with chronic lead poisoning is 96.7%, and there may be atrophic gastritis and atrophic gastritis. It has been reported that patients with chronic, moderate or severe lead poisoning are initially diagnosed as superficial gastritis, and 91% turn to atrophic gastritis after three years. Lead "colic" is characterized by extremely severe, poorly localized abdominal pain.

4) Kidneys lesions. Lead can affect the function of mitochondria in renal tubular epithelial cells, inhibit the activities of Na^+ and K^+-ATP enzymes, and cause renal tubular dysfunction and even damage. Acute poisoning mainly affects the proximal convoluted tubules, which can cause cell membrane damage, cell swelling, mitochondria swelling and rupture, and particle loss in the matrix. There is an inclusion body in the nucleus of glomeruli, which is a complex of lead and protein. Its nature is not completely clear. It is generally believed that this is a kind of defense function of cells, so that the lead in cells can be stored in the inclu-

sion body, thus preventing the direct toxicity of lead to cells. In addition to damaging the renal tubules, chronic poisoning mainly manifested as progressive interstitial fibrosis, which first appeared around the renal tubules and then gradually is expanded outward. Microtubule atrophy and fibroblast proliferation can be seen simultaneously.

5) The cardiac lesions. Long term lead exposure can lead to elevated blood pressure, toxic myocarditis and myocardial damage. Lead exposure can increase the oxygen free radicals in the body, which results in lipid peroxidation damage, including myocardial cell membrane and myocardial microsomal membrane, and affects the cation transfer enzyme of myocardial microsomal membrane, with overloading the Ca^{2+} ion in the aorta and other vascular cells, which leads to accumulation of the Ca^{2+} in the cardiac myocytes and makes the myocardial cell work disorder.

6) To those poor oral hygiene, blue black lead line can be visible on the incisors, canine gingival margin.

6.3 Injury by Physical Agents

Physical injury refers to human injuries caused by various physical factors. These include radiation injury, high and low temperature injury, and electric injury, and so on.

6.3.1 Injury by Radiation

Radiation is divided into two categories: ionizing radiation and non-ionizing radiation. Ionizing radiation includes cosmic rays, X-rays and radiation from radioactive substances. Non-ionizing radiation includes ultraviolet, thermal radiation, radio waves and microwaves. The energy of non-ionizing radiation, such as ultraviolet(UV) and infrared light, microwaves, and sound waves, can move atoms in a molecule or cause them to vibrate but is not sufficient to displace electrons from atoms. By contrast, ionizing radiation has sufficient energy to remove tightly bound electrons. Collision of these free electrons with other atoms releases additional electrons, in a reaction cascade referred to as ionization. The main sources of ionizing radiation are ①X-rays and gamma rays, which are electromagnetic waves of very high frequencies, and ②high-energy neutrons, alpha particles(composed of two protons and two neutrons), and beta particles, which are essentially electrons. At equivalent amounts of energy, alpha particles induce heavy damage in a restricted area, whereas X-rays and gamma rays dissipate energy over a longer, deeper course, and produce considerably less damage per unit of tissue.

Radiation injury refers to acute, delayed or chronic tissue damage caused by ionizing radiation. Acute, chronic, and long-term effects were observed, among which acute injury was most commonly seen in nuclear radiation accidents.

The main sources of ionizing radiation are ①X-rays and gamma rays, which are electromagnetic waves of very high frequencies, and ②high-energy neutrons, alpha particles(composed of two protons and two neutrons), and beta particles, which are essentially electrons. At equivalent amounts of energy, alpha particles induce heavy damage in a restricted area, whereas X-rays and gamma rays dissipate energy over a longer, deeper course, and produce considerably less damage per unit of tissue.

6.3.1.1 Main Determinants of the Biologic Effects of Lonizing Radiation

In addition to the physical properties of the radiation, its biologic effects depend heavily on the following variables:

1) Radiation sources and radiographic conditions: the type of radiation, the dose of radiation, the loca-

tion and area of the radiation, the fractionation and the single irradiation, all have different damage effects. In general, the damage effects of the radiation penetration and the size of the ionization density are different; the radiation dose is the main factor of the image damage effect, and there is a certain dependence between the two. The general rule is that the greater the dose, the more significant the effect, but not the linear relationship.

2) The sensitivity of different parts of the body to radiation is different. The abdomen is most sensitive to radiation, in turn, the pelvic cavity, head, chest and limbs. When the other conditions are the same, the larger the irradiated area is, the greater the damage effect. If the total radiation dose is constant, the damage effect caused by multiple radiation is lower than that caused by a full dose of radiation. Moreover, the more the frequency of the radiation and the longer the interval time is, the smaller the damage effect, which may be related to the compensation and repair of the body.

Because ionizing radiation damages DNA, rapidly dividing cells are more vulnerable to injury than are quiescent cells. Except at extremely high doses that impair DNA transcription, DNA damage is compatible with survival in nondividing cells, such as neurons and muscle cells. Understandably, therefore, tissues with a high rate of cell turnover, such as gonads, bone marrow, lymphoid tissue, and the mucosa of the GI tract, are extremely vulnerable to radiation, and the injury is manifested early after exposure

3) Rate of delivery. When the total radiation dose is the same, the damage effect of multiple radiation is lower than the damage effect of a full dose of radiation, and the more the division times, the longer the interval, the smaller the damage effect, which may be related to the compensation and repair of the body.

4) Hypoxia. The production of ROS by the radiolysis of water is the most important mechanism of DNA damage by ionizing radiation. Tissue hypoxia, may exist in the center of rapidly growing, poorly vascularized tumors, this may thus reduce the extent of damage and the effectiveness of radiotherapy directed against tumors.

6.3.1.2　DNA Damage and Carcinogenesis

The ionizing radiation damage DNA can be divided into two types: direct and indirect effects. The direct effect is DNA directly absorbing radiation energy and is damaged. The indirect effect is that other molecules around DNA(mainly water molecules) absorb ray energy to produce highly reactive free radicals and then damage DNA. Ionizing radiation can cause many types of damage in DNA, including single-base damage, single-and double-strand breaks, and crosslinks between DNA and protein. In surviving cells, simple defects may be reparable by various enzyme repair systems contained in mammalian cells. However, double-strand breaks may persist without repair, or the repair of lesions may be imprecise(error prone), creating mutations. Damage to DNA caused by ionizing radiation that is not precisely repaired leads to mutations. If cell-cycle checkpoints are not functioning(for instance, because of mutations in *TP*53), cells with abnormal and unstable genomes survive and may expand as abnormal clones to form tumors eventually.

6.3.1.3　Morphological Changes of Radiation Injury

When the radiation dose is large, vessels may show dilation only during acute injury stage. Necrosis is the most important lesion, followed by inflammatory reaction. Subsequently, endothelial cell proliferation and collagen transparency were observed in the irradiated blood vessels. With the thickening of the media layer, the vascular lumen was obviously narrow or occluded. At this time, the increase of collagen in the irradiation field leads to scar formation and contraction, usually becoming obvious. Later, or higher doses, a variety of changes, including endothelial cell swelling and vacuolization, and even necrotic small blood vessels, such as capillaries and small veins. The affected vessels may rupture or develop thrombosis.

When the radiation dose is relatively small, cells cansurvive radiation damage, showing extensive changes in the structure of chromosomes, including deletion, fragmentation, translocation and fragmentation. Mitotic spindles are often disordered, and polyploidy and aneuploidy may be encountered. The nuclear swelling, condensation and agglutination of chromatin may occur, and the breakage in the nuclear membrane can also be noticed. In addition to affecting DNA and nucleus, radiative energy may cause multiple cytoplasmic changes, including cytoplasmic swelling, mitochondrial aberration and ER degeneration. The rupture of the plasma membrane and the focal defect may occur. Of course, apoptosis may also occur.

The structure of radiation injury is similar to that of cancer. It is characterized by cellular pleomorphic, giant cell formation, nuclear changes and mitosis. Cells with abnormal nuclear morphology can be produced for several years, including giant cells with polymorphonuclear nuclei or more than one nucleus.

6.3.1.4 Effects on Organ Systems

The most sensitive organs and tissues are gonads, hematopoietic and lymphatic systems, and the lining of the gastrointestinal tract. Changes in hematopoietic and lymphatic systems, as well as cancer caused by environmental or occupational exposure to ionizing radiation, are summarized below:

(1) Hematopoietic and Lymphoid Systems

It is worth noting that hematopoietic and lymphatic systems are extremely sensitive to radiation damage. Hematopoietic precursors in bone marrow are also sensitive to radiant energy, resulting in dose dependent bone marrow aplastic anemia. Radiation directly destroys lymphocytes, both in circulating blood and tissues(lymph nodes, spleen, thymus, intestines). High dose and large area of exposure, severe lymphocytic reduction may occur in the time of irradiation, along with shrinkage of the lymph nodes and spleen. With sublethal doses of radiation, the regeneration of surviving progenitor cells is rapid, leading to a return to normal lymphocyte counts. The acute influence of bone marrow irradiation on the peripheral blood count reflects the turnover kinetics of granulocytes, platelets and red cells of the components, and their half-life is less than 1 days, 10 days and 120 days, respectively.

Neutropenia occurred within a few days after circulating neutrophil counts increased briefly. Neutrophil counts reaches the lowest point, usually at near zero counts, at the second weeks. If the patient survives, a complete recovery of granulocytes may take 2 to 3 months. Thrombocytopenia occurs at the end of the first week. The lowest point of platelet counts occurs behind granulocytes, and the recovery of platelets is later than the recovery of granulocytes. Anemia occurs after 2 to 3 weeks of radiation exposure and may last for several months. High doses of radiation will result in more severe cell loss and longer recovery. Very high doses kill marrow stem cells and induce permanent aplasia(aplastic anemia) marked by a failure of blood counts recovery, whereas with lower doses the aplasia is transient.

(2) Gonads

Testicular atrophy in males and destruction of ovaries, which can cause infertility. According to the dosage, it is divided into temporary and permanent infertility.

(3) Gastrointestinal Injury

Radiation injury to the intestine can be divided into 3 periods, namely, acute phase, subacute stage and chronic stage. The acute phase occurs in the early stage of radiation, subacute phase occurs 2–12 months after radiation, and chronic phase occurs after 12 months of radiation.

Acute phase injury is most obvious in the cells with strong metabolism and active mitosis, especially the crypt cells and mucosal epithelial cells in the basal mucosa of the intestinal mucosa. The intestinal mucosa decayes, the villi of the intestinal wall became shorter, and the surface area of the intestinal epithelium became smaller. When the cell regeneration system is further damaged, tiny ulcers are formed, and as time goes on, small ulcers fuse with each other to form an eye-visible ulcer. At the same time, there is edema, inflammatory cell infiltration, telangiectasia, and even bleeding in the submucosa. The endothelial cells of the submucosal arterioles can be swollen and separate from the basement membrane and undergo degeneration. Progressive vascular and connective tissue lesions can cause obliteration arterio-phlebitis and microvascular insufficiency. The intestinal mucosa may be ulcerated by plaque like ischemia. Large foam cells can be seen under the intima of the vessels. Because of ischemia, there are fibrous tissue hyperplasia in the submucosa and large gigantic shape fibroblasts often appear.

Chronic injury is caused by the indirect effect of radiation, mainly due to progressive occlusive arterioles and extensive collagen deposition and fibrosis. As the number of blood vessels in the intestinal wall gradually decreases, the blood supply of the intestinal wall gradually decreases, so that the intestinal wall is ischemic. Then progressive intestinal mucosal atrophy and mucosal telangiectasia occurres. As the vasculitis progressively worsens, necrosis, ulceration and perforation of the intestinal wall can occur. Among them, ulcer is the most common, which can cause perforation of intestinal wall and cause peritonitis or abdominal abscess. Healing and repair of ulcers can lead to fibrosis and scarring, resulting in intestinal stenosis and intestinal obstruction. Some patients can form fistula. Cancer can also be induced by radiation in the later period.

(4) Heart

The damaged sites include pericardium, epicardium, endocardium, and even heart valves, conduction systems and coronary arteries. General damage is closely related to the area of radiotherapy, and pericardium and myocardial damage are most common. Pericardial effusion and thickening were seen in the cases of radiation heart injuries, and thickening of the endocardium and epicardium. Myocardial fibrosis was seen in all layers of the ventricular wall. The changes can be diffuse or focal, but the right or right ventricle is more obvious, which may be related to the right ventricle from the chest wall. At the end of the course, some people have left ventricular contraction with one or more valvular thickening, among which tricuspid and aortic valve injuries are most common. However, mitral atresia and mural thrombosis are rare. About 40% of the people can find serious stenosis in the coronary artery. The main reason is the formation of atherosclerotic plaque. The plaque is mainly fibrous lesions, and the proximal end is more significant than the distal end. Under the light microscope, transient granulocyte infiltration and edema around the blood vessels can be observed during the acute stage of radiological heart damage, and cardiomyocyte edema, hyaline change, and fatty degeneration can be seen later. Subsequently, the lesions were spotted or spotted fibrosis foci and necrotic foci, scattered. Fibroplasia was seen in the interstitium and surrounding vessels, and the number of smooth muscle cells in the blood vessels decreased. Under electron microscope, cardiomyocytes arranged in disorder, broken and atrophied cardiac muscle fibers, nuclei deformed, mitochondrial sarcoplasmic reticulum and nuclear structure destroyed. There are high density particles deposition under the cell membrane, interruption of continuity, but not all cases.

(5) Kidney

Early lesions were not obvious. Four to six days after irradiation, epithelial cell degeneration and fusion of foot processes could be seen. The lesions continued to develop, endoplasmic reticulum dilatation, and a large number of lipid particles, autophagic vacuoles, extensive fusion of podocytes, and swelling of endothelial cells. In some areas, the capillary lumen was completely obstructed, the endothelial cells were separated from the basement membrane, the basement membrane was wrinkled and twisted, the mesangial cells were swollen and the matrix increased. The lesion of renal tubules mainly appeared in the proximal convoluted tubules, showing atrophy and necrosis of the renal tubules. The basement membrane of the renal tubules showed focal diffuse thickening, distortion and widening of the intercellular space.

Chronic histopathological changes: Obvious renal atrophy was observed at two months after exposure to naked eye. The endothelial cells of the glomeruli were swollen and the endothelial cells were separated from the basement membrane, which was filled with cytoplasmic fragments and low electron density and lipid particles. The mesangial cells were swollen and the cytoplasm contained a large amount of lysosomes in the cytoplasm. In 2 and 3 months after irradiation, the glomerular capillaries collapsed so that the lumen disappeared, and some glomeruli showed fibrinogen like necrosis at 4 months after irradiation, and the glomerulus became a "transparent substance" mass for nearly 6 and 9 months. In addition, severe and extensive injury of renal tubules, including atrophy, denaturation, necrosis and canalicular collapse of renal tubular epithelial cells were found. The injured renal tubules contained many lipofuscin particles. There were many transparent and granular tubules in the lumen. Interstitial edema is accompanied by infiltration of many monocytes, histiocytes and fibroblasts. Obvious fibrosis was observed at 5 months after radiation, and fibroblasts, histiocytic cells and collagen fibers gathered around renal tubules and vessels. The damage of the arteries and arterioles occurred later. The endothelial cells were swollen, the intima was thickened, fibrin deposition and thrombosis, and the middle layer was involved, and fibrin like necrosis was seen at 3 to 4 months after irradiation.

(6) Eyes

Radiation can cause radiation cataract, radiation retinopathy or optic neuropathy, keratitis or iriliary ciliary body inflammation.

(7) Skin

Acute radiation skin injury refers to the acute radiation dermatitis and radiation-induced skin ulcer caused by a number of large doses(X-ray, gamma ray and beta ray) in the part of the body in a short time(a few days). The incubation period is several days, and it is divided into 3 degrees according to the severity of the damage. Generally, the damage to epidermal cells was initially manifested as a decrease in cell proliferation. If the dose exceeds the threshold dose, local temporary inflammatory reaction can be seen, which is characterized by hair follicle papules and temporary hair loss, that is, the first-degree damage. In the first degree, there is a clear line of erythema, which is the most obvious within 2−6 weeks, burning and itching, hair loss, erythema fade and pigmentation after the decline. With the increase of radiation dose, other symptoms develop from dry dermatitis(erythema) to exudative reaction, that is second-degree injury. One to three weeks of local formation of flush, swelling, blisters, then form a superficial surface of erosion, erythema, conscious burning or pain, later scab, the healing of pigmentation, permanent hair loss and so on. Severe lesions can involve deep or subcutaneous tissue of the dermis and form carrion and necrotic ulcers, that is the third-degree injuries.

Chronic radiation-induced skin injuries were also divided into 3 degrees. In the first-degree, there is dry skin, pigmented or lost, rough, nail dark or longitudinal ridge color bar; in the second degree, there is skin hyperkeratosis, chapped or atrophy, capillary dilatation, nail thickening deformation and so on; in the third degree, there is necrotic ulcer, horny protuberance, finger end keratinization fusion, tendon contracture, joint deformation, dysfunction and so on. Chronic radiation damage can cause flat or verrucous hyperplasia of the skin, or form intractable ulcers, which can be secondary to basal cell carcinoma or squamous cell carcinoma.

6.4 Nutritional Diseases

Nutritional disease is a kind of disease caused by excessive or too little nutrients in the body, or imbalances that cause excess nutrition or nutrition deficiency and abnormal nutrition metabolism. Nutritional diseases include nutritional disorders, obesity, vitamin deficiency and hypervitamine.

Too much energy is often stored in the form of fat in our subcutaneous tissue, around the internal organs, and on the abdominal omentum. The excess fat not only ruins our body out of shape, but also increases the burden of the body, reduces the function of the heart and lungs, and causes great pressure on the body, especially the joints of the lower extremities, which maybe induce the degenerative arthropathy. At the same time, too much fat can also interfere with the absorption of other nutrients such as protein, calcium and iron.

Excessive intake of certain nutrients, which cannot be promptly metabolized in the body, may cause poisoning. Vitamin A, vitamin D, vitamin E and vitamin K, which are fat soluble nutrients, are not easily expelled from the body and can cause poisoning. Too much protein intake will also increase the liver and kidney metabolic burden and prevent iron absorption.

6.4.1 Pathogenesis of Deficiency Diseases

Nutritional deficiency is a kind of malnutrition due to inadequate intake of nutrients with various clinical manifestations. In recent years, a variety of subclinical nutritional deficiencies have been paid attention to because of the increasingly complete functional examination of nutrients. Therefore, nutritional deficiency also includes this part. The nutritional deficiency may be of 2 types: ①Primary deficiency This is due to either the lack or decreased amount of essential nutrients in diet. The most common reason is inadequate intake of food, which can be either primary or secondary. The deficiency of food caused by social factors such as disaster or war is often lacking in primary intake of food, but it is mainly characterized by malnutrition of heat energy protein. Dietary bias can cause a deficiency of nutrients. Sometimes a group's habit bias can even lead to the prevalence of a kind of nutritional deficiency disease. As the food is unreasonably cooked, it destroys nutrients. For example, in the lack of water-soluble vitamins, eating white rice noodles and dropping rice soup is often the main cause of the foot disease. After the vegetables are cut first and washed, hot drifting and squeezing will destroy most of the vitamin C. ②Secondary or conditioned deficiency Secondary or conditioned deficiency is malnutrition occurring as a result of the various factors. The secondary causes of inadequate food intake are inanorexia, coma, insanity or anorexia, oral and maxillofacial surgery, esophagus cancer and cardia cancer, which cause obstruction of the esophagus and stomach. Nasogastric feeding or parenteral nutrition are often used in these diseases, but if the amount of recharge cannot meet the needs of patients, there will still be symptoms of nutritional deficiency.

6.4.2 Obesity

Obesity is a common group of metabolic disorders. When the body eats more calories than the consumption of heat, the excess heat is stored in the body in the form of fat, which tends to be more than normal physiological needs, and then becomes obesity when a certain value is reached. The weight of adipose tissue in normal male adults is 15% to 18% of body weight and 20% to 25% for females. The proportion of body fat increases with age. The most widely used method to gauge obesity is body mass index(BMI), a measure of the ratio of body weight to height as expressed by body weight in kilograms divided by the square of the height in meters. A cut-off BMI value of 30 is used for obesity in both men and women.

6.4.2.1　Etiology

The main external cause is too much diet and too little activity. Calorie intake is more than caloric consumption, and fat synthesis is the material basis of obesity. The internal factor is the disorder of fat metabolism.

(1) Genetic Factors

There is a certain genetic background in the pathogenesis of simple obesity in humans. Studies have shown that it one side of the parents is obese, then their children's obesity rate increases by about 50%. If both parents are obese, the obesity rate of their children will rise to 80%. Human obesity is generally considered to be a polygenic inheritance, and heredity plays an important role in its pathogenesis.

(2) Neuropsychic Factors

It is known that there are two pairs of neural nuclei related to feeding behavior in the hypothalamus of humans and animals. One pair is the ventral contralateral nucleus, also known as the satiety center; the other is the ventral lateral nucleus, also known as the hunger center. When satiety centers are excited, they feel full and refrain from eating. When they are destroyed, their appetite increases. The hungry center works opposite to the satiety center. The two factors regulate each other, restrict each other, and are in a dynamic balance under physiological conditions, so that the appetite is regulated in normal range and maintains normal body weight. When the thalamus changes, whether it is the sequelae of inflammation (such as meningitis, encephalitis), or the occurrence of trauma, tumor and other pathological changes, if the lateral nucleus of the abdomen is destroyed, the function of the ventral nucleus is relatively hyperactive and gluttony is not tired, causing obesity. Conversely, when the ventrolateral nucleus is destroyed, the ventromedial nucleus is relatively hyperfunctional and anorexia, resulting in emaciation.

(3) Endocrine Factors

Many hormones, such as thyroxine, insulin and glucocorticoids, can regulate the intake of food. Therefore, it is assumed that these hormones may be involved in the pathogenesis of simple obesity. Obese people have insulin resistance and cause hyperinsulinemia which can regulate the insulin receptor and increase insulin resistance. Increased insulin secretion stimulates food intake and inhibits lipolysis, resulting in fat accumulation in the body. Sex hormones may play a role in the pathogenesis of simple obesity.

Too much intake can produce an excess of gastric inhibitory polypeptide (GIP) by stimulating the small intestine, which stimulates the release of insulin from islet beta cells. When the pituitary function is low, the secretion of growth hormone, gonadotropin and thyroid stimulating hormone is reduced, which causes the hypofunction of the gonadal and thyroid glands, and a special type of obesity can occur at this time. This may be related to decreased fat mobilization and increased synthesis. Clinically obese are more likely to occur in women, especially by parturients or by women who take oral contraceptives, suggesting that estrogen is related to the metabolism of fat. When the adrenal cortex is hyper-functional, the secretion of cortisol increases, which promotes glucoplasma and increases blood sugar, which in turn stimulates the increase of insulin secretion and increases the composition of fat.

(4) Other Factors

Lifestyle, feeding behavior, hobbies, climate and social psychological factors may lead to obesity.

6.4.2.2　Pathogenesis

The lipid storing cells, adipocytes comprise the adipose tissue, and are present in vascular and stromal compartment in the body. Besides the generally accepted role of adipocytes for fat storage, these cells also release endocrine-regulating molecules. These molecules include: energy regulatory hormone (leptin), cytokines(TNF-α and interleukin-6), insulin sensitivity regulating agents(adiponectin, resistin and RBP4), prothrombotic factors(plasminogen activator inhibitor), and blood pressure regulating agent(angiotensinogen).

Adipose mass is increased due to the enlargement of adipose cells due to excess of intracellular lipid deposition as well as due to increase in the number of adipocytes. The most important environmental factor is excess consumption of nutrients which can lead to obesity. However, underlying molecular mechanisms of obesity are beginning to unfold based on observations that obesity is familial and is seen in identical twins. Recently, two obesity genes have been found: *ob* gene and its protein product leptin, and *db* gene and its protein product leptin receptor.

6.4.2.3   Morphologic Features

Obesity is associated with increased adipose stores in the subcutaneous tissues, skeletal muscles, internal organs such as the kidneys, heart, liver and omentum; fatty liver is also more common in obese individuals. There is an increase in both size and number of adipocytes i. e. there is hypertrophy as well as hyperplasia.

6.4.2.4   Consequences of Obesity

Being obese is bad for health(Table 6-7). As a result of housing and job discrimination, poor body image, and low self-esteem, obese people are at greater risk for social, economic, and psychological problems, including diagnosed mental illness. For example, obese people are more often poor and less likely to be employed. What's more, the ill effects of obesity are pervasive and appear in unexpected ways. Obese people are more prone to home accidents because they are less fit and unable to manage their bulk; on average, they are twice as likely to suffer from hearing loss, poor eyesight, and mobility disorders of the arms or legs.

Table 6-7   Relative risk of body mass index(BMI) to cancer, cardiovascular disease and diabetes in population

Body Mass Index Classification	Increased Cardiovascular Risk	Increased Diabetes Risk	Increased Cancer Risk
18.5-24.9 Normal	None	None	None
25-29.9 Overweight	20%	100%	10%
30-40 Obese	90%	250%	30%
≥40 Morbidly obese	140%	550%	70%

The physical consequences of obesity are the following:

1) Hyperinsulinaemia. The increase in the volume and number of adipocytes leads to the enhancement or weakening of the expression of secretory hormone, which affects insulin level and leads to insulin resistance and hyperinsulinemia. Excessive storage of fat leads to the enhancement of lipid degradation, which results in a large amount of free fatty acids(FFA). Large amounts of FFA are transported into the liver and peripheral tissues, resulting in liver sugar utilization and neoglycogenesis disorder. At the same time, the decrease of insulin intake results in the increase of circulating insulin concentration, which leads to the decrease of insulin receptor expression and the production of insulin resistance. In addition, the activity of insulin receptor tyrosine kinase is inhibited in the high FFA environment, which inhibits the expression and activity of the insulin receptor substrate-1(IRS-1) and leads to insulin resistance

2) Type 2 diabetes mellitus. The study found a positive correlation between obesity and diabetes, the more obese the peoples, the higher the incidence of type 2 diabetes, and 90% of patients with type 2 diabe-

tes showed a state of obesity. Obesity often exacerbates the diabetic state and in many cases weight reduction often leads to amelioration of diabetes.

3) Hypertension. In a large sample survey, it was found that if body mass index increased by 10%, systolic blood pressure increased by 2–6 mmHg, while diastolic blood pressure increased by 1–3 mmHg on average. A strong association between hypertension and obesity is observed which is perhaps due to increased blood volume.

4) Hyperlipoproteinaemia. Obesity is strongly associated with VLDL and mildly with LDL. Also, obesity is associated with low blood HDL cholesterol and high triglyceride; both are risk factors in coronary artery disease.

5) Atherosclerosis. Obese patients are often associated with lipid metabolism disorders. The most common result of lipid metabolism disorders is lipoid deposition, mainly manifested by low density lipoprotein (LDL) elevation and high density lipoprotein(HDL) level. Obesity predisposes to development of atherosclerosis. As a result of atherosclerosis and hypertension, there is increased risk of myocardial infarction and stroke in obese individuals.

6) Hypoventilation syndrome(Pickwickian syndrome). The bulge of abdominal fat and the thick pelt of fat on the chest and breasts limit ventilation. This is characterised by hypersomnolence, both at night and during day in obese individuals along with carbon dioxide retention, hypoxia, polycythaemia and eventually right-sided heart failure. Chronic hypoxia causes vasoconstriction in the systemic and pulmonary circulation, causing high blood pressure, pulmonary hypertension, and right heart failure.

7) Osteoarthritis. These individuals are more prone to develop degenerative joint disease due to wear and tear following trauma to joints as a result of large body weight.

8) Cancer. Obesity can promote the development of cancer by changing the metabolic state of the body, releasing a large amount of inflammatory factors, changing the fat factor, and damage of the immune system. In men, obesity is strongly associated with increased risk for cancers of the esophagus, thyroid, colon, and kidney. In women, the risk is for cancer of the endometrium, gallbladder, and kidney.

6.4.3　Starvation

Starvation refers to the nutritional state of the body, such as oxygen, heat or nutrients, which can not meet the needs of the organism. General term starvation mainly refers to insufficient heat. The broad sense of starvation also includes oxygen hunger and water starvation. Protein starvation, calcium starvation, and vitamin starvation are synonymous in scientific terms with deficiency or deficiency in protein nutrition, deficiency of calcium nutrition and deficiency of vitamin nutrition or deficiency. The causes of starvation are varied, such as natural disasters, poverty, captives, imprisonment, hunger, specific religious activities, food or physical function, and so on. What is more noteworthy is the nutritional imbalance caused by inadequate food or partial insufficiency, due to economic conditions, cultural scientific literacy, religious and custom concepts, and special physiological or pathological reasons. These people are in a semi-starvation of certain nutrients, which are not uncommon in the poor, backward areas and classes. Some diseases affect the absorption of nutrients, such as wasting diseases(infections, inflammatory conditions, liver disease), cancer, etc, leading to starvation. Cancer results in malignant cachexia as a result of which cytokines are elaborated e. g. tumour necrosis factor-α, elastases, proteases etc.

6.4.3.1　Metabolic Changes

The metabolic characteristics of the starvation process under the regulation of insulin reduction and glucagon increase are as follows:

1) Muscle decomposition increases, and most of the released amino acids change to alanine and glutamine.

2) The effect of sugar isogenesis is strengthened. Glucose stores of the body are sufficient for one day's metabolic needs only. During fasting state, insulin independent tissues such as the brain, blood cells and renal medulla continue to utilise glucose while insulin-dependent tissues like muscle stop taking up glucose. This results in release of glycogen stores of the liver to maintain normal blood glucose level. Subsequently, hepatic gluconeogenesis from other sources such as breakdown of proteins takes place. It can be seen that gluconeogenesis is mainly carried out in the liver during the starvation process (about 80% of the exogenous sugar and the remaining 20% in the renal cortex). Proteins breakdown to release amino acids which are used as fuel for hepatic gluconeogenesis so as to maintain glucose needs of the brain. This results in nitrogen imbalance due to excretion of nitrogen compounds as urea.

3) Fat decomposition accelerated, glycerol and fatty acid content increased in plasma, and the result is gluconeogenesis. Starvation can then continue till all the body fat stores are exhausted following which death occurs. After about one week of starvation, protein breakdown is decreased while triglycerides of adipose tissue are brokendown to form glycerol and fatty acids. Glycerol can produce sugar directly, and fatty acid can not only provide the energy of sugar isogenesis, but also produce acetyl coenzyme A and promote the isogenesis of amino acid, pyruvic acid, lactic acid and so on. About 1/4 of fatty acids decomposed by fat can transform into ketone bodies in the liver, so the plasma ketone bodies can increase several hundred times when starving.

6.4.3.2   Clinical Presentation

The clinical manifestations of starvation include weakness, tatigue and depression; haggard, wasted and indifferent. The eyes are dull and the skin is rough and hangs in fold due to the loss of fat. The face is often pigmented. The bones protrude. A shrunken limb resembles a stick. On the face and abdomen, there is an incongruous edema. If the starvation continues for long time, it will cause hair to fall off. For children, hunger leads to growth retardation. For women, hunger often leads to amenorrhea.

6.4.3.3   Morphological Changes

Most organs shrink due to atrophy. The fat disappeared and the muscles are wasted. The heart is also smaller, and the blood pressure and heart output are low. The pulse is slow. The liver first appeares fatty degeneration, but long starved, the fat and protein stored in the liver are decomposed and absorbed, and the liver cells became very small, with few organelles. Hypoalbuminemia developed later only in the disease. The pancreas and other exocrine glands atrophy. Edema is common in the face and extremities, and ascites is also common. The wall of the intestines is so thin that it is transparent. The erythrocyte of the patient is reduced and anaemia appeares. Hemosiderosis is common. Lymphoid tissue atrophies. T-cell function and neutrophil phagocytosis become impaired, but B-cell function is preserved. Opportunistic infections or pneumonia occurs and often lead to death.

6.4.4   Disorders of Vitamins

Vitamin is a kind of nutrients necessary to maintain the health of the human body. It is a low molecular organic compound. Most of them can not be synthesized in the body, or the amount of the synthesis is difficult to meet the needs of the body. It must be supplied by food. Such substances have the following common characteristics: ①Found in natural food; the overwhelming majority can not be synthesized in the body (vitamin D, K and other few vitamins exceptions); ②it is not the structural component of the body and does not provide energy, but it plays an important role in regulating the metabolic process of the substance. The body needs only a small amount of vitamins a day to meet the metabolic needs, but it must not be lacking, Otherwise, it will cause vitamin deficiency if it is deficient to a certain extent. Vitamins can be classified into two groups according to their solubility: fat soluble vitamins and water soluble vitamins. Fat soluble vitamins include vitamin A, vitamin D, vitamin E and vitamin K, which dissolve in fat and go into the body with fat; water-soluble vitamins include vitamin C and vitamin B (B_1, B_2, B_6, B_{12}, niacin, pantothenic acid, folic acid, biotin, etc.), which can dissolve in water. Because of the different solubility of the two kinds of vitamins, their absorption, excretion and accumulation in the body are different, resulting in different symptoms of different vitamin deficiency. Table 6−8 sums up the various clinical disorders that were produced by vitamin deficiencies.

6.4.4.1 Etiology of Vitamin Deficiencies

There are many reasons for vitamin deficiency, which are common in the following aspects:

1) The supply of vitamins is insufficient. It not only includes the deficiency of food itself, but also the deficiency of food intake. It may also be in the process of food processing, due to improper use of cooking methods which cause vitamin damage and loss, resulting in insufficient dietary supply.

2) The ability of the body to absorb and utilize vitamins is reduced. Including excessive intake of dietary fiber and other factors cause vitamin absorption reduction. In addition, gastrointestinal dysfunction leads to a decrease in vitamin absorption and utilization.

3) The physiological needs of vitamins are relatively increased. The need for multivitamins in certain periods of pregnancy such, lactation, and growth is increased. In the cold, hot and other special environmental conditions or diseases, the body will also increase the demand for vitamins.

4) Vitamins excretion is increased. Vomiting, diarrhea and other conditions may lead to an increase in the elimination of multiple vitamins, especially water-soluble vitamins.

Table 6−8　Disorders caused by Vitamin deficiencies

Vitamins	Deficiency Disorders
FAT-SOLUBLE VITAMINS	
Vitamin A(Retinol)	Ocular lesions(night blindness, xerophthalmia, keratomalacia, Bitot's spots, blindness)
	Cutaneous lesions(xeroderma)
	Other lesions(squamous metaplasia of respiratory epithelium, urothelium and pancreatic ductal epithelium, subsequent anaplasia; retarded bone growth)
Vitamin D(Calcitriol)	Rickets in growing children
	Osteomalacia in adults
	Hypocalcaemic tetany
Vitamin E	Degeneration of neurons, retinal pigments, axons of peripheral nerves; denervation of muscles
	Reduced red cell lifespan
	Sterility in male and female animals
Vitamin K	Hypoprothrombinaemia(in haemorrhagic disease of newborn, biliary obstruction, malabsorption, anticoagulant therapy, antibiotic therapy, diffuse liver disease)
WATER-SOLUBLE VITAMINS	
Vitamin C(Ascorbic acid)	Scurvy(haemorrhagic diathesis, skeletal lesions, delayed wound healing, anaemia, lesions in teeth and gums)

Continue to Table 6-8

Vitamins	Deficiency Disorders
Vitamin B Complex	
(i)Thiamine(Vitamin B_1)	Beriberi('dry' or peripheral neuritis, 'wet' or cardiac manifestations, 'cerebral' or Wernicke-Korsakoff's syndrome)
(ii)Riboflavin(Vitamin B_2)	Ariboflavinosis(ocular lesions, cheilosis, glossitis, dermatitis)
(iii) Niacin/Nicotinic acid (Vitamin B_3)	Pellagra(dermatitis, diarrhoea, dementia)
(iv)Pyridoxine(Vitamin B_6)	Vague lesions(convulsions in infants, dermatitis, cheilosis, glossitis, sideroblastic anaemia)
(v)Folate/Folic acid	Megaloblastic anaemia
(vi) Cyanocobalamin (Vitamin B_{12})	Megaloblastic anaemia Pernicious anaemia
(vii)Biotin	Mental and neurological symptoms
Choline	Fatty liver, muscle damage
Flavonoids	Preventive of neurodegenerative disease, osteoporosis, diabetes

6.4.5　Vitamin A(Retinol) Deficiency

Vitamin A is necessary to maintain the integrity of all epithelial tissues. If vitamin A is deficient, the epithelial cells of the eye, respiratory, digestive, urethra and reproductive organs are significantly affected, manifested in epithelial xerosis, hyperplasia and desiccation. In addition, vitamin A can promote growth and development. During vitamin A deficiency, human bone growth is bad, growth and development are blocked, or even a reproductive decline. Vitamin A is a component of the photoreceptor in visual cells. When vitamin A is deficient, the sensitivity to weak light will be reduced, which leads to dark adaptation disorder, and even night blindness occurs in severe cases.

In short, vitamin A deficiency is a nutritional disorder caused by vitamin A deficiency, characterized by dry and rough skin, night blindness, xerosis corner and extensor conical follicular keratosis papules of the extremities.

6.4.5.1　Lesions in Vitamin A Deficiency

Nutritional deficiency of vitamin A is common in countries of South-East Asia, Africa, Central and South America whereas malabsorption syndrome may account for conditioned vitamin A deficiency in developed countries. Consequent to vitamin A deficiency, following pathologic changes are seen:

(1)Ocular Lesions

Lesions in the eyes are most obvious. The onset of ocular lesions is characterized by dry conjunctiva and cornea, loss of luster and tear loss. Night blindness is usually the first sign of vitamin A deficiency. As a result of replacement metaplasia of mucus secreting cells by squamous cells, there is dry and scaly scleral conjunctiva(xerophthalmia). The lacrimal duct also shows hyperkeratosis. Keratinized epithelium accumulating into foam like leukoplakia is called conjunctival dry spot or Bitot's spots, which are focal triangular areas of opacities. Then the cornea is dry, cloudy, softened, conscious photophobia, impeding transmission of light. Corneal ulcers may occur which may get infected and cause keratomalacia. Serious cases even have corneal perforation, leading to iris and lens prolapse. Ultimately, infection, scarring and opacities lead to blindness.

(2) Cutaneous Lesions

Skin lesions are characterized by dry skin, desquamation, epithelial keratosis, and keratosis filling hair follicles to form hair follicles and papules. When touching the skin, there is a rough sand feeling. It can develop an the neck, back and even the face with the extension of the extremities and shoulder. The hair follicle keratinization causes the hair to be dry, losing luster and being easy to fall off. Nails, toenails are brittle and easy to break.

(3) Other Lesions

1) Squamous metaplasia of respiratory epithelium of bronchus and trachea may predispose to respiratory infections.

2) Squamous metaplasia of pancreatic ductal epithelium may lead to obstruction and cystic dilatation.

3) Squamous metaplasia of urothelium of the pelvis of kidney may predispose to pyelonephritis and perhaps to renal calculi.

4) Long-standing metaplasia may cause progression to anaplasia under certain circumstances.

5) Bone growth in vitamin A deficient animals is retarded.

6) Immune dysfunction may occur due to damaged barrier epithelium and compromised immune defenses.

7) Pregnant women may have increased risk of maternal infection, mortality and impaired embryonic development.

6.4.6　Hypervitaminosis A

Vitamin A poisoning(Vitamin A toxicity) is a toxic syndrome caused by excessive intake of vitamin A. According to the study, infants and young children take vitamin A, such as a dose of more than 300 thousand international units(a gram of common cod liver oil containing vitamin A 850 international units per gram), can cause acute poisoning. Taking 50 thousand-100 thounds units per day for 6 months or so can cause chronic poisoning. In addition, the child's sensitivity and tolerance to vitamin A can be significantly different, and some children may also have mild symptoms of poisoning even if they do not exceed the above range.

6.4.6.1　Acute Toxicity

This results from a single large dose of vitamin A. Usually, vitamin A injected with 300,000 IU can produce toxic symptoms within a few days. It is manifested as loss of appetite, irritability or lethargy, vomiting, anterior fontanelle enlargement, head circumference enlargement, craniofacial dehiscence, papillary edema, etc. Increased intracranial pressure is common in acute type, which is due to increased cerebrospinal fluid volume or absorption disorders.

6.4.6.2　Chronic Toxicity

The effects of toxicity usually disappear on stopping excess intake of vitamin A.

The dosage of vitamin A reaches tens of thousands of units per day, such as vitamin A per kilogram of body weight 1,500 IU for infants and young children.

Early manifestations are irritability, anorexia, low fever, sweating and alopecia, followed by typical symptoms of bone pain, metastatic pain, soft tissue swelling, pain point without red, heat signs, more common in the long bones of the extremities.

Because of long bone epiphysis involvement, it can cause short stature. Some cases have swelling and pain in the temporal and occipital regions, which can be misdiagnosed as cranial osteomalacia. The symptoms of increased intracranial pressure such as headache, vomiting, wide anterior fontanelle, separation of cranial seams, strabismus in the eyes, nystagmus and diplopia are another feature of this disease, but they are rarely seen in the acute type. In addition, there are skin pruritus, desquamation, rash, chapped lips, dryhair, hepatomegaly, splenomegaly, abdominal pain, myalgia, bleeding, kidney disease, and regenerative anemia with leukocyte reduction. The blood alkaline phosphatase increased. It has been reported in other countries that chronic hepatomegaly and splenomegaly can cause cirrhosis, increased portal hypertension and even death.

6.4.7   Vitamin D(Calcitriol) Deficiency

Vitamin D deficiency is a disease characterized by abnormal calcium and phosphorus metabolism and poor calcification of bone like tissue. The clinical manifestations are vitamin D deficiency rickets and vitamin D deficiency tetany in adults and osteomalacia in adults.

6.4.7.1   Etiology

1) Lack of sunlight. In China, due to the long winter in the north and the long rainy season in the south, people's outdoor activities are reduced, resulting in a significant reduction in the chances of people receiving sunlight.

2) Low intake of vitamin D. Low vitamin D content in breast milk or other dairy products cannot meet the growth and development needs of infants, which can lead to vitamin D deficiency in infants. Also, unreasonable diet can lead to vitamin D deficiency.

3) Fast growth rate of the baby. Since the bones of babies grow very fast, vitamin D is in great demand. Premature infants and multiple births have insufficient vitamin D reserves. In addition, rapid growth after birth causes vitamin D demand and leads to vitamin D deficiency.

4) The influence of some diseases. Severe chronic kidney disease, hepatic disease, and gastrointestinal tract disorders can affect the absorption of vitamin D or affect the synthesis of 1,25-dihydroxy vitamin D_3.

5) Effect of some drugs. If the metabolism of vitamin D were interfered by phenobarbital and glucocorticoids, which should cause in vitamin D deficiency.

6.4.7.2   Lesions in Vitamin D Deficiency

Lesions in deficiency of vitamin D from any of the above mechanisms includes: ①rickets in growing children; ②osteomalacia in adults; ③hypocalcaemic tetany due to neuromuscular dysfunction.

6.4.7.3   Rickets

Rickets is a systemic, chronic and nutritional disease characterized by bone damage. The reason is that vitamin D deficiency in infants, children and adolescents leads to disorder of calcium and phosphorus metabolism. The main feature of rickets is the growth of the epiphyseal plate cartilage and the incomplete calcification of bone tissue. It occurs mainly in infants under 2 years of age, especially within 3-18 months, and can be prevented by taking adequate vitamin D. The pathogenesis of lesions in rickets is better understood by contrasting them with sequence of changes in normal bone growth as outlined in Table 6-9.

Morphologic features: The main lesions is the deformity of skeleton.

1) Craniotabes. In 6 months old infants, rickets is mainly caused by skull changes. The front fontanelle margin is soft and thin. At 6 months of age, table tennis-like toughness is felt by touching the bone seams, but the central frontal and parietal bones tend to thicken gradually. At 7-8 months, the head will become a "square skull" appearance and the head circumference becomes larger than that of the normal skull.

2) Rachitic rosary is a deformity of chest due to cartilaginous overgrowth at costochondral junction. The epiphyseal end is enlarged because of the accumulation of bone like tissue. Along the ribs, the rounded protuberance can be touched at the junction of ribs and costal cartilage, from upper to lower like beaded protuberances, and the most obvious seventh to 10 ribs are called rachitic rosary.

3) Harrison's sulcus appears due to indrawing of soft ribs on inspiration. In children with severe rickets, a horizontal depression is formed at the lower edge of the thorax, namely the costal phrenic groove or Harrison's sulcus.

4) Pigeon-chest deformity is the anterior protrusion of sternum and adjacent cartilage due to action of respiratory muscles. The funnel chest is the inward depression of the sternum and looks like a deep hopper.

5) As a result of osteomalacia and muscle and joint relaxation, the bone is not enough to support the weight of the body, resulting in femoral and tibiofibular bending deformation, which forms a serious genu varus("O") or genu valgus("X") deformity.

6) In patients with serious illness, the wrist, ankle and foot can also form a blunt circular rise, called the hand and foot bracelet.

7) Lumbar lordosis is due to spinal and pelvic involvement.

Table 6-9　The difference between rickets and normal bone growth

Normal bone growth	Rickets
Endochondral ossification(Occurring in long tubular bones)	
1) Normal vascularisation of bone	1) Irregular overgrowth of small blood vessels in disorganised and weak bone
2) Proliferation of cartilage cells at the epiphyses followed by provisional mineralisation	2) Proliferation of cartilage cells at the epiphyses followed by inadequate provisional mineralisation
3) Cartilage resorption and replacement by osteoid matrix	3) Persistence and overgrowth of epiphyseal cartilage; deposition of osteoid matrix on inadequately mineralised cartilage resulting in enlarged and expanded costochondral junctions
4) Mineralisation to form bone	4) Deformed bones due to lack of structural rigidity
Intramembranous ossification(Occurring in flat bones)	
Mesenchymal cells differentiate into osteoblasts which develop osteoid matrix and subsequent mineralisation	Mesenchymal cells differentiate into osteoblasts with laying down of osteoid matrix which fails to get mineralised resulting in soft and weak flat bones

Chapter 7

The Blood Vessel and Heart

Cardiovascular disease is a class of diseases, which refers to any disease that affects the cardiovascular system, principally cardiac disease, vascular diseases of the brain and kidney, and peripheral arterial diseases. There are many causes of cardiovascular disease, but atherosclerosis and/or hypertension are the most common. In addition, aging, changes in cardiovascular function, and many subsequent physiological and morphological changes, even in healthy symptomatic individuals also lead to an increased risk of cardiovascular disease.

7.1 Atherosclerosis

Atherosclerosis is a generic, inclusive term that describes thickening and hardening of the arterial wall. The term includes three pathological entities: atherosclerosis (ATH), arteriosclerosis and arterial calcification.

Atherosclerosis is a multifactorial degenerative disease characterized by the formation of plaques on the intima. Atheromatous plaques are raised lesions composed of soft gummous lipid cores covered by fibrous caps. Plaques weaken the underlying media, sometimes cause aneurysms. Atherosclerotic plaques can mechanically obstruct vascular lumina and are prone to rupture, resulting in catastrophic vessel thrombosis. This disease is commonly found in adult over the age of 40 and in many younger individuals. Large and medium arteries are usually involved.

7.1.1 Etiology and Pathogenesis

7.1.1.1 Etiology

So far, the causes of ATH are not very clear. The prevalence and severity of atherosclerosis are correlated with a number of risk factors. Some risk factors are constitutional, but others are acquired or related to modifiable behaviors. These risk factors have roughly multiplicative effects.

(1)Constitutional Risk Factors

1)Age: Atherosclerosis is usually clinically silent until lesions reach a critical threshold in middle age or later. Therefore, the incidence of myocardial infarction increases five-fold between the ages of 40 and 60.

2)Genetics: Family history is the most important independent risk of factor for atherosclerosis. Certain

Mendelian disorders are closely related to atherosclerosis, but these account for only a small percentage of cases. The most familial risk is related to polygenic traits coexisting with atherosclerosis, such as hypertension and diabetes, and other genetic polymorphisms.

3) Gender: All other factors being equal, premenopausal women are relatively protected against atherosclerosis (and its consequences) compared with age-matched men. Thus, myocardial infarction and other complications of atherosclerosis are uncommon in premenopausal woman in the absence of other predisposing factors such as diabetes, hyperlipidemia, or severe hypertension. However, after menopause, the incidence of atherosclerosis—related diseases increases and even exceeds that of men among the elderly. Although it has long been proposed to use estrogen to explain this gender difference, clinical trials have shown that hormone therapy is not beneficial in preventing vascular diseases. Moreover, estrogen replacement after menopause seems to increase.

cardiovascular risk. In addition to atherosclerosis, gender also affects other factors that may affect the prognosis of patients with IHD, such as hemostasis, infarct healing, and myocardial remodeling.

(2) Modifiable Major Risk Factors

1) Hypertension: Hypertension, especially increased diastolic blood pressure, is a major risk factor for the development of atherosclerosis. Hypertension can increase the risk of IDH by approximately 60%. Hypertension is also the major cause of left ventricular hypertrophy (LVH), which can also contribute to myocardial ischemia.

2) Diabetes: Diabetes is associated with raised circulating cholesterol levels and markedly increases the risk of atherosclerosis. Other factors being equal, the incidence of myocardial infarction is twice as high in diabetics as in nondiabetics. In addition, the disease is associated with an increased risk of stroke and a 100 —fold increase in atherosclerosis-induced gangrene of the lower extremities.

3) Hyperlipidemia: Hypercholesterolemia is another major risk factor for the development of atherosclerosis and is sufficient to induce lesions in the absence of other risk factors. The main cholesterol component associated with increased risk is low-density lipoprotein (LDL) cholesterol, which distributes cholesterol to peripheral tissues. By contrast, high-density lipoprotein (HDL) mobilizes cholesterol from developing and existing vascular plaques and transports it to the liver for biliary excretion. Consequently, higher levels of HDL correlates with reduced risk. Recognition of these relationships has spurred the development of dietary and pharmacologic interventions that lower total serum cholesterol or LDL, and/or raise serum HDL.

4) Cigarette smoking: It is a well-established risk factor in men and probably accounts for the increasing incidence and severity of atherosclerosis in women. Prolonged (years) smoking of one or more packs of cigarettes a day doubles the rate of IDH-related mortality, while smoking cessation reduces the risk.

(3) Additional Risk Factors

Roughly 20% of cardiovascular events occur in the absence of identifiable risk factors. For example, in previously healthy women more than 75% of cardiovascular events occur in those with LDL cholesterol levels below 160 mg/dL (a cut-off value generally considered to connote low risk). Other factors that contribute to risk include the following:

1) Metabolic syndrome: It is associated with central obesity, and is characterized by dyslipidemia, hypertension, hypercoagulability, insulin resistance, and a pro-inflammatory state, which may be triggered by cytokines released from adipocytes. Hypertension, dyslipidemia, and hyperglycemia are all cardiac risk factors, while the systemic hypercoagulable and pro-inflammatory state may contribute to endothelial dysfunction and/or thrombosis.

2) C-reactive protein (CRP) levels: CRP is an acute phase reactant, mainly synthesized by the liver

based on a variety of inflammatory cytokines. Locally, CRP secreted by cells within atherosclerotic plaques can activate endothelial cells, increase adhesiveness and remain in a prethrombotic state. Its clinical importance lies in its value as a circulating biomarker: CRP levels can predict the risk of stroke, peripheral arterial disease, myocardial infarction, and sudden cardiac death, in among apparently healthy persons. Statins can reduce CRP levels, and have nothing to do with lowering LDL cholesterol, suggesting that these drugs may have anti-inflammatory effects. In addition, although there is no direct evidence that lowering CRP can reduce cardiovascular risk, it is of concern that smoking cessation, weight loss and exercise can reduce CRP.

3) Inflammation: Inflammatory cells are present during all stages of atheromatous plaque formation and are intimately linked with plaque progression and rupture. With increasing recognition of the role of inflammation, measures of systemic inflammation have become important in risk stratification. Determination of CRP has emerged as one of the simplest and most sensitive systemic markers of inflammation correlate with IDH risk.

4) Elevated levels of procoagulants: It is the potent predictor of risk for major cardiovascular events. Excessive activation of thrombin, which can initiate inflammation through cleavage of protease-activated receptors (PARs) on endothelium, leukocytes, and other cells, may be particularly atherogenic.

5) Hyperhomocysteinemia: Serum homocysteine levels are related to stroke, coronary atherosclerosis, venous thrombosis, and peripheral vascular disease. Homocystinuria, due to a rare congenital metabolilerror, causes elevated circulating homocysteine (more than 100 μmol/L) and is associated with early-onset vascular disease. Although low folate and vitamin B_{12} levels can increase homocysteine levels, supplemental vitamin ingestion does not affect the incidence of cardiovascular disease.

6) Lipoprotein A levels: Lipoprotein A is an LDL-like particle that contains apolipoprotein B-100 linked to apolipoprotein A. Lipoprotein A levels are correlated with the risk of coronary and cerebrovascular disease, independent of total cholesterol or LDL levels.

7) Other factors: They are associated with difficult-to-quantify risks including lackage of exercise and a competitive, stressful life style ("type A personality").

7.1.1.2   Pathogenesis

Pathogenesis of the characteristic lipid plaques in ATH is uncertain, so far several hypotheses have been proposed. Historically, there have been two dominant theories regarding atherogenesis: one focusing on repeated formation and organization of thrombi, and the other emphasizing intimal cellular proliferation in response to endothelial injury. The contemporary view of atherogenesis incorporates elements of both theories and also integrates the risk factors previously discussed.

(1) Response to Injury Hypothesis (Endothelial Injury)

Endothelial cell injury is the cornerstone of the response to injury hypothesis. Endothelial cell loss due to any kind of injury-induced experimentally by irradiation, immune complex deposition, hemodynamic forces, mechanical denudation, or chemicals, results in intimal thickening in the presence of high-lipid diets. The importance of hemodynamic factors in atherogenesis is illustrated by the observation that plaques tend to occur at ostia of exiting vessels, at branch points, and along the posterior wall of the abdominal aorta, where there is turbulent blood flow. Suspected triggers of early atheromatous lesions include toxins from cigarette smoke, homocysteine, hypertension, and hyperlipidemia, can stimulate proatherogenic patterns of endothelial cell gene expression. Nevertheless, the two most important causes of endothelial dysfunction are hypercholesterolemia and hemodynamic disturbances. These dysfunctional endothelial cells exhibit enhanced leukocyte adhesion, altered gene expression, and increased permeability, all of which may contribute to the development of atherosclerosis.

(2) Lipid Infiltration

Lipids typically transported in the blood-stream are bound to specific apoproteins. Dyslipoproteinemias can result from mutations in genes that encode apoproteins or lipoprotein receptors, or from disorders that derange lipid metabolism, e. g. , alcoholism, nephritic syndrome, hypothyroidism, or diabetes mellitus. Common lipoprotein abnormalities in the general population(and indeed, present in many myocardial infarction survivors) include: ①decreases HDL cholesterol levels; ②increased LDL cholesterol levels; ③and increased levels of lipoprotein.

The mechanisms by which dyslipidemia contributes to atherogenesis include the following:

1) Chronic hyperlipidemia, particularly hypercholesterolemia, can directly impair endothelial cell function by increasing local oxygen free radical production; among other things, oxygen free radicals accelerate NO decay, damping its vasodilator activity.

2) With chronic hyperlipidemia, lipoproteins accumulate within the intima, where they are hypothesized to generate two pathogenic derivatives, cholesterol crystals and oxidized LDL. Oxidized LDL stimulates the local release of growth factors, cytokines, and is also cytotoxic to endothelial cells and smooth muscle cells. LDL is oxidized through the action of oxygen free radicals generated locally by macrophages or endothelial cells and ingested by macrophages through the scavenger receptor, resulting in foam cell formation. And recently, it has been shown that minute extracellular cholesterol crystals found in early atherosclerotic lesions serve as "danger" signals that activate innate immune cells.

(3) Smooth Muscle Proliferation and ECM Synthesis

Intimal smooth muscle cell proliferation and ECM deposition lead to conversion of the earliest lesion, a fatty streak, into a mature atheroma, thus contributing to the progressive growth of atherosclerotic lesions. Several growth factors are implicated in smooth muscle cell proliferation and matrix synthesis, including platelet-derived growth factor (PDGF), Fibroblast growth factor (FGF), and TGF-α. The recruited smooth muscle cells synthesize ECM, which stabilizes atherosclerotic smooth muscle cell apoptosis and breakdown of matrix, leading to the development of unstable plaques. Intimal smooth muscle cells can originate from the media or from circulating precursors; regardless of their source, they have a proliferative and synthetic phenotype distinct from that of the underlying medial smooth muscle cells.

(4) Inflammation

Inflammation contributes to the initiation, progression, and complications of atherosclerotic lesions. Normal vessels do not bind inflammatory cells. Early in atherogenesis, dysfunctional endothelial cells express adhesion molecules that promote leukocyte adhesion; vascular cell adhesion molecule-1 (VCAM-1), in particular, binds monocytes and T cells. After these cells adhere to the endothelium, they migrate into the intima under the influence of locally produced chemokines.

Monocytes differentiate into macrophages and avidly engulf lipoproteins, including small cholesterol crystals and oxidized LDL. Activated macrophages also produce toxic oxygen species that drive LDL oxidation and elaborate growth factors that stimulate smooth muscle cell proliferation. Cholesterol crystals appear to be particularly important instigators of inflammation through activation of the inflammasome and subsequent release of IL-1.

T lymphocytes recruited to the intima interact with the macrophages and also contribute to a state of chronic inflammation. It is not clear whether the T cells are responding to specific antigens(e. g. , bacterial or viral antigens, heat-shock proteins, or modified arterial wall constituents and lipoproteins) or are nonspecifically activated by the local inflammatory milieu. Nevertheless, activated T cells in the growing intimal lesions elaborate inflammatory cytokines (e. g. , IFN-γ) , which stimulate smooth muscle cells, endothelial cells, and macrophages.

Because of the chronic inflammatory state, vascular wall cells release growth factors and activated leukocytes that promote smooth muscle cell proliferation and matrix synthesis.

(5) Infection

There are circumstantial evidences linking infections to atherosclerosis. Cytomegalovirus, *Chlamydia pneumonia* and Herpesvirus, have all been found in atherosclerotic plaque, and seroepidemiologic studies show increased antibody titers to *Chlamydia pneumonia* in patients with more severe atherosclerosis. Infections with these organisms, however, are exceedingly common (as is atherosclerosis) , making it difficult to draw conclusions about causality.

It is important to recognize that atherosclerosis can be induced in germ-free mice, indicating that there is no obligate role for infection in the disease process.

7.1.2　Morphology

According to the development of the plaque, the basic pathological changes are as follows:

7.1.2.1　Fatty Streaks

Fatty streaks begin as flat, minute yellow macules that coalesce into elongated lesions, 1 cm or more in length, which are composed of lipid-filled foamy cells. In electron microscopy, there are two kinds of foamy cells: one is smooth muscle-derived foam cells, and the other is macrophage-derived foam cells. Fatty streaks can appear in the aortas of infants younger than 1 year of age and are present in virtually all children older than 10 years, regardless of dietary risk factors, genetics, or clinical factovs.

The link of fatty streaks to atherosclerotic plaques is uncertain; although fatty streaks may evolve into plaques, not all are destined to progress. Nevertheless, it is notable that coronary fatty streaks form during adolescence at the same anatomic sites that are prone to plaques later in life.

7.1.2.2　Fibrous Plaque

The term fibrous plaque refers to the gross morphologic appearance of the lesion that is the hallmark of the ATH. In gross observation, the lesions are raised, pearly white to gray, smooth-surfaced, plaque-like structures in the intima that vary in diameter form a few millimeters to over a centimeter. Microscopically, the surface of plaque is hyperplastic collagen fibers. The fibrous cap is composed of elongated smooth muscle cells and avascular connective tissues. The connective tissue contains glycosaminoglycans, elastic and collagen fibers synthesized by the smooth muscle cells. The collagen of the fibrous cap could be dense and hyalinized. In the central plaque consists of some smooth muscle cells, extracellular matrix, inflammatory cells and foam cells.

7.1.2.3　Atheromatous Plaque (Atheroma)

Atheromatous plaques are white to yellow raised lesions; they range from 0. 3 to 1. 5cm in diameter but coalesce to form larger masses. Atherosclerotic plaques are patchy, usually involving only a portion of any given arterial wall; on cross-section, therefore, the lesions appear "eccentric". The focal nature of atherosclerotic lesions may be related to the vagaries of vascular hemodynamics (Figure 7 – 1) . Atherosclerotic plaques have three principal components:

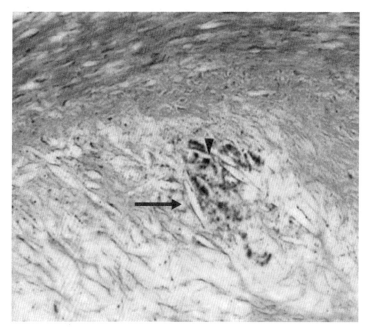

Figure 7-1　Atherosclerotic plaques internal bleeding

1) Intracellular and extracellular lipid;

2) Cells, including smooth muscle cells, macrophages, and T cells;

3) Extracellular matrix, including collagen, elastic fibers, and proteoglycans.

The proportion and configuration of each component varies from lesion to lesion. Most commonly plaques have a superficial fibrous cap composed of dense collagen and smooth muscle cells. Where the cap meets the vessel wall (the "shoulder") there is a more cellular area containing smooth muscle cells, T cells, and macrophages. Deep to the fibrous cap is a necrotic core, containing variably organized thrombus, lipid, necrotic debris, lipid-laden macrophages and smooth muscle cells (foam cells), fibrin, and other plasma proteins. The extracellular cholesterol frequently takes the forms of crystalline aggregates that are washed out during routine tissue processing, leaving behind empty "cholesterol clefts". The periphery of the lesions shows neovascularization (proliferating small blood vessels). The media deep to the plaque may be attenuated and exhibit fibrosis secondary to smooth muscle atrophy and loss.

Typical atheromas contain relatively abundant lipid, but some so-called fibrous plaques are almost entirely composed of fibrous tissue and smooth muscle cells.

Plaques generally continue to change and progressively enlarge through cell degeneration and death, thrombus organization, and synthesis and degradation of ECM. Moreover, atheromas also often undergo calcification.

In descending order, the most extensively involved vessels are the coronary arteries, the popliteal arteries, infrarenal abdominal aorta, the vessels of the circle of Willis, and the internal carotid arteries. Even in the same patient, atherosclerosis is typically more severe in the abdominal aorta than in the thoracic aorta. Vessels of the upper extremities are usually spared. The mesenteric and renal arteries tend to be spared except at their ostia. Nevertheless, in any individual case, the severity of atherosclerosis in one artery does not predict its severity in another. Moreover, in any given vessel, lesions at various stages often coexist.

7.1.3　Clinical Consequences

Large elastic arteries (e. g. , aorotic, carotid, and iliac arteries) and large and medium-sized muscular arteries(e. g. ,coronary,renal,and popliteal arteries)are the vessels most commonly involved in atherosclerosis. Accordingly,atherosclerosis is most likely to present with signs and symptoms related to ischemia in the kidneys,brain,heart,and lower extremities. Myocardial infarction,cerebral infarction,aortic aneurysms, and peripheral vascular disease are the major clinical consequences of atherosclerosis.

The principal pathophysiologic outcomes depend on the size of the affected vessel,the stability and size of the plaques,and the degree to which plaques disrupt the vessel walls.

7.1.3.1   Atherosclerotic Stenosis

At early stages,remodeling of the media tends to preserve the luminal diameter by increasing the vessel circumference. Owing to limits on remodeling,however,eventually the expanding atheroma may impinge on blood flow. Critical stenosis is the tipping point at which chronic occlusion limits flow so severely that tissue demand exceeds supply. In the coronary artery(and other)circulations,this typically occurs at approximately 70% fixed occlusion. At rest,affected patients have adequate cardiac perfusion,but with even modest exertion,demand exceeds supply,and chest pain develops because of cardiac ischemia. The toll of chronic arterial hypoperfusion due to atherosclerosis in various vascular beds includes intermittent claudication,bowel ischemia,chronic IHD,sudden cardiac death,and ischemic encephalopathy.

7.1.3.2   Acute Plaque Changes

Plaque erosion or rupture typically triggers thrombosis,leading to partial or complete vascular obstruction and often tissue infarction. The causes of acute plaque changes are complex and include both intrinsic (e. g. ,plaque structure and composition)and extrinsic factors(e. g. ,blood pressure). These factors combine to weaken the integrity of the plaque,making it unable to withstand vascular shear forces. Certain types of plaques are believed to be at particularly high risk of rupturing. These include plaques that contain abundant extracellular lipid and large numbers of foam cells,plaques that contain clusters of inflammatory cells, and plaques that have thin fibrous caps containing few smooth muscle cells. Plaques at high risk for rupture are referred to as "vulnerable plaques".

Atherosclerotic plaques are susceptible to several clinically important changes:

1) Rupture,ulceration,or erosion. They occur in the luminal surface of atheromatous plaques leading to expose highly thrombogenic substances and induce thrombus formation. Thrombi may partially or completely occlude the lumen,leading to tissue ischemia(e. g. ,in the heart). If the patient survives,thrombi become organized and incorporated into the growing plaque.

2) Hemorrhage into a plaque. Rupture of the overlying fibrous cap or of the thin-walled vessels in the areas of neovascularization can cause intra-plaque hemorrhage;the resulting hematoma may cause rapid plaque expansion or plaque rupture.

3) Atheroembolism. Ruptured plaque can discharge debris into the blood,producing microembolis composed of plaque contents leading to distant embolism and infarction.

4) Aneurysm formation. Atherosclerosis-induced pressure or ischemic atrophy of the underlying media, with loss of elastic tissue,causes structural weakening that can lead to aneurysmal dilation and rupture.

7.2   Ischemic Heart Disease

Ischemic heart disease(IHD) refers to a group of closely related syndromes caused by an imbalance between the myocardial oxygen demand and cardiac blood supply. Although ischemia can result from increased demand(e. g. ,increased heart rate or hypertension) ,or diminished oxygen-carrying capacity(e.

g. , anemia, carbon monoxide poisoning) , in the vast majority of cases, IHD is due to a reduction in coronary blood flow caused by obstructive atherosclerotic disease. Thus, IHD is often called coronary artery disease (CAD) or coronary heart disease. Despite dramatic improvement over the past 3 to 4 decades, IHD in its various forms still represents the leading cause of death in the United States and other industrialized nations. There are four types: acute myocardial infarction(MI) , angina pectoris, sudden cardiac death(SCD) and chronic IHD with congestive heart failure.

In most cases, IHD occurs because of inadequate coronary perfusion due to atherosclerotic occlusion of coronary arteries and new superimposed thrombosis and/or vasospasm. A lesion obstructing 70% to 75% or more of a vessel lumen-so-called critical stenosis-generally causes symptomatic ischemia(angina) only in the setting of increased demand; a fixed 90% stenosis can lead to inadequate coronary blood flow even at rest. Importantly, if a coronary artery develops atherosclerotic occlusion at a sufficiently slow rate, it may be able to stimulate collateral blood flow from other major epicardial vessels; such collateral perfusion can then protect against MI even in the setting of a complete vascular occlusion. But acute coronary occlusions cannot do so and will lend to infarction.

7.2.1　Angina Pectoris

Angina pectoris is intermittent chest pain caused by transient, reversible myocardial ischemia. There are three variants.

7.2.1.1　Unstable Angina

Unstable angina also called crescendo angina, is characterized by increasing frequency of pain, precipitated by progressively less exertion; it is more intense and longer lasting than stable angina. This is due to plaque disruption and superimposed partial thrombosis, distal embolization of the thrombus, and/or vasospasm. Unstable angina is the harbinger of more serious, potentially irreversible ischemia(due to complete luminal occlusion by thrombus) and is therefore sometimes called pre-infarction angina.

7.2.1.2　Typical Angina

Typical angina also called stable angina, is episodic chest pain associated with less exertion or some other form of increased myocardial oxygen demand(e. g. , tachycardia or hypertension due to fever, anxiety, fear). The pain is classically described as a crushing or squeezing substernal sensation, which can radiate down the left arm or to the left jaw(referred pain). Stable angina pectoris is usually associated with a fixed atherosclerotic narrowing(⩾75%) of one or more coronary arteries. With this degree of critical stenosis, the myocardial oxygen supply may be sufficient under basal conditions but cannot be adequately augmented to meet any increased requirements. The pain is usually relieved by rest(reducing demand) or by drugs, such as nitroglycerin, which cause peripheral vasodilation and reduce venous blood delivered to the heart(hence reducing cardias work).

7.2.1.3　Prinzmetal Angina

Prinzmetal angina also called variant angina, usually occurs at rest due to coronary artery spasm. The etiology is not clear, but Prinzmetal angina typically responds promptly to the administration of vasodilators such as nitroglycerin or calcium channel blockers.

7.2.2　Myocardial Infarction

Myocardial infarction(MI) , popularly called heart attack, is necrosis of heart muscle resulting from ischemia. Roughly more that 1 million people in China die of MI every year. MI is extremely common, accounting for 10% to 15% of all deaths and about 60% sudden unexpected deaths. The major underlying cause of MI is atherosclerosis and therefore the frequency of MIs rises progressively with increasing age and presence of other risk factors such as smoking, diabetes, and hypertension. Approximately 10% of MIs occur in people younger than 40 years, and 45% occur in people younger than age 65. In general, women are remarkably protected against MI during their reproductive years. Nevertheless, menopause and presumably declining estrogen production is associated with exacerbation of coronary atherosclerosis. Men are at significantly greater risk than woman, although the gap progressively narrows with age.

MIs are caused by acute coronary artery thrombosis. In most cases, disruption of an atherosclerotic plaque results in the formation of thrombus. Only severe ischemia lasting at least 20 to 40 min causes irreversible injury and myocyte death. Clinical features are chest pain accompanied by breathlessness, vomiting and collapse or syncope. Pain occurs in the same sites as angina but is usually more severe and lasts for longer.

7.2.2.1 Morphology

Nearly all transmural infarcts affect at least a portion of the left ventricle and/or ventricular septum. Roughly 15% to 30% of MIs affecting the posterior or posteroseptal wall also extend into the adjacent right ventricular wall. Other coronary occlusions are occasionally encountered. These include the left main coronary artery or secondary branches, such as the diagonal branches of the left anterior descending(LAD) artery or marginal branches of the left circumflex(LCx) artery. In contrast, significant atherosclerosis or thrombosis of penetrating intramyocardial branches of coronary arteries rarely occurs. Severe coronary occlusion without associated myocardial damage suggests the prior formation of protective collateral connections.

According to the area and depth of MI, MI can be divided into two types: subendocardial and transmural myocardial infarction.

1) MIs less than 12 hours old are usually not grossly apparent.

2) Infarcts more than 3 hours old: an infarcted area is revealed as an unstained pale zone(old scars appear white and glistening).

3) By 12 to 24 hours after MI, an infarct can usually be grossly identified by a reddish blue discoloration caused by stagnant, trapped blood. Then, an infarct becomes more sharply delineated as a yellow-tan, softened area.

4) By 10 to 14 day infarcts become rimmed by hyperemic granulation tissue.

5) Over the succeeding weeks the MI evolve to a fibrous scar.

The microscopic appearance also undergoes a characteristic sequence of changes:

1) Within 4 to 12 hours typical features of coagulative necrosis becomes detectable. "Wavy fibers" at the edges of an infarct reflect the stretching and buckling of noncontractile dead fibers but are considered "soft" findings of acute infarction. Sublethal ischemia can also induce myocyte vacuolization. These are large cleared intracellular spaces, probably containing water.

2) 1–3 days after MI   Necrotic myocardium elicits acute inflammation.

3) 5–10 days after MI   A wave of macrophages to remove necrotic myocytes and neutrophil fragment.

4) 2–3 weeks after MI   The infarcted zone is progressively replaced by granulation tissue.

5) By the end of the sixth week dense collagenous scar is formed.

MI heals from its borders toward the center, and a large infarct may not heal as readily or as completely as a small one. Once MI is completely healed, it is impossible to distinguish its age(i. e. , the dense fibrous scars of 8-week-old and 10-year old lesions look similar).

7.2.2.2 Clinical Features

MI is usually heralded by severe, crushing substernal chest pain or discomfort that can radiate to the neck, jaw, epigastrium, or left arm. In contrast to the pain of angina pectoris, the pain of an MI typically lasts from 20 min to several hours and is not significantly relieved by nitroglycerin or rest. In a substantial minority of patients (10% to 15%), MIs can be entirely asymptomatic. Such "silent" infarcts are particularly common in patients with underlying diabetes mellitus (with peripheral neuropathies) and in the elderly.

The pulse is generally rapid and weak, and patients can be diaphoretic and nauseated particularly with posterior-wall MIs. Dyspnea is common and is caused by impaired myocardial contractility and dysfunction of the mitral valve apparatus, with resultant pulmonary congestion and edema. With massive MIs (>40% of the left ventricle) cardiogenic shock develops.

Electrocardiographic abnormalities include Q weaves (indicating transmural infarcts), and ST-segment abnormalities and T-wave inversion (representing abnormalities in myocardial repolarization). Arrhythmias caused by electrical abnormalities of the ischemic myocardium and conduction system are common, and indeed, sudden death due to a lethal arrhythmia accounts for the vast majority of deaths occurring before hospitalization.

Laboratory evaluation of MI is based on measuring the blood levels of creatine kinase (CK, and more specifically the myocardial-specific isoform, CK-MB), cardiac troponins T and I (TnT, TnI) and myoglobin, lactate dehydrogenase, and many others. Troponins and CK-MB have high specificity and sensitivity for myocardial damage. TnI and TnT are not normally detectable in the circulation, but after acute MI both troponins become detectable after 2 to 4 h and peak at 48 h; their levels remain elevated for 7 to 10 days. CK-MB is the second best marker after the cardiac-specific troponins. Since various forms of CK are found in brain, skeletal muscle, and myocardium, total CK activity is not a reliable marker of cardiac injury. Thus, the CK-MB isoform principally derived from myocardium but also present at low levels in skeletal muscle-is the more specific indicator of heart damage. CK-MB activity begins to rise within 2 to 4 h of MI, peaks at 24 to 48 h, and returns to normal within approximately 72 h.

7.2.2.3 Consequences and Complications of MI

Nearly three-fourths of patients have one or more complications after acute MI, illustrated as follows:

1) Pericarditis. A fibrinous or hemorrhagic pericarditis usually develops within 2 to 3 days of a transmural MI and typically spontaneously resolves with time.

2) Mural thrombus. With any infarct, the combination of a local loss of contractility with endocardial damage can foster mural thrombosis and, potentially, thromboembolism.

3) Contractile dysfunction. Typically, there is some degree of left ventricular failure, with hypotension, pulmonary vascular congestion, and fluid transudation into the pulmonary interstitial and alveolar spaces. Severe "pumpfailure" occurs in 10% to 15% of patients after acute MI, generally with a large infarct (often > 40% of the left ventricle). Cardiogenic shock has a nearly 70% mortality rate and accounts for two-thirds of in-hospital deaths.

4) Ventricular aneurysm. Aneurysms of the ventricular wall most commonly result from a large transmural anteroseptal infarct that heals with the formation of thin car tissue. Complications of ventricular aneurysms include mural thrombus, arrhythmias, and heart failure, but rupture of the fibrotic wall does not occur.

5) Arrhythmias. Following MI, many patients develop arrhythmias, which undoubtedly are responsible for many of the sudden deaths. MI-associated arrhythmias include heart block, ventricular premature contractions or ventricular fibrillation, tachycardia or sinus bradycardia.

6) Myocardial rupture. Rupture complicates somewhere between 1% and 5% of MIs but is a frequent

cause of MI-associated death. Complications include ①papillary muscle rupture, resulting in severe mitral regurgitation;②rupture of the ventricular free wall, with hemopericardium and cardiac tamponade, usually fatal;③rupture of the ventricular septum, leading to a new VSD and left-to-right shunt. Rupture can occur at almost any time after MI but is most common 3 to 7 days after infarction.

7) Papillary muscle dysfunction. More frequently, postinfarct mitral regurgitation results from ischemic dysfunction of a papillary muscle and underlying myocardium, and later from papillary muscle fibrosis and shortening, or ventricular dilation.

The risk of developing complications and the prognosis after MI depends on infarct site, size, and fractional thickness of the myocardial wall that is damaged. Large transmural infarcts have a higher probability of cardiogenic shock, arrhythmias, and late CHF(congestive heart failure).

Long-term prognosis after MI depends on many variables, the most important of which are the extent of vascular obstructions in vessels that perfuse the remaining viable myocardium and the quality of left ventricular function. The overall total mortality within the first year is about 30% , including those who die before reaching the hospital. Thereafter, there is a 3% to 4% per year mortality.

8) Infarct expansion. Because of the weakening of necrotic muscle, there may be disproportionate stretching, thinning, and dilation of the infarct region(especially with anteroseptal infarcts) ; this is often associated with mural thrombus.

7.2.3   Chronic Ischemic Heart Disease

Chronic IHD, also called ischemic cardiomyopathy, is essentially progressive heart failure as a consequence of ischemic myocardial damage.

7.2.3.1   Morphology

Hearts from patients with chronic IHD are usually enlarged and heavy from left ventricular dilation and hypertrophy. There is moderate to sever atherosclerosis of the coronary arteries, sometimes with total occlusion. Discrete, gray-white scars of healed infarcts are usually present. The endocardium generally shows patchy, fibrous thickening, and mural thrombi may be present. The major microscopic findings include myocardial hypertrophy, diffuse subendocardial myocyte vacuolization, and fibrosis from previous infarcts.

7.2.3.2   Clinical Features

Chronic IHD is characterized by the development of severe, progressive heart failure, sometimes punctuated by episodes of angina or MI. Arrhythmias are common and, along with CHF and intercurrent MI, account for many deaths.

7.2.4   Sudden Cardiac Death

Sudden cardiac death(SCD) is most commonly defined as unexpected death from cardiac causes either without symptoms or within 1 to 24 h of symptom onset(different authors use different time points).

Coronary artery diseaseis the most common underlying cause, and in many adults SCD is the first clinical manifestation of IHD. With younger victims, the following non-atherosclerotic causes of SCD become more common:①hereditary or acquired abnormalities of the cardiac conduction system;②congenital coronary arterial abnormalities;③isolated hypertrophy, hypertensive or unknown cause;④mitral valve prolapse; ⑤aortic valve stenosis;⑥dilated or hypertrophic cardiomyopathy;⑦myocarditis or sarcoidosis;⑧pulmonary hypertension. The most important cause is the autosomal dominant long-QT syndrome, due to mutations in various cardiac ion channels. Increased cardiac mass is an independent risk factor for SCD, thus, some young individuals who die suddenly(including athletes) have unsuspected hypertrophic cardiomyopathy, myocarditis, or congenital abnormalities of coronary arteries.

The ultimate mechanism of SCD is most often a lethal arrhythmia, such as ventricular fibrillation. Although ischemic injury, as well as other pathologies, can directly affect the conduction system, most cases of fatal arrhythmia are triggered by electrical irritability of myocardium distant from the conduction system. The prognosis of patients who are vulnerable to SCD, especially those with chronic IHD, is markedly improved by automatic cardioverter defibrillators, which sense and electrically terminate episodes of ventricular fibrillation.

Severe coronary atherosclerosis with critical(≥75%) stenosis involving one or more of the three major vessels is present in 80% to 90% of SCD victims; acute plaque disruption is found in only 10% to 20% of these. A healed MI is present in about 40% , but in those who were successfully resuscitated from sudden cardiac arrest, new MI is found in only 25% or less. Subendocardial myocyte vacuolization indicative of severe chronic ischemia is common. Only a minority(10% to 20%)of cases of SCD are of non-atherosclerotic origin.

7.3 Hypertension

Hypertension is one of the most common serious cardiovascular diseases. Arterial hypertension is defined as a sustained rise of the systemic blood pressure above 140 mmHg(18. 4 kPa) systolic and/or 90 mmHg(12. 0 kPa)diastolic. Hypertension can be classified into two main types according to its etiology. Primary(essential or idiopathic)hypertension refers to elevation of blood pressure with age but with no apparent cause; secondary hypertension refers to elevated blood pressure due to an identifiable cause. It is also called symptomatic hypertension. Hypertension disease means primary hypertension.

With the development of the economy, cardiovascular diseases incidence are increased by the change of life style, mental stress and malfunction.

Primary hypertension is one of the most common cardiovascular diseases in China. Unfortunately, in the vast majority of patients with systemic hypertension the underlying cause is unknown. Primary hypertension tends to be familiar and develops in later adult life. The incidence of hypertension and its complication is different between gender and race. Males tend to have higher blood pressure than females at the same age before 55 years old. But at the age of 75, females tend to have higher hypertension incidence.

Secondary hypertension accounts for 5% – 10% of hypertension. There is an identifiable background abnormality precipitating the hypertension. These diseases may be divided into renal, endocrine, cardiovascular and neurologic types. Special types of hypertension include intracranial hemorrhage, unstable angina pectoris, acute myocardial infarction (AMI), pregnancy-associated hypertension and hypertension crisis by hypertensive encephalopathy, aortic dissection and eclampsia.

7.3.1 Etiology and Pathogenesis

So far the causes of hypertension are not clear. It is believed that hypertension is the result of interaction of genetic and environmental factors.

7.3.1.1 Risk Factors

(1)Dietary Factors

1)Drinking is one of the pathogenesis factors of hypertension. Alcohol could activate the sympathetic nervous-catecholamine(CA)system.

2) Obesity is a major medical and public health problem world-wide and by consequences like hypertension and other cardiovascular diseases. What makes us to be overweight, by high-fat or by high-calorie? That is controversy.

3) Mutations in proteins may affect sodium resorption. On the other hand, heavy consumption of salt has been implicated as exogenous factors in hypertension.

(2) Environmental Factors

Environmental factors could modify expression of the genetic determinants of increased pressure. Stress, physical inactivity has been as exogenous factors in hypertension. Environmental factors affect the variables that control blood pressure in the genetically predisposed individual. Susceptibility genes for essential hypertension are currently unknown but may well include genes that levels of pressor substances, govern responses to an increased renal sodium load, reactivity of vascular smooth muscle cell growth. In established hypertension, both increased peripheral resistance and increased blood volume contribute to the increased pressure.

(3) Genetic and Familial Aggregation

Genetic factor play a role in determining pressure levels, as is evidenced by studies comparing blood pressure in monozygotic and dizygotic twins and by studies of familial aggregation of hypertension. Moreover, several single-gene disorders that affect specific pathways that control normal blood pressure cause relatively rare forms of hypertension. However, it is unlikely that a mutation at a single gene locus will engage as a major cause of essential hypertension. More likely, the combined effect of mutations or polymorphisms at several gene loci influences blood pressure.

7.3.1.2   Pathogenesis

Although the specific triggers are unknown, it appears that both altered renal sodium handing and increased vascular resistance contribute to essential hypertension.

(1) Genetic Factors

It play an important role in determining blood pressure, as shown by familial clustering of hypertension and by studies of monozygotic and dizygotic twins. Polymorphisms of the renin-angiotensin system also may contribute to the known racial differences in blood pressure regulation; Hypertension has been linked to specific angiotensinogen polymorphisms and angiotensin II receptor variants. Susceptibility genes for essential hypertension in the larger population are currently unknown but probably include those that govern renal sodium handling, smooth muscle cell growth, and pressors.

(2) Environmental Factors

They include physical inactivity, obesity, stress, smoking, and high levels of salt consumption which modify the impact of genetic determinants. Evidence linking dietary sodium intake with the prevalence of hypertension in different population groups is particularly strong.

(3) Increased Vascular Resistance

It may stem from vasoconstriction or structural changes in vessel walls. These are not necessarily independent factors, as chronic vasoconstriction may result in permanent thickening of the walls of affected vessels.

(4) Reduced Renal Sodium Excretion

It is probably a key pathogenic feature; indeed, this is a common etiologic factor in most forms of hypertension. Decreased sodium excretion causes an obligatory increase in fluid volume and increased cardiac output, thereby elevating blood pressure. At the new higher blood pressure, the kidneys excrete additional sodium. Thus, a new steady state of sodium excretion is achieved, but at the expense of an elevated blood pressure.

7.3.2 Morphology

According to pathological features, primary hypertension can be divided into two types: benign and malignant hypertension.

7.3.2.1 Benign Hypertension

Benign hypertension is also called chronic hypertension. It is encountered in about 95% of hypertensive subjects. The patients are usually asymptomatic, and the diagnosis is often made incidentally. The course is a stable one(slow rise in blood pressure). With regard to the development of diseases, these patients fall into three phases.

(1) Dysfunction

It is the early changes of hypertension. Arterioles show interval spasm. Blood pressure is increased accompanied by headache. However, blood pressure can return to normal after easing spasm.

(2) Artery Lesion

It is the characteristic lesion of hypertension. Under microscopy, the intimal smooth muscle cells proliferate and elastic tissue fibers are deposited between the proliferating cells. Such intimal proliferation is most often observed in renal arteries over 50 μm in diameter and occasionally in arterioles(Figure 7-2). One of the earliest changes noted in the wall of arteries and arterioles in hypertension is medial hypertrophy due to work hypertrophy of medial smooth muscle cells and media, and the accumulation of acid mucopolysaccharides, water, and electrolytes also contributes to the medical thickening. Above all, these lesions can be called hyaline arteriolosclerosis. The same lesions also are common in diabetic microangiopathy; in this disorder, the underlying etiology is hyperglycemia associated endothelial cell dysfunction.

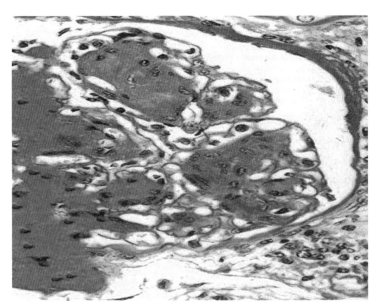

Figure 7-2   Kidney arteriole sclerosis

(3) Viscera Lesion

1) Brain: There are three main types   ①Softening of brain: small artery arteriosclerosis leads to cerebral ischemia and results in microinfarct formation. It can affect small regions and be clinically silent. Over weeks or months, there is a gradual resolution of the dead tissue and is repaired with the glial scar. ②Hy-

pertensive encephalopathy: the clinical features of acute hypertensive encephalopathy include reduced consciousness, headache, vomiting, nausea, and variable neurological signs. It is also called hypertensive crisis. Two reasons can explain the pathogenesis of acute hypertensive encephalopathy. Firstly, it is caused by overstretching of the arteriolar walls with extravasation of plasma proteins and developments of focal cerebral edema. Secondly, it is due to cerebral vasospasm with subsequent focal cerebral ischemia. ③Cerebral hemorrhage: it is the serious and life-threatening complication.

Hypertension is the most common underlying cause of intraparenchymal hemorrhages, and brain hemorrhage accounts for roughly 15% of deaths among individuals with chronic hypertension. Hypertensive intraparenchymal hemorrhages typically occur in the basal ganglia, thalamus, pons, and cerebellum. Intracerebral hemorrhage can be clinically devastating when it affects large portions of the brain and extends into the ventricular system. Rupture of the small artery arteriosclerosis or microaneurysm lead to cerebral hemorrhage with the increased blood pressure.

2) Heart

An increase in myocardial wall tension results in increased myocardial oxygen consumption, and this initiates a series of biochemical events that results in left ventricular hypertrophy. The essential feature of hypertensive heart disease is left ventricular hypertrophy. The weight of the heart usually exceeds 400 g. The hypertrophy typically involves the ventricular wall in a symmetric, circumferential pattern termed concentric hypertrophy, with free wall thicknesses exceeding 2. 0 cm. Musculi papillares and adductor are thickened. Microscopically, myocardial cell become thick and long, accompanied by more branches. Nucleus of myocardial is large, round and dark.

3) Retina: Central artery of retina may be arteriosclerosis. The serious case is papilloedema, retinal hemorrhage and cause significant vision loss.

4) Kidney: The hyaline and fibrous changes blood vessels cause vascular narrowing and consequently leading to glomerulus ischemic atrophy and fibrosis, as well as tubular atrophy and interstitial fibrosis. Also you can find glomerular compensatory hypertrophy and renal tubular compensatory enlargement. Crossly, the kidneys may be normal in size or moderately reduced. The cortical surfaces have a fine even granularity, also called primary granular atrophy of the kidney.

7.3.2.2 Malignant Hypertension

Malignant hypertension is characterized by severe hypertension of rapidly increasing severity. The blood pressure often exceedes to 230/130 mmHg. The malignant phase may be superimposed on benign hypertension; less then, it may start de novo. The pathognomonic lesions of malignant hypertension are proliferative endarteritis and fibrin onion-skin lesions. Vessels exhibit "onionskin" concentric, laminated thickening of arteriolar walls and luminal narrowing. The laminations consist of smooth muscle cells and thickened, reduplicated basement membrane. In malignant hypertension, these changes are accompanied by fibrinoid deposits and vessel wall necrosis which are particularly prominent in the kidney.

7.4   Rheumatism

Rheumatism, also called rheumatic fever(RF), is an acute, immunologically mediated, multisystem inflammatory disease. It usually occurs a few weeks after an episode of group A β-hemolytic streptococcal pharyngitis. Acute RF appears most often in children aged 5 to 15 years with peaks between 6 and 9 years. About 20% of first attacks occur in adults. There is no difference in the prevalence of RF between men and women. The connective tissue is involved mainly in blood vessels, heart and skin. So it is also called connective tissue disease or collagen disease.

Acute RF is closely related to infection with group A streptococci. It is a hypersensitivity reaction induced by host antibodies elicited by group A streptococci. However, many details of the pathogenesis remain uncertain despite many years of investigation. It appears that the M proteins of certain streptococcal strains induce host antibodies that cross-react with glycoprotein antigens in the heart, joints and other tissues. This explains the typical 2–to 3–weeks delay in symptom onset after the original infection, and the absence of Streptococci in the lesions. Because the nature of cross-reacting antigens has been difficult to define, it has also been suggested that the streptococcal infection evokes an autoimmune response against self-antigens. The chronic sequelae result from progressive fibrosis due to healing of the acute inflammatory lesions.

7.4.1 Basic Pathological Changes

According to the pathological features, the course of disease development is divided into three phases described as follows.

1) Alterative and exudative phase. This is the early stage of acute RF. Discrete inflammatory lesions are found in the connective tissues throughout the body, including skin, synovium, the heart, and joints. There is focal mucoid degeneration and fibrinoid necrosis of the collagen with surrounding polymorphs, plasma cell and monocytes. This phase can last for 1 month.

2) Proliferative or granulomatous phase. The hallmark of acute RF is the presence of multiple foci of inflammation called aschoff bodies. Aschoff bodies consist of a central zone of degenerating, hypereosinophilic extracellular matrix infiltrated by lymphocytes(primarily T cells), occasional plasma cells, and plump activated macrophages called Anitschkow cells. The Anitschkow cells have abundant cytoplasm and central nuclei with chromatin arrayed in a slender, wavy ribbon(so-called caterpillar cells); these activated macrophages can also fuse to form giant cells. This phase lesions is sustainable for 2–3 months.

3) Fibrous phase or healed phase. Progressive fibrosis of Aschoff body results in the formation of small scar. This phase is sustainable for 2–3 months.

7.4.2 Rheumatic Heart Disease

Rheumatic heart disease(RHD) can involve myocardium, endocardium, and pericardium. Chronic valvular deformities are the most important consequences of RHD; characterized by diffuse and dense scarring of valves resulting in permanent dysfunction(mitral stenosis being most common).

7.4.2.1 Rheumatic Endocarditis

Of the heart valves, the mitral valve is mostly attacked, followed by mitral and aortic combined involvement, aortic, and tricuspid valve, while pulmonary valve is rarely involved.

Valve involvement results in fibrinoid necrosis along the lines of closure forming 1–2 mm vegetations (verrucae) that have little effect on cardiac function. These irregular, warty projections probably arise from the precipitation of fibrin at sites of erosion caused by underlying inflammation and collagen degeneration. The vegetations consist of platelets and fibrin, with fibrinoid necrosis and occasional little Aschoff bodies. Chronic RHD is characterized by organization of the acute inflammation and subsequent scarring. The cardinal anatomic changes of the mitral(or tricuspid) valve include leaflet thickening, commissural fusion and shortening, and thickening and fusion of the chordae tendineae. Fibrous bridging across the valvular commissures and calcification create "fish mouth" or "buttonhole" stenosis.

7.4.2.2 Rheumatic Myocarditis

The rheumatic myocarditis takes the form of scattered Aschoff bodies within the interstitial connective tissue of the left atrial and left ventricular myocardium, particularly in the subendocardial fibrous tissues and around blood vessels in the intermuscular fibrous septa. The Aschoff bodies often lie in close proximity to a small vessel and may encroach on its wall.

7.4.2.3 Rheumatic Pericarditis

The rheumatic pericarditis is characterized with fibrinous or serous exudation. Hydropericardium results from serous exudation, while "shaggy heart" or "cor villosum" refers to that fibrinous exudates are heavily layered on the epicardial surface of the heart. Large amount of fibrinous exudation can not be completely absorbed, leading to organization with consequence of constrictive pericarditis.

7.4.2.4 Clinical Features

Typically, the symptoms occur two to three weeks after an episode of streptococcal pharyngitis. The predominant clinical manifestations are carditis and arthritis. Clinical features of the carditis include pericardial frictional rubs and arrhythmias. Myocarditis can be so severe that resulting cardiac congestive dilation causes functional mitral insufficiency and even heart failure. Nevertheless, fewer than 1% of patients die of acute RE.

After an initial attack, there is increased vulnerability to disease reactivation with subsequent pharyngeal infections. Carditis is likely to worsen within each recurrence, and damage is cumulative. Other hazards include embolization from mural thrombi, primarily within the atria or their appendages, and infective endocarditis superimposed on deformed valves. Chronic rheumatic carditis usually does not cause clinical manifestations for years or even decades after the initial episode of RF. The signs and symptoms of valvular disease depend on which valve is involved. In addition to various cardiac murmurs, cardiac hypertrophy and dilation, and CHF, patients with chronic RHD often have arrhythmias(particularly atrial fibrillation in the setting of mitral stenosis), thromboembolic complications, and an increased risk of subsequent infective endocarditis.

7.4.3 Rheumatic Arthritis

About 75% of patients with rheumatic fever in the early stages have the clinical manifestations of rheumatic arthritis. It typically begins with migratory polyarthritis accompanied by fever in which one large joint after another becomes painful and swollen for a period of days and then subsides spontaneously, leaving no residual disability. Large joints such as ankle, shoulder, wrist, elbow and knee are most frequently involved. Redness, swelling, heat(Figure 7-3), pain and dysfunction are found with the joints. Fibrinous and serous exudation fills in the articular cavity. The atypical Aschoff bodies can be seen in the adjacent soft tissue.

7.4.4 Rheumatic Arteritis

Any arteries can be involved, and the small artery involvement is common, such as renal artery, cerebral artery,

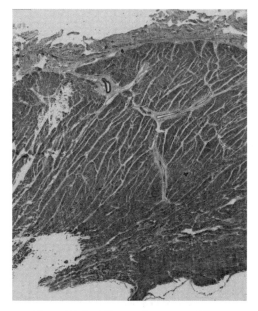

Figure 7-3 **Rheumatic myocarditis**

coronary artery, pulmonary artery and mesenteric artery, etc. In the acute phase, fibrinoid necrosis, mucous degeneration and lymphocyte infiltration of the vascular wall are prominent accompanied by formation of Aschoff body. In the late stage, the vascular wall changes are thickening with fibrosis, and the vascular cavity become narrow accompanied with thrombosis.

7.5 Infective Endocarditis

Infective endocarditis(IE) is a serious infection requiring prompt diagnosis and intervention. It is characterized by microbial invasion of heart valves or mural endocardium, often with destruction of the underlying cardiac tissues and results in bulky, friable vegetations composed of necrotic debris, thrombus, and organisms. Although fungi, chlamydiae and rickettsiae(Q fever) can cause endocarditis, the vast majority of cases are caused by extracellular bacteria.

7.5.1 Etiology and Pathogenesis

Infection occurs when organisms are implanted on the endocardial surface during episodes of bacteremia. In some instances, the cause of the hematogenous infection is obvious, as in the case of intravenous drug abuses who inject contaminated materials directly into bloodstream; an infection elsewhere or a previous dental, surgical, or other interventional procedure may also seed the bloodstream. In other cases, however, the source of bacteremia is occult and presumably related to trivial injuries to the skin or mucosal surfaces, as may be encountered.

The causative organisms differ depending on the underlying risk factors: ①prosthetic heart valves; ②preexisting cardiac abnormalities; ③intravenous drug abuse. Endocarditis of previously damaged or otherwise abnormal valves is caused most commonly(50% to 60% of cases) by Streptococci viridans. In contrast, the more virulent S. aureus(common to skin) can attack deformed and healthy valves and is responsible for 10% to 20 of cases overall; it is also the major offender in intravenous drug abusers. Additional bacterial agents include enterococci and the so-called HACEK group(Actinobacillus, Haemophilus, Eikenella, Cardiobacterium and Kingella), all commensals in the oral cavity. More rarely, gram negative bacilli and fungi are involved. In about 10% of cases, no organism can be isolated from the blood("culture-negative" endocarditis). This is attributed to previous antibiotic therapy or difficulties in isolating the offending agents, or because deeply embedded organisms within the enlarging vegetation are not released into the blood.

IE is traditionally classified into acute and subacute forms, mostly dependent on the basis of clinical tempo and severity; the distinctions are attributable to the intrinsic microbial virulence and whether underlying cardiac disease is present.

The disease typically appears insidiously and follows a protracted course of weeks to months with most patients recovering after appropriate antibiotic therapy.

7.5.2 Acute Infective Endocarditis

Acute infective endocarditis usually suggests a destructive, tumultuous infection, frequently involving a highly virulent organism attacking a previously normal valve, and causing death within days to weeks in more than 50% of patients, despite antibiotics and surgery.

In acute infective endocarditis, bulky, friable, and potentially destructive vegetations containing fibrin, inflammatory cells, and microorganisms are present on the heart valves. The mitral and aortic valves are the most common sites of infection.

The vegetations may cause rapid destruction of the valves, often resulting in rupture of the leaflets, or papillary muscles. The infection may eventually extend through the valve into the adjacent myocardium to produce abscesses in the perivalvular tissues known as ring abscesses. Systemic emboli may occur at any time because of the friable nature of the vegetations, and they may cause infarcts in the brain, myocardium, kidney and other tissues, and abscesses often develop at the site of such emboli.

7.5.3   Subacute Infective Endocarditis

Subacute infective endocarditis refers to infections by organisms of low virulence colonizing of a previously abnormal heart, especially when there are deformed valves.

The vegetations of subacute endocarditis tend to be somewhat firmer and are associated with less valvular destruction than those of acute endocarditis. The aortic and mitral valves are the most common sites of infection too. Microscopically, the vegetations of typical subacute infective endocarditis are distinguished from those of acute disease by the presence of granulation tissues at their bases, suggesting chronicity. As time passes, calcification, fibrosis and a chronic inflammatory infiltrate may develop.

Subacute infective endocarditis classically presents clinically with fever, a heart murmur, raised white cell count, anemia, hematuria and splenomegaly. Other features, which may variably be present, include Osler's nodes, petechia, Roth spots, Janeway lesions, and splinter hemorrhages in nails. Over a period of days to months, progressive valvular destruction results in valvular regurgitation and valvular stenosis and congestive heart failure.

7.6   Valvular Heart Disease

Valvular heart disease is valve abnormalities caused by congenital disorders or a variety of acquired diseases. The valve abnormalities can result in stenosis or insufficiency(regurgitation or incompetence), or both. Stenosis is the failure of a valve to open completely, obstructing forward flow. Valvular stenosis is almost always a chronic process caused by a primary cuspal abnormality. Insufficiency results from failure of a valve to close completely, thereby allowing reversed flow. Valvular insufficiency may result from either intrinsic disease of the valve cusps(e. g. , valve destruction)or distortion of the supporting structures without primary changes in the cusps. It can appear acutely, as with chordal rupture, or chronically due to leaflet scarring and retraction.

Stenosis or regurgitation can occur in pure forms, or may coexist in the same valve. Valvular disease may affect only a single valve(the mitral valve is most commonly affected), or more than one valve. The outcome of valvular disease depends on the valve involved, the degree of impairment, the tempo of its development, and the rate and quality of compensatory mechanisms.

7.6.1   Mitral Stenosis

The most common causes of mitral stenosis(MS)are postrheumatic or postinflammatory diseases and account for 99% of cases. Rare causes include congenital valvular or supravalvular stenosis, SLE(systemic lupus erythematosus), Whipple endocarditis, and extensive calcification of the mitral annulus.

7.6.1.1   Morphology

The mitral valve leaflets are swollen, and tiny flat vegetations that can be seen along the lines of closure at the acute stage. Microscopically, chronic inflammation, edema and platelet-fibrin thrombi are present; Aschoff bodies are present in a minority of cases. The valve leaflets are thickened, retracted, and calcificied, and chordae are fused and shortened, and the orifice is reduced to an oval, narrow "fish mouth" opening in chronic RHD. Microscopically, the typical findings include fibrosis, calcification with or without ossification, neovascularization, and a variable chronic inflammatory cell infiltrate containing lymphocytes, monocytes, and mast cells.

7.6.1.2 Hemodynamic Phenomena

When the mitral orifice is reduced, blood can flow from the left atrium into the left ventricle only if it is propelled by a pressure gradient. In order to double the flow through the stenotic mitral valve, the pressure gradient has to be increased 4 times. The left atrium progressively dilates and may harbor mural thrombi. Such an increase in atrial pressure will be transmitted to the pulmonary veins and capillaries and cause breathing difficulties; if it is severe enough, it may give rise to frank pulmonary edema. The left atrial hypertension resulting in dilatation, hypertrophy, and fibrosis of the atrial wall can lead to atrial fibrillation. Long-standing congestive changes in the lungs may induce pulmonary vascular and parenchymal changes and in time lead to right ventricular hypertrophy. With pure mitral stenosis, the left ventricle is generally normal.

7.6.1.3 Clinical Features

In patients whose mitral orifices are large enough to accommodate a normal blood flow with only mild elevations of left atrium pressure, marked elevations of the pressure leading to dyspnea and cough may be precipitated by sudden change in the heart rate, volume status, or CO. As MS progresses, the patients become limited in daily activities, and orthopnea and paroxysmal nocturnal dyspnea. The characteristic physical finding in MS is a rumbling diastolic murmur, which is heard at the cardiac apex. Liver congestion, jugular filing, serous cavity effusion and edema of lower limbs can be present. The chest X-ray showing enlarged left atrium, and pear-shaped heart.

7.6.2 Mitral Insufficiency

A variety of different pathological entities can lead to regurgitation or incompetence of the mitral valve. Rheumatic heart disease is still the commonest cause of the mitral regurgitation followed by myxomatous degeneration, mitral valve prolapse (MVP), ischemic heart disease, infective endocarditis, postinflammatory disease, ruptured chordae tendineae, and annular calcification.

7.6.2.1 Morphology

The valve associated with mitral insufficiency (MI) from rheumatic valves is often thickened, shortened, and has fused chordae, anchoring the posterior cusp of the mitral valve to the wall of the left ventricle.

7.6.2.2 Hemodynamic Phenomena

In patients with mitral regurgitation, the left ventricle ejects blood via two routs: ①through the aortic valve to the systemic circulation; ②through the mitral valve into the left atrium. In order to maintain normal systemic cardiac output, more complete systolic emptying of the left ventricle is required. Over many years, the additional burden imposed by mitral regurgitation on the myocardium leads to dilatation and hypertrophy of the left ventricle. Then, after many decades, left ventricular failure develops. Eventually, it leads to dilatation and hypertrophy of right ventricle and right atrium, or right ventricular failure.

7.6.2.3 Clinical Features

Patients with chronic mild-to-moderate isolated MI are usually asymptomatic. Orthopnea, exertional dyspnea, and fatigue are the most prominent complaints in patients with chronic severe MI. In patients with chronic severe MI, a whiffing systolic murmur is often heard at the cardiac apex. The chest X-ray may show ball-shaped heart.

7.6.3　Aortic Stenosis

Aortic stenosis(AS) is usually the result of rheumatic valvular injury and a congenital abnormality of the valve that leads to fibrosis and calcification of the valve. Other less common causes are unicuspid/unicommissural valve, dysplastic valvular formation and a group of rare metabolic disorders.

7.6.3.1　Morphology

The classic gross appearances of aortic valve leaflets are thickening, rigidity, calcification, fusion, and the orifice is reduced to a narrow opening. The histopathologic changes reflect the extensive calcific changes that begin in the fibrosa layer and expand into the sinuses(Figure 7-4).

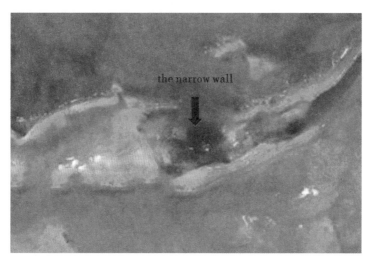

Figure 7-4　Stenotic aorta

7.6.3.2　Hemodynamic Phenomena

The hemodynamic burden imposed by critical aortic valve stenosis is systolic overloading of the left ventricle. In order to overcome the impedance to emptying imposed by the stenotic valve, the left ventricle increases its contractile mass. Dilatation of the left ventricular chamber and the hypertrophy of muscles may results in elevated left ventricular end-diastolic pressure. Then, left ventricular failure develops. Eventually, it leads to dilatation and hypertrophy of right ventricle and right atrium, or right ventricular failure.

7.6.3.3　Clinical Features

In severe aortic stenosis, the left ventricular outflow obstruction leads to left ventricular pressures as high as 200 mmHg or more; cardiac output is maintained only by virtue of concentric left ventricular hypertrophy. The hypertrophied myocardium tends to be relatively ischemic, and can develop into angina. Syncope may develop due to poor perfusion of the brain. Syncope may be caused by poor cerebral perfusion. The combination of systolic and diastolic dysfunction leads to CHF, which ultimately leads to cardiacdecompensation. The chest X-ray may show boot-shaped heart.

7.6.4　Aortic Insufficiency

Regurgitation of blood back through the aortic valve during diastole occurs as a result of a number of different pathological entities: bicuspid aortic valve, rheumatic heart disease, myxomatous degeneration, infective endocarditis and Marfan syndrome or septal myomectomy.

7.6.4.1 Morphology

In root dilatation associated with Marfan syndrome, the leaflets display a range of myxomatous expansion of the spongiosa layer that is highlighted by stains of glycosaminoglycans such as colloidal iron. Aortic insufficiency caused by postrheumatic lesions contains limited amounts of calcific deposits and fibrosis. In age-related aortic root dilatation, the leaflets show minimal or no degenerative features under the microscope.

7.6.4.2 Hemodynamic Phenomena

Aortic regurgitation produces a volume overload of the ventricle. Left ventricular end-diastolic volume is increased by the quantity of regurgitant blood flow. Initially, compensatory left ventricular hypertrophy and dilatation maintain cardiovascular homeostasis. Over the years, left ventricular function deteriorates and signs and symptoms of heart failure ensue. Left ventricular diastolic pressure rises and is transmitted to the pulmonary capillaries cauing lung congestion and difficulty breathing. Thus, it leads to dilatation and hypertrophy of right ventricle and right atrium, or right ventricular failure.

7.6.4.3 Clinical Features

Symptomatic aortic valve regurgitation is characterized by the presence of one or more of a triad of symptoms: orthopnea, dyspnea and angina. The characteristic physical finding in aortic valve regurgitation is a whiffing diastolic murmur, which is usually best heard along the left sternal border. The carotid pulsation, Corrigan's pulse, capillary pulsation and vascular shot sound phenomenon can be present.

7.7 Cardiomyopathy

Most cardiac diseases are secondary to some other conditions(e. g. , hypertension, coronary atherosclerosis, or valvular heart disease). However, there are some cardiac diseases that are attributable to intrinsic myocardial dysfunction. Such myocardial diseases are termed cardiomyopathies. In many cases, cardiomyopathies are of unknown etiology(termed idiopathic); however, several previously "idiopathic" cardiomyopathies have been shown to be caused by specific genetic abnormalities in cardiac energy metabolism or structural and contractile proteins.

Cardiomyopathies can be subdivided by a variety of criteria. The 2006 American Heart Association classification divides them into two major groups: ①primary it includes those entities in which the disease is solely or predominantly confined to the heart muscle and ②secondary, in which heart is involved as a part of a generalized multiorgan disorder. Within both of the two groups, some diseases are genetic, others are acquired, and many are idiopathic. A more clinical and functional classification of cardiomyopathies are as follows: dilated cardiomyopathy(90% of cases), hypertrophic cardiomyopathy, restrictive cardiomyopathy, Keshan disease and arrhythmogenic right ventricular cardiomyopathy.

7.7.1 Dilated Cardiomyopathy

Dilated Cardiomyopathy(DCM), also called congestive cardiomyopathy is defined clinically by global left ventricular systolic dysfunction and increased left ventricular cavity diameter in the absence of hypertension, value disease, or significant coronary artery disease. Approximately 25% to 35% of DCM cases have a familial(genetic)basis. Others result from a variety of acquired myocardial insults including toxic exposures

(e. g. ,chronic alcoholism) ,myocarditis,and pregnancy-associated changes. In some patients,the cause of DCM is unknown. Such cases are appropriately called idiopathic dilated cardiomyopathy.

7.7.1.1 Morphology

Because of the wall thinning that accompanies dilation,the ventricular thickness may be less than,e-qual to,or greater than normal. Mural thrombi are common and may be a source of thromboemboli. The heart in DCM is characteristically enlarged (increase two to three times compared with its normal weight) and flabby,with dilation of all chambers.

The histologic abnormalities in DCM are nonspecific. Microscopically most myocytes are hypertrophied with enlarged nuclei,but many are irregular,stretched and attenuated. There is variable interstitial and en-docardial fibrosis;scattered scars are also often present,probably marking previous myocyte ischemic necro-sis caused by reduced perfusion (due to poor contractile function) and increased demand (due to myocyte hypertrophy). The extent of the changes frequently does not reflect the degree of dysfunction or the patient's prognosis.

7.7.1.2 Pathogenesis

The causes of DCM can be grouped into four broad categories:family history of cardiomyopathy,idio-pathic dilated (no known association) ,acquired DCM includes viral coxsackievirus B and other enterovirus-es,peripartum cardiomyopathy,alcohol or other toxic exposure,and secondary DCM includes IHD,autoim-mune diseases,endocrine,metabolic,and nutritional disorders.

7.7.1.3 Clinical Features

DCM can occur at any age,but it most commonly occurs between ages of 20 and 50. The fundamental defect in DCM is ineffective contraction. Fifty percent of patients die within 2 years,and only 25% survive longer than 5 years. Death is usually due to progressive cardiac failure or arrhythmia. In most cases cardiac transplantation is the only definitive treatment.

7.7.2 Hypertrophic Cardiomyopathy

Hypertrophic cardiomyopathy (HCM) (also known as idiopathic hypertrophic subaortic stenosis) is characterized by abnormal diastolic filling,myocardial hypertrophy,and in a third of cases ventricular out-flow obstruction. The heart is heavy,thick-walled,and hypercontracting,in striking contrast to the flabby, poorly contractile heart in DCM.

7.7.2.1 Morphology

The essential gross feature of HCM is massive myocardial hypertrophy without ventricular dilation. The classic pattern of HCM involves disproportionate thickening of the ventricular septum relative to the left ven-tricle free wall (so-called asymmetrical septal hypertrophy) ;but in about 10% of cases there is concentric hypertrophy. On longitudinal sectioning,the ventricular cavity loses its usual round-to-ovoid shape and is compressed into a "banana-like" configuration. Often present is an endocardial plaque in the left ventricular outflow tract,as well as a thickening of the anterior mitral leaflet. Both findings reflect contact of the anterior mitral leaflet with the septum during ventricular systole and correlate with functional left ventricular outflow tract obstruction.

The characteristic histologic features in HCM are severe myocyte hypertrophy,myocyte (and myofiber) disarray,and interstitial and replacement fibrosis.

7.7.2.2 Pathogenesis

Almost all cases of HCM are caused by missense point mutations in one of several genes encoding the sarcomeric proteins that form the contractile apparatus of striated muscle. Greater than 100 causal mutations have been identified in at least 12 sarcomeric genes, with the β-myosin heavy chain being most frequently affected, followed by myosin-binding protein C and troponin T. These three genes account for 70% to 80% of all cases of HCM.

7.7.2.3 Clinical Features

High left ventricular pressures, the massive hypertrophy, and compromised intramural coronary arteries often lead to myocardial ischemia(with angina), even without coronary artery disease. Major clinical problems include atrial fibrillation with mural thrombus, IE of the mitral valve, CHF, arrhythmias, and sudden death. Most patients improve by therapy that promotes ventricular relaxation; occasionally, partial surgical excision of septal muscle is necessary to relieve the outflow tract obstruction.

7.7.3 Restrictive Cardiomyopathy

Restrictive cardiomyopathy(RCM) is characterized by a primary decrease in ventricular compliance, resulting in impaired ventricular filling during diastole, RCM can be idiopathic or associated with systemic diseases that also happen to affect the myocardium, for example, radiation fibrosis, amyloidosis, hemochromatosis, sarcoidosis, or products of inborn errors of metabolism.

7.7.3.1 Morphology

In idiopathic restrictive cardiomyopathy, the ventricles are of approximately normal size or slightly enlarged, the cavities are not dilated, and the myocardium is firm. Biatrial dilation is commonly observed. Microscopically there is interstitial fibrosis, varying from minimal and patchy to extensive and diffuse. Restrictive cardiomyopathy of disparate causes may have similar gross morphology. However, endomyocardial biopsy can reveal disease-specific features.

Two other forms of restrictive cardiomyopathy merit brief mention:

1) Endomyocardial fibrosis is principally a disease of children and young adults in Africa and other tropical areas; it is characterized by dense fibrosis of the ventricular endocardium and subendocardium extending from the apex up to the tricuspid and mitral valves. The fibrous tissue markedly diminishes the volume and compliance of affected chambers and so causes a restrictive physiology. Worldwide, this is the most common form of restrictive cardiomyopathy.

2) Loeffler endomyocarditis also causes endocardial fibrosis, typically with large mural thrombi. However, Löeffler's endomyocarditis is not geographically restricted. These is often an associated peripheral hypereosinophilia; the circulating eosinophils are abnormal, and many are degranulated. Release of the eosinophil granule contents, especially major basic protein, is speculated to initiate endocardial damage, with subsequent endomyocardial necrosis followed by scarring of the necrotic area.

7.7.3.2 Clinical Features

Because of increased ventricular stiffness, there is reduced diastolic ventricular volume with normal or near-normal systolic function(ejection fraction) and wall thickness. The atria are dilated with non-hypertrophied, nondilated ventricles.

7.7.4 Keshan Disease

Keshan Disease(KD) is an endemic cardiomyopathy found in Keshan, north-east China. The first patient was identified in 1935. This disease is characterized by a blood circulation disorder, endocardium abnormality and myocardium necrosis. Selenium(Se) deficiency is thought to be a major factor by Chinese scientists. However, the exact etiology has not been clarified up to now. The government decided to apply sodium selenite to growing crops, and the incidence of disease decreased dramatically. The largest prevalence age rates are boys under 15 years old and women of childbearing age. There are several hypotheses; acute carbon monoxide poisoning, virus infection, malnutrition, or selenium deficiency.

Scar lesions are scattered on ventricular wall, and mural thrombus are found on ventricular trabecular muscles or left or right atrial appendage. Microscopically, different degrees of cellular granular degeneration, vacuole degeneration and fatty degeneration, coagulation and fatty degeneration, coagulation necrosis can be seen. Scar formation is prominent with the chronic cases. The pathological features of Keshan disease are severe myocardial degeneration, necrosis and scarring. Crossly, heart is large, spherical, increased weight. Both sides of the heart chamber are expanded with ventricular wall thinning, especially in the apex area.

7.7.5　Arrhythmogenic Right Ventricular Cardiomyopathy

Arrhythmogenic right ventricular cardiomyopathy is a unique (albeit uncommon) entity with a clinical presentation involving right-sided heart failure and various rhythm disturbances (including SCD). Morphologically, the right ventricular wall is severely thinned as a result of myocyte replacement by massive fatty infiltration and lesser accounts of fibrosis. Most cases are sporadic, but familial forms do occur with gene defects localized to chromosome 14 (autosomal dominant inheritance with variable penetrance). Most of the mutations seem to involve desmosomal junctional proteins.

7.8　Myocarditis

Myocarditis refers to generalize inflammation of the myocardium associated with necrosis and degeneration of myocytes. The term is generally used only for diffuse myocardial inflammation that results in symptoms, although focal myocarditis has been described. In myocarditis there is inflammation of the myocardium with resulting injury. Myocarditis can occur at any age and is one of the few heart diseases that can produce acute heart failure in previously healthy adolescents or young adults. Although unusually, it can occur with the sudden onset of arrhythmias and even sudden cardiac death. According to etiology myocarditis can be divided into infective and noninfective myocarditis. The causes of former type include virus, bacteria, parasites, fungi, etc. The later type is usually caused by allergic reaction, drugs, physical or chemical factors. However, most cases are caused by viral infection.

7.8.1　Viral Myocarditis

It is also called lymphocytic myocarditis and idiopathic, is most common. The most frequently implicated agents are coxsackie A and B, ECHO, Polio, and influenza viruses. The pathogenesis of myocyte injury is complex, involving myocyte receptors specific for enter and adenoviruses, and immune-regulated myocyte cell death.

Crossly, myocarditis reveals nonspecific findings ranging from normal to dilatation of all four chambers, depending on specific agents and the duration of illness. The histology changes of viral myocarditis vary with the clinical severity of the disease. Most cases show a patchy of a diffuse interstitial infiltrate composed principally of lymphocytes and macrophages. Multinucleated giant cells often surround individual myocytes, and there is focal or patchy acute myocyte necrosis associated with the inflammatory cell infiltrate. In the early stage, necrosis and accumulation of interstitial proteinaceous material are prominent, whereas during the resolving phase, fibroblast proliferation and interstitial collagen deposition become predominant.

Most viruses that cause myocarditis also cause pericarditis. Most patients present with symptoms of concomitant pericardial inflammation, chest pain, and palpitations. The clinical diagnosis is made on the basis of electrocardiographic changes, myocardial damage evidenced by elevated troponin, evidence of systemic inflammation, lack of epicardial coronary artery disease, and generally mild and transient ventricular dysfunction.

7.8.2 Bacterial Myocarditis

Myocarditis involvement is most commonly encountered with meningococcal, diphtheritic, and leptospiral infections amongthe bacteria. The exotoxin of the diphtheria bacillus causes cardiac damage by inhibiting protein synthesis, since it specifically interferes with a transferase involved in the delivery of amino acid to elongating polypeptide chains. Myocardium may be affected in any bacterial infection when the causative agent is blood borne, for example, with salmonellosis or any form of bacterial endocarditis.

Bacterial myocarditis is characterized by a different mixed inflammatory cell infiltrate, with neutrophils as the major component. Organisms can often be marked by special stains. Micro abscesses can occur when septic emboli lodge in the coronary circulation, often as a consequence of infective endocarditis.

7.8.3 Isolated Myocarditis

Isolated myocarditis refers to those sporadic cases of myocarditis which occur without discernible cause in previously healthy individuals. A fatal type of isolated myocarditis is also known as idiopathic giant cell myocarditis of Fiedler's myocarditis. This type affects males more than females.

Crossly, the heart is flabby, dilated and may contain mural thrombi. Microscopically, focal necrosis associated with a granulomatous reaction containing multinucleate giant cells, and interspersed with lymphocytes, plasma cells, eosinophils and macrophages.

Whatever the pattern of histological changes during the acute phase of the disease, all inflammatory lesions either resolve, leaving no residuals, or undergo progressive fibrosis. Often the persistent connective tissue is sufficiently scattered and subtle to be virtually in apparent at a later date. With more severe damage, focal minute scars may remain. Transient ECG abnormalities may be the only indication of its presence, particularly abnormalities of the ST segment and T wave, point to a diffuse myocardial lesion.

Acute symptomatic myocarditis often manifests itself as malaise, dyspnea and low grade fever, with tachycardia more marked than the fever alone would warrant. Most patients recover from acute myocarditis, although a few die of congestive heart failure or arrhythmias. The patients of isolated myocarditis usually die of congestive heart failure or sudden death from arrhythmias.

7.9 Aneurysm and Dissections

Aneurysm is congenital or acquired localized abnormal dilations of blood vessels or the heart. The two most important causes of aneurysms are atherosclerosis and cystic medial degeneration of the arterial media. Arterial aneurysms can also be caused by systemic diseases, such as vasculitis. Other causes that weaken vessel walls include trauma, congenital defects, infections (mycotic aneurysms), and syphilis.

"True" aneurysms involve all three layers of the artery (intima, media, and adventitia) or the attenuated wall of the heart; these include atherosclerotic and congenital vascular aneurysms, as well as ventricular aneurysms resulting from transmural myocardial infarctions. Aneurysms and dissections are important causes of stasis and subsequent thrombosis; they also have a propensity to rupture often with catastrophic results.

Aneurysms can be classified by the shape:

1) Fusiform aneurysms are circumferential dilations up to 20 cm in diameter; these most common involve the aortic arch, the abdominal aorta, or the iliac arteries.

2) Serpentine aneurysms are asymmetric expend. Look like serpentine distention.

3) Saccular aneurysms are discrete outpouchings ranging from 5 to 20 cm in diameter, often with a contained thrombus.

4) Dissecting aneurysms refer to the arterial dissection, when blood enters the wall of the artery leading a hematoma dissection between its layers.

5) Navicular aneurysms outstand in one-side wall, but the opposite wall is alright.

6) False aneurysms are the breach in the vascular wall leading to an extravascular hematoma that freely communicates with the intravascular space (pulsating hematoma), most commonly a post-myocardial infarction rupture that has been contained by a pericardial adhesion or a leak at the junction (anastomosis) of a vascular graft with a natural artery.

Chapter 8

Respiratory Diseases

The respiratory system includes nose, pharynx, larynx, trachea, bronchus and lung. Usually, the respiratory tract is divided into two parts of the upper and lower parts according to the laryngeal cricoid. The upper respiratory tract includes the nose, pharynx and larynx; the lower respiratory tract includes the trachea and bronchus.

The major function of the lung is to replenish oxygen and excrete carbon dioxide from blood. The midline trachea develops two lateral outpocketings, the lung buds. The right lung bud eventually divides into three main bronchi, and the left into two main bronchi, thus giving rise to three lobes on the right and two on the left. The main bronchi branch (left and right) further branching smaller airways, termed bronchioles, which are distinguished from bronchi by the lack of cartilage and submucosal glands within their walls. Additional branching of bronchioles leads to terminal bronchioles; the part of the lung distal to the terminal bronchiole is called an acinus. Pulmonary acini are composed of respiratory bronchioles which proceed into alveolar ducts immediately branching into alveolar sacs, the blind ends of the respiratory passages, whose walls are formed entirely of alveoli which is the ultimate site of gas exchange. The microscopic structure of the alveolar walls (or alveolar septa) consists of the following components:

➡ The capillary endothelium.

➡ Abasement membrane.

➡ The pulmonary interstitium is most prominent in thicker portions of the alveolar septum, composed of fine elastic fibers, small bundles of collagen, a few fibroblast-like cells, smooth muscle cells, mast cells, and rare mononuclear cells.

➡ Alveolar epithelium contains a continuous layer of two principal cell types: type I pneumocytes and type II pneumocytes. Type I pneumocytes which are flattened, platelike cover 95% of the alveolar surface, and rounded type II pneumocytes only cover 5%. The latter which secret pulmonary surfactant are the main cell type involved in repair of alveolar epithelium when type I are injured. There are numerous pores of Kohn in alveolar walls, which permit passage of air, bacteria, and exudates between adjacent alveoli.

➡ A few alveolar macrophages.

8.1   Respiratory Tract and Pulmonary Infections

The respiratory system communicates directly with the outside world. Harmful substances and pathogenic microorganisms can enter the respiratory tract with breathing and cause inflammatory diseases of the respiratory tract. Infections are the most common diseases of respiratory system. This section will introduce acute tracheobronchitis, acute bronchiolitis and pneumonia.

8.1.1   Acute Tracheobronchitis

Acute tracheobronchitis is a common disease of the respiratory system, usually occurring in children and elderly people. It happens after cold and upper respiratory tract infection, more easily in cold season.

8.1.1.1   Etiology

The major cause of this disease is virus infection, such as rhinovirus, influenza virus, respiratory syncytial virus, adenovirus, and by secondary bacterial infection like influenza bacillus, streptococcus pneumonia. In addition, in a few cases inhalation of harmful dust or gas(such as sulfur dioxide, chlorine, etc.) can also cause acute tracheal bronchitis.

8.1.1.2   Morphology

The tracheobronchial mucosa is red and swollen, and there are white or yellowish mucous secretions in the surface adheres, even necrosis and ulcers happening on mucous in severe cases. According to the features of the disease, it is divided into: ①acute catarrhal tracheobronchitis: the mucosa and submucosa become congested with edema, accompanied by neutrophils infiltration; the luminal surface covered with yellow sticky secretions. The secretions can be coughed up or it can cause obstruction. ②acute suppurative tracheobronchitis: it is suppurative inflammation. a large number of neutrophils infiltrate in mucosa and submucosa, and inflammation can involve alveoli near bronchioles. Patients often produce yellow sticky purulent sputum. ③acute ulcerative tracheobronchitis: the disease is serious, most of which are caused by virus and pyogenic bacteria at the same time. In the early stage, superficial necrosis, erosion and ulcers were formed in the mucosa of the lumen. After the inflammation subsided, the mucous epithelium was repaired by the proliferation of basal cells, the structure and the function of trachea and bronchus returned to normal.

8.1.2   Acute Bronchiolitis

Acute bronchiolitis(acute bronchiolitis)is an acute inflammation of the bronchioles with a diameter of <2 mm. It is common in infants under 4 years old, especially in 1 year olds which about represents 90%. Most of the cases are caused by virus infection in winter, mainly respiratory syncytial virus, adenovirus and parainfluenza virus.

8.1.2.1   Morphology

bronchial mucous causes hyperemia, edema. Columnar epithelium and simple squamous epithelium replace pseudostratified ciliated columnar epithelium, which are necrosic. The number of goblet cell is increased, highly mucus secretion. lymphocytes and mononuclear cell infiltrate. The lumen full of inflammatory exudates, making the lumen partially or completely blocked, resulting in acute focal atelectasis or obstructive emphysema. Because the bronchial is thin, the inflammation can easily extend to the surrounding pulmonary interstitium and alveoli, forming peribronchiolitis or focal pneumonitis.

8.1.3 Pneumonia

Pneumonia can be very broadly defined as any infection in the lung, which is most common disease of the respiratory system. According to a survey of WHO, pneumonia mortality accounted for 75% of the mortality of acute respiratory infection. In China, among all the causes of death, pneumonia accounts for the fifth. The clinical presentation of pneumonias may be as an acute, fulminant clinical disease or as a chronic disease with a more protracted course. Pneumonia can be caused by different pathogenic factors. According to the etiology, bacterial pneumonia, viral pneumonia, mycoplasma pneumonia, fungal pneumonia and parasitic pneumonia are caused by biological factors; radiation pneumonia, aspiration pneumonia, lipoid pneumonia and allergic pneumonia are caused by physicochemical factors. According to the site of the lesion, it can be divided into alveolar pneumonia(most of pneumonia) and interstitial pneumonia. According to the extent of the lesion, it can be divided into lobar pneumonia, lobular pneumonia and interstitial pneumonia. The histologic spectrum of pneumonia may range from a fibrinopurulent alveolar exudate seen in acute bacterial pneumonias, to mononuclear interstitial infiltrates in viral and other atypical pneumonias, to granulomas and cavitation seen in many of the chronic pneumonias.

8.1.3.1 Bacterial Pneumonia

Among the different types of pneumonia, bacterial pneumonia is the most common, accounting for about 80%. Acute bacterial pneumonias can manifest as one of two anatomic and radiographic patterns, referred to as lobar pneumonia and lobular pneumonia(also called bronchopneumonia).

(1)Lobar Pneumonia

Lobar pneumonia is mainly caused by pneumococcal infection, which is characterized by acute pulmonary fibrinous inflammation. The onset usually is abrupt, with high fever, shaking chills, pleuritic chest pain and a productive mucopurulent cough; occasional patients may have hemoptysis. More than 90% of the lobar pneumonia are caused by the pneumococcus, especially the strongest of type Ⅲ.

1)Morphology and Clinical features: The lower lobes or the right middle lobe is most frequently involved. Before antibiotics used, pneumococcal pneumonia involves entire or almost entire lobes and evolves through four stages: congestion, red hepatization, gray hepatization, and resolution. Early antibiotic therapy alters or halts this typical progression. The first stage is congestion, the affected lobe(s)is(are)heavy, red, and boggy; histologically, vascular congest, with proteinaceous fluid, scattered neutrophils, and many bacteria in the alveoli. Because of toxemia, patients take on chills, high fever, the number of white blood cells increases. The auscultation can be heard and wet rales, and the chest film shows a flaky shadow. After one or two days, the second stage of red hepatization ensues. In this stage the affected lobe is still red and has a liverlike consistency; the alveolar spaces are packed with neutrophils, red cells, and fibrin(Figure 8−1). A large number of bacteria can be detected in the exudate. Because of reduced PaO_2, patients can appear dyspnea, cyanosis following hypoxia. The erythrocyte in the exudate is swallowed by alveolar macrophage, which makes the rusty sputum. This is a diagnostic significance. When the lesion is involved in the pleura, it causes fibrinous pleurisy and chest pain, aggravated with breathing and coughing. The X-ray shows a large area of dense shadow. The next stage is gray hepatization. The affected lobes become dry, gray, and firm(liverlike consistency), because the red cells are lysed, while the fibrinosuppurative exudate can be seen still, within the alveoli(Figure 8−2). Because the alveolar capillaries are pressed in the ischemic state, the anoxia is relieved, but the signs of pulmonary consolidation still exist. The sputum turnes to mucous purulent sputum, and the rest of the symptoms are relieved. Last stage resolution follows in uncomplicated cases, as exudates within the alveoli are enzymatically digested to produce granular, semifluid debris that is resorbed, ingested by macrophages, coughed up, or organized by fibroblasts growing into it. The pleural reaction (fibrinous or fibrinopurulent pleuritis) may similarly resolve or undergo organization, leaving fibrous thickening or permanent adhesions.

2) Complication: With appropriate therapy, complete restitution of the lung is the rule for both forms of pneumococcal pneumonia, but occasionally in a few cases complications may occur: ①organization of the intraalveolar exudate may convert areas of the lung into solid fibrous tissue, called pulmonary carnification; ②tissue destruction and necrosis may lead to abscess formation; ③suppurative material may accumulate in the pleural cavity, leading to empyema; ④bacteremic dissemination may lead to meningitis, arthritis, or infective endocarditis; ⑤Septic shock is the most serious complication that can cause death of the patient.

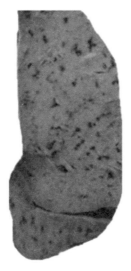

Figure 8-1 **Lobar pneumonia**
The affected lobe become dry, gray, and firm

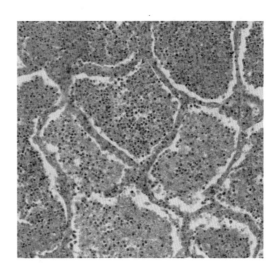

Figure 8-2 **Lobar pneumonia**

(2) Lobular Pneumonia

It is mainly caused by pyogenic infection, such as *staphylococcus aureus*, *streptococcus hemolyticus*, and so on. The lesions begin in the bronchioles and develop to the periphery or peripheral lung tissues, forming a pyogenic inflammation in the lung lobules as a unit. Lobular pneumonia is also known as bronchopneumonia because of its lesion in the bronchus. It occurs mainly in the children and the elderly.

1) Morphology and clinical features: In the bronchopneumonic pattern, foci of inflammatory consolidation are distributed in patches throughout one or several lobes, most frequently bilateral and basal. Well-developed lesions up to 3 or 4 cm in diameter are slightly elevated and are gray-red to yellow; confluence of these foci may occur in severe cases, leading the appearance of a lobar consolidation (confluent bronchopneumonia). The lung substance immediately surrounding areas of consolidation is usually hyperemic and edematous, but the large intervening areas are generally normal. Pleural involvement is less common than in lobar pneumonia. Histologically, the reaction consists of focal suppurative exudate that fills the bronchi, bronchioles, and adjacent alveolar spaces (Figure 8-3, Figure 8-4).

2) Clinical features: Although lobular pneumonia is a complication of other diseases, its clinical symptoms are often obscured by primary diseases. The main symptoms are cough, expectoration and fever. The inflammation of the bronchial mucosa causes coughing and sputum, and the phlegm is purulent. The lesions often appear to be focally distributed, and the physical signs of the lung are generally not obvious (except confluent bronchopneumonia). Chest X-ray shows irregular small flaky or spotted blurred shadows. If the disease is found in time and the treatment is proper, the exudate in the lungs can be completely absorbed

and the patients recover. However, the prognosis is mostly poor in young children and elderly. The risk of complications of lobular pneumonia is much greater than that of lobar pneumonia. It can be complicated with heart failure, respiratory failure, sepsis, pulmonary abscess and empyema.

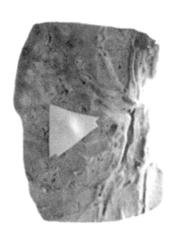

Figure 8-3　**Lobular pneumonia**

Foci of inflammatory consolidation are distributed in patches, gray-red to yellow

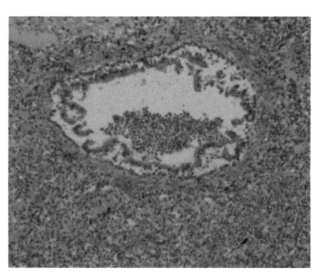

Figure 8-4　**Lobular pneumonia**

3) Other Important Bacterial Pneumonia

1) Haemophilus in-fluenzae: Both encapsulated and unencapsulated forms are important causes of pneumonias. The former can cause a particularly life threatening form of pneumonia for children, often following respiratory viral infection. Adults at risk for developing infections include those with chronic pulmonary diseases such as chronic bronchitis, cystic fibrosis, and bronchiectasis. H. in-fluenzae is the most common bacterial cause of acute exacerbation of COPD. Encapsulated H. in fluenzae type b was formerly an important cause of epiglottitis and suppurative meningitis in children, but vaccination against this organism in infancy has significantly reduced the risk.

2) Klebsiella pneumoniae: K. pneumoniae is the most frequent cause of gram negative bacterial pneumonia. Klebsiella-related pneumonia frequently affects debilitated and malnourished persons, especially chronic alcoholics. Because the organism produces an abundant viscid capsular polysaccharide, thick and gelatinous sputum is characteristic, which make the patient have difficulty coughing up.

(3) Legionella pneumophila: L. pneumophila is the agent of legionnaire disease, an eponym for the epidemic and sporadic forms of pneumonia caused by this organism. Pontiac fever is a related self-limited upper respiratory tract infection caused by L. pneumophila, without pneumonic symptoms. L. pneumophila flourishes in artificial aquatic environments, such as water-cooling towers and within the tubing system of domestic(potable) water supplies. The mode of transmission is thought to be either inhalation of aerosolized organisms or aspiration of contaminated drinking water. Legionella pneumonia is common in persons with some predisposing condition such as cardiac, renal, immunologic, or hematologic disease. Organ transplant recipients are particularly susceptible. Legionella pneumonia can be quite severe, frequently requiring hospitalization, and immunosuppressed persons may have a fatality rate of 30% to 50%. Rapid diagnosis is facilitated by demonstration of Legionella antigens in the urine or by a positive fluorescent antibody test on sputum samples; culture remains the standard diagnostic modality. PCR-based tests can be used on bronchial

secretions in atypical cases.

8.1.3.2　Atypical Pneumonia(Interstitial Pneumonia)

The primary atypical pneumonia initially was applied to an acute febrile respiratory disease characterized by patchy in flammatory changes in the lungs, largely confined to the alveolar septa and pulmonary interstitium. The word "atypical" means the moderate amounts of sputum, absence of physical findings of consolidation, only moderate elevation of white cell count, and lack of alveolar exudates.

(1)Etiology and Pathogenesis

Atypical pneumonia is caused by a variety of pathogens. Mycoplasma pneumoniae is the most common. Mycoplasma infections are particularly common in children and young adults. Others are viruses, such as in fluenza types A and B, the respiratory syncytial viruses, human metapneumovirus, adenovirus, rhinoviruses, rubeola virus, and varicella virus. Nearly all of these agents can also cause a primarily upper respiratory tract infection. The common pathogenetic mechanism is attachment of the organisms to the respiratory epithelium followed by necrosis of the cells and an in flammatory response. When the process extends to alveoli, there is usually interstitial in flammation, but some outpouring of fluid into alveolar spaces may also occur, so that on chest X-ray the changes may mimic those of bacterial pneumonia. Damage to and denudation of the respiratory epithelium inhibits mucociliary clearance and predisposes to secondary bacterial infections. Viral infections of the respiratory tract are well known for this complication. More serious lower respiratory tract infection is more likely to occur in infants, elderly persons, malnourished patients, alcoholics, and immunosuppressed persons. Not surprisingly, viruses and mycoplasmas frequently are involved in outbreaks of infection in hospitals.

(2)Morphology

Regardless of cause, the morphologic patterns in atypical pneumonias are similar. The process may be patchy, or it may involve whole lobes bilaterally or unilaterally. Grossly, the affected lobes are red-blue, and congested. Histologically, the inflammatory reaction is largely confined within the walls of the alveoli. The septa are widened and edematous; they usually contain a mononuclear inflammatory infiltrate of lymphocytes, histiocytes, and occasionally plasma cells. In contrast to bacterial pneumonias, alveolar spaces in-atypical pneumonias are distinctly free of cellular exudate. In severe cases, however, full-blown diffuse alveolar damage with hyaline membranes may develop. In less severe, uncomplicated cases, subsidence of the disease is followed by reconstitution of the native architecture. A mixed histologic picture is caused by co-infection with bacteria.

(3)Clinical Features

The clinical features of primary atypical pneumonia is extremely varied. It may masquerade as a severe upper respiratory tract infection, or it may manifest as a fulminant, life-threatening infection in immunocompromised patients. The initial presentation usually is that of an acute, nonspecific febrile illness characterized by fever, headache, malaise, later cough with minimal sputum. Because the edema and exudation are both in a strategic position to cause an alveolocapillary block, there may be respiratory distress seemingly out of proportion to the physical and radiographic findings. Identifying the causative agent can be difficult. Tests for Mycoplasma antigens and polymerase chain reaction(PCR)testing for Mycoplasma DNA are available. As a practical matter, patients with community-acquired pneumonia for which a bacterial agent seems unlikely are treated with a macrolide antibiotic effective against Mycoplasma and Chlamydia pneumoniae, because these are the most common pathogens producing treatable disease.

8.1.3.3　Severe Acute Respiratory Syndrome

Severe acute respiratory syndrome(SARS) is a viral respiratory disease of zoonotic origin caused by the SARS coronavirus(SARS-CoV). Between November 2002 and July 2003, an outbreak of SARS in southern China caused an eventual 8,098 cases, resulting in 774 deaths reported in 37 countries, with the majority of cases in China(9. 6% fatality rate) according to the WHO. No cases of SARS have been reported worldwide since 2004.

The primary route of transmission for SARS is contact of the mucous membranes with respiratory droplets or fomites. The initial symptoms are flu-like and include fever, myalgia, lethargy symptoms, cough, sore throat, and other nonspecific symptoms. The only symptom common to all patients appears to be a fever above 38 °C(100 °F). SARS may eventually lead to shortness of breath and/or pneumonia; either direct viral pneumonia or secondary bacterial pneumonia. The lungs of dying patient usually demonstrate diffuse alveolar damage and multinucleated cells.

8.2 Chronic Obstructive Pulmonary Disease

Chronic obstructive pulmonary disease(COPD) is a type of obstructive lung disease characterized by long-term breathing problems and poor airflow, including chronic bronchitis, emphysema, asthma and bronchiectasis. The main symptoms include shortness of breath and cough with sputum production. COPD is a progressive disease, meaning it typically worsens over time.

8.2.1　Chronic Bronchitis

Chronic bronchitis is a chronic nonspecific inflammation occurring in the tracheal mucosa and its surrounding tissues, it is a common disease. It is common among cigarette smokers and urban dwellers in smog-ridden cities; The diagnosis of chronic bronchitis is made on clinical grounds; it is defined by the presence of a persistent productive cough for at least 3 consecutive months in at least 2 consecutive years.

8.2.1.1　Etiology and Pathogenesis

Chronic bronchitis is the result of a long and comprehensive effect of a variety of factors. The distinctive feature of chronic bronchitis is hypersecretion of mucus, beginning in the large airways. The most important cause is smoking, other air pollutants, like sulfur dioxide and nitrogen dioxide also contribute. These environmental irritants cause hypertrophy of mucous glands in the trachea and main bronchi, resulting in a marked increase in mucin-secreting goblet cells in the surface epithelium of smaller bronchi and bronchioles. In addition, these irritants cause inflammation with infiltration of CD_8^+ lymphocytes, macrophages, and neutrophils. Whereas the defining feature of chronic bronchitis is primarily a reflection of large bronchial involvement, the morphologic basis of airflow obstruction in chronic bronchitis is more peripheral and results from coexistent emphysema and small airway disease, which are induced by goblet cell metaplasia with mucous plugging of the bronchiolar lumen, inflammation, and bronchiolar wall fibrosis. Generally, a small airway disease(also known as chronic bronchiolitis) is an important component of early and relatively mild air flow obstruction, chronic bronchitis with significant air flow obstruction is almost always complicated by emphysema.

8.2.1.2　Morphology

In gross specimens, the mucosal lining of the larger airways usually is hyperemic and swollen by edema fluid. It is often covered with a layer of mucinous or mucopurulent secretions. The smaller bronchi and bronchioles also may be filled with similar secretions. Histologically, the diagnostic feature of chronic bronchitis in the trachea and larger bronchi is enlargement of the mucus-secreting glands. Inflammatory cells, lymphocytic and plasma cell, infiltrate. For chronic bronchiolitis, the number of goblet cells are increased and squamous metaplasia occurs. In the most severe cases, there may be complete obliteration of the lumen as a consequence of fibrosis. It is the submucosal fibrosis that leads to luminal narrowing and airway obstruction.

8.2.1.3   Clinical Features

In early stages of the disease, the productive cough raises mucoid sputum, but air flow is not obstructed. Some patients with chronic bronchitis may demonstrate hyper-responsive airways with intermittent bronchospasm and wheezing. Some patients develop significant COPD with out flow obstruction. This clinical syndrome is accompanied by hypercapnia, hypoxemia, and (in severe cases) cyanosis. Differentiation of this form of COPD from that caused by emphysema can be made in the classic case, but many such patients have both conditions. Developing chronic bronchitis is complicated by pulmonary hypertension and cardiac failure.

8.2.2   Emphysema

Emphysema is a chronic obstructive airway disease characterized by permanent enlargement of air spaces distal to terminal bronchioles.

8.2.2.1   Pathogenesis

Emphysema is most often caused by smoking but can be caused by other diseases or have no known cause at all. Current opinion favors emphysema as a consequence of two critical imbalance: the protease-anti protease imbalance and oxidant-antioxidant imbalance.

8.2.2.2   Types of Emphysema

Emphysema is divided into four major types, according to its anatomic distribution within the lobule; There are: ①centriacinar; ②panacinar; ③distal acinar; ④irregular. Only the first two types cause clinically significant airway obstruction, with centriacinar emphysema being about 20 times more common than panacinar disease.

(1) Centriacinar Emphysema

This type of emphysema is most commonly seen as a consequence of cigarette smoking in people who do not have congenital deficiency of $\alpha 1$-antitrypsin. The distinctive feature of centriacinar emphysema is the pattern of involvement of the lobules: The central or proximal parts of the acini are affected, formed by respiratory bronchioles, while distal alveoli are spared. The lesions are more common and severe in the upper lobes, especially in the apical segments.

(2) Panacinar (Panlobular) Emphysema

In panacinar emphysema, the acini are uniformly enlarged, from the level of the respiratory bronchiole to the terminal blind alveoli. Compared to centriacinar emphysema, panacinar emphysema tends to happen more commonly in the lower lung zones and is the type of emphysema that occurs in $\alpha 1$-antitrypsin deficiency.

(3) Distal Acinar Emphysema

The cause of this type of emphysema is unknown; it is seen most often in cases of spontaneous pneumothorax in young adults. In distal acinar emphysema, the distal part is primarily involved, but the proximal portion of the acinus is normal. The emphysema is more striking adjacent to the pleura, along the lobular connective tissue septa, and at the margins of the lobules. It is usually more severe in the upper half of the lungs. The characteristic finding is the presence of multiple, contiguous, enlarged air spaces ranging in diameter from less than 0.5 mm to more than 2.0 cm, sometimes forming cystic structures that, with progressive enlargement, lead to bullae.

(4) Irregular Emphysema

Because the acinus is irregularly involved, so named irregular emphysema, which is almost invariably associated with scarring, such as that resulting from healed inflammatory diseases. Although clinically a-symptomatic, this may be the most common form of emphysema.

1) Morphology: The diagnosis and classification of emphysema depend largely on the macroscopic appearance of the lung. Panacinar emphysema, when the pathologic process is well developed, produces pale and big lungs. For centriacinar emphysema, the lungs are a deeper pink than in panacinar emphysema and less voluminous, unless the disease is well advanced. Generally, in centriacinar emphysema the upper two thirds of the lungs are more severely affected than the lower lungs. Histologically, alveolar walls are destructed, leading to enlarged air spaces. In addition to alveolar loss, the number of alveolar capillaries is diminished. Terminal and respiratory bronchioles may be deformed because of the loss of septa. With the loss of elastic tissue in the surrounding alveolar septa, radial traction on the small airways is reduced. As a result, they tend to collapse during expiration, which is an important cause of chronic air flow obstruction in severe emphysema (Figure 8–5, Figure 8–6).

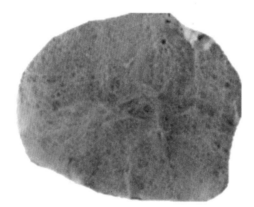

Figure 8–5　**Emphysema**

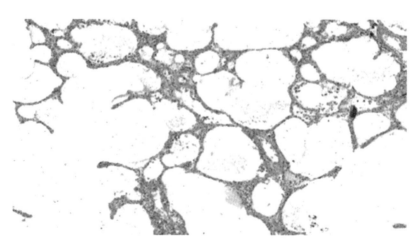

Figure 8–6　**Emphysema**

2) Clinical features: Usually, dyspnea is the first symptom; it begins insidiously but is steadily progressive. Cough and wheezing may be the initial complaint, for patients with underlying chronic bronchitis or chronic asthmatic bronchitis. Weight loss is common and may be so severe as to suggest a hidden malignant

tumor. Pulmonary function tests reveal reduced FEV1 with normal or near-normal FVC. Hence, the ratio of FEV1 to FVC is reduced.

The classic presentation in emphysema with no "bronchitic" component is one in which the patient is barrel-chested and dyspneic, with obviously prolonged expiration. In these patients, air space enlargement is severe and diffusing capacity is low. Dyspnea and hyperventilation are prominent, so that until very late in the disease, gas exchange is adequate and blood gas values are relatively normal. Because of prominent dyspnea and adequate oxygenation of hemoglobin, these patients sometimes are called "pink puffers".

The other extreme of the clinical presentation in emphysema is a patient who also has pronounced chronic bronchitis and a history of recurrent infections with purulent sputum. Dyspnea usually is less prominent, with diminished respiratory drive, so the patient retains carbon dioxide, becomes hypoxic, and often is cyanotic. For reasons not entirely clear, such patients tend to be obese hence the designation "blue bloaters." They often seek medical help after the onset of CHF(cor pulmonale) and associated edema. Death from emphysema is related to either pulmonary failure, with respiratory acidosis, hypoxia, and coma, or right-sided heart failure(cor pulmonale).

8.2.3   Asthma

Asthma is a chronic inflammatory disorder of the airways that causes recurrent episodes of wheezing, breathlessness, chest tightness, and cough, particularly at night and/or early in the morning. The hallmarks of the disease are intermittent and reversible airway obstruction, chronic bronchial in flammation with eosinophils, bronchial smooth muscle cell hypertrophy and hyperreactivity, and increased mucus secretion. Some of the stimuli that trigger attacks in patients would have little or no effect in persons with normal airways. Many cells can be found in the inflammatory response, particularly eosinophils, mast cells, macrophages, lymphocytes, neutrophils, and epithelial cells. The major etiologic factors of asthma are genetic predisposition to type I hypersensitivity(atopy), acute and chronic airway inflammation, and bronchial hyperresponsiveness to a variety of stimuli. The inflammation involves many cell types and numerous inflammatory mediators, but the role of type 2 helper T(TH2)cells may be critical to the pathogenesis of asthma.

8.2.3.1   Morphology

Grossly, the lungs are overdistended because of overin flation, and there may be small areas of atelectasis. The most striking macroscopic finding is occlusion of bronchi and bronchioles by thick, tenacious mucous plugs. Histologically, the mucous plugs contain whorls of shed epithelium. Amount of eosinophils and CharcotLeyden crystals also appear. Other characteristic morphologic changes in asthma, collectively called "airway remodeling," include: ①Thickening of the basement membrane of the airway wall; ②Increased vascularity in submucosa; ③An increase in size of the submucosal glands; ④Hypertrophy and/or hyperplasia of the bronchial muscle.

8.2.3.2   Clinical Features

An attack of asthma is characterized by severe dyspnea with wheezing; the chief difficulty lies in expiration. In the usual case, attacks last from 1 to several hours and subside either spontaneously or with therapy, usually bronchodilators and corticosteroids. The associated hypercapnia, acidosis, and severe hypoxia may be fatal, although in most cases the condition is more disabling than lethal.

8.2.4   Bronchiectasis

Bronchiectasis is the permanent dilation of bronchi and bronchioles caused by destruction of the muscle and the supporting elastic tissue, resulting from or associated with chronic necrotizing infections. It is not a primary disease but rather secondary to persisting infection or obstruction caused by a variety of conditions. Once developed, it gives rise to a characteristic symptom complex dominated by cough and expectoration of copious amounts of purulent sputum. Diagnosis depends on an appropriate history along with radiographic demonstration of bronchial dilation. In these conditions, bronchiectasis easily happen, which are bronchial obstruction, congenital or hereditary conditions, necrotizing or suppurative pneumonia.

8.2.4.1 Morphology

The disease usually affects the lower lobes bilaterally, particularly those air passages that are most vertical. When caused by tumors or aspiration of foreign bodies the involvement may be sharply localized to a single segment of the lungs. Usually, the most severe involvement is found in the more distal bronchi and bronchioles. The airways may be dilated to as much as four times their usual diameter, and grossly, the lung can be followed almost to the pleural surfaces. Compared to normal lungs, the bronchioles cannot be followed by ordinary gross examination beyond a point 2 to 3 cm from the pleural surfaces. Histologically, findings vary with the activity and chronicity of the disease. In typical case, an intense acute and chronic inflammatory exudate within the walls of the bronchi and bronchioles and the desquamation of lining epithelium cause extensive areas of ulceration. In the usual case, a mixed flora can be cultured from the involved bronchi, including staphylococ-

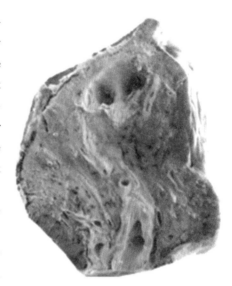

Figure 8-7 Bronchiectasis

ci, streptococci, pneumococci, enteric organisms, anaerobic and microaerophilic bacteria, and (particularly in children) Haemophilus in fluenzae and Pseudomonas aeruginosa. Fibrosis of the bronchial and bronchiolar walls and peribronchiolar fibrosis develop in more chronic cases. Sometimes, the necrosis destroys the bronchial or bronchiolar walls resulting in the formation of an abscess cavity within which a fungus ball may develop (Figure 8-7).

8.2.4.2 Clinical Features

The clinical manifestations consist of severe, persistent cough with expectoration of mucopurulent, sometimes fetid sputum. The sputum may contain flecks of blood; frank hemoptysis can occur. The patients may take on clubbing of the fingers. In severe cases, widespread bronchiectasis, with significant obstructive ventilatory defects are usual, with hypoxemia, hypercapnia, pulmonary hypertension, and (rarely) cor pulmonale.

8.3 Pneumoconiosis

Pneumoconiosis is originally coined to describe the non-neoplastic lung reaction to inhalation of mineral dusts. The term has been broadened to include diseases induced by organic as well as inorganic particulates, and some experts also regard chemical fume-and vapor-induced non-neoplastic lung diseases as pneumoconioses. with mineral dust pneumoconioses—the three most common of which result from exposure to coal dust, silica, and asbestos-nearly always result from exposure in the workplace. However, the increased risk of cancer as a result of asbestos exposure extends to happen to family members of asbestos workers and to other persons exposed to asbestos outside of the workplace.

8.3.1   Pathogenesis

The reaction of the lungs to mineral dusts depends on many factors, including size, shape, solubility and reactivity of the particles. For example, particles greater than 5–10 μm are unlikely to reach distal airways, whereas particles smaller than 0.5 μm move into and out of alveoli, often without substantial deposition and injury. Particles that are 1–5 μm in diameter are the most dangerous, because they get lodged at the bifurcation of the distal airways. Coal dust is relatively inert, and large amounts must be deposited in the lungs before lung disease is clinically detectable. Silica, asbestos, and beryllium are more reactive than coal dust, resulting in fibrotic reactions at lower concentrations. Most inhaled dust is entrapped in the mucus blanket and rapidly removed from the lung by ciliary movement. But some of the particles become impacted at alveolar duct bifurcations, where macrophages accumulate and engulf the trapped particulates. The pulmonary alveolar macrophage is a key cellular element in the initiation and perpetuation of lung injury and fibrosis. Many particles activate the in flammasome and induce IL-1 production. The more reactive particles trigger the macrophages to release a number of products that mediate an in flammatory response and initiate fibroblast proliferation and collagen deposition. Some of the inhaled particles may reach the lymphatics either by direct drainage or within migrating macrophages and thereby initiate an immune response to components of the particulates and(or) to self-proteins that are modified by the particles. This then results in an amplification and extension of the local reaction. Tobacco smoking worsens the effects of all inhaled mineral dusts, more so with asbestos than with any other particle.

8.3.2   Silicosis

Silicosis is the most common pneumoconiosis in the world, and crystalline silica is the usual cause, mostly in occupational settings. Workers in several occupations especially those involved in sandblasting and hard-rock mining are at particular risk. Silica occurs in both crystalline and amorphous forms, but crystalline forms are by far the most toxic and fibronectin. Of these, quartz is most commonly implicated in silicosis. After inhalation the particles, 1–5 μm in diameter, interact with epithelial cells and macrophages. Ingested silica particles cause activation and release of mediators by pulmonary macrophages, including IL-1, TNF, fibronectin lipid mediators, oxygen-derived free radicals, and fibronectin cytokines.

8.3.2.1   Morphology

Grossly silicotic nodules are characterized in their early stages by tiny, barely palpable, discrete, pale-to-blackened(if coal dust is also present)nodules in the upper zones of the lungs(Figure 8–8). Histologically, the silicotic nodule is concentrically arranged hyalinized collagen fibers surrounding an amorphous center. The "whorled" appearance of the collagen fibers is quite distinctive for silicosis(Figure 8–9). Examination of the nodules using polarized microscopy reveals weakly birefringent silica particles, primarily in the center of the nodules. With the disease developing, the individual nodules may coalesce into hard, collagenous scars, with eventual progression to PMF(progressive massive fibrosis). The intervening lung parenchyma may be compressed or over-expanded, and a honeycomb pattern may develop. Fibrotic lesions may be seen in the hilar lymph nodes and pleura. Sometimes, the lymph nodes take on the thin sheets of calcification, and radiographically as "eggshell" calcification.

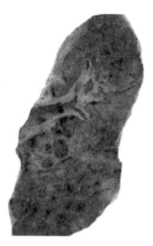

Figure 8-8　Silicosis

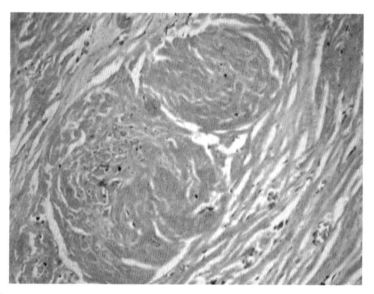

Figure 8-9　Silicosis(silicotic nodule)

8.3.2.2　Clinical Features

Usually, silicosis is detected on routine chest radiographs obtained in asymptomatic workers. The radiographs typically show a fine nodularity in the upper zones of the lung, but pulmonary function is either normal or only moderately affected. Most patients do not develop shortness of breath until in later stage of the disease, after PMF is present. Even if the person is no longer exposed, the disease may be still progressive. Many patients with PMF develop pulmonary hypertension and cor pulmonale, as a result of chronic hypoxia-induced vasoconstriction and parenchymal destruction. The disease is slow to kill, but impaired pulmonary function may severely limit activity. Silicosis is easily associated with an increased susceptibility to tuberculosis(silico-tuberculosis), and other infections. It is postulated that silicosis results in a depression of cell-mediated immunity, and crystalline silica may inhibit the ability of pulmonary macrophages to kill phagocytosed mycobacteria.

8.3.3   Coal Worker's Pneumoconiosis

The spectrum of lung findings in coal workers is wide, ranging from asymptomatic anthracosis, in which pigment accumulates without a perceptible cellular reaction, to simple coal worker's pneumoconiosis (CWP), in which accumulations of macrophages occur with little to no pulmonary dysfunction, to complicated CWP or PMF, in which fibrosis is extensive and lung function is compromised. Although statistics vary, it seems that less than 10% of cases of simple CWP progress to PMF. Of note PMF is a generic term that applies to a con fluent fibrosing reaction in the lung; this can be a complication of any one of the pneumoconioses discussed here. Although coal is mainly carbon, coal mine dust contains a variety of trace metals, inorganic minerals, and crystalline silica. The ratio of carbon to contaminating chemicals and minerals ("coal rank") increases from bituminous to anthracite coal; in general, anthracite mining has been associated with a higher risk of CWP.

8.3.3.1   Morphology

Pulmonary anthracosis is the most innocuous coal induced pulmonary lesion in coal miners and also is commonly seen in all urban dwellers and tobacco smokers. Inhaled carbon pigment is engulfed by alveolar or interstitial macrophages, which then accumulate in the connective tissue along the lymphatics, including the pleural lymphatics, or in lymph nodes. Simple CWP is characterized by coal macules and the somewhat larger coal nodule. The coal macule consists of dust-laden macrophages; in addition, the nodule contains small amounts of collagen fibers arrayed in a delicate network. The lesions are scattered in the upper lobes and upper zones of the lower lobes are more (Figure 8-10).

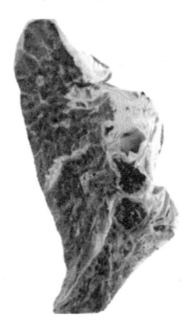

Figure 8-10   Coal Worker's Pneumoconiosis

8.3.3.2   Clinical Features

CWP is usually a benign disease that produces little decrement in lung function. If patients develop PMF, pulmonary dysfunction, pulmonary hypertension, and cor pulmonale may occur. Progression from CWP to PMF has been linked to a variety of conditions including coal dust exposure level and total dust burden. Unfortunately, PMF has a tendency to progress even in the absence of further exposure.

8.3.4 Asbestosis

Asbestos is a family of crystalline hydrated silicates with a fibrous geometry. On the basis of epidemiologic studies, occupational exposure to asbestos is linked to ①parenchymal interstitial fibrosis(*asbestosis*) ; ②localized fibrous plaques or, rarely, diffuse fibrosis in the pleura; ③pleural effusions; ④lung carcinomas; ⑤malignant pleural and peritoneal mesotheliomas; ⑥laryngeal carcinoma. An increased incidence of asbestos-related cancers in family members of asbestos workers has alerted the general public to the potential hazards of asbestos in the environment.

8.3.4.1 Pathogenesis

Concentration, size, shape, and solubility of the different forms of asbestos dictate whether inhalation of the material will cause disease. There are two distinct forms of asbestos: serpentine, in which the fiber is curly and flexible, and amphibole, in which the fiber is straight, stiff, and brittle. The serpentine chrysotile accounts for most of the asbestos used in industry. Amphiboles, even though less prevalent, are more pathogenic than the serpentine chrysotile, but both types can produce asbestosis, lung cancer, and mesothelioma.

8.3.4.2 Morphology

Diffuse pulmonary interstitial fibrosis, visceral pleura thickening, pleural plaques in parietal pleura, asbestos bodies are the main feature in asbestosis. Asbestos bodies apparently are formed when macrophages attempt to phagocytose asbestos fibers, the iron is derived from phagocyte ferritin. Asbestos bodies sometimes can be found in the lungs of normal persons, but usually in much lower concentrations and without an accompanying interstitial fibrosis. Asbestosis begins in the lower lobes and subpleural, but the middle and upper lobes of the lungs become affected with fibrosis progressing. Contraction of the fibrous tissue distorts the normal architecture, creating enlarged air spaces enclosed within thick fibrous walls. Simultaneously, fibrosis develops in the visceral pleura, causing adhesions between the lungs and the chest wall. The scarring may trap and narrow pulmonary arteries and arterioles, causing pulmonary hypertension and cor pulmonale. Pleural plaques in parietal pleura are the most common manifestation of asbestos exposure and are well-circumscribed plaques of dense collagen, often containing calcium. They do not contain asbestos bodies, and only rarely do they occur in persons with no history or evidence of asbestos exposure. Uncommonly, asbestos exposure induces pleural effusion or diffuse pleural fibrosis.

8.3.4.3 Clinical Features

The clinical findings in asbestosis are indistinguishable from those of any other chronic interstitial lung disease. Typically, progressively worsening dyspnea appears 10 to 20 years after exposure. The dyspnea is usually accompanied by a cough associated with production of sputum. The disease may remain static or progress to congestive heart failure, cor pulmonale, and death. Pleural plaques are usually asymptomatic and are detected on radiographs as circumscribed densities. Both lung carcinoma and malignant mesothelioma develop in workers exposed to asbestos. The risk of lung carcinoma is increased about five times for asbestos workers.

8.4　Pulmonary Hypertensive Heart Disease—Cor Pulmonale

Cor pulmonale consists of right ventricular hypertrophy and dilation frequently accompanied by right heart failure that is caused by pulmonary hypertension attributable to primary disorders of the lung parenchyma or pulmonary vasculature.

Morphology

Chronic cor pulmonale is characterized by right ventricular (and often right atrial) hypertrophy. It results from pulmonary hypertension due to primary lung parenchymal or vascular disorders. Hypertrophy of both the right ventricle and the right atrium is characteristic. When ventricular failure develops, the right ventricle and atrium are often dilated. Because chronic cor pulmonale occurs in the setting of pulmonary hypertension, the pulmonary arteries often contain atheromatous plaques and other lesions, reflecting long-standing pressure elevations (Figure 8-11).

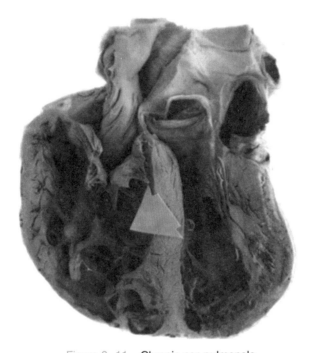

Figure 8-11　**Chronic cor pulmonale**

The right ventricle (shown on the left side of this picture) is markedly dilated and hypertrophied with a thickened free wall and hypertrophied trabeculae. The shape and volume of the left ventricle have been distorted by the enlarged right ventricle

Disorders Predisposing to Cor Pulmonale

Diseases of the Pulmonary Parenchyma

Chronic obstructive pulmonary disease

Diffuse pulmonary interstitial fibrosis

Pneumoconiosis

Cystic fibrosis

Bronchiectasis

Diseases of the Pulmonary Vessels

Recurrent pulmonary thromboembolism

Primary pulmonary hypertension

Extensive pulmonary arteritis (e. g. , Wegener granulomatosis)

Drug-, toxin-, or radiation-induced vascular obstruction

Extensive pulmonary tumor microembolism

Disorders Affecting Chest Movement

Kyphoscoliosis

Marked obesity(pickwickian syndrome)

Neuromuscular diseases

Disorders Inducing Pulmonary Arterial Constriction

Metabolic acidosis

Hypoxemia

Obstruction to major airways

Idiopathic alveolar hypoventilation.

8.5   Acute Respiratory Distress Syndrome(ARDS)

Acute respiratory distress syndrome(ARDS)is a clinical syndrome caused by diffuse alveolar capillary and epithelial damage. The usual course is characterized by rapid onset of life-threatening respiratory insufficiency,cyanosis,and severe arterial hypoxemia that is refractory to oxygen therapy and may progress to multisystem organ failure. The histologic manifestation of ARDS in the lungs is known as diffuse alveolar damage(DAD). It should be recalled that respiratory distress syndrome of the newborn is pathogenetically distinct;it is caused by a primary deficiency of surfactant.

8.5.1   Morphology

In the acute phase of ARDS,the lungs are dark red,firm,airless,and heavy. Microscopic examination reveals capillary congestion, necrosis of alveolar epithelial cells, interstitial and intra-alveolar edema and hemorrhage,and(particularly with sepsis)collections of neutrophils in capillaries. The most characteristic finding is the presence of hyaline membranes,particularly lining the distended alveolar ducts. Such membranes consist of fibrin-rich edema fluid admixed with remnants of necrotic epithelial cells. In the organizing stage,vigorous proliferation of type Ⅱ pneumocytes occurs in an attempt to regenerate the alveolar lining. Resolution is unusual;more commonly,there is organization of the fibrin exudates,with resultant intra-alveolar fibrosis. Marked thickening of the alveolar septa ensues,caused by proliferation of interstitial cells and deposition of collagen.

8.5.2   Pathogenesis

The alveolar-capillary membrane is formed by two separate barriers:the microvascular endothelium and the alveolar epithelium. In ARDS,the integrity of this barrier is compromised by either endothelial or epithelial injury,or,more commonly,both. The acute consequences of damage to the alveolar capillary membrane include increased vascular permeability and alveolar flooding,loss of diffusion capacity,and widespread surfactant abnormalities caused by damage to type Ⅱ pneumocytes. Although the cellular and molecular basis of acute lung injury and ARDS remain an area of active investigation,recent work suggests that in ARDS, lung injury is caused by an imbalance of pro-inflammatory and anti-inflammatory mediators. As early as 30 minutes after an acute insult,there is increased synthesis of interleukin 8(IL-8),a potent neutrophil chemotactic and activating agent,by pulmonary macrophages. Release of this and similar mediators,such as IL-1 and tumor necrosis factor(TNF),leads to endothelial activation as well as sequestration and activation of neutrophils in pulmonary capillaries. Neutrophils are thought to have an important role in the pathogenesis of

ARDS. Histologic examination of lungs early in the disease process shows increased numbers of neutrophils within the vascular space, the interstitium, and the alveoli. Activated neutrophils release a variety of products (e. g. , oxidants, proteases, platelet-activating factor, leukotrienes) that cause damage to the alveolar epithelium and endothelium. Combined assault on the endothelium and epithelium perpetuates vascular leakiness and loss of surfactant that render the alveolar unit unable to expand. Of note, the destructive forces unleashed by neutrophils can be counteracted by an array of endogenous antiproteases, antioxidants, and anti-inflammatory cytokines (e. g. , IL-10) that are upregulated by pro-inflammatory cytokines. In the end, it is the balance between the destructive and protective factors that determines the degree of tissue injury and clinical severity of ARDS.

8.6   Respiratory Distress Syndrome of the Newborn

There are many causes of respiratory distress in the newborn, including excessive sedation of the mother, fetal head injury during delivery, aspiration of blood or amniotic fluid, and intrauterine hypoxia secondary to compression from coiling of the umbilical cord about the neck. The most common cause, however, is respiratory distress syndrome (RDS), also known as hyaline membrane disease because of the formation of "membranes" in the peripheral air spaces observed in infants who succumb to this condition.

8.6.1   Morphology

The lungs in infants with RDS are of normal size but are heavy and relatively airless. They have a mottled purple color, and on microscopic examination the tissue appears solid, with poorly developed, generally collapsed (atelectatic) alveoli. If the infant dies within the first several hours of life, only necrotic cellular debris will be present in the terminal bronchioles and alveolar ducts. Later in the course, characteristic eosinophilic hyaline membranes line the respiratory bronchioles, alveolar ducts, and random alveoli. These "membranes" contain necrotic epithelial cells admixed with extravasated plasma proteins.

8.6.2   Pathogenesis

RDS is basically a disease of premature infants associated with male gender, maternal diabetes, and delivery by cesarean section. The fundamental defect in RDS is the inability of the immature lung to synthesize sufficient surfactant. Surfactant is a complex of surface-active phospholipids, principally dipalmitoyl phosphatidylcholine (lecithin) and at least two groups of surfactant-associated proteins. The importance of surfactant-associated proteins in normal lung function can be gauged by the occurrence of severe respiratory failure in neonates with congenital deficiency of surfactant caused by mutations in the corresponding genes. Surfactant is synthesized by type Ⅱ pneumocytes and, with the healthy newborn's first breath, rapidly coats the surface of alveoli, reducing surface tension and thus decreasing the pressure required to keep alveoli open. In a lung deficient in surfactant, alveoli tend to collapse, and a relatively greater inspiratory effort is required with each breath to open the alveoli. The infant rapidly tires from breathing, and generalized atelectasis sets in. The resulting hypoxia sets into motion a sequence of events that lead to epithelial and endothelial damage and eventually to the formation of hyaline membranes.

8.7 Carcinomas of the Lung

Carcinoma of the lung(also known as "lung cancer")is without doubt the single most important cause of cancer related deaths in industrialized countries. The incidence among males is gradually decreasing, but it continues to increase among females, with more women dying each year from lung cancer than from breast cancers, since 1987. These statistics undoubtedly reflect the causal relationship of cigarette smoking and lung cancer. The peak incidence of lung cancer is in persons in their 50 s and 60 s. At diagnosis, more than 50% of patients already have distant metastatic disease, while a fourth have disease in the regional lymph nodes. The prognosis of lung cancer is dismal: The 5−year survival rate for all stages of lung cancer combined is about 16% , a figure that has not changed much over the last 30 years; even with disease localized to the lung, a 5−year survival rate of only 45% is typical.

The four major histologic types of carcinomas of the lung are adenocarcinoma, squamous cell carcinoma, small cell carcinoma, and large cell carcinoma. In some cases there is a combination of histologic patterns(e. g. , small cell carcinoma and adenocarcinoma). Of these, squamous cell and small cell carcinomas show the strongest association with smoking. Until recently, carcinomas of the lung were classified into two broad groups: small cell lung cancer(SCLC)and non-small cell lung cancer(NSCLC) , with the latter including adenocarcinomas and squamous and large cell carcinomas.

Histologic Classification of Malignant Epithelial

Lung Tumors

Adenocarcinoma *

Acinar, papillary, micropapillary, solid, lepidic predominant, mucinous subtypes

Squamous cell carcinoma

Large cell carcinoma

Large cell neuroendocrine carcinoma

Small cell carcinoma

Combined small cell carcinoma

Adenosquamous carcinoma

Carcinomas with pleomorphic, sarcomatoid, or sarcomatous elements

Spindle cell carcinoma

Giant cell carcinoma

Carcinoid tumor

Typical, atypical

Carcinomas of salivary gland type

Unclassified carcinoma

* Adenocarcinoma and squamous cell and large cell carcinoma are collectively referred to as non-small cell lung carcinoma(NSCLC).

8.7.1 Morphology

Carcinomas of the lung begin as small mucosal lesions that typically are firm and gray-white. They may arise as intraluminal masses, invade the bronchial mucosa, or form large bulky masses pushing into adjacent lung parenchyma. Some large masses undergo cavitation secondary to central necrosis or develop focal areas of hemorrhage. Finally, these tumors may extend to the pleura, invade the pleural cavity and chest wall, and spread to adjacent intrathoracic structures. More distant spread can occur by way of the lymphatics or the hematogenous route.

8.7.1.1   Squamous cell carcinomas

They are more common in men than in women and are closely correlated with a smoking history; they tend to arise centrally in major bronchi and eventually spread to local hilar nodes, but they disseminate outside the thorax later than do other histologic types. Large lesions may undergo central necrosis, giving rise to cavitation. Squamous cell carcinomas are often preceded by the development, over years, of squamous metaplasia or dysplasia in the bronchial epithelium, which then transforms into carcinoma in situ, a phase that may last for several years. By this time, atypical cells may be identified in cytologic smears of sputum or in bronchial lavage fluids or brushings, although the lesion is asymptomatic and undetectable on radiographs. Eventually, the small neoplasm reaches a symptomatic stage, when a well-defined tumor mass begins to obstruct the lumen of a major bronchus, often producing distal atelectasis and infection. Simultaneously, the lesion invades surrounding pulmonary parendyma (Figure 8 – 12A). On histologic examination, these tumors range from well differentiated squamous cell neoplasms showing keratin pearls (Figure 8 – 12B) and intercellular bridges to poorly differentiated neoplasms exhibiting only minimal residual squamous cell features.

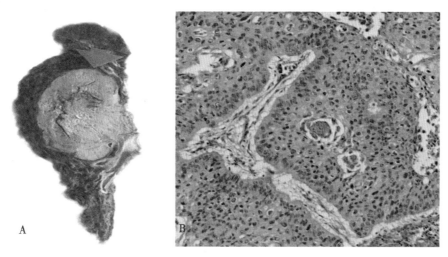

Figure 8–12   A: Squamous cell carcinoma usually begins as a central (hilar) mass and grows contiguously into the peripheral parenchyma as seen here. B: Well-differentiated squamous cell carcinoma showing keratinization and pearls

8.7.1.2   Adenocarcinomas

They may occur as central lesions like the squamous cell variant but usually are more peripherally located, many with a central scar. Adenocarcinomas are the most common type of lung cancer in women and nonsmokers. In general, adenocarcinomas grow slowly and form smaller masses than do the other subtypes, but they tend to metastasize widely at an early stage. On histologic examination, they may assume a variety of forms, including acinar (gland-forming), papillary, mucinous (formerly mucinous bronchioloalveolar carcinoma, which often is multifocal and may manifest as pneumonia-like consolidation), and solid types. The solid variant often requires demonstration of intracellular mucin production by special stains to establish its adenocarcinomatous lineage (Figure 8 – 13).

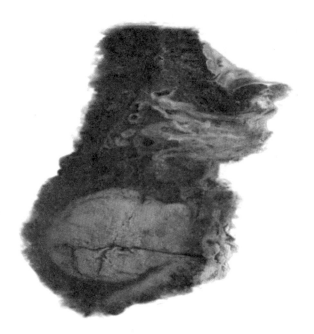

Figure 8−13 Adenocarcinomas are common in more
women than man, and almost are Gland-forming

8.7.1.3 Adenocarcinoma in Situ(AIS)

Formerly called bronchioloalveolar carcinoma, often involves peripheral parts of the lung, as a single nodule. The key features of AIS are diameter of 3 cm or less, growth along preexisting structures, and preservation of alveolar architecture. The tumor cells, which may be nonmucinous, mucinous, or mixed, grow in a monolayer along the alveolar septa, which serve as a scaffold(this has been termed a "lepidic" growth pattern, an allusion to the resemblance of neoplastic cells to butterflies sitting on a fence). By definition, AIS does not demonstrate destruction of alveolar architecture or stromal invasion with desmoplasia, but has features that would merit the diagnosis of frank adenocarcinoma. By analogy to the adenoma-carcinoma sequence in the colon, it is proposed that some invasive adenocarcinomas of the lung may arise through an atypical adenomatous hyperplasia-adenocarcinoma in situ-invasive adenocarcinoma sequence.

8.7.1.4 Large Cell Carcinomas

They are undifferentiated malignant epithelial tumors that lack the cytologic features of small cell carcinoma and have no glandular or squamous differentiation.

The cells typically have large nuclei, prominent nucleoli, and a moderate amount of cytoplasm. Large cell carcinomas probably represent squamous cell or adenocarcinomas that are so undifferentiated that they can no longer be recognized by means of light microscopy. On ultrastructural examination, however, minimal glandular or squamous differentiation is common.

8.7.1.5 Small Cell Lung Carcinomas(SCLCs)

Generally appear as pale gray, centrally located masses with extension into mediastinal nodes. These cancers are composed of tumor cells with a round to fusiform shape, scant cytoplasm, and finely granular chromatin. Mitotic figures frequently are seen. Despite the appellation of small, the neoplastic cells are usually twice the size of resting lymphocytes. Necrosis is invariably present and may be extensive. The tumor cells are markedly fragile and often show fragmentation and "crush artifact" in small biopsy specimens. Another feature of small cell carcinomas, best appreciated in cytologic specimens, is nuclear molding resulting from close apposition of tumor cells that have scant cytoplasm. These tumors often express a variety of neuroendocrine markers in addition to secreting a host of polypeptide hormones that may result in paraneoplastic syndromes.

8.7.1.6　Combined patterns

Require no further comment. Of note, however, a significant minority of lung carcinomas reveal more than one line of cellular differentiation, sometimes several, suggesting that all are derived from a multipotential progenitor cell. For all of these neoplasms, ent of successive chains of nodes about the carina, it is possible to trace involvement of successive chains of nodes about the carina, in the mediastinum, and in the neck (scalene nodes) and clavicular regions and, sooner or later, distant metastases. Involvement of the left supraclavicular node (Virchow node) is particularly characteristic and sometimes calls attention to an occult primary tumor. These cancers, when advanced, often extend into the pleural or pericardial space, leading to inflammation and effusion. They may compress or infiltrate the superior vena cava to cause either venous congestion or the vena caval syndrome. Apical neoplasms may invade the brachial or cervical sympathetic plexus to cause severe pain in the distribution of the ulnar nerve or to produce Horner syndrome (ipsilateral enophthalmos, ptosis, miosis, and anhidrosis). Such apical neoplasms sometimes are called Pancoast tumors, and the combination of clinical findings is known as Pancoast syndrome. Pancoast tumor often is accompanied by destruction of the first and second ribs and sometimes thoracic vertebrae. As with other cancers, tumornode-metastasis (TNM) categories have been established to indicate the size and spread of the primary neoplasm.

8.7.2　Pathogenesis

Smoking-related carcinomas of the lung arise by a stepwise accumulation of a multitude of genetic abnormalities (estimated to be in the thousands for small cell carcinoma) that result in transformation of benign progenitor cells in the lung into neoplastic cells.

With regard to carcinogenic influences, there is strong evidence that cigarette smoking and, to a much lesser extent, other environmental insults are the main culprits responsible for the genetic changes that give rise to lung cancers. About 90% of lung cancers occur in active smokers or those who stopped recently. A nearly linear correlation has been recognized between the frequency of lung cancer and pack-years of cigarette smoking. The increased risk becomes 60 times greater among habitual heavy smokers (two packs a day for 20 years) than among nonsmokers. Since only 11% of heavy smokers develop lung cancer, however, other predisposing factors must be operative in the pathogenesis of this deadly disease. For reasons not entirely clear, women have a higher susceptibility to carcinogens in tobacco than men. Although cessation of smoking decreases the risk of developing lung cancer over time, it may never return to baseline levels.

Other influences may act in concert with smoking or may by themselves be responsible for some lung cancers; witness the increased incidence of this form of neoplasia in miners of radioactive ores; asbestos workers; and workers exposed to dusts containing arsenic, chromium, uranium, nickel, vinyl chloride, and mustard gas. Exposure to asbestos increases the risk of lung cancer fivefold in nonsmokers. By contrast, heavy smokers exposed to asbestos have an approximately 55 times greater risk for development of lung cancer than that for nonsmokers not exposed to asbestos.

The sequential changes leading to cancer have been best documented for squamous cell carcinomas, but they also are present in other histologic subtypes. In essence, there is a linear correlation between the intensity of exposure to cigarette smoke and the appearance of ever more worrisome epithelial changes that begin with rather innocuous basal cell hyperplasia and squamous metaplasia and progress to squamous dysplasia and carcinoma in situ, before culminating in invasive cancer. Among the major histologic subtypes of lung cancer, squamous and small-cell carcinomas show the strongest association with tobacco exposure.

8.8   Nasopharyngeal Carcinoma

Nasopharyngeal carcinoma is a rare neoplasm that merits comment because of ①the strong epidemiologic links to EBV and ②the high frequency of this form of cancer among the Chinese, which raises the possibility of viral oncogenesis on a background of genetic susceptibility. It is thought that EBV infects the host by first replicating in the nasopharyngeal epithelium and then infecting nearby tonsillar B lymphocytes. In some persons this leads to transformation of the epithelial cells. In infectious mononucleosis, EBV directly infects B lymphocytes, after which a marked proliferation of reactive T lymphocytes causes atypical lymphocytosis, seen in the peripheral blood, and enlarged lymph nodes. Similarly, in nasopharyngeal carcinomas, a striking influx of mature lymphocytes often can be seen. These neoplasms are therefore referred to as "lymphoepitheliomas"-a misnomer, because the lymphocytes are neither part of the neoplastic process, nor the benign tumors. The presence of large neoplastic cells in a background of reactive lymphocytes may give rise to an appearance similar to that in non-Hodgkin lymphomas, and immunohistochemical stains may be required to prove the epithelial nature of the malignant cells. Nasopharyngeal carcinomas invade locally, spread to cervical lymph nodes, and then metastasize to distant sites. They tend to be radiosensitive, and 5-year survival rates of 50% are reported even for patients with advanced cancers.

8.9   Carcinoma of the Larynx

Carcinoma of the larynx represents only 2% of all cancers. It most commonly occurs after age 40 years and is more common in men than in women (with a gender ratio of 7 : 1). Environmental influences are very important in its causation; nearly all cases occur in smokers and alcohol and asbestos exposure may also play roles. Human papillomavirus sequences have been detected in about 15% of tumors, which tend to have a better prognosis than other carcinomas.

Carcinoma of the larynx manifests itself clinically with persistent hoarseness. The location of the tumor within the larynx has a significant bearing on prognosis. For example, about 90% of glottic tumors are confined to the larynx at diagnosis. First, as a result of interference with vocal cord mobility, they develop symptoms early in the course of disease; second, the glottic region has a sparse lymphatic supply, and spread beyond the larynx is uncommon. By contrast, the supraglottic larynx is rich in lymphatic spaces, and nearly a third of these tumors metastasize to regional (cervical) lymph nodes. The subglottic tumors tend to remain clinically quiescent, usually manifesting as advanced disease. With surgery, radiation therapy, or combination treatment, many patients can be cured, but about one third die of the disease. The usual cause of death is infection of the distal respiratory passages or widespread metastases and cachexia.

8.10   Pleural Lesions

Pathologic involvement of the pleura is, with rare exceptions, a secondary complication of an underlying pulmonary disease. Evidence of secondary infection and pleural adhesions are particularly common findings at autopsy. Important primary disorders are ①primary intrapleural bacterial infections and ②a primary neoplasm of the pleura known as malignant mesothelioma.

8.10.1   Pleural Effusion and Pleuritis

In pleural effusion(the presence of fluid in the pleural space)the fluid can be either a transudate or an exudate. When the pleural fluid is a transudate, the condition is termed hydrothorax. An exudate, characterized by protein content greater than 2.9gm/dL and, often, inflammatory cells, suggests pleuritis. The four principal causes of pleural exudate formation are ①microbial invasion through either direct extension of a pulmonary infection or blood-borne seeding(suppurative pleuritis or empyema); ②cancer(lung carcinoma, metastatic neoplasms to the lung or pleural surface, mesothelioma); ③pulmonary infarction; ④viral pleuritis. Other, less common causes of exudative pleural effusions are systemic lupus erythematosus, rheumatoid arthritis, and uremia, as well as previous thoracic surgery. Malignant effusions characteristically are large and frequently bloody(hemorrhagic pleuritis). Cytologic examination may reveal malignant and inflammatory cells.

8.10.2   Malignant Mesothelioma

Malignant mesothelioma is a rare cancer of mesothelial cells, usually arising in the parietal or visceral pleura, although it also occurs, much less commonly, in the peritoneum and pericardium. It has assumed great importance because it is related to occupational exposure to asbestos in the air. Approximately 50% of persons with this cancer have a history of exposure to asbestos. Those who work directly with asbestos (shipyard workers, miners, insulators) are at greatest risk, but malignant mesotheliomas have appeared in persons whose only exposure was living in proximity to an asbestos factory or being a relative of an asbestos worker. The latent period for developing malignant mesothelioma is long, often 25 to 40 years after initial asbestos exposure, suggesting that multiple somatic genetic events are required for neoplastic conversion of a mesothelial cell.

▶▶ *Morphology*

Malignant mesotheliomas are often preceded by extensive pleural fibrosis and plaque formation, readily seen on computed tomography scans. These tumors begin in a localized area and over time spread widely, either by contiguous growth or by diffusely seeding the pleural surfaces. At autopsy, the affected lung typically is ensheathed by a yellow-white, firm, sometimes gelatinous layer of tumor that obliterates the pleural space. Distant metastases are rare. The neoplasm may directly invade the thoracic wall or the subpleural lung tissue. Normal mesothelial cells are biphasic, giving rise to pleural lining cells as well as the underlying fibrous tissue. Therefore, histologically, mesotheliomas conform to one of three patterns: ①epithelial, in which cuboidal cells line tubular and microcystic spaces, into which small papillary buds project; this is the most common pattern and also the one which most likely to be confused with the pulmonary adenocarcinoma; ② sarcomatous, in which spindled and sometimes fibroblastic-appearing cells grow in nondistinctive sheets; ③ biphasic, having both sarcomatous and epithelial areas.

Chapter 9

Degistive System Diseases

❯ Introduction

The digestive system consists of two main parts: digestive tract and digestive gland. Digestive tract includes oral, pharynx, esophagus, stomach, small intestine (duodenum, jejunum, ileum) and large intestine (cecum, appendix, colon, rectum, anal canal). Four of the ten most serious malignancies in China are from the digestive system, including esophageal carcinoma, gastric carcinoma, liver carcinoma, colorectalcarcinoma. Inflammation of the digestive system is also common, such as appendicitis, cholecystitis, cholelithiasis, acute pancreatitis. This chapter will discuss diseases of gastrointestinal tract, the liver and biliary tract, and pancreas.

9.1 Esophagitis

9.1.1 Reflux Esophagitis

Reflux esophagitisis is defined as chronic inflammation in the lower esophageal mucosa caused by reflux of gastric juice. It is also known as gastroesophageal reflux disease(GERD).

Pathological changes of local hyperemia is common and severe damage cause obvious hyperemia. Epithelial hyperplasia and infiltration of neutrophils and eosinophils can be found at early stage, sometimes local epithelial necrosis may develop into superficial ulcers; fibrosis occurs when inflammation spreads to the esophageal wall. Barrett esophagus can develop as a result of chronic inflammation.

Clinical features the clinical manifestations include nausea, heartburn, pain and dysphagia, sometimes vomiting and melena. However, the severity of the clinical symptoms is not necessarily consistent with histological changes of esophagitis.

9.1.2 Barrett Esophagus

Barrett esophagus is defined as the replacement of the normal stratified squamous epithelium of the lower oesophagus by metaplastic columnar epithelium containing goblet cells. Ulceration and canceration may happen.

Pathological changes Barrett esophageal mucosa presents visible orange-red, velvet-like irregular shaped lesions, a patch-like island or ring on the background of normal esophageal mucosa. Esophagus stenosis and hiatus hernia may be secondary to erosiveulcers.

Barrett esophageal mucosa has similar mucosal epithelial cells and glands of gastric intestinal. It can be diagnosed when intestinal goblet cells are found in columnar epithelial cells. In Barrett esophagus, columnar epithelial cells have the ultrastructural and cytochemical characteristics of both squamous and columnar epithelial cells.

Clinical features: The major complications of Barrett esophagus include peptic ulcer, stricture, bleeding, which are similar to reflux esophagitis. Sometimes, atypical hyperplasia and adenocarcinomamay occur.

9.2   Gastritis

Gastritis is defined as inflammatory disease of the gastric mucosa. It is common and can be divided into acute and chronic gastritis. Acute gastritis often has definite causes, while the causes and pathogenesis of chronic gastritis are complex and unclear by far.

9.2.1   Acute Gastritis

It is often caused by physical and chemical factors and microbial infections. Usually, it has four types as follows:

1) Acute irritant gastritis. It isusually caused by having too much hot or excitant food, or drinking strong alcohol. Under gastroscope, red mucosa, congestion and edema, mucus covering the surface, and sometimes erosion can be found.

2) Acute hemorrhagic gastritis. It is often caused by improper medication or excessive consumption of alcohol, in addition to stress response to trauma and surgery. Mucosal acute bleeding, mild erosion and multiple superficial stress may be seen.

3) Corrosive gastritis. It is often caused by corrosive chemical agent. Mucosa is necrotic and dissolved. The lesion may involve deep tissue or even lead to perforation.

4) Acute infective gastritis. Pyogenic bacteria such as *staphylococcus aureus*, *streptococcus*, *Escherichia coli* infect the stomach through the blood or due to stomach trauma. It can cause acute phlegmonous gastritis.

9.2.2   Chronic Gastritis

Chronic gastritis is a chronic non-specific inflammation of the gastric mucosa and has a high incidence.

The pathogenesis of chronic gastritis is still unknown. The causes can be divided into four types: ①H. pylori infection. H. pylori is a gram-negative bacillus which exists in the gastric epithelial surface or the mucous layer in glands of the patients. It can secrete urease, cytotoxin-related proteins and vacuolating cytotoxin and so on, which can cause chronic gastritis. ②Chronic stimulus, such as long-term drinking and smoking, abuse of salicylic acid, eating hot or spicy food, acute gastritis recurrent and so on. ③The destruction of gastric mucosa with duodenal liquid reflux. ④Autoimmune injury.

According to different pathological changes, it can be divided into four types:

9.2.2.1   Chronic Superficial Gastritis

It is also known as chronic simple gastritis and commonly occurs in the antrum. It can be multifocal or diffuse. It is one of the most common gastric mucosa diseases. Congestion, edema, sometimes slight bleeding or erosion can be seen under gastroscope. Grayish yellow or white mucous exudates cover the surface. Chronic inflammatory cells such as lymphocytes and plasma cells infiltrate in lamina propria. Most patients can be cured with therapy or reasonable diet. A few cases can develop into chronic atrophic gastritis.

9.2.2.2 Chronic Atrophic Gastritis

Gastric mucosa becomes atrophic and thinning, and mucosal glands are partial or complete loss with intestinal metaplasia. Lymphocytes and plasma cells infiltrate into lamina propria.

There are complex causes for the disease. Some may be associated with smoking, drinking or improper drug use; some may originate from chronic superficial gastritis; some belong to autoimmune diseases. Depending on whether it is associated with autoimmunity or accompanied by pernicious anemia, it can be divided into types A and B(Table 9−1). Type A belongs to autoimmune diseases, mainly in the body and fundus of stomach, with pernicious anemia. The antibodies against parietal cell and intrinsic factor are positive. Type B is more common in the gastric antrum, without pernicious anemia. In China, type B is more common. Mucosa lesions are similar in these two types of gastritis.

Under gastroscope, the mucosa turns into gray or gray-green; mucosal folds become thin or disappear; the mucosa is finely granular; submucosal blood vessels are visible. Hemorrhage and erosion are rare.

Microscopically: lymphocytes and plasma cells infiltrate in lamina propria with the formation of lymphatic follicles; stomach mucosa becomes thinner and glands are atrophic with sparsely distributed cystic dilatation(Figure 9−1); fibrous tissue hyperplasia can be observed in the gastric mucosa; pseudopyloric gland metaplasia and intestinal metaplasia can be found. Intestinal metaplasia refers to the replacement of gastric mucosal epithelium by intestinal epithelium. Atypical hyperplasia can be found in intestinal metaplasia. If there are both goblet cells and absorptive epithelial cells paneth cells, we call it complete metaplasia. If there are only goblet cells, we call it incomplete metaplasia. It has been reported that large intestine incomplete metaplasia is closely related with intestinal type carcinoma of stomach.

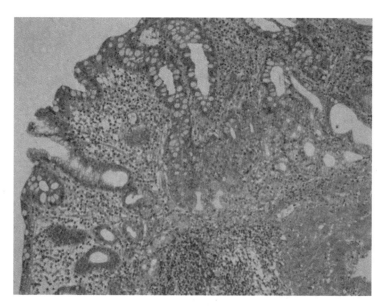

Figure 9−1　Chronic atrophic gastritis(HE)

Gastric mucosa becomes atrophic and thinning. Mucosal glands become fewer or disappear with intestinal metaplasia. Lymphocytes and plasma cells infiltrate into lamina propria

Pseudoplyloric gland metaplasia refers to the replacement of the parietal cells and the chief cells in the fundus and body of the stomach by the mucin-producing cells.

Clinico-pathological relationship: Secretion of gastric juice is reduced because of the decrease or disappearance of parietal cells and chief cells. Patients suffer from dyspepsia, poor appetite and upper abdominal discomfort. Type A patients are prone to have pernicious anemia because of the obvious destruction of parietal cells, the lack of internal factors and malabsorption of vitamin B_{12}. Atrophic gastritis is usually accompanied with varying degrees of intestinal metaplasia. In the derelopment of metaplasia, it will be inevitably accompanied with the proliferation of local epithelial cells, which may lead to carcinoma of stomach.

Table 9-1   Comparison of two types of chronic atrophic gastritis

	Type A	Type B
Etiology and pathogenesis	Autoimmunity	Infection with *H. pylori* (60% -70%)
Location	Gastric body or fundus	Gastric antrum
Anti-parietal cell and anti-intrinsic factor antibody	Positive	Negative
Serum gastrin level	High	Low
Hyperplasia of G cells	Yes	No
Autoantibody	Positive (>90%)	Negative
Secretion of gastric acid	Significant reduction	Moderate reduction or normal
Serum vitamin B_{12} level	Reduction	Normal
Pernicious anemia	Common	None
Peptic ulcer	None	Common

9.2.2.3   Chronic Hypertrophic Gastritis

It is also known as giant hypertrophic gastritis, Menetrier's-like disease. The pathogenesis is unknown. It often occurs in the body and fundus of stomach. Under gastroscopy, mucosal folds become deepened, widened and coarse, gyrus-like; transverse cracking on mucosal folds is visible with numerous verrucous protrusion; the top of mucosal protrusion is often accompanied by erosion. Gland hypertrophy and hyperplasia, and lumen extension are visible. Sometimes, hyperplasia glands break through the muscularis mucosa. The mucus secretion on mucosal surface is increased dueto increasing number of mucin-producing cells. In the lamina propria, inflammatory cell infiltration is unconspicuous.

9.2.2.4   Gastritis Verrucosa

Its etiology is unknown. It is a characteristic lesion, which usually occurs in the antrum. A lot of verrucous lesions with depressed centre appear on the gastritis mucosa. Under microscope, gastric epithelial degeneration, shedding and necrosis, accompanied by acute inflammatory exudate are noted.

9.3   Peptic Ulcer Disease

It is characterized by chronic ulcer in gastric or duodenal mucosa and is related to the self digestion of gastric juice. It is more common in adults (20-50 years old). Usually, it is a chronic recurrent disease. Duodenal ulcer is more common than gastric ulcer. The former accounts for 70%, the latter 25%, and the compound ulcer only 5%. Patients are prone to have periodic abdominal pain, acid reflux, and belching.

9.3.1 Causes and Pathogenesis

The causes are thought to be related to factors as follows:

1) The infection of helicobacter pylori. A large number of studies have shown that helicobacter pylori (Figure 9-2) play an important role in the pathogenesis of ulcers in the following aspects. ①They can release a bacterial platelet activating factor, which promotes the formation of thrombosis in the capillary, then lead to blood vessel obstruction, mucosal ischemia and so on. All of those may destroy gastric and duodenal mucosal defense barrier. ②They secrete urease that catalyzes the production of free ammonia and proteinase, which contribute to the cleavage of glycoprotein in the gastric mucosa. All those things result in the direct contact for gastric acid to the epithelium and mucous membrane, promoting the proliferation of G cells in the gastric mucosa and increasing the secretion of gastric acid. ③They also have the chemotaxis for neutrophils. Neutrophils can release myeloperoxidase and then produce hypochlorous. Ammonia chloride is synthesized if ammonia exists. Hypochlorous acid and ammonia chloride destroy mucosal epithelial cells and induce peptic ulcer.

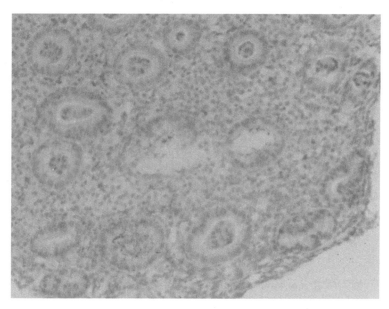

Figure 9-2 **Helicobacter pylori(IHC)**

Pyloric helicobacter pylori can be seen in chronic active inflammation of the gastric antrum. (Immunohistochemical detection of HP)

2) Decrease of mucosal anti-digestive ability. Under normal condition, the mucus is secreted by the gastric mucosa(mucus barrier) and the lipoprotein of mucosal epithelial cells(mucosa barrier) protect mucous membrane from being digested by the gastric juice. When gastric mucus secretion is insufficient or mucosa is damaged, barrier functions are weakened, reducing the resistance to digestion. Hydrogen ions in gastric juice reversely diffuse into the gastric mucosa, bring damage to capillaries in the mucosa and induce mast cells to release histamine, leading to local blood circulation disorder and gastric mucosa damage. Secretion of pepsinogen increases, which strengthens the digestive function of gastric juice, and leads to ulcers formation. The diffusing capacity of hydrogen ions in gastric antrum is 15 times higher than in gastric fundus, while in duodenum it is 2-3 times higher than in gastric antrum. That may explain the higher morbidity in duodenum and gastric antrum compared to other parts.

In addition, long term usage of non steroidal anti-inflammatory drugs, smoking and other factors that damage mucous membrane barrier can induce peptic ulcers disease.

3) Digestive effect of gastric juice. It has been proved that the disease is the result of stomach and duodenal mucosa tissue digestion by gastric acid and pepsin. In duodenal ulcer, the number of parietal cells increases significantly, and the increased gastric acid digests the mucous membrane. The environment of the jejunum and ileum is alkaline, in which ulceration rarely occurs. But after gastrojejunostomy, ulcers may occur in the anastomosis due to the digestion of gastric juice.

4) Neuroendocrine dysfunction. Mental stimulation causes functional dysfunction of cerebral cortex, which leads to dysfunction of autonomic nervous system. When duodenal ulcer occurs, vagus hyperfunction increases gastric acid secretion. But in gastric ulcer, vagus nerve excitation decreases, gastric peristalsis weakens, secretion of gastric acid increases induced by gastrin.

5) Genetic factors. Ulcers have a high tendency in some families, revealing that the occurrence of this disease may also be associated with genetic factors.

9.3.2   Pathological Changes

Grossly, gastric ulcer occurs at lesser curvature of the stomach near the pylorus side, most commonly in the gastric antrum area; more closer to the stomach pylorus, the more common it occurs. Usually, the ulcer is single, round or ellipse, two centimeters in diameter, with neat edges, clean flat bottom, often deep into myometrial layer, even to serosa. Generally the ulcer is deep in the side of the cardia, and shallow at the edge. The mucosal folds turn to radial owing to traction of scar formation at the bottom of the ulcer.

Undermicroscope, ulcers can be divided into four layers form mucosa to serosa: inflammatory exudate such as leukocyte and cellulose, necrotic tissue, granulation tissue, and scar tissue (Figure 9-3).

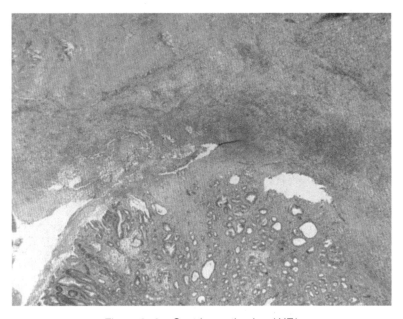

Figure 9-3   **Gastric peptic ulcer(HE)**

The most superficial layer is covered by a little inflammatory exudate such as leukocyte
and cellulose; the next is necrotic tissue; fresh granulation tissue can be seen in the third
layer; in the fourth layer, granulation tissue turns into old scar tissue

Duodenal ulcer is similar to gastric ulcer, but it occurs mainly in duodenal anterior or posterior wall. The ulcers are small, less than 1cm in diameter and easier to heal.

9.3.3 Outcomes and Complications

1) Healing. Exudates and necrotic tissues will be gradually absorbed or expelled if they do not recur. The damaged muscle layer can't regenerate, and will be filled with scar tissue formed by hyperplasia of the granulation tissue at the bottom. The surrounding mucosa epithelium will regenerate and cover the ulcers.

2) Complications. Hemorrhage(accounts for about 10% –35%): Fecal occult blood tests of the patients are positive due to the rupture of the capillaries at the bottom of ulcer. If the big blood vessel ruptures, hematemesis and tarry stools even hemorrhagic shock may be seen.

Perforation(accounts for about 5%): Duodenal ulcer is more prone to perforate because of the thinner wall. Gastrointestinal contents leak into the abdominal cavity causing peritonitis. If the perforation occurs in the posterior wall of the stomach, the contents of the stomach leak into lesser omentum sac.

Pyloric stenosis(accounts for about 3%): Prolonged ulcers tend to form large number of scars. Shrinking of the scars cause pyloric stenosis, making it difficult for gastric contents to pass through, and then secondary gastric dilatation. Patients vomit a lot and even develop alkalosis.

Cancerization(accounts for less than 1%): Cancerization is commonly seen in patients with long-term gastric ulcer and rarely seen in duodenal ulcer.

9.3.4 Clinico-pathological Relationship

Gastric acid stimulates local nerve endings in gastric ulcer, resulting in periodic upper abdominal pain. In addition, pain is also related to the spasm of smooth muscle in gastric wall. In duodenal ulcer, increased excitation of the vagus nerve increases secretion of gastric acid, so pain often occurs at night. Belching and acid regurgitation are related to factors such as pyloric sphincter spasm, gastric antiperistalsis, early pyloric stenosis.

9.4 Appendicitis

Appendicitis is a common disease. Its main clinical manifestations include metastatic right lower abdominal pain, vomiting accompanied with elevated body temperature and peripheral blooding neutrophils wunt. According to the course of disease, it can be divided into acute and chronic appendicitis.

9.4.1 Causes and Pathogenesis

Appendix is a slender blind tube with a narrow cavity. Feces and bacteria from the intestinal cavity canget easily trapped. The wall of appendix is rich in nerve tissue such as myenteric plexus. The end of appendix has a structure similar to the sphincter, so it is easy to shrink and the cavity become narrower when it is stimulated.

Appendicitis is caused by bacterial infection, but there is no specific pathogenic bacterium. 50% –80% of appendicitis is accompanied with the obstruction of appendix cavity. Feces and parasites cause mechanical obstruction. Various stimuli induce the contraction of appendix, resulting in blood circulation disorder of the appendix wall and injury of mucosa. Which changes are conducive to bacterial infection.

9.4.2　Pathological Changes

(1)Acute Appendicitis

It mainly has three subtypes. Acute simple appendicitis:It happens in early stage. Mild swelling of the appendix and serosal hyperemia are noted. Neutrophil infiltration, fibrin exudates and inflammatory edema can be seen, especially severe in the mucosa and submucosa.

Acute phlegmonous appendicitis:It is usually a developed ment of simple appendicitis. There are significant swelling and serosal hyperemia. The surface of the appendix is covered with purulent exudation. Microscopically, neutrophils, inflammatory edema and fibrous exudation extend from mucosa to deep layer, directly to the muscular and serous layer(Figure 9-4). Patients may have periappendicitis or localized peritonitis.

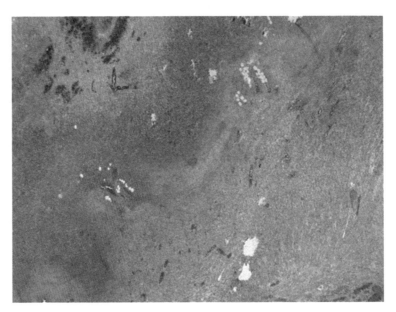

Figure 9-4　**Suppurative appendicitis(HE)**

The inflammatory lesions extend form the surface layer to the deep layer. Every layer is infiltrated by a large number of neutrophils. Inflammatory edema and fibrous exudation are noted

Acute gangrenous appendicitis:It is a serious kind of appendicitis. Obstruction, empyema, increased pressure in the cavity, and thrombophlebitis induced by appendicular vein inflammation contribute to the disturbance of blood circulation and appendix necrosis. The appendix looks dark red or black and perforation can lead to periappendicitis or localized peritonitis.

(2)Chronic Appendicitis

The main lesions are varying degrees of fibrosis and infiltration of chronic inflammation cells. Patients may have right lower abdominal pain. It can clevelop acute attack sometimes.

9.4.3　Outcomes and Complications

Acute appendicitis has a good prognosis with surgical treatment. Acute diffuse peritonitis and periappendiceal abscess are the main complications. Sometimes there is thrombophlebitis or liver abscess. Liver abscess occurs when bacterial or detached bacterial embolus flow into the liver. If the proximal end of the appendix is blocked, the distal end of the appendix is highly expanded and appendiceal abscess or appendiceal mucocele may occur. If the mucocele ruptures, the mucus on the peritoneum and pseudomyxoma will be formed.

9.5　Inflammatory Bowel Disease

Inflammation bowel disease(IBD)can occur in any age. Regional enteritis and ulcerative colitis are two main IBDs.

9.5.1　Regional Enteritis

Regional enteritis is also known as Crohn's disease. It is a systemic disease, which mainly involve terminal ileum. Patients have abdominal pain, diarrhea, abdominal mass, perforated ulcer, intestinal fistula and intestinal obstruction. Immune diseases outside intestine such as migrating polyarthritis and ankylosing spondylitis may exist.

9.5.1.1　Causes and Pathogenesis

Anticolonic antibody can be detected in the blood of patients. Immune complex deposit can be detected in the site of lesion by immunofluorescence and ELISA. Though the causes are unclear, it may be related to immune disorder.

9.5.1.2　Pathological changes

1)Gross appearance. The lesions mostly occur in the segment of terminal ileum and/or colon, though any part of the gastrointestinal tract may be involved. Well demarcated segmental bowel lesion are intervened with uninvolved 'skip areas'. Because of fibrosis and stenosis, the wall of the affected bowel segment is thick and hard. The lumen of the affected segment is markedly narrowed.

2)Microscopic changes. The lesions are complex and diverse. The characteristic features are as follows: ①Transmural inflammatory cells are chronic inflammatory cells(lymphocytes, plasma cells and macrophages). ②Non-caseating, sarcoid-like granulomas are present in all the layers of the affected bowel wall in 50% of cases. ③Patchy ulceration of the mucosa may form deep fissures, accompanied by lymphocytes and plasma cells infiltrating. ④Due to edema and aggregations of foci lymphoid, the submucosa is widening. ⑤ In chronic cases, fibrosis becomes increasingly prominent in all the layers.

9.5.2　Ulcerative Colitis

Ulcerative colitis is a chronic inflammation affecting mainly the mucosa and submucosa of the rectum and descending colon, though sometimes it may involve the entire length of the large bowel, and occasionally it may involve ileum. The disease is often accompanied by immune disease of external intestine, such as roving polyarthritis, uveitis and primary sclerosing cholangitis. Patients may have abdominal pain, diarrhea, and bloody mucus feces.

9.5.2.1　Causes and Pathogenesis

The exact etiology of ulcerative colitis remains unknown. However, it is mainly considered as an autoimmunity disease. Antibodies to colonic cells can be detected in less than half of patients' serum.

9.5.2.2　Pathological Changes

Gross changes: Compared to Crohn's disease, the characteristic feature is the continuous involvement of the rectum and colon without any uninvolved skip areas. The varying appearance of colon depends upon the stage and intensity of the disease because of remissions and exacerbations. Initially, hyperaemia, punctate hemorrhage and small abscess are seen in colonic mucosa. Abscess turns into shallow ulcers due to necrosis and abscission of the mucosa. Shallow ulcers merge with each other to form deep ulcers, and may even cause abscess beside colon, peritonitis or adhesion with the adjacent organs. Due to hyperaemia, edema and hyperplasia, inflammatory 'pseudopolyps' may form in the intervening intact mucosa. Microscopically, superficial mucosal ulcerations can be seen in the intestinal mucous fossa in the early stage, and penetrate into the muscle coat in severe cases, accompanied by nonspecific inflammatory cell infiltration of neutrophils, lymphocytes, plasma cells, and eosinophils in the mucous and submucosa. In the late stage, fibrous tissue proliferates. In long-standing cases, atypic epithelium(pseudopolyp) may develop into carcinoma in situ and adenocarcinoma.

9.5.2.3   Complications

Complications of Ulcerative colitis include malabsorption, formation of fistula and stricture, toxic megacolon and the development of malignancy in late cases. If the lesion is limited to the left colon, it has low cancerous rate. If the lesion expands to the whole colon within 20 years course, the rate of canceration increases to 17%, and 30 years increases to 50%.

9.5.3   Acute Hemorrhagic Enteritis

Acute hemorrhagic enteritis(AHE), is a pediatric emergency characterized by acute necrotizing hemorrhagic inflammation. The main clinical manifestations are abdominal pain, hematochezia, fever, vomiting, diarrhea and even shock to death.

9.5.3.1   Causes and Pathogenesis

Exact etiology of AHE is not known. But it has been reported that the disease is a severe allergic diseases(Schwartzman) caused by nonspecific infection such as bacterium, virus, or their decomposed product.

9.5.3.2   Pathological Changes

It is characterized by obvious hemorrhage and necrosis. It's often segmental, and usually involves jejunum and ileum. The bowel wall is thickened, edema, distinctive from the normal, with surface covered by pseudomembrane. Secondary ulcers can cause intestinal perforation. Inflammatory cells infiltrate in submucosa. Smooth muscle fiber ruptures in muscle layer.

9.5.4   Dysplastic Enteritis

It is also known as antibiotic enteritis and often caused by long-term use of broad-spectrum antibiotics.

9.6   Viral Hepatitis

Viral hepatitis is a common infectious disease caused by a group of hepatitis viruses. It's main pathological changes are liver parenchyma cell degeneration and necrosis. It has been confirmed that viral hepatitis is caused by hepatitis virus A and B, C, D, E and G(Table 9-2). Among them, Hepatitis B caused by Hepatitis B virus is more common. Studies have shown that it is caused by cellular immune response, and the humoral immune response may not be significant. Viral hepatitis has a high incidence and a rising trend. Epidemic areas are widespread, and all ages and genders can all suffer from it, which seriously endangers human health.

Table 9-2   Characteristics of each type of hepatitis virus and the corresponding hepatitis

Types of Hepatitis virus	Size andcharacter	Incubation period (Week)	Channel of infection	Chance of turning into chronic hepatitis	Fulminant hepatitis
HAV	27 nm, single strand	2-6	Intestinal tract	None	0.1%-0.4%
HBV	43nm, DNA	4-26	Intimate contact, blood transfusion, injection	5%-10%	<1%
HCV	30-60 nm, single strand	2-26	The same as above	>70%	Seldom
HDV	Defective RNA	4-7	The same as above	<5% whencoinfection 80% when Overlapping infection	3%-4% when coinfection 7%-10% when overlapping infection
HEV	32-34 nm, single strand	2-8	Intestinal tract	None	20% concurring during pregnancy
HGV	Single strand	Unknown	Blood transfusion, injection	None	Unknown

9.6.1 Etiology and Pathogenesis

The pathogenesis of viral hepatitis is complex and has not yet been fully elucidated, depending on a variety of factors, especially the immune state of the body.

9.6.1.1 Hepatitis A Virus(HAV)

HAV is a benign, self-limited disease with an incubation period of 2-6 weeks. It is characterized by infection of the digestive tract, which can be scattered or endemic. The hepatitis A virus reaches the liver through the portal vein system from the intestinal tract, the virus replicates in the liver cells and lsshed in the bile. Therefore, the virus can be discovered in the feces. Hepatitis A virus itself does not damage the cell, but may cause liver cell damage through the cellular immune mechanism. HAV does not lead to chronic hepatitis or a carrier state and only rarely causes acute hepatic failure.

9.6.1.2 Hepatitis B Virus(HBV)

HBV was first linked to hepatitis in the 1960s when the Australia antigen(later known as HBV surface antigen) was identified. The mature HBV virion is a spherical double-layered "Dane particle" that has an outer surface envelope of protein, lipid, and carbohydrate. The genome of HBV is a partially double-stranded circular DNA molecule having 3 200 nucleotides with four open reading frames which are S, C, P and X genes. S gene codes for the surface envelope protein, hepatitis Bsurface antigen(HBsAg); HBsAg is major protein. HBsAg consist of three related proteins: large, middle, and small HBsAg. Infected hepatocytes are capable of synthesizing and secreting massive quantities of noninfective surface protein(mainly small HBsAg). C gene codes for two nucleocapsid proteins, HBeAg and a core protein termed HBcAg. P gene is the largest and codes for DNA polymerase. X gene codes for HBxAg which plays an important role in the occurrence of hepatocellular carcinoma.

There is strong evidence linking immunepathogenesis with hepatocellular damage. HBV generally does not cause direct hepatocyte injury. Instead, viral antigens(in particular nucleocapsid proteins HbcAg and HbeAg)are attacked by host cytotoxic CD_8^+ T lymphocyte. HBV is the main cause of chronic hepatitis in China, which eventually leads to liver cirrhosis. It also can cause acute hepatitis B, acute severe hepatitis and asymptomatic carriers state. HBV is mainly transmitted by blood flow, blood contaminated items, drug use or close contact. Maternal-neonatal transmission is also common in high incidence areas.

Ground glass-like hepatocytes: HBsAg carriers and chronic hepatitis patients show hepatocyte change such as presence of finely granular, groundglass, eosinophilic cytoplasm, which are called ground glass-like hepatocytes and were positive for HBsAg by immunohistochemistry and immunofluorescence test. Under electron microscopy, the smooth endoplasmic reticulum hyperplasia and more HBsAg particles were found in the endoplasmic reticulum.

9.6.1.3　Hepatitis C Virus(HCV)

The main route of transmission is taken by injection or transfusion. HCV is a single-stranded RNA virus and has six main genotypes. The main genotypes are 1a,1b,2a and 2b. 1b is closely related to hepatocellular carcinoma. Drinking can promote HCV replication, activation and liver fibrosis. HCV virus can destroy the liver cells directly. Numerous experiments show that the immune factors are also the important cause of liver cell injury. Chronic disease occurs in the majority of HCV-infected individuals (80% to 90%)and cirrhosis eventually occurs in as many as 20% of individuals with chronic HCV infection. Hepatocellular carcinoma(HCC)may occur in some cases.

9.6.1.4　Hepatitis D Virus

Hepatitis D virus(HDV)is a replication-defective RNA virus that must rely on coinfection or superinfection with HBV to replicate. HDVinfection and hepatitis B may be simultaneous(co-infection), or HDV may infect a chronic HBsAg carrier(superinfection). It is self-limited and is usually followed by clearance of both viruses. However, there is a higher rate of acute hepatic failure, in intravenous drug users. HBV/HDV complex chronic hepatitis may be responsible for about 80% cases. , and acute severe hepatitis may occur.

9.6.1.5　Hepatitis Evirus

HEV is a single-stranded RNA virus. Hepatitis E is mainly transmitted through the digestive tract and prevalent in the rainy season and after the flood. It often appears in autumn and winter(10−11 months). Sporadic cases occur throughout the year in poor environmental and water hygiene conditions. HEV sometimes is prevalent in middle aged and older people over 35 years old. The proportion of severe HEV hepatitis in pregnancy is high. HEV is mainly prevalent in developing countries such as Asia and Africa, especially in India and other countries. HEV infection has a particularly high mortality in pregnant women(account for 20%)but is otherwise a self-limited disease and has not been associated with chronic liver disease.

9.6.1.6　Hepatitis G virus

HGV infection primarily occurs in dialysis patients, mainly transmitted through contaminated blood or blood products, and may also be transmitted through sexual contact. In some patients it may become chronic disease. Whether HGV is the hepatitis virus is still controversial. It is believed that HGV can be replicated in mononuclear cells, so it is not necessarily hepatitis virus.

9.6.2　Basic Pathological Changes

All types of hepatitis have similar changes: hepatocellular degeneration, necrosis, varying degrees of inflammatory cell infiltration, hepatocellular regeneration and interstitial fibrosis.

9.6.2.1 Hepatocyte Degeneration

1) Cellular swelling: It is the most common lesion. Under light microscope, the hepatocyte is obviously enlarged, and the cytoplasm is reticular and translucent, which is called "cytoplasm loosening". With further development, the size of hepatocytes expands from polygon to round. The cytoplasm is almost completely transparent, called ballooning degeneration. Under electron microscope, the endoplasmic reticulum showes different degrees of expansion, mitochondria swelling and lysosomes increase sosomes.

2) Acidophilic degeneration: This type of degeneration generally involves only a single or several hepatocytes and is scattered within the hepatic lobules. Under light microscope, the cytoplasm becomes intensely eosinophilic and the nucleus becomes small and pyknotic.

9.6.2.2 Hepatocyte Necrosis and Apoptosis

1) Lytic necrosis: It develop from severe cell edema. The range and distribution of this kind of necrosis of different types of viral hepatitis can be divided into:

Spotty necrosis: It refers to the necrosis of a single or several hepatocytes and is common in acute common hepatitis(Figure 9-5).

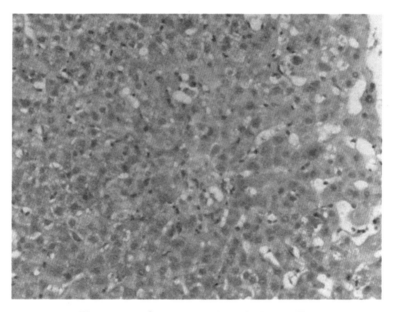

Figure 9-5   **Spotty necrosis in the liver(HE)**

It refers to the necrosis of a single or several hepatocytes, common in acute common hepatitis

Piecemeal necrosis: The focal necrosis and disintegration of the liver cells at the periphery of the hepatic lobule are common in chronic hepatitis.

Bridging necrosis: It is characterized by bands of necrosis linking portal tracts to central hepatic veins, one central hepatic vein to another, or a portal tract to another tract, which is commonly seen in moderate and severe chronic hepatitis.

Massive necrosis: It refers to a large area of hepatocyte necrosis that is almost involved the whole hepatic lobule and is common in severe hepatitis(Figure 9-6).

2) Apoptosis: It was considered considered to be eosinophilic necrosis in the past. With acidophilic degeneration development, cytoplasm becomes intensely eosinophilic and the nucleus is eventually extruded from the cell, leaving behind necrotic, acidophilic mass called acidophil body by the process of apoptosis.

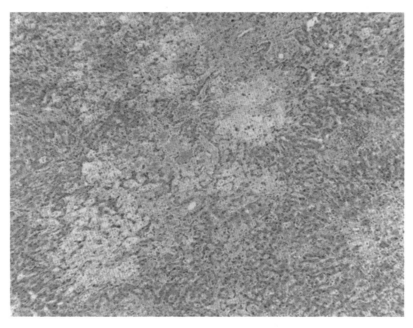

Figure 9-6   Massivenecrosis in the liver(HE)

It refers to a large area of hepatocyte necrosis that is almost involved in the whole hepatic
lobule and is common in severe hepatitis

9.6.2.3   Inflammatory Cell Infiltration

Lymphocytes and mononuclear cells are mainly infiltrated in the hepatic lobule or the portal tracts(Figure 9-7).

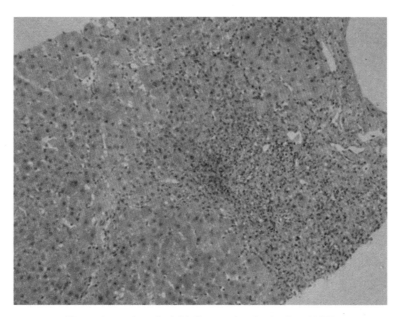

Figure 9-7   Interfacial inflammation in the liver(HE)

Significant plasma cell infiltration of chronic inflammation was found at the junction
of hepatic lobulesand portal area

9.6.2.4   Regeneration

1)Hepatocyte regeneration: Necrotic hepatocytes are repaired by direct or indirect division of the surrounding liver cells. The regenerated hepatocytes are large in size with basophilic cytoplasm, and large and deeply dyed nucleus, sometimes binuclear. The regenerated hepatocytes can arrang along the original net frame. But if the necrosis is serious, the reticular scaffold in the primary lobule collapses, then the regenerated hepatocytes are organized in a bulky mass, called nodular regeneration.

2) Interstitial reactive hyperplasia and small bile duct hyperplasia: Kupffer cells proliferate, and can be transferred into the sinus cavity to become phagocytic cells that migrate and participate in inflammatory cells infiltration. Mesenchymal stem cells and fibroblast proliferation are also involved in the injury repair. In cases of severe hepatocellular necrosis, hepatic fibrosis and hepatic cirrhosis may develop due to proliferation of a large number of fibroblasts, and small bile duct hyperplasia can be seen in the portal area or large necrotic foci.

9.6.2.5　Fibrosis

In general, fibrosis is mostly irreversible, but now some researches suggested think that liver fibrosis can be absorbed in certain cases, so it is reversible. The deposition of collagen in fibrosis has a significant effect on the liver's blood flow and hepatocyte perfusion. Early fibrosis distributs around the portal area or the central vein, or collagen directly deposits within the Disse cavity. With the continuous progress of fibrosis, the liver is directly divided into fibrous nodules, which eventually develop into liver cirrhosis.

9.6.3　Clinicopathological Types

9.6.3.1　Common Viral Hepatitis Divided into two Types Including Acute and Chronic

(1) Acute Common Hepatitis

According to whether the patients had jaundice, it is divided into anicteric type and icteric type. In our country, there are more non-jaundice type cases, among which hepatitis B virusis is the main type. The jaundice type hepatitis is heavier and the course of the disease is shorter. It is more common in type A, D and E hepatitis. The pathological changes of jaundice type and non-jaundice type hepatitis are basically the same.

Macroscopically, the liver is swollen, the texture is soft and the surface is smooth.

Microscopically, hepatocytes show extensive degeneration, mainly with cellular swelling, and appeared to be hepatocytes with loose and light staining and ballooning like changes. As a result, the hepatocytes increase in size, arrange in a disorderly and crowded manner, and the hepatic sinusoids are compressed and narrowed, and cholestasis can be observed in liver cells. Slight cell necrosis, and eosinophilic bodies are found in the hepatic lobule. Mild inflammatory cell infiltration is found in the hepatic lobule and portal area. The jaundice type necrosis is often heavier, with cholestasis and embolus formation in the capillary bile duct.

Clinicopathological relationship: Diffuse hepatocytes swelling causes liver size to increase and capsule to tighten, causing liver pain. The degeneration of liver cells causing the release of liver enzymes into the blood and the increase of serum alanine aminotransferase(SGPT), but also can cause abnormal liver function, severe jaundice.

Outcome Most hepatitis patients can be cured within 6 months, and spottynecrotic hepatocytes can be completely regenerated and repaired. However, hepatitis B and C often recover slowly, of which about 5% – 10% of hepatitis B and about 70% of hepatitis C can be converted into chronic hepatitis.

(2) Chronic(Common) Hepatitis

Chronic hepatitis is defined as continuing or relapsing hepatic disease for more than 6 months. The factors leading to chronic hepatitis are as follows: the type of virus infection, improper treatment, malnutrition, and suffering from other infectious diseases, drinking, drug damage to the liver, and immune factors, which the clinician should pay attention to. In the past, chronic hepatitis was divided into chronic persistent hepatitis and chronic active hepatitis. At present, it has been noted that the percentage of HCV patients who develope chronic hepatitis later developed into cirrhosis is extremely high, regardless of the degree of the initial liver disease. Therefore, the pathogenesis of chronic hepatitis is more important. According to the degree of inflammation, necrosis and fibrosis, chronic hepatitis can be divided into three types:

1) Mild chronic hepatitis: There are spotty necrosis, few chronic inflammatory cell infiltrations in the portal area, and a small number of fibrous tissue proliferation around. Hepatic plate of lobule is integrated and the structure of the lobule is clear.

2) Moderate chronic hepatitis: Liver cell degeneration and necrosis are obvious. There are moderate fragment necrosis, and characteristic bridging necrosis. There is a fibrous septum in the lobule, but the structure of the lobule is mostly preserved.

3) Severe chronic hepatitis: There are the severe fragmented necrosis and extensive bridging necrosis. In the necrotic area, the hepatocytes were irregularly regenerating, and the fibrous septum separats the hepatic lobule structure.

In the late chronic hepatitis may stage gradually transformed into liver cirrhosis. If a large area of fresh necrosis occurs on the basis of chronic hepatitis, it will turn into severe hepatitis.

9.6.3.2　Severe Viral Hepatitis

This is the most serious type of viral hepatitis and it is rare. According to the disease course and the severity of disease, it is divided into two categories, including acute fulminant and subacute fulminant hepatitis:

(1) Acute Severe Hepatitis

A rare, abrupt onset, short duration, mostly for about 10 days, severe lesions, high mortality disease. Clinically, this type of hepatitis is called an outbreak type, an electric shock type or a malignant hepatitis.

Macroscopically, the size of the liver is significantly reduced, especially in the left lobe. The capsules are wrinkled with soft texture, yellow or reddish brown cuts, and some areas show red and yellow stripes. So it is also called acute yellow atrophy or acute atrophy of red liver.

Microscopically, the necrosis of hepatocyte is extensive and serious, the liver cell cords are dissociated, the liver cells are dissolved. Hepatocyte necrosis starts from the center of the hepatic lobule and spreads rapidly to the periphery. Only a few degenerated hepatocytes remain around the lobule. The necrotic hepatocytes are quickly removed and only reticulated stents remain. The hepatic sinusoids dilate. There are hyperemia and even bleeding. Kupffer cells proliferated and hypertrophy, and phagocytosis is active. A large number of lymphocytes and macrophages in filtrat in the hepatic lobule. Several days later, the reticular scaffold collapse and the residual hepatocytes have no obvious regeneration. A large number of liver necrosis cells can cause: a large amount of bilirubin to enter the blood and cause severe hepatocellular jaundice; the synthesis obstacles of coagulation factors lead to obvious bleeding tendency; the liver failure, the detoxification function of various metabolites presents disorders leading to hepatic encephalopathy. In addition to bilirubin metabolic disorders and blood circulation disorders, it can also induce renal failure(hepatorenal syndrome).

Outcome: Most patients die in short term. The main cause of death is liver failure(hepatic encephalopathy), followed by massive hemorrhage of the digestive tract, renal failure and DIC. A small number of patients with delayed healing turned to suffer subacute severe hepatitis.

(2) Subacute Severe Hepatitis

the onset is slower than the acute severe hepatitis, and the duration is longer(weeks to months). Most cases are migrated from severe acute hepatitis, and a few are caused by the worsening of acute common hepatitis.

Macroscopically, the size of the liver is smaller, the surface of the envelope is inhomogeneous, the quality of the texture is different, and regions are nodular capsule. The necrotic area is red brown or yellow, and the regenerated nodule is yellow green because of the cholestasis.

Microscopically, it is characterized by large necrosis of both hepatocytes and nodular regeneration of hepatocytes. In the necrotic area, reticular fiber scaffolds collapsed and collagenate (sclerotic free). Therefore, the remnant hepatocytes can not be arranged along the original scaffolds but nodules. Obvious infiltration of inflammatory cells is seen inside and outside the hepatic lobules, mainly lymphocytes and monocytes. There are small bile ducts in the periphery of the lobules, and connective tissue hyperplasia is seen in the older lesions.

Outcome: If treated reasonably and timely, the disease can stop developing and possibly be cured. Most cases often developed into necrotic cirrhosis.

9.6.4   Characteristics of Various Types of Viral Hepatitis

9.6.4.1   Pathological Changes of Hepatitis

It mainly causes acute hepatitis, sometimes also causes cholestatic hepatitis and severe hepatitis. The main pathological changes are as follows: ①degeneration and necrosis of liver cells. The most common are early hepatocyte swelling and ballooning degeneration, accompanied by the formation of eosinophilic and eosinophilic bodies of hepatocytes, and the disappearance of hepatic sinusoids, resulting in disorder of liver cells in lobules. The liver cells in the central vein of the hepatic lobules are dissolved and necrotic. ②infiltration of inflammatory cells in the portal area, mainly large mononuclear cells and lymphocyte cells. ③the proliferation of Kupffer cells in the hepatic sinusoids. The above lesions are reversible.

9.6.4.2   Pathological Changes of Hepatitis B

Groud glassy-like cells are a special morphological feature of hepatitis B.

9.6.4.3   Pathological Changes of Hepatitis C

Microscopically, in addition to the typical characteristics of chronic hepatitis, there are some unique changes in chronic hepatitis C: the fatty degeneration of liver cells, which are caused by changes in lipid metabolism of infected hepatocytes or insulin resistance, so-called metabolic syndrome; the periportal lymphocyte cells infiltration, sometimes lymph follicles formation can be observed; the bile duct injury may be associated with direct viral infection of bile duct epithelial cells.

9.6.4.4   Pathological Changes of Hepatitis D

The liver cells are eosinophilic with vesicular fatty degeneration, coupled with infiltration of inflammatory cells and inflammatory reaction in the confluence area. Patients with chronic HBV infection have severer liver tissue lesions after overlapping infection with HDV.

9.6.4.5   Pathological Changes of Hepatitis E

There are inflammation changes in the portal area, showing a large number of Kupffer cells and polymorphonuclear leukocytes, but rare lymphocytes; There are hepatocyte cytoplasm and bile capillary cholestasis; Hepatocellular necrosis shows focal or patchy to sub-area or large area necrosis, especially in the area around the portal vein.

9.6.4.6   Pathological Changes of Hepatitis G

Hepatitis G pathologies characterized by a single HGV infection are generally less damaging. Acute hepatitis is mainly hepatocyte swelling and portal inflammatory cell infiltration. Chronic hepatitis has hepatocyte swelling, lobular or focal necrosis, portal area inflammatory cell infiltration and fibrosis.

9.6.5   Other Types of Hepatitis

9.6.5.1   Hepatitis Caused by Other Viral Infections

1) Epstein-Barr virus infection can cause mild hepatitis in the acute stage.

2) Cytomegalovirus infection, involving in almost all liver cells, including hepatocytes, bile duct epithelial cells and endothelial cells, can cause virus related giant cell changes.

3) Yellow fever virus infection is a major and serious cause of hepatitis in tropical countries. It can cause massive hepatocyte apoptosis, and the apoptotic of liver cells show strong eosinophilic changes. This phenomenon is known as Councilman body.

4) Herpes simplex virus infection of the liver cells of newborns or immunosuppressed lead to characteristic pathological changes of cells and necrosis of liver cells.

9.6.5.2   Drug/toxin-mediated Injury Mimicking Hepatitis

Many drug effects can mimic the characteristics of acute or chronic virus or autoimmune hepatitis.

9.6.5.3   Autoimmune Hepatitis

It is a chronic, progressive hepatitis. Its histological features are difficult to distinguish from chronic viral hepatitis. Although the damage pattern of autoimmune hepatitis is the same as that of acute and chronic viral hepatitis, its histologic progress is different. In the early stage, there are severe cells damage, inflammation and scar formation. The mortality of patients with severe untreated autoimmune hepatitis is approximately 40% within six months of diagnosis and cirrhosis develops in at least 40% of survivors.

9.7   Alcoholic Liver Disease

Alcoholic liver disease is one of the main manifestations of chronic alcoholism. According to the statistics of foreign countries, patients with alcoholic liver disease caused by alcoholism accounted for 25% – 30%. There is no definite statistical data on the incidence of alcoholic liver disease in our country but there is a tendency to increase obviously in recent years.

9.7.1   Pathological Change

Chronic alcoholism mainly causes three types of liver damages: hepatocellular steatosis or fatty change, alcoholic hepatitis, and alcoholic cirrhosis. They three can appear individually or simultaneously or successively.

9.7.1.1   Fatty Liver

The most common liver disease of alcoholism is steatosis. Macroscopically, the fatty liver in individuals with chronic alcoholism is a large soft organ that is yellow. Hepatocytes are swollen and round, and when the hepatocytes contain large lipid droplets, the nucleus can be pushed to the side of the cells. The central lobules are significantly affected, sometimes accompanied by various degrees of hydropic degeneration of hepatic cells. The simple fatty liver is often asymptomatic. If the lesion does not develop to fibrosis, the abstinence can restore the fatty liver.

9.7.1.2 Alcoholic Hepatitis

There are three kinds of pathological changes in patients with clinical symptoms of liver: steatosis, alcoholic hyaline, focal hepatocyte necrosis with neutrophil infiltration.

9.7.1.3 Alcoholic Cirrhosis

It is believed that this cirrhosis is caused by the progression of fatty liver and alcoholic hepatitis. If continued exposure, fatty liver develops alcoholic hepatitis followed by cirrhosis. Alcoholic hepatitis is often accompanied by prominent activation of sinusoidal stellate cells and portal fibroblasts, giving rise to fibrosis. Liver fibrosis results in the division and destruction of the normal structure of the hepatic lobules and the formation of alcoholic cirrhosis.

9.7.2 Pathogenesis

The liver is the main place for alcohol metabolism and degradation. Alcohol has a direct damage to the liver. The following mechanisms are as follows:

Alcohol into the liver is transformed into ethanol under the action of ethanol dehydrogenase and microsomal ethanol oxidase, and then into acetic acid. The latter reaction converts NAD to NADH, resulting in an increased effect of NADH on the ratio of NAD, thereby inhibiting the mitochondrial tricarboxylic acid cycle three, causes liver cells to reduce the oxidation of fatty acids, and the accumulation of fat in the liver; Increased NADH can also cause increased lactic acid, and increased oxygen consumption affects liver metabolism. Alcohol plays a role of free radical damage in the membrane system by the action of microsome oxidation system in hepatocytes. Acetaldehyde has strong lipid peroxidation and toxicity, which can destroy liver cells structure and induce immune response. In addition, alcoholism often causes malnutrition, especially protein and vitamin deficiency.

9.8 Liver Cirrhosis

Liver cirrhosis is a common chronic liver disease caused by diffuse degeneration and necrosis of liver cells, fibrous tissue hyperplasia and nodular regeneration of hepatocytes. The advanced patients often have different levels of portal pressure increased and liver dysfunction, which are very harmful to the human body. Most of the onset ages ranged from 20 to 50 years old, with no significant difference in the incidence of males and females. Due to the cause of liver cirrhosis and the complexity of its pathogenesis, there is no unified classification yet. It is generally classified according to the size of the nodules or the cause of the formation of nodules. The international classification of liver cirrhosis is divided into four types: mnacronodulor type, small nodule type, micronodular mixed nodulay type and incomplete segmentation type. The following three types of liver cirrhosis common in our country are introduced.

9.8.1 Portal Cirrhosis

Portal cirrhosis is the most common type of liver cirrhosis all over the world. It is equivalent to small nodular cirrhosis in the international morphological classification.

9.8.1.1 Etiology and Pathogenesis

It is not yet fully understood. Most studies have shown that many different factors can cause liver cell damage and then develop into liver cirrhosis. The common factors are:

1) Viral hepatitis: This is the main cause of liver cirrhosis in China, especially hepatitis B and C. There are many convincing data in the epidemiology, clinical and pathological forms. It is worth paying attention to the viral hepatitis.

2) Chronic alcoholism. Chronic alcoholism is another important factor for liver cirrhosis, which is more prominent in some countries in Europe and America. The acetaldehyde produced during the metabolism of alcohol in the body has a direct toxic effect on the liver cells, making the liver cells fatty change, to degeneratie and gradually developing to liver cirrhosis.

3) The damage effect of toxic substances. Many chemicals can damage liver cells, such as carbon tetrachloride, cinchophen, and so on. The long-term effects can cause liver damage and cirrhosis of the liver.

4) Malnutrition. If there is a long-term lack of methionine or choline in food, the liver can synthesize phosphatidylcholine impaired and develop liver cirrhosis through fatty liver.

All of the above factors can cause diffuse damage to the liver cells. If the long-term effects and repeated attacks continue, it can cause extensive proliferation of collagen fibers in the liver. There are two sources of this increased collagen fiber: The first is that after hepatocyte necrosis, the original mesh scaffold in the hepatic lobule collapses, accumulates, collagen (no cell sclerosis), or the hepatic stellate cells transform into myofibroblast-like cells to produce collagen fibrosis. The second is that fibroblasts in the portal area proliferate and secrete collagen fibers. After the collapse of the hepatic lobule, the regenerated hepatocytes can not be arranged along the original scaffold, and the irregular regenerated hepatocyte nodules are formed. On one hand, extensive proliferating collagen fibers extend to the lobules and divide the liver lobules. On the other hand, it connects with collagenous fibers in the hepatic lobules, forming the fibrous septum that surrounds the original or regenerative liver cell clusters and forming pseudolobules. These lesions are repeated with the continuous necrosis and regeneration of liver cells, eventually forming pseudolobules that pervade the whole liver, and lead to hepatic blood circulation remodeling and hepatic dysfunction and liver cirrhosis.

9.8.1.2   Pathological Change

Macroscopically, the early liver size is normal or slightly increased, the weight increases, the texture is normal or slightly hard. The size of the advanced liver is obviously reduced, the weight is reduced, and the hardness is increased. Small nodules diffuse the whole liver. The nodules are similar in size, with a diameter between 0.15-0.5 cm, and generally not more than 1cm. The liver is thickened by the membrane. There are round or circular island-like shaped structures with the same size as the nodules on the surface, surrounded by gray white fibrous tissue cord (Figure 9-8).

Microscopically: The structure of normal lobule is destroyed and replaced by pseudolobul. The extensively-proliferated fibrous tissue divides the original hepatic lobules, encircling the round or round-shaped hepatocyte masses of varying sizes to form pseudolobules. The liver cells in the false lobule are arranged disorderlly, and there is degeneration, necrotic and regenerated hepatocytes. The central vein is often absent, or not incentral, or more than two. Regenerated hepatocyte nodules are also seen, characterized by disordered arrangement of hepatocytes with large size, large nuclear and deep staining, and visible dual-nuclei. A small number of fibrous spacers wrapped around the pseudo lobule are similar, with a small number of lymphocytes and mononuclear cells infiltrated, and the small bile duct hyperplasia is seen (Figure 9-9).

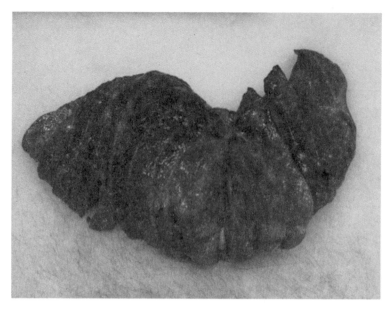

Figure 9-8　**Nodular cirrhosis**

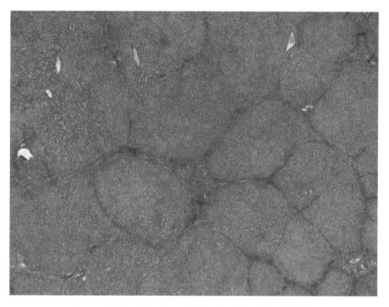

Figure 9-9　**Nodular cirrhosis of the liver(HE)**
The structure of normal lobule is destroyed and replaced by. The liver cells in the
false lobule are arranged in disorder. The central vein is often absent, or more than two

9. 8. 1. 3　Clinicopathological Relationship

1) Portal Hypertension. The causes of increased portal pressure as follows: ①A wide range of connective tissue hyperplasia in the liver causes hepatic sinusoid occlusion and impedes portal circulation; ②The pseudolobule compresses the sublobular veins and affects the portal vein blood flowing into the hepatic sinusoids; ③Intrahepatic small branches of the hepatic artery and small branches of the portal vein form abnormal anastomosis before entering the hepatic sinusoids, allowing high-pressure arterial blood to flow into the portal vein. Because of the elevated portal vein pressure, a series of symptoms and signs are often present in the patients. The main manifestations are as follows:

Splenomegaly: Long-standing congestion may cause splenomegaly. The degree of splenic enlargement varies widely and may reach as much as 1 000 mg. About 70% to 85% of patients with cirrhosis have splenomegaly. The splenomegaly may cause hematologic abnormalities, such as hypersplenism, thrombocytopenia or even pancytopenia. The dilatation of the splenic sinus, the proliferation and enlargement of the sinusoidal endothelial cells, the atrophy of the splenic corpuscle, the proliferation of the fibrous tissue in the red pulp, and some nodules with, iron are seen.

Ascites: The accumulation of excess fluid in the peritoneal cavity are called ascites. Ascites is the translucent yellowish transudate, which can lead to bulging of the abdomen. In 85% of cases, ascites is caused by cirrhosis. The pathogenesis of ascites is complex, involving the following mechanisms: The elevation of portal vein pressure increases the hydrostatic pressure of the capillary fluid in the portal system, the permeability of the vessel wall increases, and the liquid leaks into the abdominal cavity. Liver dysfunction reduces the inactivation of aldosterone and antidiuretic hormone, which increase in the blood and causes the formation of ascites by water and sodium retention. Due to the presence of hypoproteinemia in the patient, the plasma colloid osmotic pressure is reduced and it is also contributes to the formation of ascites.

Portosystemic Shunts: With the rising pressure in portal system, the flow is reversed from portal to systemic circulation by dilation of collateral vessels and development of new vessels. Venous bypasses develop because the systemic and portal circulation share common capillary beds. Principal sites are veins around and within the rectum(manifest as hemorrhoids), the esophagogastric junction(producing varices), the retroperitoneum, and the falciform ligament of the liver(involving periumbilical and abdominal wall collaterals). Although hemorrhoidal bleeding may occur, it is rarely massive or life-threatening. Much more important are the esophagogastric varices that appear in about 40% of individuals with advanced cirrhosis of the liver and cause massive hematemesis and death in about half of them. Each episode of bleeding is associated with a 30% mortality. Abdominal wall collaterals appear as dilated subcutaneous veins extending from the umbilicus toward the rib margins(caput medusae) and constitute an important clinical hallmark of portal hypertension.

Gastrointestinal congestion and edema: The portal vein pressure is increased, and the drainage of the gastrointestinal venous blood is blocked, resulting in congestion and edema of the gastrointestinal wall which affect the digestion and absorption functions of the stomach. The patients may have symptoms such as abdominal distension and loss of appetite.

2) Hepatosis. Hepatosis is mainly caused by repeated injury of liver cells for a long time. When the liver cells can not completely regenerate and compensate for the function of the injured liver cells, the following symptoms and signs of liver dysfunction may appear.

Protein synthesis disorder: When the liver cells are damaged, the function of the synthesizing protein is reduced and the plasma protein is decreased. At the same time due to absorption from the gastrointestinal tract some antigenic substance without treatment of liver cells directly through the collateral circulation and enter the systemic circulation, stimulate the immune system synthesis globulin increased, and serological examination can appear lower albumin, albumin/globulin ratio decreased or inverted phenomenon.

Bilirubin metabolic disorder: It is mainly related to hepatocyte necrosis and capillary cholestasis. Patients often have hepatocyte jaundice in the clinic.

Hemorrhagic tendency: Patients with cirrhosis may have skin, mucous, or subcutaneous bleeding, mainly due to the reduction of the liver's synthesis of coagulation factors. In addition, it is also related to splenomegaly, hypersplenism and excessive destruction of platelets.

Abating the inactivation of hormone: Patients with chronic liver failure may develop palmar erythema(a reflection of local vasodilatation) or spider angiomas of the skin. The spider angiomas is due to the obstacle of the inactivation of estrogen in the liver the dilation of peripheral arterioles. It often appears on the patient's neck, chest, and face. In men, hyperestrogenemia also leads to hypogonadism and gynecomastia. In women, oligomenorrhea, amenorrhea, and sterility as a result of hypogonadism are frequent.

Hepatic encephalopathy (hepatic coma): This poses the most serious consequences. It is the manifestation of extreme liver function failure. And it is also another important cause of death in patients with liver cirrhosis.

9.8.2 Postnecrotic Cirrhosis

Postnecrotic cirrhosis is equivalent to the large nodular type and large nodules mixed cirrhosis in international classification. It is formed on the basis of massive necrosis of hepatocytes.

9.8.2.1 Etiology and Pathogenesis

1) Viral hepatitis. Most of them are delayed by subacute severe hepatitis. In the course of repeated episodes of chronic hepatitis, if the necrosis is serious, it can also develop into this type of liver cirrhosis.

2) Drug and chemical poisoning. Some drugs or chemicals can cause diffuse toxic liver necrosis in liver cells, and then nodular regeneration develops into postnecrotic cirrhosis.

9.8.2.2 Pathological Change

Macroscopically, the liver is narrowed and hardened in the left lobe. The difference from portal cirrhosis is that the liver is deformed obviously, and the size of the nodules is very large. The diameter of the largest nodule is up to 5-6 cm, and the connective tissue space of the section is wide and the thickness becomes uneven.

Microscopically, the scope of liver cell necrosis and irregular shape, so the pscuololobule morphological size may be semilunar shape, map shape, and can also be seen as round and nearly-circular shape. Large pseudo lobules can sometimes be seen as a few complete liver lobules, and some can be seen in the focus of the remaining portal area; within the false lobule of liver cells have varying degrees of degeneration and necrosis, if there is viral hepatitis, hepatocyte edema, eosinophilic, or formation of eosinophilic bodies are often seen. Wide fiber spacing, which has a large number of inflammatory cells infiltration and small bile ducts hyperplasia.

Ending Hepatic necrosis of postnecrotic cirrhosis is more severe, and the course of disease is shorter. Therefore, liver dysfunction is more obvious and earlier than portal cirrhosis. Portal hypertension is mild and late. The canceration rate of this type of liver cirrhosis is also higher than that of portal cirrhosis.

9.8.3 Biliary Cirrhosis

Biliary cirrhosis is a rare disease due to biliary obstruction and cholestasis of liver cirrhosis. According to the different causes, it is divided into two types: primary and secondary.

Primary biliary cirrhosis is rare in China. The cause is unknown. It may be related to the autoimmune reaction, because autoantibodies can be detected in patients' blood. It can be caused by chronic non suppurative cholangitis of the small bile duct in the liver.

The causes of secondary biliary cirrhosis are associated with two factors such as long-term extrahepatic bile duct obstruction and upper biliary tract infection. Long term obstruction of bile duct, cholestasis, liver cells degeneration and necrosis, secondary connective tissue proliferation can lead to liver cirrhosis.

Pathological changes

Macroscopically, the liver shrinkage is not as obvious as that of the first two types of cirrhosis. The texture is medium hard, and the surface is smooth with small nodules or no obvious nodules. The color is dark green or green brown.

Microscopically, primary lobar biliary cirrhosis have early edema and necrosis of interlobular bile duct epithelial cells, surrounded by lymphocytic infiltration. The destruction of the small bile duct eventually results in hyperplasia of the connective tissue and then extends into the hepatic lobules. The pseudo lobules are incompletely divided. Microscopic examination of secondary biliary cirrhosis shows obvious hepatocytes degeneration and necrosis, and the necrotic hepatocytes are swollen with loose cytoplasm, reticular formation and nuclear disappearance, keticular or feathery necrosis, and incomplete segmentation of connective tissue around the pseudo lobule can be seen.

9.9 Metabolic Liver Disease and Circulatory Disorders

9.9.1 Metabolic Liver Disease

9.9.1.1 Hepatolenticular Degeneration

Hepatolenticular degeneration is also called Wilson disease. It is a hereditary disease transmitted by the recessive gene on chromosome 13 with many familial characteristics. Most of the patients are children and adolescents. The characteristic of this disease is copper metabolism disorder. Copper cannot be discharged normally and accumulates in various organs. The liver is usually the fist to be affected. After the liver is saturated, the copper is redeposited in the central nervous system, so neurologic symptoms occur. Copper can also accumulate in the cornea, causing is a green brown ring around the cornea(Kayser-Fleischer ring). Liver disease: the liver cells have visible lipofuscin and copper binding protein, iron and other. Copper or copper binding proteins(such as rhodamine, rubeanic acid, etc.) can be detected by histochemical staining. In the early stages, large particles or crystal sediments can be seen in the mitochondrial matrix of hepatocytes. Patients can also have acute, chronic hepatitis and liver cirrhosis. The central nervous system is most prominent in the striatum, thalamus and globus pallidus.

9.9.1.2 Hemosiderosis

Hemosiderosis refers to the hemochromatosis of dyeable iron in the liver tissue. The etiology of hemosiderin deposition is mainly caused by massive erythrocyte destruction and hemoglobin decomposition, such as chronic hemolytic anemia caused by hemolysis and intrahepatic hemorrhage. The hemosiderin is mainly deposited in the liver cells, and is often seen in Kupffer cells. The pigmentation of Kupffer cells caused by blood transfusion is more obvious.

Hemochromatosis is a systemic disease with congenital iron metabolism abnormalities. The pathogenesis is unknown. Liver disease is a part of the systemic lesion, which is characterized by severe hemosiderin deposition in the liver, and the whole liver is rusty. In the later period, there is liver fibrosis or cirrhosis of the liver.

9.9.1.3 Glycogenosis

Glycogenosis is the deposition of abnormal qualities and increased amounts of glycogen in the tissue, caused by congenital autosomal recessive inheritance. Glycogenosis is mainly involving the liver, heart, kidney and muscle tissue, with hypoglycemia, retardation and ketonuria performance. According to the abnormal glucose metabolism during different stages and different enzymes, now the disease is divided into O-XI type, including more subtypes.

There is visible hepatomegaly, some up to 3 times more than the normal liver, lighter in color. Microscopically, the liver cells were obviously swollen and the pulp was pale, with loose granules and bright areas. PAS staining can discover the red glycogen granules in the liver cells with frozen section. The digestive reaction of amylase is stable. In the later period, many types can be accompanied by liver fibrosis or cirrhosis. It should be pointed out that the diagnosis of glycogenosis and its classification classification cannot be based based solely on histopathological changes and must be combined with clinical and liver biopsy samples for enzyme analysis.

9.9.1.4　Lipoidosis

Lipoidosis is the accumulation and deposition of intra-tissue lipids caused by congenital defective lipid metabolism disorders. It is mainly deposited with glycolipid, phospholipid and cholesterol. The mechanism is mostly due to the genetic deletion of enzymes involved in some aspects of lipid metabolism, leading to the corresponding substrate(lipid)catabolism cannot be deposited in tissues.

1)Phosphatide lipoidosis. The increase and accumulation of phosphatidylcholine without glycerin, also known as Niemann-Peake disease, or neuro-phosphatidylcholine. The nervous phospholipase deficiency caused by the autosomal recessive heredity makes the phospholipid unable to be hydrolyzed, as a resuct deposits in the tissue. It can also be accompanied by other lipid storage. This disease mainly involves the liver, spleen, bone marrow and lymph nodes and so on. In children, the nervous system is also violated. The main lesion is hepatomegaly. Under the microscope, a large number of Kupffer cells and macrophages accumulate in the hepatic sinusoid and in the portal area. The cell size is enlarged and the cytoplasm is foamed. The nucleus is small and centered, called the Pick cell. There is also fat in the liver cells, mainly neutral fat and cholesterol. Under the electron microscope, the Pick cells are filled with many spherical inclusion bodies arranged like rings. This disease often occurs in young children, and the prognosis is poor.

2)Glycogenosis disease. Glycolipid refers to the lipids such as brain glucoside and nervon, which do not contain phosphoric acid. Their metabolic disorders can cause cerebral glucosides(such as Gaucher disease)and ganglioside deposition, respectively.

Gaucher disease, also known as brain glycoside deposition disease, is the disorder of cerebroside catabolism due to the deficiency of β-glucosidase in the body, caused by autosomal recessive inheritance. It mainly involves the mononuclear phagocyte system such as liver, spleen, lymph node and bone marrow. It often occurs in babies and it is a fatal disease. The main lesions are liver and spleen enlargement, and the splenomegaly is obvious, 20 times the normal weight of spleen. Microscopically, a large number of highly swollen lipid carrier macrophages accumulate in the liver. Some cytoplasm is foamed, and some cytoplasm appeares to have red stripes. The latter is arranged in wrinkled pattern. The nucleus is small, round or oval in the center of cells, called Gaucher's cells. These cells are mainly distributed in the hepatic sinuses and portal areas near the central vein of the lobule. Occasionally, liver fibrosis and cirrhosis of the liver occur(Figure 9-10).

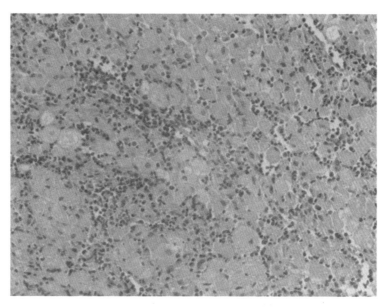

Figure 9-10   **Gaucher disease of the liver(HE)**

A large number of highly swollen lipid carrier macrophages were found in the liver.
Some cytoplasm was foamed, or red stripe, arranged in wrinkled pattern. The nucleus
was small, round or oval in the center of cells

9.9.2   Circulatory Disorders

9.9.2.1   Portal Vein Obstruction

It is rare. It is due to liver cirrhosis, liver carcinoma, pancreatic carcinoma, and other liver or pancreatic diseases invading the intrahepatic portal vein, and purulent peritonitis, neonatal umbilical cord suppurative infections cause portal vein thrombosis or embolism. The thrombosis does not cause ischemic infarction but instead results in a sharply demarcated area of red-blue discoloration called the infarct of Zahn. There is no necrosis, only severe hepatocellular atrophy and marked stasis in distended sinusoids. The lesion is round or rectangular, dark red and clear. The local hepatocytes are atrophic, necrotic or disappearing. A new anastomosis was found around the occlusion of the portal vein in the recovery period. This disease has no great influence on the body, and it can be a source of intraperitoneal bleeding.

9.9.2.2   Hepatic Venous Obstruction

Hepatic venous obstruction is generally divided into two types. One is the obstruction of hepatic vein to inferior vena cava. It is called Budd-Chiari syndrome. The other is intrahepatic small hepatic vein obstruction which is called veno-occlusive disease.

The obstruction of two or more major hepatic veins produces liver enlargement, pain, and ascites, a condition known as Budd-Chiari syndrome. Hepatic vein thrombosis is associated with myeloproliferative disorders such as polycythemia vera, inherited disorders of coagulation, antiphospholipid antibody syndrome, paroxysmal nocturnal hemoglobinuria, and intraabdominal cancers, particularly hepatocellularcarcinoma. In pregnancy or with oral contraceptive use, it occurs through interaction with an underlying thrombogenic disorder. The main pathological changes are the atrophy, degeneration and necrosis of the liver cells. In addition, there is hepatic hemorrhage, which is the deposition of the red blood cells in the hepatic sinusoids entering into the Disse cavity with a lower pressure outside the sinus and the atrophy of the hepatic plate. Chronic cases develop into congestive of liver cirrhosis.

9.10 Cholecystitis and Cholelithiasis

9.10.1 Cholecystitis

Cholecystitis is often caused by bacteria, and often based on cholestasis. The main bacteria are E. coli, staphylococcus and so on. If the inflammation mainly involves includes gallbladder, we call it Cholecystitis. If it mainly involve bile duct, we call it cholangitis.

9.10.1.1 Pathological Changes

1) Acute cholecystitis and cholangitis. It is characterized by mucosal hyperemia and edema, epithelial cells denaturation, necrosis and exfoliation neutrophils infiltratation. If it occurs in the gallbladder, it is catarrhal cholecystitis, which can develop into honeycombed cholecystitis. Gangrenous cholecystitis occurs when there is disturbance of blood circulation in bile ducts or gallbladder wall caused by spasm, edema, obstruction and cholestasis. If the wall is perforated, then bile peritonitis may be seen.

2) Chronic cholangitis and cholecystitis. It often developes from recurrent acute cholangitis and cholecystitis. The mucosa of bile ducts and gallbladder wall are atrophic. Lymphocytes, monocyte infiltration and obvious fibrosis can be seen in each layer.

9.10.2 Cholelithiasis

In the biliary system, some elements of the bile (bile pigment, cholesterol, mucosa substance calcium and so on) can be precipitated and form calculus. Calculus formed in the bile duct are called bile duct calculus, those formed in the gallbladder are called cholelithiasis (Figure 9-11).

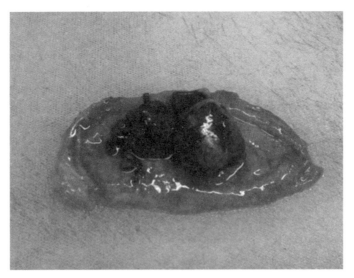

Figure 9-11 Cholecystolithiasis

9.10.2.1 Causes and Pathogenesis

1) Changes in physical and chemical properties of bile Bilirubin is mostly combined with glucuronic acid to from esters in normal bile. The glucuronidase in intestinal bacteria such as *H. coli* decomposes the above esters to free the bilirubin. Too much dissociated bilirubin combines with calcium in the bile to form

insoluble bilirubin calcium. Too much cholesterol is prone to form cholesterol calculus. The loss of bile salts in certain intestinal disease promotes the formation of cholesterol.

2) Stagnation of bile stasis. If the water in bile is absorbed too much, bile pigment or cholesterol will be concentrated and form gallstone.

3) Infection. The inflammatory edema and chronic fibroplasia due to infection thicken the biliary wall, resulting in cholestasis. The cells transudatory during inflammation, deciduous epithelium, the worm residue and insect eggs can be the core of the stone to promote the formation of cholelithiasis.

9.10.2.2   Types and Characteristics of Gallstones

1) Pigmentary gallstone: It is muddy or arenaceous gallstone, multiple, mostly in the bile duct.

2) Cholesterol gallstone: It is often single in the gall bladder, large and round-like.

3) Mixed gallstone: It consists of more than two main components. In china, the most common is the mixed gallstone whose main component is bilirubin. It is unsingle, in the gallbladder or in the bolder tube, mostly polyhedron and colorful. The outer layer is often very hard and has many layers on the section.

9.11   Pancreatitis

Pancreatitis is the pancreatic self digestion caused by abnormal activation of the pancreatic enzyme.

9.11.1   Acute Pancreatitis

It often occurs in middle-aged men after binge eating or biliary disease.

9.11.1.1   Pathological Type and its Pathological Features

1) Acute edematous(interstitial) pancreatitis. Acute edematous pancreatitis is more common with better prognosis, mostly confined to the tail of the pancreas. The disease is characterized by swelling of the pancreas, hyperemia and edema tous interstitial tissuc and infiltration of neutrophils and mononuclear cells. Sometimes localized fat necrosis may occur. A small amount of exudate can be found in the abdominal cavity.

2) Acute hemorrhagic pancreatitis. The onset is rapid, in critical condition. It is characterized by extensive bleeding and necrosis.

Grossly, the pancreas is soft, swelling, dark red, with disappeared original lobulated structure. Scattered muddy yellow white spots(fat is hydrolyzed into glycerol and fatty acid, and combined with calcium ions to form insoluble calcium soap), or small focal fatty necrosis(adipose tissue is necrotic and catabolized by pancreatic juice) can be seen in pancreas, omentum and mesentery.

Microscopically, it is characterized by massive coagulation necrosis and unclear cell structure. Necrosis of interstitial small vessel wall makes massive hemorrhage. Around the necrotic pancreas tissue, there are mild inflammatory cells infiltration. If the patient survive the crisis, inflammatory exudation and bleeding can be absorbed, be cured by fibrosis, or develop to chronic pancreatitis.

9.11.1.2   Clinicopathological Relationship

1) Shock the main causes are as follow: severe abdominal pain caused by stimulation to peritoneum from extravasated pancreatic juice; massive body fluid loss and electrolyte disorder caused by massive bleeding and vomiting; poisoning caused by tissue necrosis and protein decomposition.

2) Peritonitis it is usually caused by stimulation of extravasated pancreatic juice, so the pain is severe and radiates to the back.

3) Enzyme changes. The extravasated pancreatic juice contains a lot of amylase and lipase, which can be absorbed into the blood and expelled in urine, which can be detected to help diagnose.

4) Serum ion change. The levels of calcium, potassium and sodium ions in the serum of the patients are decreased. When pancreatic islet A cells are stimulated, the secretion of glucagon causes lead to secret cal-citonin, which inhibits calcium to dissociate from the bone. Because of persistent vomiting, the level of potassium and sodium in blood is reduced.

9.11.2 Chronic Pancreatitis

It is developed from recurrent acute pancreatitis, and often accompanied with biliary tract diseases, sometimes diabetes. In addition, chronic alcoholism is also the cause.

Grossly, the pancreas is nodular atrophied and hard. On the section, diffuse fibrotic interstitial hyper-plasia, pancreatic duct dilatation, and stone formation can be seen. There are sometimes focal necrosis or pseudocysts wrapped by fiber.

Microscopically, chronic pancreatitis is characterized by fibrosis, atrophy and infiltration of lymphocytes and plasma cells.

9.12 Common Tumors in the Digestive System

9.12.1 Carcinoma of Esophagus

Carcinoma of esophagus is defined as malignant tumor of the esophageal mucosa epithelium or glands. In the whole world, about 300,000 people die from it each year. It is more common in men and adults older than 40 years of age. Clinically, it is characterized by different degrees of dysphagia.

9.12.1.1 Causes

Its etiology is not clear now; The related factors are as follow:

1) Life style: Long term drinking and consumption of overheated, harsh diet, smoking and nitriteis are related to carcinoma of esophagus.

2) Chronic inflammation: Unhealed chronic esophagitis may cause precancerous lesions of carcinoma of esophageal.

3) Genetic factor: In high incidence area, the familial aggregation of the disease is more obvious. The relationship between the gene diversity of metabolic enzymes and the susceptibility of the disease has attrac-ted the attention of scholars.

9.12.1.2 Pathological Changes

It often occurs in three physiological strictures, of which the most common is the middle, the next in the fodowed by distal and upperpart in descending order.

1) Early cancer: There is no obvious clinical symptoms in early stage. The lesion is limited, and often in situ or intramucosal, without muscle layer invading or lymph node metastasis.

Grossly, cancerous mucosa is mild erosive grainy or tiny papillary. X-ray barium meal examination shows normal or mild limited rigid wall.

Microscopically, most of them are squamous cell carcinoma.

2) Middle and advanced cancer: Typical clinical symptoms such as dysphagia appear in this stage. According to gross changes, it can be divided into four types:

Medullary type: It is the most common type. The invasive growth of the carcinoma tissue involves the whole or most of the esophagus. The wall of the tube thickens and the lumen becomes smaller. The section of cancer is soft like brains. Its color is gray and sometimes ulcers cover the surface.

Fungating type: The cancer is a flat round lump, protruding to the esophagus, with superficial ulcers and an ectropion of the edge. The cancer tissue invades part or most of the esophagus wall.

Ulcerated type: There are deep ulcers that cover the surface the surface of the cancer, even to the muscle layer, the bottom is uneven.

Narrow type: The cancer tissue is hard. There are obvious connective tissue proliferating and infiltrating to the wall of esophagus. The local esophageal wall annularly narrows, with obvious expansion above.

Microscopically, more than 95% of the Chinese patients has squamous cell carcinoma, and adenocarcinoma is the second. Most of the adenocarcinoma develops from cardia, little from gland of the esophagus mucosa.

Battle of adenocarcinoma of the esophagus developes from canceration of esophagus, the incidence of which in white people has increased in recent years.

9.12.1.3   Spread

1) Direct spread. The cancer tissue continuously and continuously infiltrates the surrounding tissue and organs after penetrating the wall of the esophagus.

2) Metastasis. Lymphatic metastasis: It metastasizes following the lymphatic drainage. In the upper, it metastasize to the upper mediastinal lymph and neck, to the paraesophageal or hilar lymph nodes in the middle segment and the lymph nodes adjacent to the esophageal or cardia and upper abdominal in the lower segment.

Hematogenous metastasis: It often metastasizes to lung or liver in later stage.

9.12.1.4   Clinicopathological relationship

There is no obvious infiltration or obvious mass in early stage, so its symptoms are not obvious. Only mild retrosternal pain, burning sensation or choking feeling can be experienced in part of the patients which are due to esophageal spasm or mucous infiltration. In the moderate or advanced stage, the wall of esophagus become narrow. Patients have dysphagia or even lose the ability to take in food, then people have cachexia and die in the end.

9.12.2   Carcinoma of Stomach

Carcinoma of stomach is a malignant cancer origining in the epithelium of gastric mucosa and glandular epithelium. The predilection site is in the lesser curvature of the gastric antrum. It often occurs in patients 40–60 years old, and more common in men.

9.12.2.1   Causes

The causes are not clear, and may be related to factors as follow:

1) Dietary and environmental factors. The incidence has some relationships to geographical distribution. For example, in Japan, Chile, Columbia, Costa Rica, Hungary and some places in China, the incidence of carcinoma of stomach is 4–6 times higher than that in United States and Western Europe. Immigration epidemiological surveys show that the incidence of the next generation is correspondingly reduced when people immigrate from areas with high incidence to low incidence areas. However, the incidence of the next generation of gastric cancer is also increased by immigrating to high incidence areas from low incidence areas.

2) Nitroso compounds. Animal experiments have proved using nitroguanidine to feed rats, mice and dogs has successfully induced carcinoma of stomach. Secondary amines and nitrite can be transformed into nitroso compound under the action of gastric acid.

3) *Helicobacter pylori*. Epidemiological studies have revealed that *Helicobacter pylori* infection may be associated with the occurrence of gastric cancer. It has been shown that Helicobacter pylori infection can lead to the CpG islandmethylation of tumor related genes in gastric epithelial cells and apoptosis, etc.

4) Some long-term unhealed chronic gastric diseases such as chronic atrophic gastritis, gastric ulcer disease with abnormal hyperplasia and intestinal metaplasia of gastric mucosa are the pathological basis of gastric cancer.

9.12.2.2　Pathological Changes

1) Early carcinoma of stomach. The cancer tissue is limited to the mucosa or submucosa, regardless of lymph node metastasis. Microcarcinoma refers to cancer less than 0.5 cm in diameter. Small carcinoma of stomach refers to carcinoma 0.6-1.0 cm in diameter.

Grossly, early carcinoma of stomach can be divided to three types as follow:

Protruded carcinoma of stomach: Carcinoma protrudes from the surface of the mucous membrane obviously like polypus. It is rare.

Superficial carcinoma of stomach: The tumor is flat, slightly swells on the mucous surface.

Concave carcinoma of stomach: It is early carcinoma in the surrounding mucosa of the ulcer, also known as cancerous erosion around ulcers. It is the most common type.

Microscopically, cancer in situ and well differentiated tubular adenocarcinoma are more common, followed by papillary adenocarcinoma, and the most rare is undifferentiated carcinoma.

The 5 years survival rate of early gastric cancer is over 90%, the 10 years survival rate is 75%, and the 5 years survival rate of small gastric cancer and microcarcinoma is 100%. Early diagnose can improve the 5 years survival rate after operation and improve the prognosis of gastric cancer.

2) Advanced carcinoma of stomach. It refers to carcinoma infiltrating byond the submucosa. The deeper it invades, the worse the prognosisis. Grossly, it can be divided to three types:

Polypoid or fungoid type: It is also known as the nodular fungoid type. The carcinoma grows forward to the surface of the mucous membrane, like polyps or mushrooms, protruding into the stomach cavity.

Ulcerated type: The necrotic carcinoma tissue exfoliates and forms ulcers. The ulcer is generally large, like a dish with the unclear boundary. It can also rise like a volcano, with clear edges and uneven bottom (Figure 9-12, Table 9-3).

Infiltrating type: Carcinoma infiltrates locally or diffusely into the gastric wall, with unclear boundary. Most of the mucous folds disappeared. When diffuse infiltrated, gastric wall thickens, hardens, gastric cavity becomes narrow, like leather, so it is called linitis plastica.

Colloid carcinoma: When cells secrete a lot of mucus, carcinoma is translucent jelly grossly. It can present as any of the three forms above.

Microscopically, the main type is adenocarcinoma, commonly tubular adenocarcinoma and mucous carcinoma. A few cases may also be adenosquamous or squamous cell carcinoma, which is common in the cardia.

More than two types can exist in the same specimen.

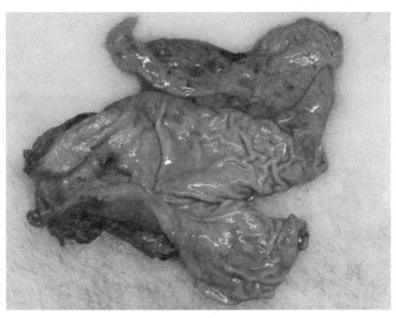

Figure 9-12   Ulcerative gastric cancer

Table 9-3   Differentiation of gross appearance between the benign uclers and malignant ulcers

	Benign ulcers (Gastric ulcer)	Malignant ulcers (Ulcerative gastric cancer)
Gross appearance	Round or ellipse	Irregular
Size (diameter)	<2 cm	>2 cm
Depth	Deep	Shallow
Marginal	Regular and flat	Irregular and bulging
Bottom	Flat	Irregular, necrosis and obvious hemorrhage
Peripheral mucous	Mucous folds concentrating to the ulcer	Mucous folds interruption and nodular hypertrophy

9.12.2.3   Spread

(1) Direct Spread

The cancer tissue can infiltrate to all layers of the stomach wall. It continues to spread to the surrounding tissue and organs such as liver, omentum majus when penetrating the wall.

(2) Metastasis

Lymphatic metastasis: This is the main metastasis way. Firstly, it metastasizes to local lymph node, the most common is lymph node of lesser curvature under the pylorus, then topara-aortic lymph node, portal or mesenteric lymph node, late to left supraclavicular lymph node (Virchow) by thoracic duct.

Hematogenous metastasis: It often metastasizes to some organs like liver, lung, brain or bone by portal vein in the later stage.

Transcoelomic metastasis: cell in carcinoma of stomach, especially inmucinouscarcinoma of stomach infiltrates to the surface of the serous membrane, falls into the abdominal cavity and grow on the serous membrane of the abdominal and pelvic organs. Krukenberg tumor refers to metastatic mucinous carcinoma in the bilateral ovaries.

9.12.2.4　Histogenesis of Gastric Cancer

1) The cell origin of gastric cancer. Carcinoma of stomach mainly occur from tissue stem cells in cervix of gastric gland and the bottom of the gastric pits where the regeneration and repair are active and canceration begins. The cells can differentiate into the epithelium of the stomach or the intestine.

2) Intestinal metaplasia and carcinogenesis. The detection rate of intestinal metaplasia in gastric carcinoma is 88. 2%. It can be found that the activity of aminopeptidase, lactate dehydrogenase and its isozyme increased in the cytoplasm of intestinal metaplastic cells and cancer cells, while those in normal gastric mucosal cells are inactive.

3) Atypical hyperplasia and carcinogenesis. Severe atypical hyperplasia are common in paracancerous mucosa, and some are associated with carcinogenesis.

9.12.3　Carcinoma of Large Intestine

Carcinoma of large intestine is a kind of malignant tumor that occurs in the epithelium or glands in intestine, including cancer of colon and cancer of rectum. It is the third common malignant tumor in the world. It is often seen in the region of Europe, North America, and other places where British ancestry live. From the whole world, China is the low incidence area of large intestine carcinoma, but large intestine carcinoma is the fifth most common malignant tumor in China. The incidence of the disease is on the rise, especially the incidence of colon carcinoma is increasing rapidly, and the growth rate is faster in big cities. In China, the incidence in the city is higher than in the country, the incidence in big cities is higher than in small cities, and the incidence in men grows faster than that in women, which may have a close relationship with the improvement of life and the change of diet.

The main clinical manifestations are anemia, weight loss, increased stool frequency, stool mucosa, abdominal pain, abdominal mass and intestinal obstruction.

9.12.3.1　Causes and Pathogenesis

1) Genetic factors. Inherited carcinoma of large intestine mainly has two types: one is canceration of familial adenomatous polyposis(FAP), which is caused by the mutation of the APC gene. The other is hereditary nonpolyposis colorectal cancer(HNPCC), which is caused by the mutation of mismatch repair genes, such as hMSH2, hMLH1 and so on.

2) Eating habits. A diet of high nutrition and low fiber is related to the occurrence of this disease. Because the highly nutritious diet is not conducive to regular defecation and prolongs the contact time between the intestinal mucosa and carcinogens that may be contained in food.

3) Some chronic intestinal diseases accompanied by intestinal mucosal hyperplasia. For example, some diseases like intestinal polypoid adenoma, proliferative polyposis, juvenile polyposis, villous adenoma, chronic schistosomiasis, chronic ulcerative colitis and so on, become cancer due to hyperplasia of mucosal epithelium.

4) Molecular biological basis of gradual canceration in large intestinal mucosa epithelium. In addition to a small number of hereditary tumors, in the process of the disease development, there are many genetic changes interactions like APC, c-myc, ras, p53, p16, DCC, mcc, DPC4 or mismatch repair genes. The overexpression of gene c-myc can be seen in 90% of large intestine carcinoma. Most of the disease has the mutation of gene p53, defect of gene von Hippel-Lindau. In recent years, studies have found that abnormal expression of some proteins may be related to the occurrence of large intestine carcinoma.

So far the pathogenesis of large intestine carcinoma mainly has four types as follows:

Adenoma canceration: The majority of colorectal carcinomas come from the preexisting adenomas, the so-called adenoma-carcinoma sequence. The occurrence of sporadic large intestine carcinoma is considered to be related to abnormal route of APC-β-catenin-Tcf, methylation cease of specific genes, dysfunction of caryomitosis checkout and so on.

Ulcerative colitis associated cancer pathway: Ulcerative colitis associated carcinoma is different from sporadic large intestine carcinoma. It has the smaller age of onset, the similar incidence rate of different intestine segments, and its molecular mechanism is also different. For example, the abnormality of gene p53 in sporadic colorectal carcinoma occurs mostly in the stage of adenocarcinoma to adenoma, but in ulcerative colitis associated carcinoma, it occurs in the early stage of epithelial proliferation. Morphologically, there were multiple lesions with flat infiltrating focus. Low differentiated adenocarcinoma and mucous adenocarcinoma are common.

Serrated route to carcinoma: Hyperplastic polyposis and malignant transformation of a serrated adenoma are caused by the inhibition of gene expression due to methylation in the promoter region of the mismatched repair gene and functional incapacitation.

Juvenile polyposis-carcinoma pathway: The occurrence of partial juvenile polyposis is due to mutation of gene Smad4.

9.12.3.2   Pathological Changes

The most common site the disease occurs is the rectum(50%), the second most common is the sigmoid colon(20%), cecum and colon(16%), descending colon(6%).

Grossly, the gress form is divided into the following four types:

1) Protruded type. The tumor is polypoid or discoid and protrudes into the lumen of the intestine, and may be accompanied by superficial ulcers. This type is mostly the well-differentiated adenocarcinoma.

2) Ulcerative type. There is a deep ulcer or crater on the surface of tumor. This type is more common.

3) Infiltrative type. Carcinoma tissue infiltrates into the deep wall of the intestinal, and often involves the whole intestine wall, resulting in thickening and stiffening.

4) Gelatinous type. The surface and section of the tumor are translucent and jelly-like. The prognosis is worse.

The gross form of the large intestine carcinoma is slightly different in the left and right colon. The left intestine colorectal carcinoma is more common in infiltrative type, which can easily cause narrowing of the intestinal wall and early symptoms of obstruction. But in the right colon, protruding type is more common.

Microscopically, the histologic types are as following. ①Papillary adenocarcinoma: The papillary tissues thin, rarely have mesenchyme. ②Tubular adenocarcinoma: It can be divided into three grades according to differentiation. ③Mucinous adenocarcinoma: It is characterized by the formation of large mucous lake. ④Undifferentiated adenocarcinoma. ⑤Adenosquamous carcinoma. ⑥Squamous cell carcinoma. The carcinoma major histologic types are highly differentiated tubular adenocarcinoma and papillary adenocarcinoma. Undifferentiated adenocarcinoma and squamous cell carcinoma are minority. Squamous adenocarcinoma often occurs near the rectum and anus.

9.12.3.3   Stage and Prognosis

The stages have a certain significance to the prognosis. The stage commonly used now is proposed by Astler-Coller in 1954, and has been revised many times after Dukes. It is based on the spread of colorectal cancer and whether there are regional lymph nodes metastasis and distant viscera metastasis.

The definition of large bowel carcinoma is clearly defined by WHO. Carcinoma of the large intestine is called as carcinoma only when invasion of the mucous layer reaches to the submucosa layer. It is called intraepithelial neoplasia when the invasion does not exceed the muscularis mucosae. The original severe atypical hyperplasia and carcinoma in situ are classified as high grade intraepithelial neoplasia, and intramural carcinoma is called intra-mucosal neoplasia. Because of the large intestine, scholars found that the 5 years survival rate of intramucosal carcinoma(not over muscularis mucosae) is as high as 100%. But once the invasion is at the submucosa, the 5 years survival rate will decrease obviously.

9.12.3.4　Spread

1) Direct spread: When the invasion is in the serous layer by muscle layer, the disease can spread to organs nearby like prostate, bladder, and peritoneum.

2) Metastasis Lymphatic metastasis: When cancerous tissue does not penetrate the intestinal muscle layer, lymphatic metastasis rarely occurs. Once the penetration can be seen there, the rate of lymphatic metastasis is obvious. It generally metastasizes to the local lymph nodes and then to the distant lymph nodes in the direction of lymphatic drainage. Rarely, it can be seen in supraclavicular lymph node by invasion to thoracic duct.

Hematogenous metastasis: Advanced carcinoma cells can be seen in the liver, or even more remote organs like lung or brain by hematogenous metastasis.

Implantation metastasis: After the carcinoma tissue breaks through the serous membrane of the intestinal wall, it reaches the surface of the intestinal wall. The carcinoma cells fall off and spread into the abdominal cavity to form the implantation metastasis.

9.12.4　Primary Carcinoma of Liver

Primary carcinoma of liver is a malignant tumor of the hepatocyte or intrahepatic bile duct epithelial cells. The incidence of this carcinoma is high in our country. It is one of the common tumors in our country. Most of them are in the middle age. There are no clinical symptoms in the early stage of liver carcinoma, so most of them are late in clinical discovery and the mortality rate is high. In recent years, extensive use of alpha fetoprotein(AFP) and imaging examination has led to the significant increase in the detection rate of early liver carcinoma. Some early tumor lump with a diameter below 1cm were found and achieved satisfactory results.

9.12.4.1　Etiology

It is not clear, but the relevant factors are as follows:

1) Hepatitis virus. Epidemiological and pathological data showes that HBV is closely related to HCC, followed by HCV. There are HBV infections in patients with primary carcinoma of the liver, with a high incidence of up to 60% –90% of liver carcinoma. At present, scholars have found that the common HBV gene is integrated into the genome of hepatoma cells. The genome of HBV encoding HBx protein can inhibit the function of P53 protein, activate mitogen activated protein kinase(MAPK) and Janus family tyrosine kinase (JAK) signal transduction. Repeated regeneration of liver cells may accumulate cell gene mutation, resulting in malignant transformation.

2) Cirrhosis liver. Carcinoma is often associated with liver cirrhosis in China, and most of them are necrotic cirrhosis. According to statistics cirrhosis can elevelop liver carcinoma generally about seven years laler.

3) Fungus and their toxins. Aspergillus flavus, Penicillium, and so on can cause experimental liver carcinoma. Especially the close relationship between aflatoxin B1 and hepatocellular carcinoma is highly valued.

4) Alcohol. It is a carcinogenic factor of liver carcinoma, indirectly via liver cirrhosis. Later live cirrhosis develops liver carcinoma during the repair process.

9. 12. 4. 2 Pathological Change

(1) Grossly

1) Early liver carcinoma(small liver carcinoma). It refers to primary liver carcinoma in which the maximum diameter of a single carcinoma nodule is less than 3 cm or the total maximum diameter of two cancer nodules is less than 3cm. Morphological characteristics: mostly spherical, clear boundary, uniform section, no bleeding and necrosis.

2) Advanced liver carcinoma. The size of the liver increased obviously and the weight increased significantly(often over 2,000-3,000g), and the general morphology is divided into the following three types:

Massive type: The tumor is huge in size, even up to the head of the child, It is round and more common in the right lobe. The central part of the section is often bleeding and necrotic. There are often many different satellite cancer nodules around the tumor. Non or only mild cirrhosis is associated with this type(Figure 9-13).

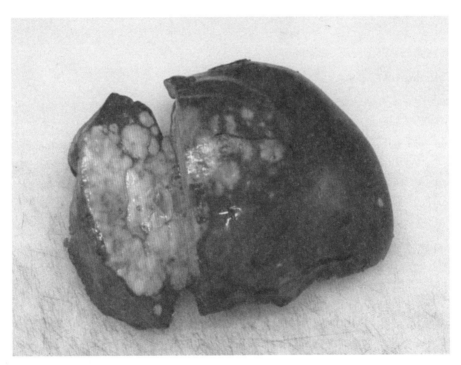

Figure 9-13 **Massive liver carcinoma**

Multiple nodule type: The tye is most common, usually accompanied by cirrhosis of the liver. Cancer nodules are scattered, round or oval, with different sizes. If it is merged, it will form larger nodules.

Diffuse type: The cancer tissue is diffused in the liver, and the nodule is not obvious. It often occurs on the basis of liver cirrhosis, and is easily confused with the liver cirrhosis. This type is rare.

(2) Microscopically, there are three Types of Tissue

1) Hepatocellular carcinoma: It origins from in the hepatocyte, most common. The differentiation degree is different. Cancer cells with higher differentiation are similar to the hepatocytes, secreting bile. The cancer cells are arranged in the nests with many blood vessels(like the hepatic sinusoids) and fewer interstitial substances. The heteromorphy of low differentiation is obvious. Cancer cells are different in size and shape.

2) Cholangiocarcinoma: It is a malignant tumor that occurs in the intrahepatic bile duct epithelium. The neoplastic cells are arranged in a tubular gland manner, which can secrete mucus and have more interstitial cancerous tissue. Liver cirrhosis is usually not complicated.

3) Mixed cell type liver carcinoma. There are two components including hepatocellular carcinoma and cholangiocarcinoma in cancer tissue, which are the most rare.

9.12.4.3 Spread

The cancer tissue first spreads directly in the liver and metastasizes along the portal vein, causing multiple metastatic nodules in the liver. Through the lymphatic passage, the extra hepatic metastasis can be transferred to the hilar lymph nodes, upper abdominal lymph nodes and retroperitoneal lymph nodes. In the late stage, through the hepatic vein is transferred to the lungs, adrenal glands, brain and kidney. After the cancerous cells on the surface of the liver have fallen off, implantable metastases can form.

9.12.5   Carcinoma of Pancreas

Carcinoma of pancreas is a rare digestive tract tumor. It accounts for 1% of the total body cancer in China. However, according to statistics from some countries, the incidence of pancreatic carcinoma is increasing in recent years. The age of patients is 60–80 years old. The main environmental impact factor is smoking, which can double the risk. About 90% of the patients have K-ras mutation. In addition, there is c-myc overexpression and P53 gene mutation.

9.12.5.1   Pathological Change

Carcinoma of the pancreas can occur in the head (60%) of the pancreas (60%), body (15%), tail (5%) or the whole pancreas.

Grossly, the size and shape of pancreatic carcinoma are different. Sometimes, the tumor is a rigid nodule that protrudes from the surface of the pancreas. Sometimes the tumor is buried in the pancreas and cannot be seen from the outside surface the pancreas. Common sclerosis of the peritumoral tissue is so hard that the entire gland becomes hard, and it is difficult to distinguish from the chronic pancreatitis even when the laparotomy is proceeded.

Microscopically, common histological types are ductal adenocarcinoma, cystadenocarcinoma, mucous carcinoma and solid carcinoma. There are also undifferentiated carcinoma or pleomorphic carcinoma, and rare types of squamous cell carcinoma or adenosquamous carcinoma.

9.12.5.2   Spread

The carcinoma of the head of the pancreas can directly spread to adjacent tissues and organs, such as the bile duct and the duodenum. Then it is transferred to the head of the pancreas and the common bile duct lymph nodes. Intrahepatic metastasis through portal vein is the most common, especially for the body or tail cancer, and then the tumor cells intrude into the celiac plexus perilymphatic space and metastasis to the lung and bone. Cancers of pancreatic body and tail are often accompanied by multiple venous thrombosis.

9.12.5.3   Clinicopathological Relationship

The main symptom of pancreatic head carcinoma is painless jaundice. The main symptoms of body and tail tumors are deep tingling caused by invasion of the celiac plexus, ascites caused by invasion of the portal vein, and splenomegaly occurring in the compression of the splenic vein. In addition, symptoms such as anemia, hematemesis and constipation can be seen without jaundice, and extensive thrombosis may form. If it cannot be diagnosed early, the prognosis is poor and most patients died within a year.

9.12.6   Tumor of Biliary Tract

9.12.6.1   Carcinoma of the Gallbladder

Pathological features: The carcinoma of the gallbladder often occurs at the bottom and neck of the gallbladder.

Grossly, the gallbladder wall is thickened, hardened and gray(mostly diffuse infiltrating growth). It can also grow in the form of polyps, and the basal part is wide.

Microscopically, most of them are adenocarcinoma, and some are adenosquamous carcinoma or squamous cell carcinoma.

Clinical manifestation: It occurs mostly in and older people. Because it is not easy to find early, the prognosis is poor. Its occurrence is related to cholelithiasis and chronic cholecystitis.

9.12.6.2   Extrahepatic Cholangiocarcinoma

Pathological features: The confluence of the common bile duct, the hepatic duct and the cystic duct is common.

Grossly, it can be polypoid, nodular, or deep infiltrated in the deep wall of the bile duct.

Microscopically, most of them are adenocarcinoma, including papillary adenocarcinoma, mucinous adenocarcinoma and sclerosing cholangiocarcinoma with abundant fibrous interstitium. A few are adenosine squamous cell carcinoma or squamous cell carcinoma.

Clinical manifestation: More common in the elderly, with obstructive jaundice, abdominal pain and abdominal mass.

9.12.7   Gastrointestinal Stromal Tumors

Gastrointestinal stromal tumors(GIST) are a class of tumors that originate from the gastrointestinal mesenchymal tissue and is mainly found in the elderly.

Pathological features: It is most common most common in the stomach, followed by the small intestine, less seen in the large intestine and the esophagus, occasionally occurs in the omentum and mesentery. Most tumors do not have the complete capsule, which can be accompanied by cystic degeneration, necrosis and focal hemorrhage. The degree of malignancy is related to the size of the tumor, the image of the mitosis and the site of its occurrence. If the diameter of the tumor is more than 5 cm, the tumor is malignant, and the risk of GIST in the small intestine is higher than that in the stomach.

Microscopical features: 70% of gastrointestinal stromal tumors are spindle cells, 20% are epithelioid cells. Immunohistochemical features of gastrointestinal stromal tumors are positive for cell surface antigen CD117. About 60% –70% of gastrointestinal stromal tumors were CD34 positive.

Chapter 10

The Diseases of Hematopoietic and Lymphoid Systems

⟫ Introduction

Disorders of the hematopoietic and lymphoid systems include a wide range of diseases that are traditionally, classified as disorders which primarily affect red cells, white cells, and the hemostatic system. Diseases of red cells and white cells the hemostatic system include anemia, leukopenia, and thrombocytopenia. On the contrary, proliferation may be reactive, such as reactive lymphadenitis, leukocytosis, and thrombocytosis, or neoplasms, such as leukemias and malignant lymphomas. The hematopoietic and lymphoid systems, unlike other organ systems, are not confine to a single anatomic site. Therefore, when diseases of the hematopoietic and lymphoid system are considered, it is important to keep in mind that the hematopoietic and lymphoid cells are spread throughout the body. Therefore, a patient with malignant lymphoma diagnosed by lymph node biopsy can also have neoplastic lymphocytes in the bone marrow and blood. Malignant lymphoid cells in the bone marrow can inhibit hematopoiesis, giving rise to cytopenias, and the further spread of tumor cells to the liver and spleen may cause hepatomegaly and splenomegaly. Thus, in benign and malignant hematolymphoid disorders, a single underlying abnormality can result in diverse systemic manifestations. In this chapter, we first briefly introduce the structure and function of hematopoietic and lymphoid system, describe some non-neoplastic conditions, and then mainly focus on white cell disorders.

10.1 Structure and Function of the Hematopoietic System and Lymphoid Systems

The hematopoietic and lymphoid systems are composed of lymphoid tissue (thymus, spleen, lymph nodes and extranodal lymphoid tissues) and myeloid tissue(bone marrow). The thymus and bone marrow are often termed central lymphoid tissues in that they are central to the prenatal development of the immune system, but they do not participate in the immune response in the adults. The remaining lymphoid organs are actively involved in the immune response, and constitute the peripheral lymphoid tissue.

The lymph nodes are surrounded by a capsule of connective tissue capsule, with trabeculae that extend into the substance of the node and provide a framework for the contained cellular elements. Beneath the capsule is a slit-like space, the subcapsular sinus. There are three distinct regions in normal lymph nodes:

①the cortex, which contains nodules of B-lymphocytes either primary or as germinal centers;②the paracortex or deep cortex, which is the T-cell dependent region of the lymph node;③medullar, containing the medullary cords and sinuses which drain into the hilum.

The appearance of the follicles varies according to their activity status. The primary follicles appear as small, round nodules with small lymphocytes. Secondary follicles appear following antigenic stimulation and are characterized by the presence of germinal centers. The cells present in these formations are B-lymphocytes known as follicles center cells, including centroblasts and centrocytes, macrophages and follicular dendritic cells(FDCs). The germinal center is surrounded by a mantle zone of small B-lymphocytes.

There are many kinds of immune cells in the lymphatic system(lymph nodes, spleen, tonsils, etc.), where lymphocytes, macrophages, and other immune cells are arranged in various ways which is conducive to the formation of immune responses. Lymphatic tissues mainly gather at the entrance of the antigen entrance: tonsillar(mouth and nose), respiratory and gastrointestinal submucosa(inhaling and ingested antigen), lymph nodes(lymphatic drainage for skin and organs) and spleen(such as blood filters). The histologic appearances of lymphoid tissue mainly depend on the degree of antigenic stimulation. Reactive follicles (foci of B-cell proliferation) appear only under antigen exposure. Similarly, immunoblasts are only present under antigenic stimulation.

In the embryos, the formation of blood may occur in various parts of the body, such as the liver and spleen. In addition to the fact that lymphocytes and large mononuclear cells continue to mature in lymphoid tissue, the main center of hematopoietic activity is located in bone marrows. After birth, the bone marrow is the only site of production of erythrocytes, granulocytes, and platelets. It also produces blood monocytes, which are part of the macrophage system. At birth, hematopoietic marrow is present in the medullary cavity of bones. In adults, the hematopoietic marrow is replaced by adipose tissue in the bones of the extremities, and hematopoietic marrow is found only in the axial skeleton.

10.2 Infection and Reactive Proliferation

10.2.1 Reactive Lymphadenitis

Lymph nodes undergo reactive changes in response to a wide variety of stimuli which include microbial infections, drugs, environmental pollutants, tissue injury, immune-complexes and malignant neoplasms. Reactive lymphadenitis is the most common benign lesion. Immune response against foreign antigens can lead to lymph node enlargement(lymphadenopathy). The histologic appearance of reactive lymphadenitis is nonspecific with a few variant forms. Microscopically, the features of 3 patterns of reactive lymphoid hyperplasia are as follows:

10.2.1.1 Follicular Hyperplasia

This is the most common pattern. There is marked enlargement and prominence of the germinal centers of the lymphoid follicles(Figure 10-1, from ROBBINS and COTRAN Pathologic Basis of Disease), consisting of numerous activated B cells, scattered T cells, and phagocytic macrophages(containing nuclear debris), and a meshwork of antigen-presenting follicular dendritic cells. The reactive follicles develop from primary follicles in the cortex of the lymph node. The first phase of follicular formation appears to be antigen capture by dendritic reticulum cells, and then play a role in stimulating B-cell proliferation, leading to the development of a group of active B-lymphocytes(the secondary or reactive follicles). Follicular hyperplasia can be found in rheumatoid arthritis, toxoplasmosis, and early HIV infection.

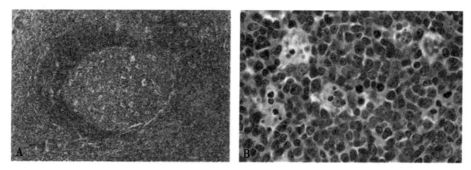

Figure 10-1   Reactive hyperplasia in lymph node shows features of a predominantly
B cell response, characterized by enlarged follicles with prominent reactive centers

A, Low-power view shows a reactive follicle and surrounding mantle zone. The dark-staining mantle zone
is more prominent adjacent to the germinal-center light zone in the left half of the follicle. The right half of
the follicle consists of the dark zone. B, High-power view of the dark zone shows several mitotic figures and
numerous macrophages containing phagocytosed apoptotic cells (tingible bodies)

10.2.1.2   Paracortical Hyperplasia

This is due to hyperplasia of T-cell-dependent area of the lymph node. When activated, parafollicular T cells transform into a large number of proliferating immunoblasts that can affect the follicles of B cells. In some instances, the T-cell response may be dominant; follicles may be inconspicuous. Paracortical hyperplasia commonly occurs in viral infections [such as Epstein-Barr virus (EBV)], vaccinations (e. g. smallpox), and drug-induced immune responses (especially phenytoin).

10.2.1.3   Sinus Histiocytosis

It is characterized by distention and prominence of the lymphatic sinuses, which are filled with macrophages (histiocytes) and hypertrophy of lining endothelial cells. It often occurs in lymph nodes draining cancers and may represent an immune response to the tumor or its products.

10.2.2   Infectious Mononucleosis

It is caused by B lymph cytotropic Epstein-Barr virus. Infected B cells express virus antigens on their surface, which results in strong immune responses of T cells. Infectious mononucleosis is characterized by a florid T-cell hyperplasia, which is so extensive that follicles are obscured. The most striking feature is the expansion of paracortical areas with a large number of immunoblasts and transformed large T cells. B-cell areas (follicles) may also be hyperplastic, but usually mild. Occasionally, EBV-infected B cells resembling Reed-Sternberg cells may be found, leading to possible misdiagnosis as malignant lymphoma. Increased number of large transformed lymphocytes can also be found in the peripheral blood (so-called Downey cells). Infectious mononucleosis is more common in adolescents and young adults and is transmitted via the upper respiratory tract. Patients are characterized by high fever, sore throat, lymphadenitis, and hepatosplenomegaly. Lymph nodes are enlarged throughout the body, principally in the posterior cervical, axillary, and groin regions. Spleen is enlarged in most cases and is usually soft and fleshy, with a hyperemic cut surface. The histologic changes of the spleen show an expansion of white pulp follicles and red pulp sinusoids due to the presence of numerous activated T cells. It may be diagnosed by the peripheral blood appearance (lymphocytosis with Downey cells). It should be noted that cytomegalovirus infection induces a similar syndrome, which can be differentiated only by serologic methods.

10.2.3　Specific Infections of Lymph Nodes

Characteristics of various special infections within the lymph node are listed as the following: ①Specific microbial antigens, special pathological features of inflammation, special staining in the diseased tissue, secretions or body fluid can be found associated with microbial pathogens. ②Special drug therapy may be required in the clincic. The presence of specific reagents in lymph nodes is often allowed to be diagnosed through the culture of lymph nodes, which should be required in the biopsy.

10.2.3.1　Tuberculosis Lymphadenitis

It usually occurs in the cervical nodes(scrofula)and is frequently associated with extrapulmonary tuberculosis. It tends to be unifocal and localized. Enlarged a group of lymph nodes can be merged together to form a big lump. The cut surface reveals cheesy material(caseation). The basic histopathological lesion is caseous necrosis of granulomatous inflammation. The centers of granulomas undergo caseation necrosis resulting in featureless areas of eosinophilic material. Langhans lump. The cut surface reveals cheesy material (caseation). The basic histopathological lesion is caseous necrot be identified with special stains.

10.2.3.2　Cat-Scratch Disease

It is a self-limited lymphadenitis caused by the bacterium Bartonella henselae. 90% of the patients are younger than 18 years of age. It presents as regional lymphadenopathy, most frequently in the axilla and the neck. The nodal enlargement appears approximately 2 weeks after a feline scratch or, less commonly, after a splinter or thorn injury. An inflammatory nodule, vesicle, or eschar is sometimes visible at the site of the skin injury. In most patients the lymph node enlargement regresses over a period of 2–4 months.

The pathological changes in the lymph node in cat scratch disease are quite characteristic. Initially sarcoid-like granulomas form, but these then undergo central necrosis associated with an infiltrate of neutrophils. These irregular stellate necrotizing granulomas are similar to those seen in a limited number of other infections, such as lymphogranuloma venereum. The microbe is extracellular and can be visualized with silver stains. The diagnosis is based on a history of exposure to cats, the characteristic clinical findings, are a positive result on serologic testing for antibodies to Bartonella, and the distinctive morphologic changes in the lymph nodes.

10.3　Lymphoid Neoplasms

Lymphoid neoplasms, both malignant lymphomas and lymphocytic leukemias, are a group of tumors with clinical manifestations and behaviors that vary widely. In fact, they are the same disease in different clinic stages, resulting in diverse manifestations. Both lymphomas and lymphocytic leukemias may initially arise from lymphoid tissues or hematopoietic tissue and then involve each other. Lymphocytic leukemia is used for neoplasms that present with widespread involvement of the bone marrow and(usually, but not always)the peripheral blood. Lymphoma is used for proliferation that arises as discrete tissue masses. Originally these terms were attached to what were considered distinct entities, but now these divisions have blurred. Many entities called "lymphoma" occasionally have leukemic presentations. Conversely, tumors identical to issue masses. Originally these terms were attached to what were considered distinct entities, but now these divisions have blurred. Many entities called "lymphoma" occasionissue distribution of each disease at presentation.

In daily medical practice, lymph nodes and bone marrow biopsy, bone marrow aspiration cytology and blood cytology are the most important methods in diagnosis of lymph hematopoietic system diseases. Many tumors also involve the gene-phenotype changes. Therefore, molecular biology, immunohistochemistry and flow cytometry have become indispensable tools in the diagnosis of blood diseases.

10.3.1　Classification of Lymphoid Neoplasms

Lymphoid neoplasms show enormous variation in clinical behavior and response to therapy. The classification aims to identify homogeneous subgroups that behave in a predictable way. Lymphoid neoplasms are derived from cells that recapitulate stages of normal B-, T-, and NK-cell differentiation and function, so to some extent they can be classified according to the corresponding normal counterpart. Several morphologic stages can be identified in the process of lymphocytes differentiation from stem cells to mature cells according to the differentiation pattern of lymphocytes proposed by Lennert et al. in 1975. However, the classification method varied greatly because lymphocytic morphology change can occur at any stage of lymphocyte differentiation.

The WHO classification of lymphoid neoplasms is based on the morphology, cell origin (determined by immunophenotyping), clinical features, and genotype (e. g. karyotype, the presence of viral genomes) of each entity. All lymphoid neoplasms can be classified on the basis of cell origin: ①Precursor lymphoid neoplasms; ②Mature B-cell neoplasms; ③Mature T-and NK-cell neoplasms; ④Hodgkin lymphomas (Table 10-1).

Table 10-1　WHO classification of Lymphoid Neoplasms (2017)

1. Precursor lymphoid neoplasms
B-lymphoblastic leukemia/lymphoma, not otherwise specified
B-lymphoblastic leukemia/lymphoma with recurrent genetic abnormalities
T-lymphoblastic leukemia/lymphoma
NK-lymphoblastic leukemia/lymphoma
2. Mature B-cell neoplasms
Chronic lymphocytic leukemia/small lymphocytic lymphoma
B-cell prolymphocytic leukemia
Splenic marginal zone lymphoma
Hairy cell leukemia
Splenic B-cell lymphoma/leukemia, unclassifiable
Lymphoplasmacytic lymphoma
IgM Monoclonal gammopathy of undetermined significance
Heavy chain diseases
Plasma cell neoplasms
Extranodal marginal zone lymphoma of mucosa-associated lymphoid tissue (MALT lymphoma)
Nodal marginal zone lymphoma
Follicular lymphoma
Pediatric-type follicular lymphoma

Continue to Table 10-1

Large B-cell lymphoma with IRF4 rearrangement
Primary cutaneous follicle center lymphoma
Mantle cell lymphoma
Diffuse large B-cell lymphoma(DLBCL) ,NOS
T-cell/histiocyte-rich large B-cell lymphoma
Primary diffuse large B-cell lymphoma of the CNS
Primary cutaneous diffuse large B-cell lymphoma,leg type
EBV-positive diffuse large B-cell lymphoma,NOS
EBV-positive mucocutaneous ulcer
Diffuse large B-cell lymphoma associated with chronic inflammation
Lymphomatoid granulomatosis
Primary mediastinal(thymic)large B-cell lymphoma
Intravascular large B-cell lymphoma
ALK-positive large B-cell lymphoma
Plasmablastic lymphoma
Primary effusion lymphoma
HHV8−associated lymphoproliferative disorders
Burkitt lymphoma
Burkitt-like lymphoma with 11q aberration
High-grade B-cell lymphoma
B-cell lymphoma,unclassifiable,with features intermediate between DLBCL and classic Hodgkin lymphoma
3. Mature T-and NK-cell neoplasms
T-cell prolymphocytic leukemia
T-cell large granular lymphocytic leukemia
Chronic lymphoproliferative disorder of NK-cells
Aggressive NK-cell leukemia
EBV-positive T-cell and NK-cell lymphoproliferative diseases of childhood
Adult T-cell leukemia/lymphoma
Extranodal NK/T-cell lymphoma,nasal type
Intestinal T-cell lymphoma
Hepatosplenic T-cell lymphoma
Subcutaneous panniculitis-like T-cell lymphoma
Mycosis fungoides
Sézary syndrome
Primary cutaneous CD30−positive T-cell lymphoproliferative disorders
Primary cutaneous peripheral T-cell lymphomas,rare subtypes
Peripheral T-cell lymphoma,NOS

Continue to Table 10-1

Angioimmunoblastic T-cell lymphoma and other nodal

Anaplastic large cell lymphoma. ALK-positive

Anaplastic large cell lymphoma. ALK-negative

Breast implant-associated anaplastic large cell lymphoma

4. Hodgkin lymphomas

Nodular lymphocyte predominant Hodgkin lymphoma

Classical Hodgkin lymphoma

    Nodular sclerosis classical Hodgkin lymphoma

    Lymphocyte-rich classical Hodgkin lymphoma

    Mixed-cellularity classical Hodgkin lymphoma

    Lymphocyte-depleted classical Hodgkin lymphoma

10.3.2 Precursor B-and T-cell Lymphoblastic Leukemia/Lymphoma

These are high-grade NHLs and composed of diffuse sheets of medium-sized immature lymphocytes (lymphoblasts). It may be B-or T-cell lineage, which are morphologically similar, presenting similar signs and symptoms, and treated similarly. Thus, precursor B-and T-cell lymphoblastic Leukemia/Lymphoma are classified together.

Acute Lymphoblastic Leukemia/Lymphoblastic Lymphoma(ALL)occurs predominantly in children and young adults. ALLs accounted for 80% of childhood leukemia, the peak age is 4 years old, and most cases are pre-B cell origin. The pre-T cell tumors are most common among male between 15 and 20 years old. Just as B cell precursors normally develop within the bone marrow, pre-B cell tumors usually present in the bone marrow and peripheral blood as leukemia. Similarly, pre-T cell tumors commonly present as masses involving the thymus, the normal site of early T cell differentiation. However, pre-T cell "lymphomas" often progress rapidly to the leukemic stage, while other pre-T cell tumors seem to involve bone marrow only. Hence, both pre-B and pre-T cell tumors usually present clinical manifestations at a certain time in their process.

10.3.2.1 Morphology

Microscopically, lymph nodes composed of small to medium-sized blast cells with scant cytoplasm and inconspicuous nucleoli. Most pre-T-cell lymphomas present as mediastinal masses and progress rapidly to leukemia stage, but other cases present as marrow involvement only. Pre-B-cell lymphoma usually presents as bone marrow involvement. Meningeal infiltration is an important feature. In the blood smear slide, the nuclei of lymphoblastsic with Wright-Giemsa staining show somewhat coarse and clumped chromatin and one or two nucleoli; myeloblasts tend to have fine chromatin and more cytoplasm, which may contain granules. It is practically essential to distinguish ALL from AML as these two diseases have different therapies.

10.3.2.2 Immunophenotypic and Genetic Features

Immunophenotyping is very useful in distinguishing ALL from AML. Terminal deoxynucleotidyl transferases(TdT), a DNA polymerase and a utility marker for these diseases, is present in more than 95% of ALL cases. It is necessary to perform specific immunologic staining to subtype further into pre-B-and pre-T-cell types, such as CD19(B cell)and CD3(T cell).

Approximately 90% of ALLs have nonrandom karyotypic abnormalities. Most common in childhood, pre-B cell tumours are hyperdiploidy(more than 50 chromosomes/cell)and the presence of a cryptic(12; 21)translocation involving the ETVL and RUNX1 genes,while about 25% of adult pre-B cell tumours harbor the(9;22)translocation involving the ABL and BCR genes. Pre-T cell tumors are associated with diverse chromosomal aberrations,including frequent translocations involving the T cell receptor loci and transcription factor genes such as TAL1.

10.3.2.3 Clinical Features

The clinical characteristics of ALL are similar to that of AML. The manifestations are anemia,bleeding (petechiae,ecchymoses,epistaxis,gum bleeding)and infection as well as related symptoms,characterized by an abrupt,clinical onset. Intensive combination chemotherapy,using several anticancer agents simultaneously in various combinations,has improved the prognosis of ALL patients dramatically. Recently,acute leukemias have been treated more aggressively with the intention of destroying all the hematopoietic cells in bone marrow,including leukemic cells,followed by bone marrow transplantation.

10.3.3 Mature B Cell Neoplasms

Many mature B cells originate from follicular growth pattern of normal B-cells. Thus,in some B cell tumors,tumor cells are clustered into identifiable nodules similar to normal follicles. These tumors are called follicular lymphomas. Other B cell tumors do not produce nodules but diffuse into lymph nodes. This structure is referred to as diffuse lymphoma. The normal structure of the lymph node disappears.

10.3.3.1 Chronic Lymphocytic Leukemia/Small Lymphocytic Lymphoma

It is a neoplasm composed of monomorphic small,round to slightly irregular B lymphocytes in the peripheral blood(PB),bone marrow(BM),spleen,and lymph nodes,admixed with prolymphocytes and paraimmunoblasts forming proliferation centers in tissue infiltrates. Chronic lymphocytic leukemia(CLL) and small lymphocytic lymphoma(SLL) are considered the same underlying disease,just with different appearances,thus termed as CLL/SLL. If the peripheral blood lymphocyte count exceeds 5000 cells/μL,the patient is diagnosed with CLL. Tumors mainly involve lymph node,spleen,or extra nodal locations are diagnosed as SLL. CLL/SLL is a disease of adults,and most(>75%)people newly diagnosed with CLL are over the age of 50,and the majority are men.

(1)Morphology

Histologically,enlarged lymph nodes in patients with CLL/SLL show effacement of the architecture, with a pseudofollicular pattern of regularly-distributed pale areas corresponding to proliferation centers containing larger cells in a dark background of small cells. The predominant cells are small,resting lymphocytes with dark,round nuclei,and scanty cytoplasm. Proliferation centers contain a continuum of small,medium and large cells. Prolymphocytes are small to medium-sized cells with relatively clumped chromatin and small nucleoli;paraimmunoblasts are larger cells with round to oval nuclei,dispersed chromatin,central eosinophilic nucleoli and slightly basophilic cytoplasm. In addition to the lymph nodes,the bone marrow,spleen, and liver are involved in almost all cases. In most patients there is an absolute lymphocytosis featuring small,mature-looking lymphocytes. The circulating tumor cells are fragile and during the preparation of smears are frequently disrupted,producing characteristic smudge cells. Variable numbers of larger activated lymphocytes are also usually found in the blood smear.

(2)Immunophenotypic and Genetic Features

CLL/SLL is a neoplasm of mature B cells expressing the pan-B cell markers CD19,CD20,and CD23 and surface immunoglobulin heavy and light chains. The tumor cells also express CD5,which is a helpful diagnostic clue since among B cell lymphomas only CLL/SLL and mantle cell lymphoma commonly express

CD5. Approximately 50% of tumors have karyotypic abnormalities, the most common of which are trisomy 12 and deletions of chromosomes 11, 13, and 17. "Deep sequencing" of CLL/SLL cell genomes has identified activating mutations in the Notch1 receptor in a subset of cases that predict a worse outcome. Unlike in other B cell neoplasms, chromosomal translocations are rare.

(3) Clinical Features

CLL/SLL is often asymptomatic. Most cases are diagnosed as a result of routine blood tests or clinical examination for some other reasons. The most common clinical signs and symptoms are nonspecific, including fatigue, weight loss, and anorexia. 50% to 60% of patients have lymphadenopathy and hepatosplenomegaly. White blood cell count may only increase slightly in SLL or may exceed 200,000 cells/μL or clinical hypogammaglobulinemia develops in more than 50% of the patients, usually in later stages, and leads to an increased susceptibility to bacterial infections. Rare autoimmune hemolytic anemia and thrombocytopenia are seen. DNA analysis has distinguished two major types of CLL/SLL, with different survival times. CLL/SLL that is positive for the marker ZAP-70 has an average survival of 8 years. CLL/SLL that is negative for ZAP-70 has an average survival of more than 25 years. Many patients, especially older ones, with slowly progressing disease can be reassured and may not need any treatment in their lifetimes. Approximately 2% – 8% of CLL/SLL patients develop DLBCL and <1% develop classic Hodgkin lymphoma.

10.3.3.2 Follicular Lymphoma

Follicular lymphoma is a tumor derived from germinal center B-cells, characterized by a follicular or nodular architecture. It accounts for about 20% of all lymphomas with the highest incidence in the USA and Western Europe. In China, it accounts for only about 10% of NHL cases.

(1) Morphology

Microscopically, the closely packed neoplastic follicles replace the normal Lymph node architectures. Neoplastic follicles are mainly composed of centrocyte(CC) and centroblast(CB) cells. CC cells are slightly larger than resting lymphocytes that have angular nuclei with prominent indentations and linear infoldings. The nuclear chromatin is coarse and condensed, and nucleoli are indistinct. CB cells are larger centroblast-like cells with vesicular chromatin, several nucleoli, and modest amounts of cytoplasm. In most tumors, CB cells are a minor component of the overall cellularity, mitoses are infrequent, and single necrotic cells(cells undergoing apoptosis) are not found(Figure 10-2, from ROBBINS and COTRAN Pathologic Basis of Disease). These features help to distinguish follicular lymphoma from reactive follicular hyperplasia, in which mitoses and apoptosis are prominent. With the progress of the disease course, the number of CB cells gradually increased. The growth pattern change from the follicular to diffuse, resulting in a more aggressive clinical behavior.

(2) Immunophenotypic and Genetic Features

These neoplastic cells express pan-B cell markers(CD19 and CD20), CD10, BCL6, and BCL2(Figure 10-3, from ROBBINS and COTRAN Pathologic Basis of Disease). Most of the cases have specific chromosome translocation involving the immunoglobulin heavy chain promoter region on chromosome 14 and the anti-apoptotic gene BCL-2 on chromosome 18, t(14;18)(q32;q21), which resulted in high expression of BCL-2 gene and protein.

(3) Clinical Features

Follicular lymphoma is more common in adults over the age of 50. Most patients present with painless and lymphadenopathy. Bone marrow is commonly involved in the diagnosis, while visceral diseases are rare. It is an indolent disease and the median survival time is 7–9 years. Approximately 40% of FL patients develop DLBCL, resulting in a more aggressive clinical behavior.

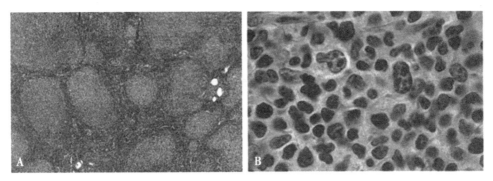

Figure 10-2   **Follicular lymphoma**

The neoplastic follicles are closely packed. Focally show an almost back-to-back pattern. A, Nodular aggregates of lymphoma cells are present throughout lymph node. B, At high magnification, small lymphoid cells with condensed chromatin and irregular or cleaved nuclear outlines(centrocytes) are mixed with a population of larger cells with nucleoli(centroblasts)

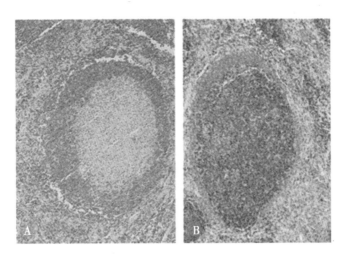

Figure 10-3   **BCL2 expression in reactive and neoplastic follicles**

In reactive follicles(A), BCL2 is present in mantle zone cells but not follicular center B cells in follicular lymphoma cells(B)show strong BCL2 staining

10.3.3.3 Mantle Cell Lymphoma

Mantle cell lymphoma is composed of monomorphic small to medium-sized cells resembling naive B cells of mantle zones. It accounts for approximately 4% of all NHLs and occurs mainly in men more than 50 years old.

(1)Morphology

Mantle cell lymphoma may involve lymph nodes in a diffuse or nodular pattern. Tumor cells usually are slightly larger than normal with an irregular nucleus, inconspicuous nucleoli, and scant cytoplasm. Bone marrow involvement occurs in most cases, but the peripheral blood involvement is rare. Sometimes it originates from extranode lymphoid tissue, such as gastrointestinal tract presenting as multifocal submucosal nodules that grossly resemble polyps(lymphomatoid polyposis).

(2)Immunophenotypic and Genetic Features

Tumor cells usually express pan-B cell antigens(CD19 and CD20), and CD5.

MCL is genetically characterized by the translocation(11;14)and cyclin D1 gene rearrangement, which resulted in high expression of cyclin D1 gene and protein.

Cyclin D1, a cell cycle regulator, is believed to be an important mediator of uncontrolled tumor cell growth.

(3) Clinical Features

Most patients present with fatigue and lymphadenopathy and are found to have generalized disease involving the bone marrow, spleen, liver, and (often) the gastrointestinal tract. The tumor is moderately aggressive and median survival time is 3–5 years.

10.3.3.4 Diffuse Large B Cell Lymphomas

Diffuse large B cell lymphomas (DLBCL) is the most common type of high-grade lymphoma, accounting for approximately 50% of adult NHLs.

(1) Morphology

DLBCL is characterized by a diffuse outgrowth of large B-cells, which may display centroblastic or immunoblastic cytology. Nuclear size is equal to or exceeds normal macrophage nuclei or more than twice the size of a normal lymphocyte.

Three common and additional minor morphological variants have been recognized. ①Centroblastic variant: this is the most common variant. Centroblasts are medium-sized to large lymphoid cells with oval to round, vesicular nuclei containing fine chromatin. There are two to four nuclear membrane-bound nucleoli. The cytoplasm is usually scanty and amphophilic to basophilic. ②Immunoblastic variant: greater than 90% of the cells in this variant are immunoblasts with a single centrally located nucleolus and an appreciable amount of basophilic cytoplasm. Immunoblasts with plasmacytoid differentiation may also be present. ③Anaplastic variant: this variant is characterized by large to very large round, oval or polygonal cells with bizarre pleomorphic nuclei that may resemble, at least in part, HRS cells.

(2) Immunophenotypic and Genetic Features

Tumor cells express pan-B cell antigens, such as CD20, CD19 and CD79a. Some cases also tumor cells express surface IgM and/or IgG. Other antigens (e.g., CD10, CD5) are variably expressed. A variety of cytogenic abnormalities can be seen in DLBCL. (14;18) translocation is the most common deregulation and about one-third of cases show rearrangement of the BCL6 gene.

(3) Clinical Features

It occurs primarily in older individuals, with a median age at diagnosis of around 70 years of age. DLBCL is an aggressive tumor which can arise in virtually any part of the body and the first sign of this illness is typically the observation of a rapidly growing mass at single or multiple nodal or extranodal sites, such as gastrointestinal tract, skin, bone, or brain. Most patients are asymptomatic but when symptoms are present they are highly dependent on the sites of involvement. Without treatment, the prognosis of DLBCL is poor. With intensive combination chemotherapy and anti-CD20 immunotherapy, complete remissions is achieved in 60%–80% patients.

10.3.3.5 Burkitt Lymphoma

It is a B-cell lymphoma with an extremely short doubling time that often presents in extranodal sites or as an acute leukemia. It is named after Denis Parsons Burkitt, a surgeon who first described the disease in 1958 while working in equatorial Africa. It is endemic in parts of Africa and occurs sporadically in other areas. The disease is associated with EBV infection.

(1) Morphology

The tumor consists of sheets of a monotonous (i.e. similar in size and morphology) population of medium size lymphoid cells with high proliferative activity and apoptotic activity. A "starry sky" pattern is usually present, which is imparted by numerous benign macrophages that have ingested apoptotic tumor cells (Figure 10-4, from ROBBINS and COTRAN Pathologic Basis of Disease). Tumor cells have round or oval nuclei, two to five distinct nucleoli and a moderate amount of basophilic or amphophilic cytoplasm.

(2) Immunophenotypic and Genetic Features

Tumor cells express CD20, CD19, CD10, and BCL6, a phenotype consistent with germinal center B cells. Tumor cells do not express BCL2. The high mitotic activity of Burkitt lymphoma is confirmed by nearly 100% of the cells staining positive for Ki-67. Most of the cases have MYC translocation at band 8q24 to the immunoglobulin heavy chain region, 14q32 or, less commonly, at the lambda, 22q11 or kappa, 2p12 light chain loci. The translocations lead to MYC protein overexpression.

(3) Clinical Features

Both the endemic and nonendemic sporadic forms affect mainly children and young adults, accounting for approximately 30% of childhood NHLs. It often occurs in mandible, skull, bones, abdominal organs and the central nervous system and forms a rapidly growing mass. Leukemic presentations are rare, which should be distinguished from ALL. Clinically, it is a highly invasive tumor. Intensive combination chemotherapy regimens result in cure rates of up to 90% in patients with low stage disease and 60% –80% in patients with advanced stage disease. The results are better in children than in adults.

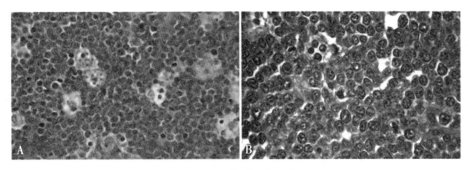

Figure 10-4   **Burkitt lymphoma**

A: At low power, numerous pale tingible body macrophages are evident, producing a "starng sky" appearance. B: At high power, tumor cells have multiple small nucleoli and high mitotic index. The lack of significant variation in nuclear shape and size lends a monotonous appearance

10.3.4   Mature-T and NK-cell Neoplasms

These categories are a heterogeneous group of neoplasms resembling mature T cells or NK cells. Peripheral T-cell tumors make up about 5% –10% NHLs in the United States and Europe, but are more common in Asian. NK-cell tumors are rare in the western countries, but more common in the Far East.

10.3.4.1   Peripheral T-Cell Lymphomas, not Otherwise Specified

T-cell lymphomas are relatively common in Asian, accounting for 20% –30% NHL in our country. Although the WHO classification includes a number of distinct peripheral T cell lymphomas, many cases are still difficult to be categorized. Furthermore, morphology is not a good indicator of clinical behaviors. Thus, a majority of these tumors have been lumped into a "wastebasket" diagnosis, peripheral T-cell lymphoma, not otherwise specified. Histologically, tumor cells diffusely infiltrate lymph nodes paracortex with angiogenesis. The cytological spectrum of tumor cells is extremely broad, from highly polymorphous to monomorphous, accompanied by numerous of non-neoplastic cells, such as eosinophils, plasma cells, macrophage, exithelioid histiocyte. The tumor cells are positive for CD2, CD3, CD5 and other mature T cell marker(i. e. $\alpha\beta$ or $\gamma\delta$ T-cell receptors). Some also express CD4 or CD8 which are considered as helper or cytotoxic T-cell origin, respectively. However, the phenotype of many tumors is not similar to any known normal T cells. The T cell receptor gene rearrangement analysis can be used to confirm the existence of a monoclonal rearrangement for distinguishing lymphoma from lymphoid hyperplasia. Most patients present with lymphadenopathy, sometimes accompanied by eosinophilia, pruritus, fever, and weight loss. These are highly aggressive lymphomas, with a poor response to therapy, frequent relapses and low 5-year overall survival(20%-30%).

10.3.4.2 Mycosis Fungoides(MF)

Mycosis fungoides(MF) is the most common form of cutaneous T-cell lymphoma. Most cases are found in people over 20 years of age, and it is more common in men than women. Histologically, the epidermis and upper dermis are infiltrated by neoplastic T cells, which often have a cerebriform appearance due to marked infolding of the nuclear membrane. The neoplastic T-cells form a band-like upper dermal infiltrate with a moderate degree of epidermal infiltration, often forming small aggregates of cells within the epidermis (termed Pautrier microabseess. It generally affects the skin, but may progress internally over time.

Clinically, the cutaneous lesions of mycosis fungoides usually undergo three different stages, the patch stage, characterized by erythematous macules usually occurring in areas not exposed to sunlight; the plaque stage, with elevated scaly plaques which may be pink or red/brown and are often intensely pruritic; the tumour phase, with dome-shaped firm tumours which may ulcerate. With the development of disease, the density of lymphoid infiltrate increases from the patch to the tumor stage. Although MF is initially confined to the skin, the involvement of lymph nodes and viscera is particularly common in the late stage of the disease. Patients with limited extent cutaneous disease have a good prognosis and mean survival time is 8-9 years. When the visceral organ is involved the median survival time is 2.5 years.

10.3.4.3 Extranodal NK/T-Cell Lymphomas

The tumors are derived from cytotoxic T-cells or NK-cells and are highly aggressive. It is closely associated with EBV. 80%-100% of cases are EBV DNA or its encoded protein positive. It occurs primarily in nasal, followed by jaw and throat, often involves nasopharynx and nasal sinuses. 10%-20% nasal NK-/T-cell lymphomas may also have skin involvement at the same time. In the advanced stage, tumors may disseminate rapidly to various sites, e.g. skin, digestive tract, testis, brain, and spleen, etc. The histological features of extranodal NK/T-cell lymphoma are similar irrespective of the site of involvement. In the coagulation necrosis background, neoplastic lymphoid cells are scattered or diffusely distributed admixed with inflammatory cells. The tumor cells vary in size and shape. The nuclear shape is irregular and hyperchromatic with one to two nucleoli. Tumor cells infiltrate into the vessel wall, also termed as angiocentric infiltration, resulting in lumen stenosis, atresia and elastic membrane rupture. Fibrinoid changes can be seen in the blood vessels even in the absence of angioinvasion. Tumor cells often express T cell antigens(CD2, cytoplasmic CD3), cytotoxic proteins(such as granzyme B) and CD56, which is a useful NK cell marker. The prognosis of nasal NK/T-cell lymphoma is variable, with some patients responding well to therapy and others dying of disseminated disease despite aggressive therapy.

10.4 Hodgkin Lymphoma

Hodgkin lymphoma(HL) is a group of primary malignant tumor of lymphoid tissues, which characterized by the presence of tumor giant cells, the Reed-Sternberg cells.

HLs have the following characteristics: ①they usually arise in lymph nodes, preferentially in cervical lymph node; ②the majority of the patients are young adults; ③large mononucleated and multinucleated tumour cells only account for a minority of the total number of cells, dispersing in an abundant heterogeneous admixture of non-neoplastic inflammatory and accessory cells;④the tumour cells are often ringed by T cells in a rosette-like manner.

(1)Morphology

Macroscopically,lymph nodes are enlarged with the homogeneously pale white cut surface,or a nodular or fibrotic appearance. Microscopically,lymph node structure is destroyed and composed of a mixed infiltrate containing lymphocytes,histiocytes,plasma cells,and eosinophils,as well as Feed-Sternbergcells,R-S cells of Hodgkin lymphoma. These large malignant cells are abundant,with slightly eosinophilic cytoplasm and a diameter of 15−45 μm. A typical R-S cell is binuclear,in a face-to-face arrangement,symmetric to each other,forming the so-called mirror cells(mirror image cell). HRS cells are generally considered as precursor cells of classical R-S cells. There are also several special types of tumor cells(Figure 10−5,from ROBBINS and COTRAN Pathologic Basis of Disease):①Reed-Sternberg cell,mononuclear variant:the cells are large and irregular in shape. Nuclei have coarse chromatin,with the obvious nucleolus. Mitotic figures are common,usually multipolar mitosis. Lacunar cells:its cytoplasm retracts when fixed in formalin,so the nuclei give the appearance of cells that lie in empty spaces(called lacunae)between them. ③Lymphocyte predominant cells:(previously,lymphocytic L&H variant R-S,cells):the cells are large and usually have one large nucleus and scant cytoplasm. The nuclei are folded or multilobated that have also been termed as and histiocells. The nucleoli are usually multiple,basophilic and smaller than those seen in classical R-S cells.

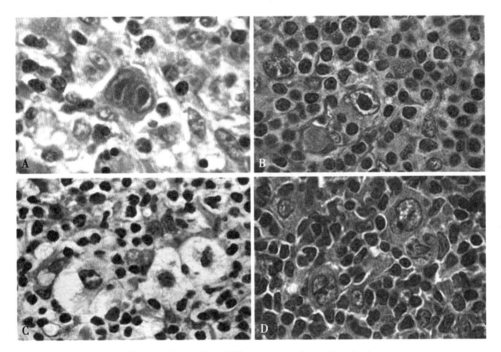

Figure 10−5   **Reed-Sternberg cells and variants**

①Diagnostic Reed-Sternberg cell,with two nuclear lobes,large inclusion-like nucleoli,and abundant cytoplasm,surrounded by lymphocytes,macrophages,and an eosinophil. ②Reed-Sternberg cell,mononuclear variant. ③Reed-Sternberg cell,lacunar variant. This variant has a folded or multilobated nucleus and lies within an open space,which is an artifact created by disruption of the cytoplasm during tissue sectioning. ④Reed-Sternberg cell,lymphohistiocytic variant. Several such variants with multiply infolded nuclear membranes,small nucleoli,fine chromatin,and abundant pale cytoplasm are present

Although the diagnosis of Hodgkin lymphoma depends upon the discovery of classic R-S cells,there is little evidence of nucleic acid synthesis or proliferative activity in these cells. Large mononuclear R-S cells (called Hodgkin's cells) are proliferating cells in Hodgkin lymphoma. The histologic feature of Hodgkin lymphoma is particularly obvious in that the neoplastic R-S cells are few and are admixed with variable numbers of lymphocytes, plasma cells, histiocytes, eosinophils, neutrophils, and fibroblasts, all of which are considered to be reactive. However, malignant cells are dominant in other tumors. Lymph node can be totally destroyed, involving spleen, liver, bone marrow, and extralymphatic tissues.

(2) Classification of Hodgkin Lymphoma

According to 2017 WHO classification, Hodgkin lymphomas is classified into two subtypes, i. e. nodular lymphocyte predominant Hodgkin lymphoma(CHL) and classic Hodgkin lymphoma. Based upon Reed-Sternberg cell morphology and the composition of the reactive cell infiltrate seen in the lymph node biopsy specimen, CHL can be subclassified into four pathologic subtypes: nodular sclerosis classical Hodgkin lymphoma(NSCHL), mixed cellularity classical Hodgkin lymphoma(MCCHL), lymphocyte-rich classical Hodgkin lymphoma(LRCHL) and lymphocyte-depleted classical Hodgkin lymphoma(LDCHL)(Table 10-2).

The subtypes of Hodgkin lymphoma are recognized as:

1) Nodular lymphocyte predominant Hodgkin lymphoma.

2) Classic Hodgkin lymphoma: ①nodular sclerosis, ②mixed cellularity, ③lymphocyte rich, and ④lymphocyte depletion.

Table 10-2　WHO classification of Hodgkin lymphoma

Histologic Subtype	Incidence	Main Pathology	R-S Cells	Prognosis
A. Nodular lymphocyte predominant HL				
	5%	Proliferation of small lymphocytes, nodular pattern of growth	Sparse number of RS cells, CD45 +, EMA +, CD20+, CD15-, CD30-	Chronic relapsing, may transform into large B cell NHL
B. Classic HL				
Lymphocyte-rich	5%	Proliferating lymphocytes, a few histiocytes	Few, classic and polyploid type, CD15transfrom in CD20 +?	Excellent
Nodular sclerosis	30%–60%	Lymphoid nodules, collagen bands	Frequent, lacunar type CD15+, CD30+	Very good
Mixed cellularity	20%–40%	Mixed infiltrate	Numerous, classic type CD15+, CD30+	Good
Lymphocyte-depletion (*Diffuse fibrotic and reticular variants*)	<2%	Scanty lymphocytes, atypical histiocytes, fibrosis	Numerous pleomorphic type CD15+, CD30+	Poor

10.4.1　Nodular Lymphocyte-Predominant Hodgkin Lymphoma(NLPHL)

It is characterized by the presence of lymphohistiocytic(L&H) variant R-S cells that have a delicate multilobed, puffy nucleus resembling popped corn("popcorn cell"). L&H variants usually are found within large nodules containing numerous mature-looking small B cells admixed with a variable number of macrophages. Other types of reactive cells, such as eosinophils, neutrophils, and plasma cells, are scanty or absent, and typical R-S cells are rare. Unlike the Reed-Sternberg variants in "classical" forms of Hodgkin lymphoma, L&H variants express B cell markers, such as CD20, CD79a, but lack CD15 and CD30. Most patients present with cervical or axillary lymphadenopathy, and have a good prognosis.

10.4.2 Classical Hodgkin Lymphoma

Classical Hodgkin lymphoma (CHL) is a monoclonal lymphoid neoplasm composed of mononuclear Hodgkin cells and multinucleated R-S cells residing in an infiltrate containing a variable mixture of non-neoplastic small lymphocytes, eosinophils, neutrophils, histiocytes, plasma cells, fibroblasts, and collagen fibers. CHL represents approximately 95% of all HLs. A bimodal age distribution is seen with peaks in the 10 −35 years old age group and more than 50 years old age group. 75% of cases involve cervical lymph node.

10.4.2.1 Nodular Sclerosis Classical Hodgkin Lymphoma(NSCHL)

It is the most common subtype. The incidence of NSCHL is similar in males and females and peaks at ages 15−34 years. It has a striking propensity to involve the lower cervical, supraclavicular, and mediastinal lymph nodes. Mediastinal involvement occurs in 80% of cases, a bulky disease in 54%, splenic involvement in 10%, and bone marrow involvement in 3%. Morphologically, it is characterized by the presence of nodular sclerosis, broad bands of collagen circumscribing nodules of involved tissue and by the presence of large R-S cell variants. This large cell, termed as the lacunar cell, has a single multilobate nucleus, multiple small nucleoli and abundant, pale-staining cytoplasm. In sections of formalin-fixed tissue, the cytoplasm often is torn away, leaving the nucleus lying in an empty space. The immunophenotype of lacunar variants is identical to that of other R-S cells found in classical subtypes.

10.4.2.2 Mixed Cellularity Classical Hodgkin Lymphoma(MCCHL)

It is more frequent in patients with HIV infection and in developing countries. A bimodal age distribution is not seen. The median age is 38 years and approximately 70% are males. Histologically, lymph nodes architecture is usually obliterated although an inner-follicular growth pattern may be seen. Interstitial fibrosis may be present, but the lymph node capsule is usually not thickened and there are no broad bands of fibrosis as seen in NSCHL. The R-S cells are typical in appearance. The background cells consist of numerous inflammatory cells, which are rich in T lymphocytes, histiocytes, eosinophils, and plasma cells. This type is most often associated with EBV infection.

10.4.2.3 Lymphocyte-rich Classical Hodgkin Lymphoma(LRCHL)

It is a subtype of CHL with scattered R-S cells and a nodular or less common diffuse cellular background consisting of small lymphocytes and with an absence of neutrophils and eosinophils.

10.4.2.4 Lymphocyte Depleted Classical Hodgkin Lymphoma(LDCHL)

It is the rarest subtype of CHL, composed of large numbers of pleomorphic RS cells with only a few reactive lymphocytes which may easily be confused with diffuse large cell lymphoma. Prior to modern therapy, the course of LDCHL was aggressive. Histologically, compared with the lymphocytes in the background, R-S cells are dominant. There are two patterns ①diffuse fibrotic pattern: Lymph node cells is significantly reduced. The irregular arrangement of reticular fibers and amorphous protein substances increases. There are a few diagnostic HRS cells, tissue cells and lymphocytes. Necrosis usually can be seen; ②reticular cell pattern, it is rich in cells, comprising lots of pleomorphic R-S cells, a small number of diagnostic R-S cells and spindle tumor cells. Mature lymphocytes, eosinophils, plasma cells, neutrophils and histiocytes are rare. Compared to other types of HL, necrosis is more obvious. R-S cells are positive for CD15 and CD30. Most cases express EBV encoded LMP-1 and EBER.

10.4.3 Staging of Hodgkin Lymphoma

Treatment of HL is based on clinical, and occasionally on the pathological staging of the disease. The modified Ann Arbor staging system is used(Table 10-3).

Table 10-3　Clinical staging of Hodgkin and non-Hodgkin lymphomas

Stage	Distribution of Disease
I	Involvement of a single lymph node region(I)or involvement of a single extralymphatic organ or tissue(I $_E$)
II	Involvement of two or more lymph node regions on the same side of the diaphragm alone(II)or with involvement of limited contiguous extralymphatic organs or tissue(II $_E$)
III	Involvement of lymph node regions on both sides of the diaphragm(III),which may include the spleen(IIIS), limited contiguous extralymphatic organ or site(III $_E$),or both(III $_{ES}$)
IV	Multiple or disseminated foci of involvement of one or more extralymphatic organs or tissues with or without lymphatic involvement

Younger patients with the more favorable subtypes tend to present with stage I or II disease,without systemic manifestations. Patients with advanced disease(stages III and IV)are more likely to have systemic complaints such as fever,weight loss,pruritus,and anemia.

10.4.4　Clinical Features of Hodgkin Lymphoma

Hodgkin Lymphoma is more common in males and shows a peak incidence in early adulthood. Like NHLs,it usually manifests as painless lymphadenopathy,most often in the upper half of the body,with involvement of cervical and/or axillary lymph nodes,and spreads to anatomically contiguous nodes. Radiological evidence of mediastinal involvement is present in over 40% of patients and on occasion may be massive. With the advancement of the disease,the involvement of spleen,liver,bone marrow,and other organs and tissues may appear. Some patients with the disease have systemic symptoms,such as weight loss,unexplained pyrexia which exceeds 39 ℃ ,anemia,and drenching night sweats. In spite of intensive research and a wealth of immunologic data,the diagnosis of Hodgkin lymphoma is still based entirely upon histologic examination-the finding of the classic R-S cell in pathologic tissue is considered essential for diagnosis.

Localized forms of Hodgkin lymphoma may be treated with either radiation or chemotherapy. Chemotherapy is highly effective when multiple agents are used and may lead to cures even in patients with disseminated disease. The 5-year survival rate of patients with stage I or II disease is close to 100%. Fifty percent of patients with advanced disease(stages III and IV)can achieve 5-year disease-free survival.

Although a definitive distinction from NHL can be made only by examination of a lymph node biopsy, several clinical features favor the diagnosis of Hodgkin lymphoma(Table 10-4).

Table 10-4　Clinical differences between Hodgkin and non-Hodgkin lymphomas

Hodgkin Lymphoma	Non-Hodgkin Lymphoma
More often localized to a single axial group of nodes (cervical,mediastinal,para-aortic)	More frequent involvement of multiple peripheral nodes
Orderly spread by contiguity	Noncontiguous spread
Mesenteric nodes and Waldeyer ring rarely involved	Mesenteric nodes and Waldeyer ring commonly involved
Extranodal involvement uncommon	Extranodal involvement common

10.5   Myeloid Neoplasms

Myeloid neoplasms arise from hematopoietic progenitors and typically give rise to clonal proliferations that replace normal bone marrow cells. There are three broad categories of myeloid neoplasia: ①acute myeloblastic leukemias (AMLs), the neoplastic cells are blocked at an early stage of myeloid cell development; ②myelodysplastic syndromes, terminal differentiation occurs but in a disordered and ineffective fashion, leading to the appearance of dysplastic marrow precursors and peripheral blood cytopenias, and ③myeloproliferative neoplasms, the neoplastic clone continues to undergo terminal differentiation but exhibits increased or dysregulated growth. Commonly, these are associated with an increase in one or more of the formed elements (red cells, platelets, and/or granulocytes) in the peripheral blood.

Although these three categories provide a useful starting point, the divisions between the myeloid neoplasms sometimes blur. Both myelodysplastic syndromes and myeloproliferative neoplasms often transform to AML, and some neoplasms have features of both myelodysplasia and myeloproliferative neoplasms. Because all myeloid neoplasms arise from early multipotent progenitors, the close relationship among these disorders is not surprising.

10.5.1   Acute Myeloblastic Leukemia (AML)

AML is a very heterogeneous neoplasm. It primarily affects older adults; the median age is 50 years. The clinical signs and symptoms closely resemble those produced by ALL and usually are related to the replacement of normal marrow elements by leukemic blasts. Fatigue, pallor, abnormal bleeding, and infections are common in newly diagnosed patients, who typically present within a few weeks of the onset of symptoms. Splenomegaly and lymphadenopathy generally are less prominent than in ALL, but on rare occasions AML mimics a lymphoma by manifesting as a discrete tissue mass (a so-called granulocytic sarcoma). The diagnosis and classification of AML are based on morphologic, histochemical, immunophenotypic, and karyotypic findings. Of these tests, the karyotype is most predictive of outcome.

(1) Morphology

By definition, AML myeloid blasts or promyelocytes make up more than 20% of the bone marrow cellular component. Myeloid blasts have delicate nuclear chromatin, which has three to five nucleoli, and fine azurophilic cytoplasmic granules. In some cases, there are red-staining rod-like structures (Auer rods) which are more often present in the promyelocytic variant. Therefore, Auer rods are specific for neoplastic myeloblasts and a helpful diagnostic clue when present.

(2) Immunophenotypic Features

The expression of immunologic markers is varied in AML. Most tumors express some combination of myeloid-associated antigens, such as CD13, CD14, CD15, CD64, or CD117 (cKIT). Because multipotent stem cells express CD33, myeloid progenitor cells are positive for CD33.

(3) Clinical Features

AML is a devastating disease. The onset is often very rapid and progresses to death because of anemia, hemorrhage, or infection occurs within weeks without treatment. Severe anemia causes pallor and hypoxic symptoms. Thrombocytopenia may lead to abnormal bleeding or purpura. Neutropenia results in infections. AMLs with t(8;21) or inv(16) have a better prognosis with conventional chemotherapy, particularly in the absence of c-KIT mutations, which have a 50% chance of long-term disease-free survival. However, the overall long-term disease-free survival is only 15% to 30% with conventional chemotherapy. Currently, allergenic marrow transplantation seems to be the only method to cure the disease.

10.5.2 Chronic Myelogenous Leukemias(CML)

CML is a myeloproliferative neoplasm characterized by the presence of a chimeric BCR-ABL gene, which is the product of a(9;22)translocation that moves the ABL gene on chromosome 9 to a position on chromosome 22 adjacent to the BCR gene. It accounts for 15% –20% of all leukemias. It peaks at ages 40– 50 years.

(1)Morphology

CML is characterized by the presence of very high peripheral blood cells counts. The leukocyte count often exceeds 300×10^9/L. The circulating cells are predominantly neutrophils, metamyelocytes, and myelocytes, but basophils and eosinophils are also prominent. A small proportion of myeloblasts, usually less than 5%, can be seen in the peripheral blood. The bone marrow is hypercellukar due to the proliferation of granulocytic and megakaryocytic precursors. Similar to bone marrow, the red pulp of the spleen present extensive extra medullary hematopoiesis. This burgeoning mass often compromises the local blood supply, leading to splenic infarcts.

(2)Clinical Features

The onset of CML often is usually slow and the initial symptoms usually are nonspecific(e. g. , easy fatigability, weakness, weight loss). Massive splenomegaly is common in CML patients. Sometimes the first symptom is a dragging sensation in the abdomen, caused by extreme splenomegaly. More than 90% of cases have(9;22)(q34;q11)translocation(the so-called Philadelphia chromosome[Ph]), which can be tested for the presence of the BCR-ABL fusion gene. In other cases, the BCR-ABL fusion gene is formed by cytogenetic complexity or recessive rearrangement. The CML patients are at the accelerated or explosive stage when bone marrow contains more than 5% myeloblasts. The natural history of CML is initially slow. The median survival is 3 years without treatment. After a variable(and unpredictable)period, approximately half of CML cases enter an accelerated phase, characterized by increasing anemia and new thrombocytopenia, with additional cytogenetic abnormalities, and finally transformation into a picture resembling acute leukemia(i. e. blast crisis).

10.6 Histocytic Neoplasms

Histocytic neoplasms originate from mononuclear phagocytes(macrophages, and dendritic cells)or histiocytes. Some are malignant tumors, such as very rare histiocytic lymphoma. Others are benign, such as the reactive histiocytic proliferations in lymph nodes. Langerhans cell histiocytic disease is relatively rare and is characterized by clonal proliferation of Langerhans' cells. Clonal proliferation of others are benign, such as the reactive histiocytic proliferations in lymph nodes.

In the past, these disorders were regarded as histiocytosis X and subdivided into three categories: Letterer-Siwe syndrome(generalized histiocytosis), Hand-Schuller-Christian disease, and eosinophilic granuloma. Based on recent studies, these three categories represent three different stages of the same disease. The proliferating Langerhans' cells are human leukocyte antigen DR(HLA-DR)and CD1 antigen positive. HX bodies(Birbeck granules)in the cytoplasm of these cells are characteristic. Under light microscopy, proliferating Langerhan cells have abundant, vacuolated cytoplasm and vesicular nuclei, which is different from their normal dendritic counterparts.

Clinically, Langerhans' cell histiocytosis can be divided into three types: acute disseminated Langerhans' cell histiocytosis, unifocal eosinophilic granuloma, or multifocal granuloma.

10.6.1   Acute Disseminated Langerhans' cell Histiocytosis

Acute disseminated Langerhans' cell histiocytosis(also called Letterer-Siwe syndrome)appear to represent the aggressive end of the spectrum, with widespread lesions of bone and lymphoid tissue, and occurs usually before 2 years of age. The dominant clinical signs are skin lesions due to Langerhans' cells infiltration. Most patients have hepatosplenomegaly lymphadenopathy, pulmonary lesions and destructive osteolytic bone lesions. Extensive infiltration of the marrow leads to anemia, thrombocytopenia, and recurrent infections. Thus, the clinical signs and symptoms may resemble that of acute leukemia. Without treatment, the prognosis is poor. With intensive chemotherapy, 50% of the patients survive 5 years.

10.6.2   Eosinophilic Granulomas

Both unifocal and multifocal eosinophilic granulomas are characterized by expanding, erosive, accumulation of Langerhans' cells, usually within the medullar cavities of bones. The proliferative Langerhans' cells are variably admixed with eosinophils, lymphocytes, plasma cells, and neutrophils. The eosinophilic component ranges from scattered mature cells to sheet-like masses of cells. The calvarium, ribs, and femur are commonly involved.

Unifocal lesion is a relatively benign disease that involves bone, particularly the skull and ribs of children and young adults, although long bones are sometimes involved. It may be asymptomatic or may cause pain and tenderness, and pathologic fracture. Radiologically, it presents as a well-demarcated lytic lesion. This disorder may heal spontaneously or may be cured by local excision or irradiation.

Multifocal lesions have a less favorable prognosis. It usually affects children presenting with fever diffuse eruptions, particularly on the scalp and in the ear canals and frequent bouts of otitis media. Lymphadenopathy, hepatomegaly, and splenomegaly presented by the infiltrate of Langerhanent cells. The base of the skull is characteristically involved, producing the triad of proptosis, lytic bone lesions in the skull, a diabetes insipidus-the last due to the destruction of the posterior pituitary. The combination of calvarial bone defects, diabetes insipidus, and exophthalmos as referred to as the Hand-Schiller-Christian triad. Most patients with this disease experience spontaneous regression and others can be treated with chemotherapy.

CD1a and S-100 protein are positive of Langerhans' cell with immunohistochemistry techniques. Birbeck bodies can be found with electron microscopy. These indicators are useful for the diagnosis of Langerhans' cell histiocytosis.

Chapter 11

Diseases of the Immune System

Immunity refers to protection against infections, and the immune system is the collection of cells and molecules that are responsible for defending organism against the countless pathogenic microbes from outside. Deficiencies in immune defences result in an increased susceptibility to infections, which can be life-threatening if the deficits are not corrected. On the other hand, the immune system is itself capable of causing great harm and is the root cause of some of the most vexing and intractable diseases of the modern world. Thus, diseases of immunity range from those caused by "too little" to those caused by "too much or inappropriate" immune activity. This chapter briefly introduces some of common types of immune diseases.

11.1 Autoimmune Diseases

Autoimmune disease is the underlying status which is indeed the result of autoimmune reactions. Comparing with other diseases, autoimmune diseases have their-self characters: ①in many of these diseases, autoimmune antibody or/and autoreactive T lymphocytes can be detected; ②in some cases, autoimmune antibody or/and autoreactive T lymphocytes are known to cause pathologic abnormalities and functional disorders; ③recurrent linger and chronic deferred.

11.1.1 Factors and Mechanisms

Autoimmune disease results from a breakdown of self-tolerance to their self-antigens and mutations of genes, therefore, understanding the pathogenesis of autoimmunity diseases requires familiarity with the mechanisms of normal immunologic tolerance and genetic factors in autoimmunity.

11.1.1.1 Immunologic Tolerance

Immunologic tolerance is unresponsiveness to an antigen that is induced by exposure of specific lymphocytes to that antigen. Self-tolerance refers to a lack of immune responsiveness to one's own tissue antigens. These mechanisms are broadly include central tolerance and peripheral tolerance.

(1) Central Tolerance

The principal mechanism is the antigen-induced death/apoptosis of self-reactive T and B lymphocytes during their mutation in generative lymphoid organs, such as in the bone marrow for B cells and the thymus for T cells. Many autologous protein antigens in the thymus are processed and presented by thymic APCs (antigen-presenting cell) in association with self-major histocompatibility complex. Any immature T cells which recognize self-antigens in the central lymphoid organs undergo deletion or called negative selection. Similarly, immature B cell lineage, in some cause may be deleted by apoptosis; while, some self-reactive B cells may not be killed but undergo a receptor editing.

(2) Peripheral Tolerance

Mature lymphocytes that recognize self-antigens in peripheral tissues lose function and become anergic, or may be suppressed by T cells, or may die by apoptosis.

11.1.2   Factors Affected Autoimmunity

11.1.2.1   Genetic Factors in Autoimmunity

Many susceptibility genes take an important part in the occurrence of autoimmune diseases. ①autoimmune diseases share a tendency to exist in families, and the incidence of the same autoimmune disease in monozygotic is greater than in dizygotic twins. ②There is proof that HLA locus, such as HLA-DR, −DQ, link with several autoimmune diseases, and is called the odds ratio or relative risk. ③Genetic polymorphisms associated and linked studies in families are revealed that they are associated with autoimmune diseases. Some loci are seemed to be linked with general mechanisms of self-tolerance and immune regulation, other loci are reported to show special self-antigens or influence organ sensitivity.

11.1.2.2   Role of Infections and Tissue Injury

A variety of bacteria, mycoplasmas, and viruses, have been indicated as triggers for autoimmunity. The underlying mechanism of microbe induced autoimmune reactions may include three factors. ①viruses and other bacteria such as streptococci, and klebsiella organisms, may have cross-reacting epitopes with self-antigens which are called molecular mimicry. ②Microbial infections with inflammation and resultant tissue necrosis may lead to upregulation of costimulatory molecules on APCs in the tissue, therefore, helping a breakdown of T cell anergy and activating subsequent T cell subsequently.

11.1.3   Systemic Lupus Erythematosus

Systemic Lupus Erythematosus(SLE) is a multisystem autoimmune disease of variable clinical behavior and labile manifestations. The prevalence of SLE is about 1 : 2,500 persons in certain populations. Similarly like other immune diseases, there is a strong(approximately 9 : 1) female preponderance, and influence 1 : 700 women of childbearing age. The onset of SLE is usually among 10−30 years old, but may manifest at any age, even in the early childhood.

11.1.3.1   Etiology and Pathogenesis

The major defect in SLE is a failure to maintain self-tolerance, leading to the production of multiple auto-antibodies which can injure tissues either directly or form immune complex deposits. Like in other autoimmune diseases, the process of pathogenesis includes a combination of environmental and genetic factors. Recent reports have demonstrated some interesting factors about the pathogenesis of this enigmatic disorder. There are many studies demonstrated that environmental factors ①Genetic Factors. Much evidence supports a genetic inclination to SLE; ②Environmental Factors, like ultraviolet radiation, cigarette smoking, sex hormones, or failure of B cell tolerance. are implicated in the pathogenesis of SLE.

11.1.3.2   Morphology

The morphologic changes are variable in SLE, and the most characteristic morphologic changes depend on natural autoantibodies and/or immune complexes deposition.

(1)Blood Vessel

Affecting arteries and arterioles present acute necrotizing vasculitis which display necrosis, fibrinoid deposits involving antibodies, DNA, fibrinogen and complement fragment, as well as leukocytic infiltrate in transmural and perivascular wall. Vessels become fibrous which thickening in the wall and narrowing in the lumen.

(2)Kidney

Kidney failure is the most common cause of death in SLE. The classical character is pathological changes on glomerular, although the pathological lesions are also displayed on interstitial and tubular. Glomerulonephritis which includes DNA-anti-DNA complexes deposition is the major forms in SLE. The pathological lesions only can be detected in 25% –30% of cases by light microscopy, although all can be examined the abnormality by immunofluorescence microscopy and electron microscopy.

According to the International Society of Nephrology/Renal Pathology Society (SNPS) morphologic classification, there are six patterns of glomerular disease in SLE: class Ⅰ, minimal mesangial lupus nephritis; class Ⅱ, mesangial proliferative lupus nephritis; class Ⅲ, focal lupus nephritis; class Ⅳ, diffuse lupus nephritis; class Ⅴ, membranous lupus nephritis; and class Ⅵ, advanced sclerosing lupus nephritis.

Class Ⅰ: Minimal mesangial lupus nephritis

It rarely structural alterations under microscopy, although immune complexes are deposited in the mesangium.

Class Ⅱ: Mesangial proliferative lupus nephritis

It is detected in 10% –25% of SLE cases and is connected with mild clinical symptoms, since immune complexes deposit in the cellularity and mesangial matrix.

Class Ⅲ: Focal lupus nephritis

It is detected in 20% –35% of SLE cases. Pathological lesions are visualized in less than half glomeruli, and they may be segmentally or globally displayed within each glomerulus. Endothelial and mesangial cells experience swelling and proliferation, neutrophils infiltration, and fibrinoid deposits distribute with capillary thrombi(Figure 11 –1A).

Class Ⅳ: Diffuse lupus nephritis

It is the most common and serious form in SLE renal biopsies, occurring in 35% –60% of cases. Endothelial and mesangial proliferation is detected in most of the glomeruli, and producing epithelial crescents that fill Bowman's space in some cases(Figure 11 –2B). Further mone, immune complexes in capillary wall subendothelial show a circum-ferential thickening with "wire loops" on light microscopy(Figure 11 –1C). Subendothelial immune complexes(between endothelium and basement membrane) display prominent electron-dense deposition(Figure 11 –1D), although immune complexes are also shown in other parts of the capillary wall and in the mesangium. Immune complexes can be detected by staining with fluorescent antibodies directed against immunoglobulins or complement, causing a granular fluorescent staining form(Figure 11 –1E). Therefore, glomerulosclerosis formed. Most SLE patients complain about hematuria, moderate to severe proteinuria, hypertension, and renal insufficiency.

Class Ⅴ: Membranous lupus nephritis

It occurs in 10% –15% of SLE cases, and the pathological lesions are on the glomerulus which characterized by widespread thickening of the capillary wall because of the deposition of subepithelial immune complexes and basement membrane-like material

Class Ⅵ: Advanced sclerosing lupus nephritis

More than 90% glomeruli display complete sclerosis, and the patient corresponds to clinical end-stage renal disease.

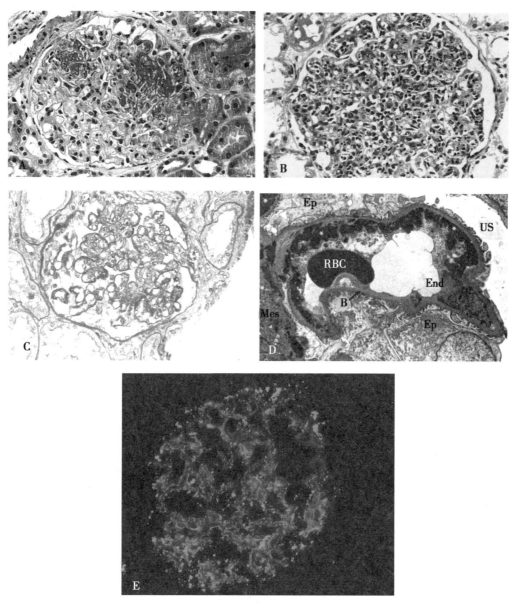

Figure 11-1   **Lupusnephritis**

A:Focal lupus nephritis,with two necrotizing lesions in a glomerulus(segmental distribution)(H&E stain). B: Diffuse lupus nephritis. Note the marked global increase in cellularity throughout the glomerulus(H&E stain). C:Lupus nephritis showing a glomerulus with several "wire loop" lesions representing extensive subendothelial deposits of immune complexes(periodic acid Schiff stain). D:Electron micrograph of a renal glomerular capillary loop from a patient with SLE nephritis. Confluent subendothelial dense deposits correspond to "wire loops" seen by light microscopy. E:Deposition of IgG antibody in a granular pattern,detected by immunofluorescence. B,basement membrane;End, endothelium;Ep,epithelial cell with foot processes;Mes,mesangium;RBC,red blood cell in capillary lumen;US,urinary space; * ,electron-dense deposits in subendothelial location

(3)Skin

Erythematous or maculopapular eruption over the malar eminences and the nose bridge are the most characteristic lesions on approximately half of the SLE patients. The similar red rash occurs on the sun-exposed area,therefore called photosensitivity. Histopathologically,basal layer of the epidermis shows liquefactive degeneration,as well edema at the dermoepidermal junction,and mononuclear infiltration around blood vessels and skin appendages. Immunoglobulin and complement deposition at the dermoepidermal junction and other apparently uninvolved skin can be observed on immunofluorescence microscopy.

(4) Joints

Joint lesion is frequent but not associated with obvious pathological changes or with joint deformity most of the time. When present, swelling and a nonspecific mononuclear cell infiltration in the synovial membranes exist. Erosion of the membranes and destruction of articular cartilage, are extremely rare.

(5) CNS

Central nervous system (CNS) lesion is also very common, accompanying with focal neurologic deficits and/or neuropsychiatric symptoms. Mostly, CNS disease is due to vascular changes causing ischemia or multifocal cerebral micro-infarcts. The most frequent pathological lesion is small vessel angiopathy with endothelial proliferation; frank vasculitis is uncommon. Premature atherosclerosis occurs and contributes to CNS ischemia.

(6) Cardiovascular System

The heart involved in is manifested major in the pattern of pericarditis. Myocarditis, in the pattern of a nonspecific mononuclear cell infiltration, and valvular lesions, called Libman-Sacks endocarditis which is less common in the current era of aggressive corticosteroid therapy. The verrucous endocarditis displays irregular, 1–3 mm warty deposits, shown as distinctive characteristic changes on either surface of the leaflets. In acute stage, small arteries and arterioles become affected by necrotizing vasculitis, moreover, necrosis and fibrinoid deposition within vessel walls involved antibody, DNA, fibrinogen and complement fragments. The transmural and perivascular leukocytic infiltrate also can be present. In chronic process, vessels display fibrous thickening with luminal narrowing.

(7) Other Organs

Many other organs, like spleen may be involved. The pathological lesions are caused by acute vasculitis of the small vessels. The effected spleen may be enlarged, capsular fibrous thickening, central penicilliary arteries thickening, and perivascular fibrosis showing onion-skin lesion.

11.1.3.3 Clinical Manifestations

SLE is a multisystem lesion disease with variable in clinical presentation. The typical manifestations include kidney nephritis, skin lesions, arthritis, and hematologic and/or neurologic abnormalities.

(A-C, courtesy of Dr. Helmut Rennke, Department of Pathology, Brigham and Women's Hospital, Boston, Massachusetts. D, Courtesy of Dr. Edwin Eigenbrodt, Department of Pathology, University of Texas Southwestern Medical School, Dallas. E, Courtesy of Dr. Jean Olson, Department of Pathology, University of California, San Francisco, California.)

11.1.4   Rheumatoid Arthritis

Rheumatoid Arthritis (RA) is a systemic chronic inflammatory disease attacking principally the joints to produce a nonsuppurative proliferative synovitis that frequently progresses to destroy articular cartilage and underlying bone with resulting disabling arthritis. The prevalence of RA approximately 1%, and the occurence is three to five times in women than in men.

11.1.4.1   Pathogenesis

RA is an immune-mediated inflammatory disease which is approved genetic predisposition. The underlying mechanism is the activation of CD4$^+$ T cells which respond to the arthritogenic agent, like microbial, self-antigen. Cytokines that are activated by T cells, firstly activate macrophages and other cells in joint space that release specific enzymes or other factors to perpetuate inflammation. Secondly, cytokines can activate B cells to produce antibodies or against self-antigens in the joint.

According to a variety of clinical and experimental observations, approximately 80% of RA patients have serum IgM and, less frequently, have IgG antibodies which bind to Fc fragment on IgG. Therefore, these antibodies are named rheumatoid factor(RF). The increased frequency of RA in first-degree relative families is suggested that genetic variables play an important role during pathogenesis process. Moreover, some specific agents activating from infectious agents, such as EBV, Mycoplasma species, mycobacteria, parvoviruses, may activate T or B cells.

11.1.4.2　Morphology

Typical RA shows assymmetri arthritis, especially affecting small joints of the feet, wrists, knees, elbows, shoulder and hands. Histopathologically, the affected joints display chronic synovitis, and the classical characters are: ①synovial cell hyperplasia and proliferation; ②dense perivascular inflammatory cell infiltrates in the synovium consist of CD4$^+$ T cells, macrophages and plasma cells; ③increased vascularity; ④neutrophils and organizing fibrin are aggregate on the synovial surface and in the joint space; ⑤increased osteoblast activity in the related bone leads to synovial penetration and bone erosion. The most characteristic appearance is the pannus, formed by proliferating synovial-lining cells mixed with inflammatory cells, granulation tissues, and fibrous connective tissue; smooth synovial membrane is transformed into lush, edematous, frond-like projections,

11.2　Rejection of Transplants

Immunologic rejection of organ transplants is the major barrier during allografts(from one individual organ to another of the same species). Transplant rejection is a complex procedure mediated by both cell and antibody reactions which injures the graft. The key point to successful transplantation is minimizing rejection or development of therapies. How grafts are recognized as foreign or rejected is discussed as follow.

11.2.1　Immune Recognition of Allografts

Rejection of allografts is mainly caused by reaction to MHC molecules, which are polymorphic that most people in an outbred population differ in at least few of the MHC molecules they express, except for identical twins. Two main underlying mechanisms which the host immune system recognizes and responds to the MHC on the graft are: ①direct recognition, host T cells recognize the foreign allogeneic MHC molecules directly; ②indirect recognition, host CD$^+$4 T cells recognize MHC molecules after the above molecules are picked up.

11.2.2　Effector Mechanisms of Graft Rejection

11.2.2.1　T-cell-Mediated Rejection

CTLs which cause parenchymal and endothelial cell death kill grafted tissue cells and result in thrombosis and graft ischemia. Furthermore, cytokine trigger DTH reactions with secreting CD$^+$4 T cells and increase vascular permeability which accumulate local mononuclear cells. Therefore, graft cells and vasculature may get injured by activated microphages, thus, graft destruction occurrs.

11.2.2.2　Antibody-mediated Rejection

Alloantibodies directed against graft MHC molecules, while other alloantigens bind to the graft endothelium, causing vascular injury through complement system activation and leukocytes recruitment.

11.2.3 Morphology

On the basis of the time course and morphology of rejection reactions, they have been classified as hyperacute, acute, and chronic rejection and each pattern is caused by a different type of dominant immunologic reaction. The morphology of all patterns is described in the context taking renal transplants as example; moreover, similar changes are demonstrated in other vascularized organ transplants.

11.2.3.1 Hyperacute Rejection

The reaction occurs within minutes to a few hours after organ transplantation in a presensitized host and classically is recognized by the surgeon finish vascular anastomosis. In comparison, a non-rejecting kidney graft, recoveres a normal red color and tissue turgor and rapidly excretes urine, a hyperacute rejecting kidney fast becomes cyanotic and mottled, and excrete only a few drops of bloody fluid as urine. The histologic change is characterized by widespread acute arteritis and arteriolitis, vessel thrombosis, and ischemic necrosis, all resulting from the binding of preformed antibodies to graft endothelium. In fact, all arterioles and arteries exhibit characteristic acute fibrinoid necrosis of the walls, with lumen narrowing or complete occlusion by precipitated fibrin and cellular debris.

11.2.3.2 Acute Rejection

Acute rejection normally occurs within a few days to weeks or months and even years later, of transplantation in a non-immunosuppressed host, even in the presence of adequate immunosuppression. The underlying mechanisms may are caused by both cellular and humoral immune reactions, and in each one patient, the two ways may predominate, or both may be controlled together. On histopathology detection, cellular rejection is determined by interstitial mononuclear cell to infiltrate accompanied with edema and parenchymal injury, whereas humoral rejection is associated with vasculitis.

(1) Acute Cellular Rejection

Generally, acute cellular rejection is detected within the first few months after transplantation and normally is accompanied by clinical renal failure. Histopathology detection shows extensive interstitial $CD4^+$ and CD^+8 T cell infiltration and mild interstitial hemorrhage. Large numbers of mononuclear cells distribute around glomerular and peritubular capillaries. Furthermore, CD^+8 T cells may injure the endothelium while tubular injury, causing an endothelium. Cyclosporine (a widely used immunosuppressive agent) is also nephrotoxic and induces so-called arteriolar hyaline deposits. Renal biopsy is useful to distinguish rejection from drug toxicity.

(2) Acute Humoral Rejection (Rejection Vasculitis)

Acute humoral rejection also may be involved in acute graft rejection. The histopathology lesions may show in the form of necrotizing vasculitis with endothelial cell necrosis; neutrophilic infiltration; deposition of antibody, complement, and fibrin; and thrombosis. Such lesions may be associated with ischemic necrosis of the renal parenchyma. Some older subacute lesions are characterized by marked thickening of intima by proliferating fibroblasts, myocytes, and foamy macrophages. The arterioles narrowing may cause renal infarction or cortical atrophy. The proliferative vascular lesions mimic arteriosclerotic thickening and are believed to be caused by cytokines that stimulate proliferation of vascular smooth muscle cells. Local deposition of complement breakdown products is used to examine antibody-mediated rejection of kidney allografts.

11.2.3.3 Chronic Rejection

Chronic rejection with a progressive rise in serum creatinine levels occurs months to years late after transplantation. Vascular changes, interstitial fibrosis, and loss of renal parenchyma are the typical characters without ongoing cellular parenchymal infiltrates. The vascular changes mainly occur in the arteries and arterioles, which exhibit intimal smooth muscle cell proliferation and extracellular matrix synthesis. These lesions finally result in renal ischemia or hyalinization of glomeruli, interstitial fibrosis, and tubular atrophy. The vascular lesion may be caused by cytokines released according to activated T cells that play on the cells of the vascular wall, and it may be the end stage of the proliferative arteritis.

11.3   Immune Deficiency Diseases

Immune deficiency diseases may be effected by inherited defects with immune system development, or result from secondary effects of other diseases, such as infection, degeneration, malnutrition, autoimmunity, chemotherapy, or immunosuppression. Clinically, individuals suffer immune deficiency present with increased susceptibility to infectious diseases as well as to certain types of cancer. Patients with immune defects on immunoglobulin, complement, or phagocytic cells easily get affected by recurrent infections by pyogenic bacteria, whereas those patients with defects in cell-mediated immunity easily cause infections by viruses, fungi, and intracellular bacteria. Discussed next are the acquired immunodeficiency syndrome (AIDS), the most devastating example of secondary (acquired) immune deficiency.

11.3.1   Acquired Immunodeficiency Syndrome (AIDS)

AIDS is a retroviral disease caused by the human immunodeficiency virus (HIV). It is characterized by infection of HIV and depletion of $CD4^+$ T lymphocytes, and by profound immune-suppression leading to opportunistic infections, secondary neoplasms, as well neurologic manifestations.

At the end of 2009, more than 33 million people were living with HIV infection and AIDS, of which approximately 70% were in Africa and 20% in Asia; there were almost 2 million cases diagnosed and almost 2 million died of the disease in that year, with a total of more than 22 million deaths since the epidemic was recognized in 1981. Africa has the largest number of HIV infections, however, the most rapid increases in HIV infection in the past decade have occurred in Southeast Asian countries, including Thailand, India, and Indonesia. By contrast, in the Western world approximately 1 million U. S. citizens are infected. Furthermore, more Americans (more than 500,000) have died of AIDS than died in both world wars combined. AIDS-related death rates continue to decline from their 1995 peak. Thus, discussed next is a summary of the currently available information on HIV epidemiology, etiology, pathogenesis, and morphological changes.

11.3.1.1   Epidemiology

Transmission of HIV occurs under conditions that facilitate the exchange of blood or body fluids that contain the HIV virus or virus-infected cells. Thus, the major ways of HIV infection are sexual contact, parenteral inoculation, as well passage of the virus from infected mothers to their newborns.

11.3.1.2   Morphology

The pathologic changes of AIDS patient in the tissues are neither specific nor diagnostic. Generally, the pathologic characters of AIDS patient are opportunistic infections, Kaposi sarcoma and lymphoma, which are discussed elsewhere since the non-specific features. Therefore, the focus here is on pathologic changes in the lymphoid organs. Biopsy specimens of early-stage HIV infection from enlarged lymph nodes approved a marked follicular hyperplasia. The medulla involves abundant plasma cells. The morphologic counterparts of the polyclonal B cell activation and hypergammaglobulinemia seen in AIDS individuals are the primarily affected B cell areas of the node. Additionally, pathologic changes in the follicles, the sinuses display increased cellularity, due mainly to increased numbers of macrophages, as well as contributing to B cell lymphoblasts and plasma cells. HIV particles can be demonstrated within the germinal centers, concentrated on the villous processes of the follicular DCs. Viral DNA also can be determined in macrophages and CD4$^+$ T cells.

With disease developed, the frenzy of B cell proliferation makes a pattern of severe follicular involution and generalized lymphocyte depletion. The organized network of follicular DCs is disrupted, and the follicles may become hyalinized. These "burnt-out" lymph nodes are atrophic and small and may harbor numerous opportunistic pathogens. Non-Hodgkin lymphomas, often involving extranodal sites such as the brain are mainly aggressive B cell neoplasms.

Chapter 12

Diseases of the Urinary System

> ### Introduction

The urinary system consists of kidneys, ureters, bladder and urethra. The main function of urinary system is to eliminate waste, excess water and inorganic salts. The kidney is the most important organ in urinary system, the main function is to generate, drain urine metabolites, regulate water, electrolyte and acid-base balance and it also has endocrine function, can secrete renin, erythropoietin, prostaglandins and so on.

The kidney unit is the basic structure and functional unit of the kidney, consisting of glomerulus and tubule. There are about 2 million kidney units on both sides of the human body, with powerful compensatory functions. The glomeruli mainly perform filtration function, and the renal tubule has the function of reabsorbing the original urine composition and excretion. The glomeruli are composed of a central vascular ball and a capsule wrapped around the kidney capsule. The blood vessel is composed of the capillary loops. The capillary wall of the glomeruli is the filtration membrane, which is composed of capillary endothelial cells, basement membrane and visceral epithelial cells (also known as foot cells). Under normal circumstances, glomerular filtration membranes are highly permeable to water and small molecular solutes, while macromolecules such as proteins are almost completely unable to pass (Figure 12-1).

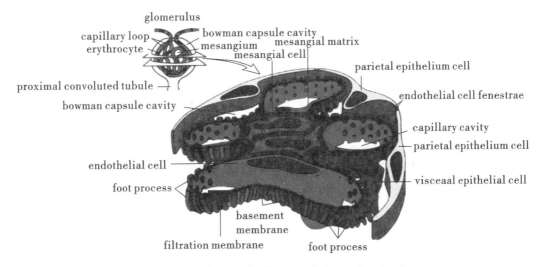

Figure 12-1 Schematic diagram of glomerular structure

The glomerular mesangium is composed of mesangial cells and mesangial matrix. The mesangium is located between the capillaries, which forms the central axis of the glomerulus and has the supporting and protective effect on the capillaries. Mesangial cells have the functions of contraction, phagocytosis, proliferation, synthetizing membrane matrix and collagen fibers. It can secrete a variety of vasoactive substances and cytokines to participate in the inflammatory response.

The renal capsule is also known as the Bowman capsule, and the inner layer is the visceral epithelial cells, the outer layer is the parietal epithelium cells, between the two layers are the balloon lumen and its urinary pole is connected with the proximal convoluted tubule.

The renal tubules including proximal convoluted tubules, thin segment, and distal convoluted tubules, constituted of a single layer of epithelium.

Diseases of the urinary system include renal and urinary tract lesions, which include inflammation, tumor, urinary obstruction, vascular disease, metabolic diseases, congenital malformations, etc. Base on the main part of the lesion, renal diseases are divided into glomerular diseases, renal tubular diseases, renal interstitial diseases and vascular diseases. This chapter mainly introduces primary glomerular disease, renal tubule-interstitial nephritis, and common neoplasms of the kidney and bladder.

12.1   Glomerular Disease

Glomerular disease is also called glomerulonephritis(GN), a group of diseases dominated by glomerular damage and change. Glomerular disease is divided into primary glomerulonephritis, secondary glomerular disease and hereditary diseases. Primary glomerulonephritis is an independent disease of the kidney, which is mainly involved in the kidneys. The secondary glomerular disease is a part of other diseases or systemic diseases, such as lupus nephritis, diabetic nephropathy, allergic purpura nephritis, etc. This section mainly discusses primary glomerulonephritis.

12.1.1   Etiology and Pathogenesis

The etiology and pathogenesis of primary glomerulonephritis have not been fully elucidated, but it has been confirmed that most of the types are caused by the immune mechanism.

There are many kinds of antigens known to cause glomerulonephritis, which can be divided into two categories: endogenous and exogenous. Endogenous antigens including glomerular antigen(glomerular basement membrane antigen, foot cells, endothelial cells and mesangial cell membrane antigen, etc.) and non-glomerular antigen(nuclear antigens, DNA, immunoglobulin, tumor antigen, thyroglobulin, etc.). Exogenous antigens include bacteria, fungi, viruses, parasites, helix, drugs, exogenous lectin and heterogeneous serum, etc.

The antigen-antibody response is the main cause of glomerular injury. The damage related to antibodies is mainly through two mechanisms: One is the reaction of antibody with glomerular antigen in situ; the other is the antigen-antibody complex formed in blood circulation, which is deposited in glomeruli and causes glomerulopathy. These two methods are the basic mechanism of glomerulonephritis. Other immunological mechanisms involved in the occurrence of nephritis include cytotoxic reactions induced by anti-glomerular cell antibodies, activation of cellular immunity and complement replacement pathways. The pathways of immune damage are not mutually exclusive. Different damage mechanisms may work together to cause glomerular lesions.

(1) Nephritis Caused by in Situ Immune Complexes

Antibody is directly interaction with the antigen components of glomerulus itself or the antigen implanted from blood circulation into the glomerulus, forming an in situ immune complexes in glomeruli, causing glomerulopathy. Different kinds of antigens can cause different types of glomerulonephritis. There are three main types: ①Nephritis caused by anti-glomerular basement membrane antibodies: this type of nephritis is caused by interaction between the antibody and the glomeruli membrane itself(Figure 12-2). The formation of glomerular basement membrane(GBM) antigen may be due to infection or other factors that change the base membrane structure and have the antigenicity, stimulate the body to produce autoantibodies. It may also be a cross-reaction due to the common antigenicity of the pathogenic microorganism and the GBM component. The antibodies are deposited along the GBM, and the immunofluorescence examination shows a characteristic continuous linear fluorescence. ②Heymann nephritis: Heymann nephritis is a classic animal model for the study of human primary membranous glomerulopathy. The brush border of proximal convoluted tubule has joint antigenic with foot cells. The former stimulates the antibody produced by the body and the cross immunoreaction with podocyte to form an immune complex to deposit in the upper subcutaneous region and cause glomerulonephritis(Figure 12-3). The immunofluorescence showed I diffuse granular immunoglobulins or complement deposition. ③The reaction of antibody and implantable antigen: some non-glomerular antigens can be combined with the components in the glomerulus, forming an implanted antigen, resulting in the formation of in situ immune complexes, causing glomerulonephritis. The immunofluorescence examination showed scattered granular fluorescence.

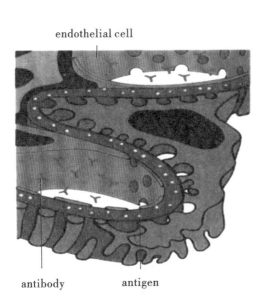

Figure 12-2   Schematic diagram of nephritis caused by anti-glomerulosa basement membrane antibodies

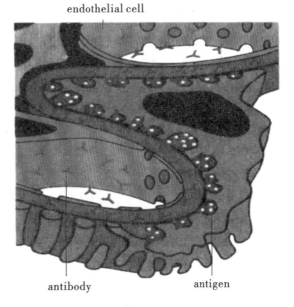

Figure 12-3   Schematic diagram of Heymann nephritis

(2) Nephritis Caused by Circulating Immune Complexes

Endogenous non-glomerular antigen or exogenous antigens stimulate the body to produce the corresponding antibody, the two combines to form an immune complex in the blood circulation, with the deposition in the glomerulus when blood flows through the kidneys, and often in combination with complement can cause glomerular lesions(Figure 12-4). Neutrophils are usually locally infiltrated, with endothelial cells, mesenchymal cells and epithelial cells proliferation.

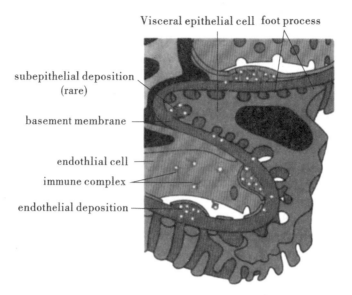

Visceral epithelial cell foot process

subepithelial deposition
(rare)

basement membrane

endothlial cell

immune complex

endothelial deposition

Figure 12-4   Schematic diagram of nephritis caused by circulating immune complexes

Whether the circulating immune complex deposition in glomerular and the location and quantity of glomerular deposition, whether it causes glomerular injury depends on many factors. The two most important
factors are the size of the complex molecule and the charge carried by the complex. Macromolecular complexes are often scavenged by phagocytes in the blood, and small molecule complexes are easy to pass through
the glomerular filtration membrane, both of which are not easily deposited in the glomeruli. The complex of
cationic ions can pass through the basement membrane, often being deposited in the epithelium through the
basement membrane. The complex of anion is not easy to pass through the basement membrane, often being
deposited under the skin. The neutrally charged complex is easily deposited in the mesangial region. Immunofluorescence examination showed discontinuous granular fluorescence in the lesion of glomerular (Figure
12-5).

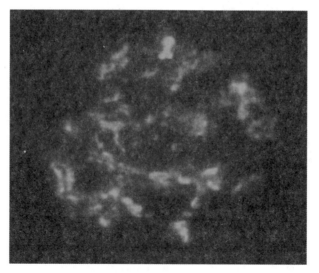

Figure 12-5   Immunofluorescence staining showed discontinuous granular fluorescence

The presence of immune complexes or sensitized T lymphocytes in glomeruli, need various media to participate in the glomerular injury, these mediators include cells and macromolecules bioactive substances, such as neutrophils, macrophages and platelets release of inflammatory mediators, intrinsic glomerular cells etc.

The formation and deposition of immune complexes is characteristic of most types of glomerulonephritis and the clinical detection of immune complexes is an important content of glomerulonephritis pathological diagnosis and research. Electron microscopy and immunofluorescence examination is a common and indispensable method at present, which is one of the pathological features of glomerulonephritis the school.

Different types of glomerulonephritis have different location of immune complex deposition and formation. Immune complexes can respectively deposit under the endothelium(basement membrane and endothelial cells), basement membrane, and under the epithelium(between the basement membrane and podocyte) or mesangial area. Under the electron microscope, the immune complex is deposited as electron dense material. Immunofluorescence confirmed that the immune complex contained immunoglobulin and complement, and showed continuous linear fluorescence or discontinuous granular fluorescence in different positions of glomeruli according to different types.

Summary, the point mechanism of glomerular injury as follows: ①Antibody mediated immune injury is an important mechanism of glomerular injury, the mechanism mainly by complement and leukocyte mediated function. ②Most antibody mediated nephritis is caused by circulating immune complex deposition, immunofluorescence examination showed the granular distribution of immune complexes. ③anti-GBM; antibodies can induce anti-GBM nephritis, immunofluorescence showed that linear distribution of antibody. ④The antibody could react with implanted glomerular antigens in situ causing the formation of immune complexes, immunofluorescence examination showed granular fluorescence.

12.1.2   Morphology

Pathological examination of renal tissue has an irreplaceable role in the diagnosis of glomerular disease. The renal puncture tissue can be routinely examined by light microscopy, immunofluorescence and transmission electron microscopy. In addition to hematoxylin(HE) staining, tissue sections were routinely stained with PAS staining, PASM staining and Masson staining. Renal biopsy tissue routine use of immunofluorescence examination immunoglobulin(IgG, IgM and IgA) and complement components(C3, C1q and C4) deposits, electron microscope observe ultrastructural changes and immune complex deposition condition and location.

The basic pathological changes of glomerulonephritis include:

1)Hypercellularity. The number of glomerular cells increased, mesangial cells, endothelial cells and epithelial cells proliferation, accompanied by neutrophils, macrophages and lymphocyte infiltration. The epithelial cell hyperplasia of the epithelium can form the inner crescent of the kidney capsule

2)Basement Membrane Thickening. The thickening of the basement membrane can be the thickening of the basement membrane itself, or it can be caused by the deposition of the immune complex in the subcutaneous, epithelium or basement membrane. PAS and PASM staining showed thickening of the basement membrane.

3)Inflammatory Exudation and Necrosis. In acute inflammation, the glomeruli can have neutrophils and other inflammatory cells infiltration and cellulose exudation, capillary wall can be cellulose like necrosis with thrombosis.

4)Hyalinization and Sclerosis. The hyalinization of the glomeruli are characterized by a homogeneous eosinophilic deposition in HE staining. In severe cases, the glomerular inherent cell decreases or disappear, the capillary tube experience stenosis and occlusion, the increase of collagen fibers, and eventually lead to glomerulosclerosis. Glomerular hyalinization and sclerosis are the final results of the development of various glomerular lesions.

5) Renal Tubules and Interstitial Changes. The epithelial cells of the renal tubule often occur degeneration, and the tubular form of protein, cell or cell debris is formed in the lumen. Hyperemia, edema and infiltration of inflammatory cells can occur in the renal interstitium. When the glomerulus appears hyalinization and sclerosis, the corresponding renal tubules atrophy or disappear, and interstitial fibrosis is occurring.

According to the lesion range, glomerulonephritis is divided into two categories, focal and diffuse. Focal glomerulonephritis involves only less than half of the glomeruli, and diffuse glomerulonephritis involves more than half or all of the glomeruli. A glomerulus, if all or most of the lesions involving the glomerular capillary loops, itis called global lesions; if the lesions only involved some capillary loops(no more than 50% of the glomerular section), itis called segmental lesions.

12.1.3　Clinical Course

The clinical course of glomerulonephritis mainly includes urine volume changes(oliguria, no urine, polyuria or nocturia), in urine characteristics changes(hematuria, proteinuria and tubular urine), edema and hypertension.

The clinical course of glomerulonephritis is closely related to the pathological type, but it is not completely corresponded. The same pathological type of pathological changes can produce different symptoms and signs, and different pathological changes can also cause similar clinical manifestations. In addition, the clinical manifestation is related to the degree and stage of the disease. The main clinical manifestations of glomerulonephritis are divided into the following types:

1) Acute Nephritic Syndrome. Acute onset, with obvious hematuria, mild to moderate proteinuria, edema and hypertension as the main clinical manifestations, severe patients can appear azotoxemia. Acute glomerulonephritis syndrome is often seen in acute diffuse proliferative glomerulonephritis.

2) Rapidly Progressive Nephritic Syndrome. Acute onset, rapid progress, manifested as edema, hematuria, proteinuria, rapid oliguria or no urine, azotaemia, and acute renal failure. Rapidly progressive nephritic syndrome mainly appears in rapidly progressive glomerulonephritis.

3) Nephritic Syndrome. The main clinical course are proteinuria(urinary protein is more than 3.5 g/d), severe edema, hypoproteinemia, hyperlipemia and lipid in urine, the so-called "three high and one low". There are many pathological types that have nephrotic syndrome, including minimal change glomerulopathy, membranous glomerulopathy, focal segmental glomerulosclerosis, membranous proliferative glomerulonephritis, mesangial proliferative glomerulonephritis, etc.

4) Asymptomatic Hematuria or Proteinuria. The main clinical course is the continuous or repeated attack of the naked eye or the microscopic hematuria, the mild proteinuria, which can also occur both at the same time. The corresponding pathological type is IgA nephropathy.

5) Chronic Nephritic Syndrome. It can be found at the end stage of various glomerulonephritis, mainly manifested as polyuria, nocturia, hypobaric urine, hypertension, anemia, azotemia and uremia, and gradually develops into renal failure.

Glomerular lesions can cause a decrease in glomerular filtration rate and increase the level of blood urea nitrogen and plasma creatinine, forming azatremia. The uremia occurs in acute and chronic renal failure late in azotemia performance. In addition to the manifestations of nitrogenemia, it also has a series of symptoms and signs of self-poisoning, namely, the pathological changes of gastrointestinal tract, nerve, muscle and cardiovascular systems, such as gastroenteritis, uremic peripheral inflammation, and fibrinous pericarditis.

12.1.4   Pathological of Type of Glomerulonephritis

The pathological types of glomerulonephritis are many, the clinical courses are complex, and the therapeutic effect and prognosis are different. In recent years, due to the application of renal biopsy technique, pathomorphological classification has practical significance for the treatment and prognosis of glomerulonephritis. This department mainly introduces common primary glomerulonephritis.

12.1.4.1   Acute Diffuse Proliferative Glomerulonephritis

The characteristics of acute diffuse proliferative glomerulonephritis are diffuse glomerular capillary endothelial cells and mesangial cell hyperplasia, with neutrophils and macrophages infiltration. Clinical abbreviate acute nephritis, which mainly manifested as acute nephritis syndrome. Acute nephritis is mainly caused by infection, also known as post infectious glomerulonephritis or endocapillary proliferative glomerulonephritis.

Group A β-hemolytic Streptococcus is the most common pathogen, and a few cases are associated with other bacterial or viral infection. Majority cases encounter angina, scarlet fever or skin streptococcal infection before 1–4 weeks of onset. moreover, the antibody titer of serum anti-streptolysin O and other anti-streptococcus antigen increased, and serum complement level decreased. The pathogenesis of this disease is nephritis mediated by circulating immune complex.

(1) Morphology

Gross appearance, bilateral kidney size increased, membrane tension, kidney surface hyperemia, color red, called red kidney. Sometimes in the surface and section of the kidney, scattered Millet size hemorrhage point, like fleas, called flea-bitten kidney. The thickness of the cortex is thicker, the demarcation of cortex and medulla is clear.

Histological changes, most of glomeruli is involved. The volume of glomerulus increased, endothelial cells and mesangial cells proliferated, endothelial cells swellt, and neutrophils and macrophages infiltrate. A significant increase in the number of cells in the glomerulus could pressure the capillaries, stenosis or occlusion of the lumen (Figure 12–6). In severe lesions, fibrous necrosis and thrombus formation in glomerular capillaries can be accompanied by significant bleeding. The epithelial cells of the renal proximal convoluted tubule are denatured, and the tubule type, red cell or white cell tube type and granular tube type are found in the renal tubule. The renal interstitial blood vessels are hyperemia, edema and infiltrated with inflammatory cells. The immunofluorescence examination showed that IgG, IgM and C3 are deposited in the glomeruli and showed granular fluorescence. Electron microscopic examination showed a hump like deposit between the visceral epithelial cells and the glomerular basement membrane.

(2) Clinical Pathological Correlation

Acute nephritis is more commonly seen in children, and clinical courses are acute nephritis syndrome. Patients often have symptoms of fever, oliguria, and hematuria in about 10 days after infection in the pharynx and other places. Hematuria and mild proteinuria are caused by increased permeability of glomerular capillaries and vascular. Hematuria is a common symptom, most of the patients appear microscopic hematuria, a few appear macroscopic hematuria. In urine, protein tube type, cell tube type, granular cast can be found. Due to the proliferation of glomerular cells, the compression of capillaries causes stenosis and occlusion reducing the glomerular filtration rate, which leads to oliguria and academia in severe cases. The patient often has edema and mild to moderate hypertension. The main cause of edema is the decrease of glomerular filtration rate, which causes water, sodium retention or hypersensitivity to increase capillary permeability. Water and sodium retention increases blood volume and causes high blood pressure.

The prognosis of the children is good, most of the children's renal disease gradually subsided, the symptoms are relieved and disappear, but less than 1% of the children could develop into acute glomerulonephritis, and the disease in a few children slowly progressed to chronic glomerulonephritis. The prognosis of the adult is poor, it can transform into acute nephritis or chronic glomerulonephritis.

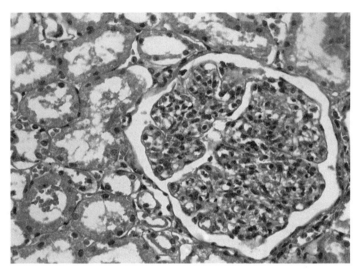

Figure 12-6   Acute diffuse proliferative glomerulonephritis

12.1.4.2   Rapidly Progressive Glomerulonephritis

The pathological changes of rapidly progressive glomerulonephritis (PRGN) are characterized by the formation of crescent in the epithelial cells of the glomerular wall layer, so it is also known as crescentic glomerulonephritis. This disease is characterized by rapid onset, rapid progress and poor prognosis. It is also called rapidly progressive glomerulonephritis. Its clinical course is rapidly progressive glomerulonephritis syndrome.

Rapidly progressive glomerulonephritis is primary, secondary or associated with other glomerular diseases. According to immunological and pathological tests, PRGN can be divided into three subtypes: ①Type Ⅰ is a glomerulonephritis caused by anti-glomerular basement membrane antibody. There is a cross reaction between the anti-GBM antibody and the alveolar basement membrane, causing pulmonary hemorrhage, accompanied by hematuria, proteinuria, hypertension and other nephritis symptoms, often developing to renal failure. This lesion is called Goodpasture syndrome. ②Type Ⅱ is immune complex nephritis, which is more common in China. It can be caused by immune complex nephritis caused by streptococcal glomerulonephritis, systemic lupus erythematosus, IgA nephropathy, anaphylactoid purpura and other causes. ③Type Ⅲ is immunoreactive deficiency type nephritis. No anti-GBM antibody or immune complex deposit is found in the glomeruli, and it is considered to be caused by glomerular vasculitis.

(1) Morphology

Gross appearance, bilateral kidney volume increased, the color is pale, the surface of the kidney can be seen scattered on the point of hemorrhage, the thickening of the cortical cortex.

Histological changes, most of the glomerulus has a characteristic crescent formation. Crescent is mainly composed of proliferating epithelial cells and mononuclear cells, neutrophils and lymphocytes infiltration, attached to the balloon wall layer formed on the outside of the capillaries ball crescent or ring structures (Figure 12-7). The early crescents are mainly cellular components, known as cellular crescents. Then the collagen fibers gradually increase, transforming into fibro-cellular crescents, and eventually the crescent is completely fibrotic and becomes fibrous crescent. The crescent often contains more cellulose, and cellulose exudation is an important reason for the formation of crescent. After the formation of the crescent or annular body, the glomerular capillaries can be compressed, and the glomerulosa can be narrowed or blocked, and the glomerular capillaries becomeied atrophy, fibrotic and hyalinization. Renal tubule epithelial cell degeneration, because of the absorption of protein and the appearance of intracellular hyalinization, partial renal tubular epithelial cells atrophy or even disappear. Renal interstitial edema and the inflammatory cell is infiltrated, late fibrosis. Immunofluorescence result is related to the type of acute nephritis. Type I is linear fluorescence. Type II is granular fluorescence. The immunofluorescence of type III is negative. Electron microscopy reveals crescentic and glomerular basement membrane defects or breakages. Electron dense deposits are found in type II cases.

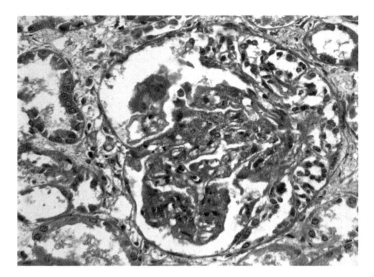

Figure 12-7   **Rapidly progressive glomerulonephritis**

(2)Clinical Pathological Correlation

The rapid progression of rapidly progressive glomerulonephritis is characterized by rapid progressive nephritis syndrome. Due to glomerular capillary necrosis, basal membrane defect and hemorrhage, the patient shows obvious hematuria and moderate proteinuria. A large number of crescent bodies are formed to block the renal capsule, which can rapidly reduce urine and anuris The retention of metabolic waste in the body leads to nitrogenemia, which eventually leads to uremia and kidney failure. Renal glomerular ischemia is caused by extensive fibrosis and hyalinization in glomerulus, which can lead to high blood pressure through the function of the renin-angiotensin system and water and sodium retention. Patients with pulmonary hemorrhagic nephritis syndrome can have recurrent hemoptysis and severe death.

Acute glomerulonephritis is a serious disease with rapid development and poor prognosis. If not treated promptly, most patients die from acute renal failure within weeks to months. The prognosis is related to the number and proportion of the formation of the crescent body, and the more the formation of the crescent, the worse the prognosis.

12.1.4.3   Nephritic Syndrome and Associated Nephritis

The main manifestation of nephrotic syndrome is a large number of proteinuria, and the protein content in urine reaches or exceeds 3. 5 g/d. Hypoalbuminemia(plasma albumin <30 g/L) ; High edema ; Hyperlipidemia and Lipid urine. The main symptoms of nephrotic syndrome are interrelated. The critical lesion is the damage of the capillary wall of the glomerulus, the filtration membrane permeability increased, and the plasma protein filtration increased. When the membrane damage is relatively light, albumin and transferrin, which are mainly low molecular weight in urine, are selective proteinuria. When the damage is serious, the protein of large molecular weight can also be filtered to form non-selective proteinuria.

Multiple primary glomerulonephritis and systemic disease can cause nephrotic syndrome. Children's nephrotic syndrome is mainly caused by primary glomerulonephritis, and adults may be associated with systemic diseases. The common types of nephrotic syndrome are as follows.

12.1.4.4 Membranous Glomerular Disease

Membranous glomerular disease is the most common cause of adult nephrotic syndrome. The lesion is characterized by diffuse thickening of glomerular capillaries. In the early stage of the lesion, the glomerular inflammatory changes are not obvious, also known as membranous nephropathy.

Membranous glomerulonephritis is a chronic immune complex mediated disease, and primary membranous glomerular disease is an autoimmune disease similar to that of Heymann nephritis. Autoantibodies and glomerular epithelial membrane antigen react, formation of immune complex deposition between the glomerular epithelial cells and basement membrane, causing the capillary wall damage and protein leakage through complement.

(1) Morphology

Gross appearance, bilateral kidney volume increases, the color is pale, present the appearance of the "white kidney", with obvious thickening of the cortex. Under microscope, early glomerulus is basically normal, with the lesion aggravating, the glomerular capillary wall diffuse thickening, the tube cavity gradually narrow, or even block, the final glomeruli sclerosis. The epithelial cells of proximal convoluted tubules often contain small drops of absorbed protein, which are infiltrated by inflammatory cells such as lymphocytes and macrophages.

Immunofluorescence examination showed that IgG and C3 were deposited along the lateral margin of the glomeruli, showing a discontinuous high intensity fine granular fluorescence. Electron microscopy observed that the epithelial cells are swelling and the footprocess disappeares, and there are a large number of electron dense deposits between the basement membrane and epithelial cells, and the basement membrane hyperplasia formes a number of spikes that are inserted between the sediments. The basement membrane is dyed black with periodic acid-silver methenamine(PASM) staining, which can show a thickened basement membrane and its vertical spike, like a comb(Figure 12-8). In the early stage of the lesion, the sediments are less, the spike is small and the depositions were gradually increased. The spike extends to the surface of the sediment and covers it, which makes the basement membrane thickened significantly. The depositions are gradually dissolved and absorbed in the thickened basement membrane, forming a worm-eaten like gap.

(2) Clinical Pathological Correlation

Membranous glomerular disease is common in adults. Clinical courses are nephrotic syndrome. Due to the serious injury of the glomerular basement membrane, the permeability of the filtration membrane is significantly increased, and it is characterized by non-selective proteinuria. Some patients have hematuria or mild hypertension.

The clinical manifestations of membranous glomerular disease are chronic, the course is long and the adrenocortical hormone is not effective. Some patients can be relieved or the controlled while some patients have renal failure due to extensive glomerular fibrosis.

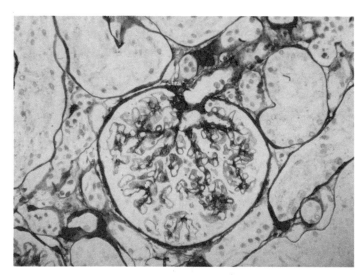

Figure 12-8   Membranous glomerular disease(PASM staining)

12.1.4.5   Minimal Change Glomerulopathy

Minimal change glomerulopathy is also known as minimal change glomerulonephritis, or minimal change nephrosis, which is the most common reason of nephrotic syndrome in children. The lesion is characterized by the diffuse disappearance of foot process of glomerular visceral epithelium cells. Under the light microscope, the glomerulus is basically normal, and lipid deposition is seen in the epithelial cells of the renal tubular epithelium, and therefore is also known as lipid nephrosis.

The occurrence of this disease may be related to abnormal immune function, especially T lymphocyte dysfunction and mutation of glomerular protein gene. Immune dysfunction causes the release of cytokines and the damage of visceral epithelial cells, causing proteinuria.

(1) Morphology

Gross appearance, bilateral kidney volume increases, yellow and white streaked due to lipid deposition in renal tubular epithelial cells. Under the microscope, the glomerular structure is basically normal, and there is a large number of lipid droplets and small proteins in the epithelial cells of the proximal convoluted tubule. Immunofluorescence examination showed no immunoglobulin or complement deposition. Under the electron microscope, the main changes are the diffuse disappearance of foot process in the visceral epithelium cells, swelling of the cytoplasm, the formation of vacuoles in the cytoplasm, and the proliferation of microvilli on the surface of the cells.

(2) Clinical Pathological Correlation

This disease occurs in children and is characterized by nephrotic syndrome, especially in highly selective proteinuria. Edema is often the earliest symptom; proteinuria is selectivity, usually without hematuria and hypertension. Corticosteroid therapy is effective for more than 90% of children. The effect of adult patients on corticosteroids is not obvious.

12.1.4.6   Focal Segmental Glomerulosclerosis

Focal segmental glomerulosclerosis is characterized by partial sclerosis of some glomeruli. The main clinical manifestation is nephrotic syndrome.

The pathogenesis of this disease has not yet been elucidated, which is mainly caused by injury and alteration of visceral epithelial cells. Due to the obvious increase of local permeability, plasma protein and lipid deposit in extracellular matrix, activate mesangial cells and cause segmental glomerulosclerosis.

(1) Morphology

Under the microscope, the lesion showed a focal distribution, early only affect the glomeruli at the junction of the skin medulla, and gradually affected the whole cortex. In the lesion of glomerular capillary loops, the mesenchymal matrix is increased, the basement membrane collapses, and the lumen is blocked, resulting in glomerular sclerosis, and renal tubular atrophy and interstitial fibrosis.

Immunofluorescence examination revealed IgM and C3 deposition in the lesion site. Electron microscopy showed that the epithelial cells of the diffuse layer of the epithelial cells disappeared, and some epithelial cells were removed from the glomeruli.

(2) Clinical Pathological Correlation

The main clinical courses of this disease are nephrotic syndrome, and a few are only proteinuria. The effect of this disease on corticosteroid is not good, the lesion is progressive, and most develop into chronic glomerulonephritis. The prognosis of children is better.

12.1.4.7 Membranoproliferative Glomerulonephritis

The pathological features of membranoproliferative glomerulonephritis are c thickening of glomerular capillaries and proliferation of glomerular cells and mesangial matrix. Due to the obvious proliferation of mesangial cells, it is also known as mesangiocapillary glomerulonephritis. The disease is characterized by nephrotic syndrome, which can also cause hematuria and proteinuria.

Primary membranoproliferative glomerulonephritis is divided into two types according to the characteristics of immunofluorescence and ultrastructure (Figure 12−9): type I is caused by cyclic immune complex deposition and complement activated. There is an autoantibody called C3 in type II patients serum, the occurrence of this type of nephritis is related to the activation of complement alternatives, significantly lower in patients with serum C3 level.

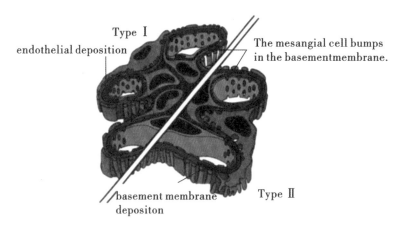

Figure 12−9   Membranoproliferative glomerulonephritis

(1) Morphology

Gross appearance, the kidneys does not change significantly. Under the microscope, the size of the glomeruli increases, the mesangial cells and endothelial cells increases, and leukocyte infiltration is observed. Increased proliferation of mesangial cell and mesangial matrix along the capillary endothelial cells under widely insert to capillary basement membrane, leading to diffuse thickening of the blood capillary basement membrane, glomus lobules separated broadening, lobulated. PASM staining showed that the thickened substrate was double-track. Type I is common, electron microscopy shows that the main sedimentary electron dense under the mesangial area and endothelial cells. Immunofluorescence examination showed C3 granular deposits, and the early components of complement, such as IgG, C1q and C4, Type Ⅱ, electron microscopy shows a large number of dense massive high electron density of sediments along the basement membrane layer shows zonal distribution and immunofluorescence examination showed C3 deposition.

(2) Clinical Pathological Correlation

This disease usually occurs in children. The clinical is chronic and the prognosis is poor. There is only mild proteinuria or hematuria in the early stage, with the progression of the disease appearance of nephrotic syndrome. In the late stage, hypertension and renal failure are caused by the narrowing and even occlusion of the glomerular capillaries, the sclerosis of the mesangium and glomerular fibrosis, and about 50% of the patients will have chronic renal failure within 10 years. The effect of hormone and immunosuppressive therapy is often not obvious. After kidney transplantation, the disease often recurs.

12.1.4.8　Mesangial Proliferative Glomerulonephritis

Mesangial proliferative glomerulonephritis is characterized by diffuse mesangial cell proliferation and increased mesangial matrix.

There may be many pathogenetic pathways, such as circulating immune complex deposition or in situ immune complex formations. Immune response stimulates mesangial cells through the action of medium, resulting in proliferation of mesangial cells and increased mesangial matrix.

(1) Morphology

Under the microscope, the mesangial area is broadened, diffuse mesangial cell proliferation and mesangial matrix increased. The hyperplastic mesangial tissue could oppresses capillary loops to lead to narrowing of the lumen, and the infiltration of a few macrophages and neutrophils in the mesangial membrane. Immunofluorescence often shows different results. In China, IgG and C3 deposits are most common, and IgM and C3 deposits are mostly in other countries. Only C3 deposition or immunofluorescence examination is negative in some cases. Electron dense deposits are observed in the mesangial area.

(2) Clinical Pathological Correlation

This disease is very common in young people. It can be characterized by asymptomatic proteinuria or hematuria and nephrotic syndrome. This disease can be treated with hormones and cytotoxic drugs, and the prognosis is generally good. If the lesion is severe, it can develop chronic sclerosing glomerulonephritis.

12.1.4.9　IgA Nephropathy

The pathological feature of IgA nephropathy is IgA deposition in mesangial area. It is characterized by recurrent microscopic or gross hematuria. The occurrence of this disease is regionally, and maybebe the most common type of glomerulonephritis worldwide. The disease was first described by Berger, so it is also known as Berger disease.

The occurrence of IgA nephropathy is related to congenital or acquired immunomodulation abnormalities. Bacterial, viral and food protein stimulates the increase of IgA synthesis in the respiratory or digestive mucosa. The immune complex of IgA or IgA deposits in the mesangial region and activates the replacement of the complement and causes the glomerular damage. The serum levels of IgA were higher in patients.

(1) Morphology

Under the microscope, there are a variety of lesions, which can show mild pathological changes, focal segmental hyperplasia or sclerosis, diffuse capillary hyperplasia, mesangial proliferative, membrane proliferative, crescent formation and even glomerulosclerosis, among which mesangial proliferative lesions are the most common. Immunofluorescence showed that there was IgA deposition in the mesangial area, often accompanied by C3 deposition, or with a small amount of IgG and IgM deposition, showing high intensity granular fluorescence. Electron microscopy showed dense deposits in the mesangial area.

(2) Clinical Pathological Correlation

IgA nephropathy often occurs in children and young people. Before occurance, there is usually upper respiratory tract infection. A few cases occur after gastrointestinal or urinary infection. The clinical manifestations of IgA nephropathy are chronic, mainly manifested as recurrent hematuria and mild proteinuria, and a few patients are characterized with a nephrotic syndrome or acute nephritic syndrome. The prognosis is related to the type of disease. The age of the disease is large, a large number of albuminuria, high blood pressure, renal biopsy, glomerulosclerosis. Severe hyperplasia or crescent formation has a poor prognosis.

12.1.4.10　Chronic Glomerulonephritis

Chronic glomerulonephritis is a common result of the development of different types of glomerulonephritis. It is characterized by a large number of glomerular hyalinization and sclerosis, so it is also called chronic sclerosing glomerulonephritis. Clinically, chronic nephritis syndrome is a typical manifestation.

Chronic glomerulonephritis is developed by different types of glomerulonephritis, with different pathogenesis. Most of the patients have a history of nephritis, but some patients have a hidden disease, no clear history of nephritis, and the lesions have entered the chronic stage when it is found. The glomerular damage caused by different causes results in glomerular fibrosis, hyalinization, sclerosis and corresponding renal tubular epithelial cell atrophy and renal interstitial fibrosis.

(1) Morphology

Gross appearance, bilateral kidneys shrink symmetry, weight decreased, hardened texture, the surface is diffuse fine granular, plane renal cortical thinning obviously, boundary is not clear between cortex and medulla, small artery wall thickening and hardening. Fat around the renal pelvis increased. The general lesion of chronic nephritis is referred to as secondary granular contracted kidney. Under the microscope, the pathological types of primary nephritis can be seen in the early stage. In the later stage, the glomerular diffusive hyalinization and sclerosis, and the renal tubule are atrophied and disappear due to ischemia. The light lesion glomeruli shows compensatory hypertrophy, and the renal tubules are dilated, with various tubular types visible in the lumen. The renal interstitial fibrous tissue is hyperplastic with lymphocytes and plasma cells infiltrating. Interstitial fibrosis brings the glomeruli of the lesion close to each other, forming glomerular concentration. Because of the high blood pressure caused by nephritis, the fine and small arteries in the kidney can produce hyalinization and sclerosis, resulting in thickening of the tube wall and stenosis of the tube (Figure 12-10). Because most glomerular sclerosis, immunofluorescence and electron microscopy are often negative. The relatively light glomeruli can sometimes be seen with immunoglobulin and complement deposition, and electron microscopy is seen in electron dense deposits.

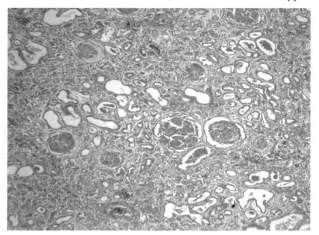

Figure 12-10　Chronic glomerulonephritis

(2) Clinical Pathological Correlation

This disease is more common in adults. Some patients have other types of nephritis history and some patients wave insidious disease. In the early stage, there may be symptoms such as poor appetite, vomiting, fatigue, anemia, etc., and some of the patients show proteinuria, edema, hypertension or azotemia. Patients with advanced stage of chronic nephritis syndrome often cause chronic renal failure. ① Polyuria, nocturia and low proportion of urine. Due to a large number of renal units structure damage and loss of function, blood through residual nephron moves fast, glomerular filtration rate increases, but renal tubular reabsorption function is limited, function of urine concentration is reduced, the patient has polyuria, nocturia and low proportion of urine. ②Hypertension. It is caused by a large number of glomerular sclerosis, which causes severe ischemia in the renal tissue and increases in the secretion of renin. High blood pressure leads to arterial sclerosis, exacerbating renal ischemia and increasing blood pressure. Chronic hypertension can lead to left ventricular hypertrophy and severe heart failure. High blood pressure can also cause cerebral hemorrhage. ③Anemia. It is caused by the destruction of kidney tissue, the reduction of erythropoietin secretion, and the accumulation of a large number of metabolites in the body to inhibit the hematopoietic function. ④Nitrogen mass concentration and uremia. A large number of renal units structure become damaged resulting in a major accumulation of metabolites in the body of water, electrolyte and acid-base balance disorders, blood urea and creatinine increased, resulting in nitrogen qualitative hematic disease and uremia.

The rate of progression of chronic glomerulonephritis is very different and the duration of the disease is different, but the prognosis is poor. Early rational treatment can control the development of disease. If dialysis or kidney transplantation cannot be performed in time, patients often die from heart failure, cerebral hemorrhage or secondary infection caused by chronic renal failure or hypertension.

It is important to note that the diagnosis and differential diagnosis of glomerulonephritis in clinic must be comprehensively analyzed in combination with the history, clinical manifestations, laboratory examination and pathological examination. The pathological types of primary glomerulonephritis, the characteristics of light microscopy and the main clinical manifestations are summarized as follows (Table 12-1).

Table 12-1　The Classification and Clinicopathologic Features of Glomerulonephritis

Pathological Types	Characteristics of Microscope	Mainly Clinical Courses
acute diffuse proliferative glomerulonephritis	diffuse glomerular capillary endothelial cells and mesangial cell hyperplasia proliferation	Acute nephritic syndrome
rapidly progressive glomerulonephritis	Crescent formation	Rapidly progressive syndrome
Membranous glomerular disease	Diffuse GBM thickening, spike formation	Nephritic syndrome
Minimal change Glomerulopathy	Normal glomeruli, the renal tubule lipid deposit	Nephritic syndrome
Focal segmental Glomerulosclerosis	Focal segmental hyalinization and Sclerosis	Nephritic syndrome, Proteinuria
Membranoproliferative glomerulonephritis	Mesangial cell proliferation, insertion, basement membrane thickening, double track	Nephritic syndrome, Hematuria, proteinuria, chronic renal failure
Mesangial proliferative glomerulonephritis	Mesangial cell proliferation and mesangial matrix increase	Albuminuria, hematuria, Nephritic syndrome
IgA nephropathy	Focal segmental hypertrophy or diffuse mesangial broadening	Repeated episodes of hematuria or proteinuria
Chronic glomerulonephritis	Glomerular hyalinization and sclerosis	Chronic nephritic syndrome

12.2   Tubulointerstitial Nephritis

Tubulointerstitial nephritis(TIN) refers to a group of inflammatory diseases that involve the renal tubules and interstitium of the kidney, and which can be divided into acute and chronic types. Acute TIN is mainly characterized by interstitial edema, tubular and interstitial neutrophil infiltration, normally combined with focal tubular necrosis; Chronic TIN manifests lymphocytic, mononuclear cells infiltration, renal interstitial fibrosis and tubular atrophy. In this section mainly talk about the pyelonephritis and tubulointerstitial nephritis caused by drugs and poisoning.

12.2.1   Pyelonephritis

Pyelonephritis is an inflammatory disease of the renal pelvis, interstitium, and renal tubules. It is a common disease of the kidney caused by bacterial infection, and the disease is more likely to affect female. According to the clinical course and pathological features, pyelonephritis can be divided into two types, acute and chronic. Acute pyelonephritis patients in clinical mainly manifest as fever, chills, low back pain, hematuria, pyuria, and irritation sign of bladder. Chronic pyelonephritis patients may have the symptoms of hypertension and renal insufficiency in addition to the changes in urine.

12.2.1.1   Etiology and Pathogenesis

Acute pyelonephritis, a common suppurative in flammation of the kidney and the renal pelvis, is caused by bacterial infection. *Escherichia coli* is by far the most common(about 60% −80%) causative pathogens. Other important pathogens are proteus, aerobacter aerogenes, staphylococcus, and fungi. Acute pyelonephritis is mostly a single bacterial infection, but the chronic pyelonephritis is mostly mixed infection of two or more bacteria.

(1) Two Main Routes of infection in Pyelonephritis

1) Hematogenous infection. Most of the causative bacteria are staphylococcus aureus. The causative bacteria invade the blood vessels from an infection site on the body, enter the kidneys with the bloodstream, stay in the glomeruli or the capillary vessels around the renal tubules and cause inflammation. Along with the spread of blood, the causative bacteria could reach to the renal medulla, calyces, and renal pelvis, so hematogenous infection also known as descending infection. Pyelonephritis caused by hematogenous infection is rare, which can occurr in some sepsis or infective endocarditis, and the lesions often involve both kidneys.

2) Ascending Infection. It is the main route to cause pyelonephritis. Most pathogens are *Escherichia coli*. Ascending infection may often occur from the lower urinary tract such as urethritis, prostatitis and cystitis, in which the bacteria could get introduced along with the ureter or periureteral lymphatic vessels up to the renal pelvis, calyces, and renal interstitial nephropathy, it is also known as retrograde infection, and the lesions could be involved with one or both kidneys.

(2) The Occurrence of Pyelonephritis

The urinary system has a defensive mechanism in the physiological status, and in the condition of simple bacterial invasion maybe not result in pyelonephritis. When the body resistance reduces or the local defense function of urinary system is weakened, the pathogenic bacteria can take advantage of the opportunity, entering and growing in the urinary tract, and finally result in pyelonephritis.

The common cause of pyelonephritis is:

1) Urethral mucosa injury: Cystoscopy, urethral catheterization, retrograde pyelography *et al*, could lead to urinary tract mucosal injury which can be brought into the pathogenic bacteria and cause infection, especially long-term indwelling catheter which is an important factor to induce this disease.

2) Urinary tract obstruction: Urinary calculi, prostatic hyperplasia, pregnant uterus, tumor compression, cicatricial stenosis, and congenital urinary tract malformation *et al*, which cause the urinary tract stenosis and the local defenses to reduced, resulting in urine retention and bacteria easily invades and breed and causes disease.

3) Vesicoureteral reflux (VUR): Congenital abnormal opening of the ureters, spinal cord injury and other reasons are the cause of relaxation of bladder, which would lead to vesicoureteral reflux. VUR can increase the residual urine volume which is good for the bacteria proliferation, the bacteria could invade into renal pelvis and calyx by the reflux.

4) Intrarenal reflux: Because of renal papillae, located in the upper or down pole of kidney, is extremely flat concave shape, while the central papillae is a convex shape, so the intrarenal reflux easily occurs in the upper and down pole of the kidney, as urine can go through the open ducts at the tips of papillae and farther into the renal parenchyma.

5) Decreased body resistance: Chronic wasting disease, paraplegia, long-term use of hormones and immunosuppressive drugs and other factors would make the body resistance decrease, which is favorable for the development of pyelonephritis.

12.2.1.2　Acute Pyelonephritis

Acute pyelonephritis, an acute suppurative inflammation of the renal pelvis, renal interstitium and renal tubules, is mainly caused by bacterial infection. It is common in children, pregnant women and elderly patients with prostatic hyperplasia.

(1) Morphology

Gross specimen. The kidney size is enlarged, the renal surface is congested and studded with discrete, yellowish, raised abscesses which are surrounded by purple-red hyperemia. They may be widely scattered or limited to one region of the kidney, or they may coalesce to form a single large area of suppuration. The mucosa of the renal pelvis is hyperemia, edema, the mucosal surface has purulent exudates, which can be accumulated in the renal calyces in the serious condition.

Histological section. The characteristic histologic feature of acute pyelonephritis is liquefactive necrosis with abscess formation within the renal parenchyma, the renal pelvis would be firstly involved in the inflammation caused by ascending infection, resulting in local mucosal hyperemia, edema, and a large number of neutrophils infiltrates. In the early stage, suppuration is limited to the interstitial tissue, but later abscesses rupture into tubules. Large masses of intratubular neutrophils frequently extend within involved nephrons into the collecting ducts, giving rise to the characteristic white cell casts found in the urine. The glomeruli of the renal cortex and the surrounding interstitium would be firstly involved in the inflammation caused by hematogenous infection, then spreads to adjacent tissues and the renal pelvis.

(2) Complication

1) Renal papillary. Necrosis is common in patients with urinary obstruction or diabetes, renal papillary necrosis due to ischemia and suppuration. The pathognomonic gross feature of papillary necrosis is sharply defined gray-white or yellow necrosis of the papillary, the papillary tips show characteristic coagulative necrosis.

2) Pyelonephrosis. In the severe urinary obstruction, especially when the upper urinary tract is blocked, the purulent exudate cannot be discharged and accumulated in the renal pelvis. In the severe pa-

tients, renal tissue would be atrophied due to the long term compression, and the entire kidney becomes filled with pus.

3) Perinephric abscess. In the severe case of renal perinephric abscess, the membrane would be breakthrough by the suppurative inflammation of the kidney and form an abscess in the perinephric tissue.

(3) Clinical Course

1) The whole body. Usually it is sudden, common with is fever, chills, peripheral blood leukocytosis and other symptoms.

2) Local manifestations. Patients often have waist and kidney pain, urinary frequency, urgency and the symptoms of bladder irritation, etc, and there are pus urine, bacteriuria, proteinuria, tube type urine, hematuria, etc. The leukocyte cast is formed in the renal tubule and is of clinical significance for pyelonephritis.

The prognosis of acute pyelonephritis is better, and most patients can be cured in time. If the treatment is not complete or the predisposing factors are present, the disease may become recurrent or chronic. Acute renal failure can occur when combined with renal papillary necrosis.

12.2.1.3 Chronic Pyelonephritis

Chronic pyelonephritis is an inflammation of the renal tubule-interstitium, which can be developed by the acute pyelonephritis. The lesion is characterized by predominantly interstitial in flammation and scarring of the renal parenchyma is associated with grossly visible scarring and deformity of the pelvicalyceal system. Chronic pyelonephritis is an important cause of chronic renal failure. It can be divided into two forms: chronic obstructive pyelonephritis and chronic reflux-associated pyelonephritis.

(1) Morphology

Gross specimen. One side or bilateral kidneys may be involved. Even when involvement is bilateral, the kidneys are not equally damaged and therefore are not equally contracted. The volume of the involved kidney is reduced and the texture is hard, the surface has uneven distribution scarring (Figure 12-11). The medullary margin of the renal cortex is not clear, the renal nipples atrophy, the renal pelvis and renal calyces are deformed by the contraction of the scar, and the mucosa of the renal pelvis is thickened and coarse.

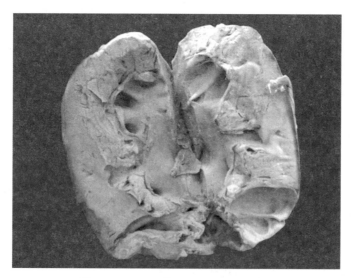

Figure 12-11 **Chronic pyelonephritis**

Histological section. Chronic pyelonephritis is a nonspecific inflammation of the renal tubules and interstitium. Histology is characterized by local lymphocytes, plasma cells infiltration and interstitial fibrosis. Renal tubule atrophy or compensatory dilation, many of the dilated tubules contain homogenous red-dyed protein, like the appearance of thyroid tissue; Renal interstitial fibrosis and lymphocytes, plasma cells infiltration, intra-renal arterial and small arterial hypertension are caused by hyaline degeneration and sclerosis. In the early stage, the glomerulus is rarely involved, fibrosis occurs around the renal capsule, and hyaline degeneration and fibrosis occur in some glomeruli in the late stage(Figure 12-12).

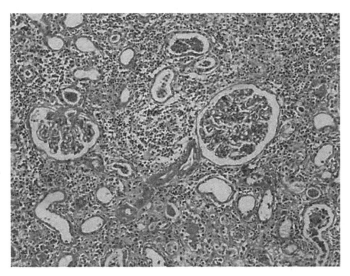

Figure 12-12   Chronic pyelonephritis

(2)Clinical Course

Many persons with chronic pyelonephritis come to medical attention relatively late in the course of the disease, because of the gradual onset of renal insufficiency or because signs of kidney disease are noticed on routine laboratory tests. Clinical manifestations of polyuria, nocturia; sodium, potassium and bicarbonate electrolytes due to excessive loss of too much urine can cause hyponatremia symptoms, hypokalemia, and metabolic acidosis. Renal tissue fibrosis and small vascular sclerosis lead to ischemia and the secretion of renin increases and then leads to hypertension. In the late stage, renal tissue is severely damaged, resulting in azotemia and uremia.

Chronic pyelonephritis can often be acute and the symptoms during the attack are similar to those of acute pyelonephritis, with fever, low back pain, pyuria, and bacteriuria. The X-ray radiologic image is characteristic: The affected kidney is asymmetrically contracted, with some degree of blunting and deformity of the calyceal system(caliectasis).

Chronic pyelonephritis has a longer duration and can often be recurrent. Better to remove the predisposing factors in time, can still control the development of lesions, renal function is in the compensatory period. Severe lesions can be life-threatening due to uremia or hypertension-induced heart failure.

12.2.2   Drug-Induced Interstitial Nephritis

In this era of widespread antibiotic and analgesic use, drugs have emerged as an important cause of renal injury. Drugs and intoxication can induce an interstitial immune response, which can cause acute hypersensitivity interstitial nephritis, and also result in renal tubular chronic injury and chronic renal insufficiency.

12.2.2.1   Acute Drug-Induced Interstitial Nephritis

Acute drug-induced interstitial nephritis can be caused by antibiotics, nonsteroidal anti-inflammatory drugs(NSAIDs), diuretics, and other drugs. The drug acts as a hapten and binds to the cytoplasm or extracellular components of the tubular epithelial cells, producing antigenicity, causing an immune response, leading to immunological damage and inflammatory reactions of the renal tubular epithelial cells and the basement membrane. The main pathological changes are severe edema of renal interstitium, infiltration of lymphocytes, macrophages, and a large number of eosinophils, neutrophils, and degeneration and necrosis of renal tubules.

The disease begins about 15 days(range, 2−40 days) after exposure to the drug and is characterized by fever, transient eosinophilia, a rash, and renal abnormalities. Urinary findings include hematuria, minimal or no proteinuria, and leukocyturia. Clinical recognition of drug-induced kidney injury is imperative, because withdrawal of the offending drug is followed by recovery, although it may take several months for renal function to return to normal.

12.2.2.2　Analgesic Nephropathy

Analgesic nephropathy is a chronic kidney disease caused by mixed administration of analgesics. The lesions are characterized by chronic tubular-interstitial inflammation with renal papillary necrosis. Most people who develop this nephropathy consume at least two analgesics, such as aspirin, phenacetin, etc, the toxic effects of drugs and ischemia would result in the kidney damage. The thickness of the renal cortex is different, and the surface of the necrotic nipple is subsidence. Necrosis, calcification and shedding can occur in the renal papilla. Microscopically, necrosis of the renal papilla appear at the early stage. In severe cases, entire renal papillary necrosis is observed and the local structure is destroyed but the preservation of tubular outlines. The renal cortex and tubules are atrophic, interstitial fibrosis and lymphocyte infiltration.

Patients often with chronic renal failure, hypertension, and anemia, renal papillary necrosis can cause hematuria and renal colic. Imaging examination revealed renal papillary necrosis and calcification. Withdrawal of analgesics can stabilize the disease the disease and may restore renal function. A small number of patients may be found to have transitional cell carcinoma of the renal pelvis.

12.2.2.3　Aristolochic Acid Nephropathy

Aristolochic acid nephropathy(AAN) is a chronic kidney interstitial disease, the incidence of AAN is closely related to the uptake of aristolochic acid-containing Chinese herbs, including Aristolochia, Tian Xian Teng, Qing Mu Xiang, Guang Fang Ji, Xun Gu Feng, Guan Mu Tong, etc.

Acute aristolochic acid nephropathy manifests as an acute renal failure and its pathological features are acute tubular necrosis. Aristolochic acid nephropathy can also cause renal tubular dysfunction, manifested as acidosis, most cases show chronic aristolochic acid nephropathy. The onset of the disease is slow and latent, a few ones rapidly developed into uremia. There is no mature treatment plan for this disease. Drugs should be withdrawn and symptomatic treatment should be used firstly. Corticosteroids may alleviate the disease in patients at the early and midterm.

12.3　Common Tumors of Kidney and Bladder

Urinary system tumors can occur at anywhere, in which the kidney and bladder tumors being common and most tumors are malignant. This section focuses on renal cell carcinoma, nephroblastoma (Wilms tumor), and urinary tract and bladder epithelial tumors.

12.3.1　Renal Cell Carcinoma

Renal cell carcinomas is a malignant tumor that is derived from the renal tubular epithelium, also called renal adenocarcinoma. Most of the tumors are yellow, and the morphology of the cells under the microscope is often similar to the adrenal cortical cells, so it was also called adrenal-like tumor. Renal cell carcinoma is the most common malignant tumor of the kidney, which represents 80% to 85% of all primary malignant tumors of the kidney in adults, and men are affected about twice as commonly as women.

12.3.1.1　Etiology and Pathogenesis

The occurrence of renal cell carcinoma is related to smoking, chemical carcinogens and genetic factors. Smoking is the most important risk factor for renal cell carcinoma. Obesity, hypertension, long-term exposure to asbestos, petroleum products, and heavy metals are also risk factors for renal cell carcinoma.

Renal cell carcinoma has two types: hereditary and sporadic. The vast majority of renal cell carcinomas are sporadic which have a high age of onset, occurring mostly on one side of the kidney. Hereditary renal cell carcinoma accounts for only 4% and is an autosomal dominant inheritance. It is characterized by a young age of onset. The tumor is often bilaterally multifocal. Hereditary renal cell carcinoma can be divided into 3 types: ①von Hippel-Lindau(VHL) syndrome, is a familial tumor syndrome. VHL disease is characterized by predisposition to a variety of neoplasms, but particularly to hemangioblastomas of the cerebellum and retina. Hundreds of bilateral renal cysts and bilateral, often multiple, clear cell carcinomas develop in 40% to 60% of affected persons. Those with VHL syndrome inherit a germline mutation of the VHL gene on chromosomal band 3p25 and lose the second allele by somatic mutation. ②Hereditary(familial) clear cell carcinoma, is a type of renal clear cell carcinoma. Patients may have the changes in VHL and related genes, but no VHL syndrome and others. ③Hereditary papillary carcinoma, these tumors are frequently multifocal and bilateral and appear as early-stage tumors, tumor cells are arranged papillary. This type tumor has no VHL gene mutation, but there are other cytogenetic abnormalities and mutations of the oncogene MET.

12.3.1.2　Morphology

(1) Gross Specimen

Renal cell carcinomas are mostly located in the two poles of the kidneys, especially in the upper poles. Usually are solitary and large when symptomatic(spherical masses 3–15 cm in diameter). The cut surface of clear cell renal cell carcinomas is yellow to orange to gray-white, with prominent areas of cystic softening or of hemorrhage, either fresh or old(Figure 12–13).

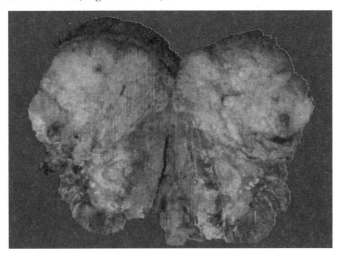

Figure 12–13　**Renal cell carcinomas**

As the tumor enlarges, it is often accompanied by hemorrhage and cystic degeneration. Tumors often have pseudo capsules with well-defined from the surrounding tissue. Advanced tumors can invade the renal pelvis, calyx and ureter, and often invades the renal vein and grows as a solid column within this vessel. Papillary carcinoma can be multifocal and bilateral.

(2)Histological Section

The main histological types of renal cell carcinoma are as follows:

1)Clear cell carcinoma, is the most common type of renal cell carcinoma, accounting for 70% to 80%. Microscopically, tumor cells are larger, round or polygonal, with clear outlines; Depending on the amounts of lipid and glycogen present, the tumor cells of clear cell renal cell carcinoma may appear almost vacuolated or may be solid. Nucleus is small and round, the tumor stroma is rich in capillaries and sinusoids (Figure 12-14).

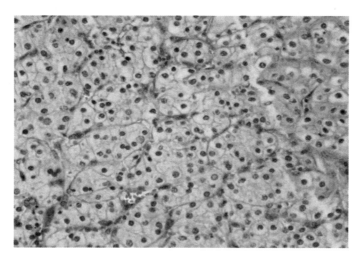

Figure 12-14　Clear cell carcinoma

Most cases are sporadic and associated with changes in the VHL gene. Immunohistochemically, tumor cells expressed low molecular weight cytokeratin, CK8, CK18, Vimentin, CD10, EMA are often positive.

2)Papillary renal cell carcinomas, account for 10% to 15% of renal cell carcinomas. Tumor cells are cubic or short columnar, arranged as papillary with fibrovascular cores, psammoma bodies and foam cells are often found in the mesenchymal of papilla, and edema can occur.

This type includes familial and sporadic. Immunohistochemical staining showed that the tumor cells are CK7 positive.

3)Chromophobe-type renal cell carcinomas, account for approximately 5% of renal cell carcinomas. Microscopically, the tumor cells are arranged in nests or alveolar, the cells usually have clear, flocculent cytoplasm with very prominent, distinct cell membranes. The nuclei are surrounded by halos of clear cytoplasm.

Cytogenetic examinations show multiple chromosome deletions and subdiploids. These patients have a good prognosis. Immunohistochemically, tumor cells show that EMA and CK positive, Vimentin negative or weak staining.

Other types of renal cell carcinoma include renal collecting duct carcinoma, unclassified renal carcinoma, multi-atrial cystic renal cell carcinoma, renal medullary carcinoma, mucinous small tubular and spindle cell carcinoma.

12.3.1.3　Tumor Spread

Renal cell carcinoma is easy to metastasize, which mostly occur commonly in the lungs and bones, but also in regional lymph nodes, liver, adrenal glands, and brain. Common spread pathways are as follows:

1)Directly spread. Cancer tissue can invade the renal calyx, pelvis, and even the ureter which would cause obstruction, resulting in hydronephrosis. It also can penetrate the renal capsule, invade the adrenal gland and surrounding soft tissue of the kidney.

2) Hematogenous metastasis. Owing to the rich blood vessels of renal cancer, hematogenous metastasis can occur in the early stage. The prevalent locations for metastases are the lungs and the bones, but also to the liver, adrenal glands, brain, etc.

3) Lymphatic metastasis. Normally, the tumor cells metastasize to the hilar and paraaortic lymph nodes.

12.3.1.4   Clinical Course

The early symptoms of renal cell carcinoma are not obvious. Three typical clinically significant symptoms are hematuria, lumbago, and renal masses. Painless hematuria is the main symptom of kidney cancer, and it is mostly caused by cancer tissue eroding blood vessels or invading renal calyx and renal pelvis. Sometimes the blood clot can cause renal colic when discharged through the ureter. When the tumor is larger or the kidney capsule is invaded, it causes pain in the kidney area and the mass can be reached.

Renal cell carcinoma can produce a variety of heterotopic hormones and hormone-like substances that cause paraneoplastic syndromes, such as: increased production of erythropoietin can cause polycythemia; increased renin production causes hypertension; increased parathyroid hormone causes hypercalcemia; increased production of adrenal glucocorticoids cause Cushing syndrome, etc.

The prognosis of patients with renal cell carcinoma is poor, and the 5-year survival rate is about 45%. If the tumor invades the renal vein and the surrounding tissue of the kidney, the 5-year survival rate is only 15% to 20%, and the patients with no metastasis can reach 70%.

12.3.2   Nephroblastoma

Nephroblastoma, also known as Wilms' tumor, originates from the kidney's residual kidney-based tissue and is the most common malignancy of childhood kidneys. The disease is more common in children and occasionally in adults.

Most nephroblastomas are sporadic and rarely inherited in an autosomal dominant manner. Its occurrence is mostly related to the deletion or mutation of the WT-1 gene (Wilms tumor-associated gene-1) located at 11p13. Some patients have different congenital malformations. The occurrence of nephroblastoma may be due to the differentiation disorder of the mesenchymal basal cells to the posterior renal tissue and the continuous proliferation.

12.3.2.1   Morphology

1) Gross Specimen. Nephroblastoma usually occurs in unilateral kidney, and a few cases are bilateral and multifocal. Most of the tumors showed a single solid mass with a large size. The tumor has a clear boundary, and the surrounding kidney tissue can form a pseudo capsule. Tumors are soft, cut surface is fish-like, gray or gray-red, may have bleeding, necrosis or cystic degeneration.

2) Histological Section. Nephroblastoma has a different histological structure at different developmental stages, and its composition and structure are complex. Histological features are naive glomerular or tubular-like structures with different stages of development. The cellular components include epithelioid cells, embryonic naive cells and cells of the mesenchymal tissue. Epithelial-like cells are small, round or polygonal, and can form small ball-like and tubular-like structures. Embryo-based naive cells are small round or ovoid primitive cells with few cytoplasm. The cells derived from the mesenchymal tissue are mostly fibrous or mucinous, and the cells are small, spindle-shaped or star-shaped, there may be differentiation of striated muscle, bone, cartilage or fat, etc.

Immunohistochemical staining showed that tumor cells could express NSE, CK, desmin, Vimentin, WT-1, and so on.

12.3.2.2　Tumor Spread

Nephroblastoma can invade the perirenal or renal veins, metastasize to the renal hilum and paraaortic lymph nodes through lymphatics, and can also metastasize to the lung or liver.

12.3.2.3　Clinical Course

Abdominal mass is the most common symptom of neoplasms, such as a mass that can compress adjacent organs and cause abdominal pain or intestinal obstruction. Some children have high blood pressure, which may be associated with tumor compression of the renal artery and the production of renin. Hematuria occurs when tumors invade the renal pelvis.

The treatment of renal tumor at present is mainly of comprehensive treatment of surgical resection combined with chemotherapy and radiotherapy. The long-term survival rate of non-metastasis is up to 90%, and the metastasis cases can also obtain satisfactory results after treatment.

12.3.3　Urinary Tract and Bladder Epithelial Tumors

Urothelial tumors can occur in the renal pelvis, ureters, bladder and urethra, but the most common is bladder. About 95% of bladder tumors originate from epithelial tissue. The vast majority of epithelial tumors consist of the urothelial epithelium, which is called a urothelial or transitional epithelial tumor. The bladder may be also squamous cell carcinoma, adenocarcinoma and mesenchymal tumors, but it is rare. Bladder cancer occurs mostly in men, with a ratio of about 3 : 1 between males and females. Most patients have an onset of age after 50 years.

12.3.3.1　Pathogenesis

The occurrence of bladder cancer is associated with smoking, long-term exposure to aromatic amines, radiation, chronic inflammation of the bladder mucosa, and schistosomiasis infection in Egypt, among which smoking is the most important risk factor for bladder cancer.

Cytogenetic and molecular changes in urothelial carcinoma are heterogeneous. In some cases, there was a single chromosome 9 deletion or a 9p or 9q deletion and deletions of 17p, 13q, 11p, and 14q. The molecular model of bladder cancer has two pathways. One way is to cause superficial papillary tumors through the loss of tumor suppressor genes located in 9p and 9q. Another way is the mutation of p53 that causes cancer in situ, and then the deletion of chromosome 9 occurs which leads to infiltrates cancer.

12.3.3.2　Morphology

According to the World Health Organization (WHO) and International Society of Urinary Pathology (ISUP) classification, urothelial tumors are classified into urothelial papilloma, papillary urothelial neoplasm of low malignant potential, low-grade papillary urothelial carcinoma and high-grade papillary urothelial carcinoma.

1) Gross specimen. Urothelial carcinoma often occurs in the bladder lateral wall and the trigone area and near the ureter opening. Tumors can be single or multiple, varying in size from a few millimeters to centimeters or more, and are mostly papillary, polypoid, or cauliflower-like protruding from the mucosal surface; or local thickening of the mucous membrane as flat plaque. Tumors may be invasive or non-invasive.

2) Histological section. Microscopically, urothelial papilloma account for about 1% of bladder tumors, more common in youth. The tumor is papillary and the center of the nipple is the axis of fibrous connective tissue and capillaries. The surface is urothelial in well differentiation and the cells are not atypia and mitotic.

The histological features of papillary urothelial neoplasm of low malignant potential are similar to those of papilloma except that the epithelial cell layer is increased, the papilla is thick, and the nucleus is generally enlarged.

The low-grade papillary urothelial carcinoma has more regular cellular and histological structures. The tumor cells are often papillary and the layer increased with normal polarity. The focal nuclei are heterogeneous with a dense staining, and a small amount of the tumor cells on the basement with nuclear mitosis and mild nuclear polymorphism. Low-grade urothelial papillary carcinoma can recur after removal and rarely invasive.

The high-grade papillary urothelial carcinoma cells are arranged in disorder, the layer increases and the polarity disappeares, the nucleus is densely stained, increased in size, some of the cells have obvious atypicality, more mitoses and may have pathological mitoses. High-grade papillary urothelial carcinomas are mostly invasive and prone to metastasis(Figure 12-15).

Immunohistochemical staining showed that tumor cellscould express CK7, CK8, CK18, CK20, EMA, survivin and so on.

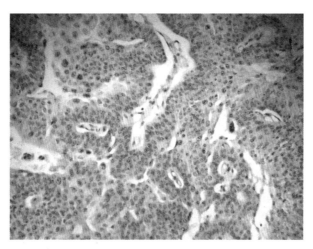

Figure 12-15   High-grade papillary urothelial carcinoma

12.3.3.3   Tumor Spread

Invasive urothelial carcinoma can affect the adjacent prostate, seminal vesicle, ureter, etc. , and can also form a fistula communicating with the vagina or rectum. About 40% of invasive urothelial carcinomas can metastasize to regional lymph nodes. Hematogenous metastasis can occur in the late stage and affects organs such as liver, lung, bone, kidney and adrenal glands, etc.

12.3.3.4   Clinical Course

The dominant clinical presentation of bladder cancer is painless hematuria. The rupture of tumor papilla, tumor surface necrosis and ulcer can cause hematuria. The tumor invading bladder wall, stimulating the bladder mucosa or concurrent infection can cause bladder irritation, such as urinary frequency, urgency, and urinary pain. Obstruction of the ureter by tumor can cause pyelonephritis, hydronephrosis and even sepsis.

Tumors of transitional cell origin of the bladder tend to recur after surgery, and the differentiation is not well in some relapsed tumors. The prognosis of patients with urothelial tumors is closely related to the grade and infiltration of tumors. The 10-year survival rate of papilloma, papillary urothelial neoplasm of low malignant potential and low-grade papillary urothelial carcinomas is 90%. The 10-year survival rate of patients with high-grade papillary urothelial carcinoma is only about 40%. Cystoscopy and biopsy are the main methods for diagnosing of bladder cancer.

Chapter 13

Female Genital System and Breast

❯ Introduction

This chapter includes common diseases of the reproductive system of men and women and the breast which are affected by endocrine and have special diseases and pathological changes. In addition to inflammation and tumors, there are some pregnancy-related diseases caused by endocrine disorders. Reproductive system inflammatory diseases are quite common, and the pathological changes are relatively simple. Therefore, the reproductive system and breast tumors and pregnancy related diseases are the focus of this chapter.

13.1   Cervix Disease

13.1.1   Cervicitis

Inflammations of the cervix are extremely common and are associated with a purulent vaginal discharge. Cytologic examination of the discharge reveals white cells and inflammatory atypia of shed epithelial cells, as well as possible microorganisms. These inflammations can be subclassified as noninfectious and infectious cervicitis.

13.1.1.1   Etiology

The major causes of this disease are streptococcus, enterococcus, staphylococcus, and special pathogenic microorganisms such as chlamydia trachomatis, neisseria gonorrhoeae, human papilloma virus(HPV), herpes simplex virus, which are encountered in sexually transmitted disease(STD) clinics. In addition, childbirth, mechanical damage is also the cause of the cervicitis.

13.1.1.2   Morphology

Nonspecific cervicitis may be either acute or chronic. The relatively uncommon acute form is limited to women in the postpartum period and usually is caused by staphylococci or streptococci. Chronic cervicitis consists of inflammation and epithelial regeneration, some degree of which is common in all women of reproductive age. The cervical epithelium may show hyperplasia and reactive changes in both squamous and columnar mucosae. Eventually, the columnar epithelium undergoes squamous metaplasia. Chronic cervicitis can be divided into three types in gross appearance: erosion, nabothian cyst, cervical polyps. Erosion can be true or pseudo. True erosion shows cervix injury, squamous cells erosion. And pseudo erosion shows columnar ectopy. Nabothian cyst with mucus can be seen in the cervix. Cervical polyp is a smooth mass of the tissue with stalks that protrude outwards from the surface of cervical mucosa.

13.1.1.3　Clinical Features

Cervicitis commonly comes to attention on routine examination or because of increased leucorrhea, vaginal bleeding, and vulva itching. Culture of the discharge must be interpreted cautiously, because (as mentioned previously) commensal organisms are virtually always present. Only the identification of known pathogens is helpful. When the lesion is severe, inflammatory changes can make differentiation from carcinoma difficult on cytologic preparations and even with colposcopy. Differentiation of inflammatory changes from premalignant dysplasia may also be difficult on cervical biopsy specimen.

13.1.2　Cervical Intraepithelial Neoplasia (CIN) and Invasive Carcinoma of the Cervix

Most tumors of the cervix are of epithelial origin. During development, the columnar, mucus-secreting epithelium of the endocervix is joined to the squamous epithelial covering of the exocervix. The exposed columnar cells, however, eventually undergo squamous metaplasia, forming a region called the transformation zone.

Cervical carcinoma was once the most frequent form of cancer in women around the world. Since the introduction of the Papanicolaou (Pap) smear 50 years ago, the incidence of cervical cancer has plummeted. The Pap smear remains the most successful cancer screening test ever developed. In populations that are screened regularly, cervical cancer mortality is reduced by as much as 99%. Many of the cases of cervical carcinoma now occur in women who have not had regular screening. Over the same period the incidence of precursor CIN has increased (this being in part attributable to better case finding) to its present level of more than 50,000 cases annually. This growing divergence is a testament to detection of precursor lesions by the Pap smear at an early stage, permitting discovery of these lesions when curative treatment is possible.

13.1.2.1　Etiology and Pathogenesis

Important risk factors which are directly related to HPV exposure for the development of CIN and invasive carcinoma include: early age at first intercourse, multiple sexual partners, smoking, and persistent infection by high-risk strains papillomaviruses. HPV is detectable by molecular methods in nearly all cases of CIN and cervical carcinoma. Although HPV infection occurs in the most immature squamous cells of the basal layer, replication of HPV DNA takes place in more differentiated overlying squamous cells. Squamous cells at this stage of maturation do not normally replicate DNA, but HPV-infected squamous cells do, as a consequence of expression of two potent oncoproteins encoded in the HPV genome called E6 and E7. The E6 and E7 proteins bind and inactivate two critical tumor suppressors, p53 gene and Rb gene, respectively. And then promoted growth rate and increased susceptibility to additional mutations, as the consequence, that may eventually lead to carcinogenesis.

Recognized serotypes of HPV can be classified as high-risk or low-risk types based on their propensity to induce carcinogenesis. High-risk HPV infection is the most important risk factor for the development of CIN and carcinoma. Two high-risk HPV strains, types 16 and 18, account for approximately 70% of cases of CIN and cervical carcinoma. In general, infections with high-risk HPV serotypes are more likely to persist, which is a risk factor for progression to carcinoma. These HPV subtypes also show a propensity to integrate into the host cell genome, an event that is linked to progression. Low-risk HPV strains (types 6 and 11), on the other hand, are associated with development of condylomas of the lower genital tract and do not integrate into the host genome, remaining instead as free episomal viral DNA (Figure 13-1). Although many women harbor these viruses, only a few develop cancer, suggesting other influences on cancer risk. Among the other well-defined risk factors are cigarette smoking and exogenous or endogenous immunodeficiency. Although HPV testing can identify the pool of women at risk for cervical cancer, most sexually active women will contact cervical HPV infections at some point in their lifetime. This limits the usefulness of HPV testing as a screening tool for cervical cancer. Thus, cervical cytology and cervical examinations (colposcopy) remain the mainstays of cervical cancer prevention. Nevertheless, women who test HPV negative with the use of molecular probes for HPV DNA are at extremely low risk for harboring a CIN, and guidelines for frequency of future screening for this group are being formulated.

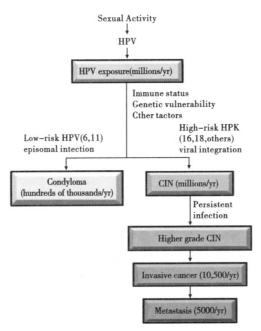

Figure 13-1   Progression of human papillomavirus (HPV) with the CIN

(from Robbins Basic Pathology 9th)

13.1.2.2   Cervical Intraepithelial Neoplasia

(1) Morphology

Cytologic examination can detect CIN long before any abnormality can be seen grossly. On the basis of histology, precancerous changes are graded as follows:

CIN I : Mild dysplasia, CIN II : Moderate dysplasia, CIN III : Severe dysplasia and carcinoma in situ (Figure 13-2).

CIN I is characterized by dysplastic changes in the lower third of the squamous epithelium and koilocytotic change in the superficial layers of the epithelium. In CIN II, dysplasia extends to the middle third of the epithelium and takes the form of delayed keratinocyte maturation. It also is associated with some variation in cell and nuclear size, heterogeneity of nuclear chromatin, and presence of mitoses above the basal layer extending into the middle third of the epithelium. The superficial layer of cells shows some differentiation and occasionally demonstrates the koilocytotic changes described. CIN III, is marked by almost complete loss of maturation, even greater variation in cell and nuclear size, chromatin heterogeneity, disorderly orientation of the cells, and normal or abnormal mitoses; these changes affect virtually all layers of the epithelium, and may extend into the endocervical glands, but the alterations are confined to the epithelial layer and its glands. These changes constitute carcinoma in situ(Figure 13-3).

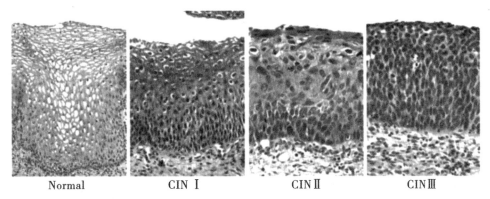

Normal　　　　CIN I　　　　CIN II　　　　CIN III

Figure 13-2　The grade of CIN(From Robbins Basic Pathology 9th)

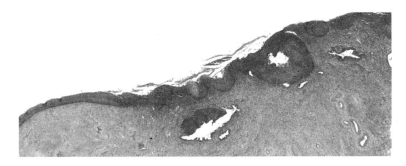

Figure 13-3　Partial replacement of endocervical glandular epithelium by CINIII

Squamous intraepithelial lesions(SIL) which is a new system based on biology and histology is more reproducible than the three-tier CIN I, CIN II and CIN III. It is divided into low-grade squamous intraepithelial lesion(LSIL) and high-grade squamous intraepithelial lesion(HSIL).

LSIL is an intraepithelial lesion of squamous epithelium that represents the clinical and morphological manifestation of a productive HPV infection. LSIL is the morphological manifestation of the differentiation-dependent expression of an HPV virion production program on the host squamous cells: koilocytosis or flat condyloma. LSIL is characterized by a proliferation of basal/parabasal-like cells that as CIN I. The mitoses are not abnormal, in the upper three-quarters to two-thirds of the epithelium, the cells differentiate and gain cytoplasm, but nuclear enlargement persists such that the nucleo-cytoplasmic ratio is increased. Cytopathic effect Koilocytosis is usually most prominent in the upper third of the epithelium. The surface cells may exhibit parakeratosis or hyperkeratosis. The finding of markedly atypical single cells in the basal third of the epithelium, or abnormal mitotic figures, should not be interpreted as LSIL, as these features correlate with DNA instability and aneuploidy and therefor represent HSIL.

HSIL is a squamous intraepithelial lesion that carries a significant risk of invasive cancer development if not treated. There is a proliferation of squamous cells most frequently in the zone of metaplasia and near the current squamocolumnar junction. The cells have abnormal nuclear features including increased nuclear size, irregular nuclear membranes, and increased nucleo-cytoplasmic ratios accompanied by mitotic figures. There is less cytoplasmic differenliation than in LSIL as the proliferating cell compartment extends up into the middle third [HSIL(CIN II)] or superficial third [HSIL(CIN III)] of the epithelium.

　(2) Clinical Features and Prognosis

CIN is asymptomatic and comes to clinical attention through an abnormal Pap smear result. These cases are followed up by colposcopy, during which acetic acid is used to highlight the location of lesions and the areas to be biopsied.

LSIL refers to the associated low risk of concurrent or future cancer. The outcome for a patient with biopsy proven LSIL is excellent as regression is expected on average within approximately one year.

HSILs are asymptomatic lesions detected by cytology and colposcopy. The size of the lesion, which correlates with the completeness of the excision/ablation, and whether HSIL reaches the margins, predict recurrence. Recent data demonstrates that testing for HPV DNA at 12 months post therapy is the best predictor of recurrent or residual disease.

13.1.2.3　Invasive Carcinoma of the Cervix

（1）Morphology

Invasive carcinomas of the cervix develop in the transformation zone and range from microscopic foci of stromal invasion to grossly conspicuous exophytic tumors. There are four types in gross appearance: erosion, exogenous cauliflower, deeply infiltration and ulcer. ①Erosion type: The mucous membrane is red, granular, brittle and easy to bleeding. Histologically, it is mostly carcinoma in situ and early invasive carcinoma. ②Exogenous cauliflower type: The cancer tissues grow mainly on the surface of the cervix, forming papillary or cauliflower-patterned masses, with necrotic and superficial ulceration on the surface. ③Deep infiltration type: The cancer tissues mainly infiltrate into the cervix, the cervical lip is thickened, and often smooth. ④Ulcer type: The carcer tissues infiltrate into the deep of cervix, there is a large necrotic lesion on the surface, forming an ulcer, which looks likes a crater.

In histology, the most common cervical carcinomas are squamous cell carcinomas (75%) (Figure 13-4), followed by adenocarcinomas and mixed adenosquamous carcinomas(20%) and small cell neuroendocrine carcinomas(less than 5%). On the basis of progress, squamous cell carcinomas are classified as early microinvasive and invasive carcinoma. The situation of early microinvasion means tumor cells infiltrating into mesenchyma with the depth less than 5mm. And the early microinvasive carcinoma has a good prognosis. The invasive cervical carcinoma is under the converse situation. On the basis of differentiation, squamous cell carcinomas are classified as keratinizing(well differentiated) and nonkeratinizing(poorly differentiated) type.

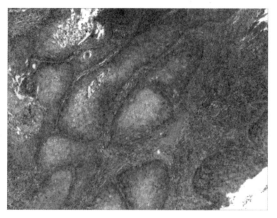

Figure 13-4　squamous cell carcinomas, cancer nests infiltrate into the cervical interstitium

（2）Spreading

Extension into the parametrial soft tissues can affix the uterus to the surrounding pelvic structures. The likelihood of spread to pelvic lymph nodes correlates with the depth of tumor invasion and the presence of tumor cells in vascular spaces.

(3)Clinical Features

Invasive cervical cancer is most often seen in women who have never had a Pap smear or who have not been screened for many years. In such cases, cervical cancer often is symptomatic, with patients coming to medical attention for unexpected vaginal bleeding, leukorrhea, painful coitus (dyspareunia), or dysuria. Treatment is surgical by hysterectomy and lymph node dissection; small microinvasive carcinomas may be treated with cone biopsy. Mortality is most strongly related to tumor stage and, in the case of neuroendocrine carcinomas, to cell type. Most patients with advanced disease die as a result of local invasion rather than distant metastasis. In particular, renal failure stemming from obstruction of the urinary bladder and ureters is a common cause of death.

13.2 Body of Uterus

13.2.1 Endometriosis

Endometriosis is defined as the presence of endometrial glands and stroma in a location which is not in the endometrium of the uterus. Sites most frequently involved are ovaries(80%), and other tissues and organs, in descending order of frequency, are uterine ligaments, rectovaginal septum, pelvic peritoneum, abdominal scar, navel, vagina, vulva and appendix. Adenomyosis refers to the endometrial glands and stroma presenting abnormally within the myometrium(2mm over the basal layer of the endometrium)(Figure 13–5).

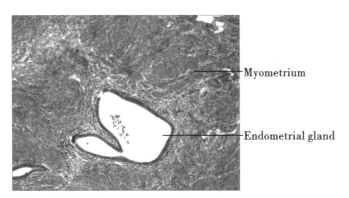

Figure 13–5   Adenomyosis(100×, hematoxylin and eosin stain). Endometrial glands and stroma presents within the myometrium

13.2.1.1 Pathophysiology

The pathogenesis of endometriosis is uncertain. Several theories are proposed to explain the origin of these dispersed lesions. The regurgitation theory proposed that the endometrium through the fallopian tube reflux to the abdominal organ during the menstrual period. The benign metastases theory suggests that endometrial tissue can implant in the surgical incision due to operation or spread to distant organ via blood vessels. The metaplastic theory holds that heterotopic endometrium arises directly from metaplasia of coelomic epithelium.

13.2.1.2 Morphology

Endometriotic bleed periodically is in response to intrinsic hormonal stimulation. The earliest lesions of endometriosis usually appear grossly as red-blue or yellow-brown nodules, with soft texture, like mulberry. When lesions are extensive, organizing hemorrhage causes fibrous adhesions with other surrounding organs. If the ovaries are involved, repeated hemorrhage enlarges lesions and may form large, blood-filled cysts that contain inspissated, chocolate-colored material("chocolate cysts").

The histologic diagnosis of endometriosis at all sites depends on finding two of the following three features within the lesions: endometrial glands, endometrial stroma, and hemosiderin pigment. Occasionally, healed foci may contain only fibrous tissue and hemosiderin-laden macrophages, which by themselves are not diagnostic.

13.2.1.3 Clinical Features

Symptoms of endometriosis depend on the distribution of the lesions. It commonly results in dysmenorrhea or menoxenia.

13.2.2 Endometrial Hyperplasia

Endometrial hyperplasia is hyperplasia of endometrial glands or stroma responding to an abnormal hormonal state of excess endogenous or exogenous estrogen. It occurs mostly in women of childbearing age and climacteric. With very similar in pathogeny and pathogenesis, endometrial hyperplasia, atypical hyperplasia and endometrial cancer are presented as a continuous process of evolution both in morphology and biology.

13.2.2.1 Morphology

Endometrial hyperplasia is divided into three types based on the cell morphology and the degree of proliferation and differentiation of the gland structure.

Simple hyperplasia: Simple hyperplasia is also called "mild hyperplasia" or "cystic hyperplasia". The morphological features(Figure 13-6) include thickening of the endometrium, increase of the glands number, and punctuated cysts. Lining epithelium is usually a single layer or a pseudo complex layer. The cells are columnar and have no heteromorphosis. The morphology and arrangement of the cells are similar to those of the endometrium in the proliferative stage. These lesions rarely progress to adenocarcinoma(approximately 1%).

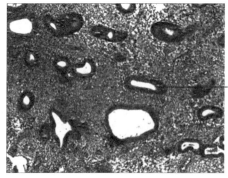

Stratified epithelial cells

Figure 13-6　Simple hyperplasia(200×, hematoxylin and eosin stain). It shows anovulatory or "disordered" endometrium containing dilated glands with multi-layer of the epithelial cells

Complex hyperplasia: Complex hyperplasia is also known as adenomatous hyperplasia. The glandular hyperplasia is obvious and crowded, and the gland structure was complex and irregular. The endometrial stroma was obviously reduced and there is no heterotypic cell (Figure 13-7).

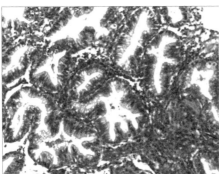

Closely packed glands

Figure 13-7 Complex hyperplasia(200×,hematoxylin and e-osin stain). It characterizes by nests of closely packed glands

Atypical hyperplasia: Atypical hyperplasia is composed of crowded aggregates of cytologically altered tubular or slightly branching glands. The proliferated glands are commonly back-to-back and often have complex outlines due to branching structures. Individual cells are rounded and lose the normal perpendicular orientation to the basement membrane. In addition, the glands display nuclear atypia and the nuclei have open chromatin and conspicuous nucleoli(Figure 13-8). The features of atypical hyperplasia have considerable overlaps with those of well-differentiated endometrioid adenocarcinoma, and accurate distinction from cancer may not be possible without hysterectomy. Approximately 1/3 of patients with atypical hyperplasia will develop adenocarcinoma.

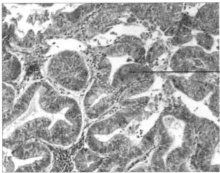

Epithelial cells with cellular atypia

Figure 13-8 Atypical hyperplasia(400×,hematoxylin and e-osin stain). It shows glandular crowing and cellular atypia

13.2.2.2 Clinical Features

The main clinical manifestations are irregular vaginal bleeding and menorrhagia, which are also called functional uterine bleeding.

13.2.3 Tumors of Uterus

13.2.3.1 Endometrial Adenocarcinoma

Endometrial adenocarcinoma is a malignant tumor derived from the epithelial cells of the endometrium. It generally appears in menopausal and postmenopausal women, between the ages of 55 and 65 years.

(1) Pathophysiology

Endometrioid adenocarcinoma accounts for 80% of cases of endometrial adenocarcinoma, which arise in association with estrogen excess. The endometrioid adenocarcinoma is designated endometrioid due to their histologic similarity to normal endometrial glands. Risk factors of this adenocarcinoma include obesity, diabetes, infertility, hypertension and smoke. Many of these risk factors result in increased estrogenic stimulation of the endometrium and are associated with endometrial hyperplasia. Microsatellite instability and mutation of the tumor suppressor gene PTEN are important events in stepwise development of endometrioid adenocarcinoma.

In addition, some endometrial adenocarcinomas appear to be irrelevant to the increase of estrogen and intimal hyperplasia, but on the basis of an inactive or atrophic endometrium. This type of endometrial adenocarcinoma, which arises in the setting of endometrial atrophy in older postmenopausal women, is much less common, accounting for roughly 15% of tumors. Some of these tumor tissues are similar to ovarian serous cystadenocarcinoma, which is called endometrial serous carcinoma. Immunohistochemistry often reveals high levels of p53 in this type, a finding that correlates with the presence of TP53 mutations. The prognosis of this type is also worse than that of estrogen related endometrial carcinoma.

(2) Morphology

Grossly, endometrial adenocarcinoma is divided into diffuse and localized type. Diffuse type is characterized by diffuse thickening of the endometrium, rough surface, gray-white, crisp, hemorrhage, necrosis or ulceration, and infiltrating the myometrium to varying degrees(Figure 13-9). The localized type is mostly located at the bottom or the corner of the uterus, often forms polyps or papillae on the uterine cavity. If the cancer tissue is small and superficial, it can be scraped out in the diagnostic curettage and the cancer tissue cannot be found in the excised uterus.

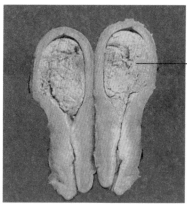

Endometrial
adenocarcinoma

Figure 13-9　Endometrial adenocarcinoma (Diffuse type). It presents as a fungating mass in the fundus of the uterus

On microscopic examination, there are three histologic grades of endometrial adenocarcinoma: well differentiated, moderately differentiated, and poorly differentiated, among which well differentiated accounts for the vast majority. In well differentiated endometrial adenocarcinoma, the glandular tubes are crowded, disorganized, the stroma reduced, and the "back-to-back" phenomenon is often found. It can also be seen that the cells have mild heterotypic structure that resemble hyperplasia of endometrial glands. The moderate differentiated endometrial adenocarcinoma shows irregular and disorder glands. The cancer tissue grows into the gland, forming a papillary or sieving structure, and cancer-foci can be seen. The cancer cells have obvious heteromorphosis, and the pathologic mitosis is often seen (Figure 13-10). The poorly differentiated adenocarcinoma: the differentiation of the cancer cells is poor, and the adenoid structure is rarely formed. The invasive lesions are composed of cells with marked cytological atypia including high nuclear-to-cytoplasmic ratio, atypical mitotic figures, hyperchromasia, and prominent nucleoli.

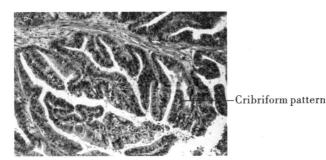

—Cribriform pattern

Figure 13-10   Endometrioid adenocarcinoma (200×, hematoxylin and eosin stain). It shows infiltrating myometrium and growing in a cribriform pattern

About 1/3 of endometrioid adenocarcinoma contain foci of squamous differentiation. Squamous elements may be histologically benign-appearing when they are associated with well differentiated adenocarcinomas. Less commonly, moderately or poorly differentiated endometrioid adenocarcinoma contains squamous elements that appear frankly malignant. Sometimes endometrioid adenocarcinoma is accompanied by metaplasia of benign squamous cell foci, called endometrioid adenocarcinoma with squamous cell metaplasia.

(3) Metastasis

Endometrial adenocarcinoma generally grows slowly, and can be confined to the uterine cavity for many years. It is easy to be detected due to irregular uterine bleeding. The prognosis of endometrial adenocarcinoma is relative better than other gynecological tumors. Metastasis occurs relatively late, in which the local infiltration and metastasis of lymph nodes are more common, and the metastasis of vascular stream is rarely.

Endometrial adenocarcinoma frequently directly spreads to the ovaries and fallopian tubes when the cancer is located in the upper part of the uterus, and the cervix when the cancer is in the lower part of the uterus. Usually, this cancer first spreads into the myometrium and the serosa, and then into other reproductive and pelvic structures. When the lymphatic system is involved, the pelvic and para-aortic nodes are usually first to be involved. More distant metastases are via blood and often occur in the lungs, as well as the liver, and bone.

(4) Clinical features

Although it may be asymptomatic for a period of time, endometrial adenocarcinoma usually manifests with excessive leucorrhea and irregular bleeding, often in postmenopausal women. With progression, the uterus enlarges and may become affixed to surrounding structures as the cancer infiltrates surrounding tissues. These tumors usually are slow to metastasize, but if left untreated, eventually disseminate to regional nodes and more distant sites. Fortunately, postmenopausal bleeding often leads to early detection, and cures are possible in most patients. The diagnosis of endometrial adenocarcinoma must be established by histologic examination of tissue obtained by biopsy or curettage. With therapy, the 5-year survival rate for early-stage tumor is 90%, but survival drops precipitously in higher-stage cacinomas. As would be anticipated, the prognosis depends heavily on the clinical stage as well as histologic grade and subtype.

13.2.3.2   Leiomyomas

Leiomyomas are the most common benign tumor in females. Including minute tumors, leiomyomas occur in 75% of women over age 30. They are rare before age 20, and most regress after menopause. Estrogens and possibly oral contraceptives stimulate their growth.

(1) Morphology

Grossly, leiomyomas are sharply circumscribed, discrete, round, firm, gray-white tumors varying in size from small, barely visible nodules to massive tumors that fill the pelvis. Their cut surface bulges, and borders are smooth and distinct from neighboring myometrium. Most leiomyomas are intramural, but some are submucosal, subserosal pedunculated. Larger neoplasms may develop foci of ischemic necrosis with areas of hemorrhage and cystic softening, and after menopause they may become densely collagenous and even calcified. Whatever their size, the characteristic whorled pattern of smooth muscle bundles on cut section usually makes these lesions readily identifiable (Figure 13-11).

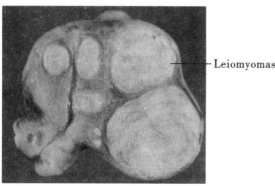

—Leiomyomas

Figure 13-11　**Leiomyomas**

The uterus is opened to reveal multiple tumors in submucosal (bulging into the endometrial cavity), intramural, and subserosal locations that display a firm white appearance on sectioning

On microscopic examination, leiomyomas are typically composed of bundles of smooth muscle cells that resemble the uninvolved myometrium. Cytoplasm is abundant, eosinophilic and fibrillar. Foci of fibrosis, calcification, ischemic necrosis, cystic degeneraion, and hemorrhage may be present.

Leiomyomas are usually benign. Benign leiomyomas rarely transform into sarcomas, and the presence of multiple lesions does not increase the risk of harboringa malignancy.

(2) Clinical Features

Leiomyomas of the uterus may be entirely asymptomatic and be discovered only on routine pelvic or post mortem examination. Many intramural leiomyomas are symptomatic because of their sheer bulk, and large ones may interfere with bowel or bladder function or cause dystocia in labor. Moreover, leiomyomas can lead to spontaneous abortion, abnormal fetal exposure, and postmenopausal bleeding.

Recurrence after removal is common with leiomyosarcomas, and many metastasize, typically to the lungs, yielding a 5-year survial rate of about 40%.

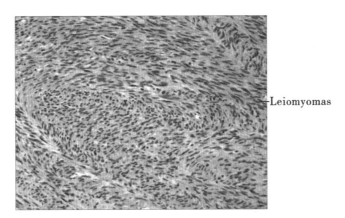

Figure 13-12　Leiomyomas (40×, hematoxylin and eosin stain). Microscopic appearance of leiomyoma reveals well-differentiated, regular, and spindle-shaped of normal-looking smooth muscle cells

13.3　Gestational Trophoblastic Diseases

The major disorders of gestational trophoblastic diseases (GTD) are hydatidiform mole (complete and partial), invasive mole, choriocarcinoma, and placental site trophoblastic tumor (PSTT). These demonstrate a range of aggressiveness from benign hydatidiform moles to high malignant choriocarcinomas. The common feature of these diseases is the abnormal proliferation of trophoblastic cells and most of them are related to pregnancy. All produce human chorionic gonadotropin (HCG), which can be detected in the blood and urine at levels considerably higher than those found during normal pregnancy and it can be used as an auxiliary index for clinical diagnosis, follow-up observation and evaluation of curative effect.

13.3.1　Hydatidiform Mole

Hydatidiform mole is a benign lesion of placental villi, with characteristics of high edema of villous stroma and different degrees of trophoblast cells hyperplasia. This disease occurs at any age during the period of childbearing, which may be related to ovarian insufficiency or recession related. There are two distinctive subtypes of hydatidiform moles: complete and partial.

13.3.1.1　Pathophysiology

The etiology and pathogenesis of hydatidiform mole have not been fully elucidated. In recent years, the study of hydatidiform chromosomes has shown that chromosomal abnormalities may play a leading role.

Complete hydatidiform moles are not compatible with embryogenesis and never contain fetal parts. It results from fertilization of an egg that has lost its female chromosomes, and as a result the genetic material is completely paternally derives. All of the chorionic villi are abnormal, and the chorionic epithelial cells are diploid (46, XX or, uncommonly 46, XY). Eighty percent have 46, XX karyotype stemming from the duplication of the genetic material of one sperm (a phenomenon called androgenesis). The remaining 10% result from the fertilization of an empty egg by two sperm; these may have 46, XX or 46, XY karyotype. In complete moles, the embryo dies very early in development and therefore is usually not identified.

Partial hydatidiform moles are compatible with early embryo formation and therefore may contain fetal parts, have some normal chorionic villi, and is almost always triploid(e. g. ,69 ,XXY) or occasionally tetraploid(92 ,XXXY).

Both types result from abnormal fertilization. In a complete mole the entire genetic content is supplied by two spermatozoa(or a diploid sperm), yielding diploid cells containing only paternal chromosomes, whereas in a partial mole, a normal egg is fertilized by two spermatozoa(or a diploid sperm), leading to a triploid karyotype with a preponderance of paternal genes.

13.3.1.2 Morphology

The uterus may be of normal size in early moles, but in more advanced cases the uterine cavity is expanded. The classic appearance of hydatidiform moles is that of a delicate, friable mass of thin-walled, translucent, cystic, grapelike structures consisting of swollen edematous(hydropic) villi(Figure 13 – 13). Fetal parts are rarely seen in complete moles but are common in partial moles.

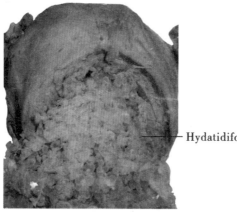

Figure 13 – 13   Hydatidiform mole. The uterus consists of numerous swollen(hydropic) villi

Microscopically, hydatidiform moles have three characteristics. ①Because of the loose, myxomatous, edematous stroma, the chorinic villi are enlarged and hydropic swelling and scalloped in shape with central cavitation. ②The blood vessels in the villous stroma disappeare, or a small amount of nonfunctional capillaries and no red blood cells are found. ③The chorionic epithelium almost always shows some degree of proliferation of both the cytotrophoblasts and syncytiotrophoblasts, which lose the normal order, display a multilayer or patchy aggregation, and mild atypia. Proliferation of trophoblast is the most important characteristic of hydatidiform mole.

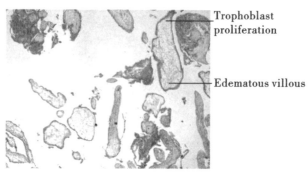

Figure 13 – 14   Complete hydatidiform mole(100×, hematoxylin and eosin stain). In this microscopic image, marked edematous villous enlargement, edema, and circumferential trophoblast proliferation are evident

13.3.1.3   Clinical Features

Most of the patients have symptoms from 11 to 25 weeks of pregnancy. Most women with partial and early complete moles present with spontaneous miscarriage or undergo curettage because of ultrasound finding of abnormal villous enlargement. Due to placental villus edema, the volume of uterine increased significantly, and exceeds that in the normal pregnancy. Because of the early embryonic death, although more than 5 months of pregnancy there is neither fetal heart, nor fetal movement.

In complete moles, human chorionic gonadotropin (HCG) levels greatly exceed those of a normal pregnancy of similar gestational age. In addition, the rate at which HCG levels rise over time in molar pregnancies exceeds those seen with normal single or even multiple pregnancies. Most moles can be successfully removed by curettage. The patients are subsequently monitored for 6 months to a year to ensure that HCG levels decrease to non-pregnant levels. Because the trophoblast cells invade the blood vessels, the uterus has repeatedly irregular bleeding, and occasionally the grapes-like substance can be seen in the outflow.

The majority of the hydatidiform mole can be cured after the complete curettage. Continuous elevation of HCG may be indicative of persistent or invasive mole, which develops in up to 10% of molar pregnancies and is seen more frequently with complete moles. In addition, 2% of complete moles give rise to subsequent choriocarcinoma. Partial moles have an increased risk of persistent molar disease, but are not associated with choriocarcinoma.

13.3.2   Invasive Mole

Invasive mole, also called malignant mole, is defined as a mole that penetrates or even perforates the uterine wall and is a borderline tumor between hydatidiform mole and choriocarcinoma. Invasive moles are complete moles that are more invasive locally but do not have the aggressive metastatic potential of a choriocarcinoma.

13.3.2.1   Morphology

There is invasion of the myometrium by hydropic chorionic villi, which penetrate the uterine wall deeply, possibly causing rupture and sometimes life-threatening hemorrhage. Hydropic villi may embolize to distant sites, such as lungs and brains, but do not grow in these organs as true metastases, and even without chemotherapy they eventually regress. On microscopic examination, the epithelium of the villi shows atypical changes, accompanied by proliferation of both cytotrophoblasts and syncytiotrophoblasts.

13.3.2.2   Clinical Features

The tumor is manifested clinically by vaginal bleeding and irregular uterine enlargement. It is always associated with a persistently elevated serum HCG. The tumor responds well to chemotherapy but may result in uterine rupture and necessitate hysterectomy.

13.3.3   Choriocarcinoma

This very aggressive malignant tumor arises either from gestational chorionic epithelium or, less frequently, from totipotential cells within the gonads or elsewhere. Women under age 20 and over age 40 are at high risk. 50% of choriocarcinomas arise in complete hydatidiform moles, 25% in previous abortions, 22% follow normal pregnancies, with the remainder occurring in ectopic pregnancies. Those instances mentioned above may suggest that choriocarcinoma origin from an abnormal ovum rather than from retained chorionic epithelium.

13.3.3.1   Morphology

Grossly, choriocarcinoma is a soft, fleshy, yellow-white tumor that usually has large pale areas of necrosis and extensive hemorrhage(Figure 13–15). Sometimes the necrosis is so extensive that little viable tumor remains. Indeed, the primary lesion may "self-destruct" and only the metastases tell the story. Very early, the tumor insinuates itself into the myometrium and into vessels.

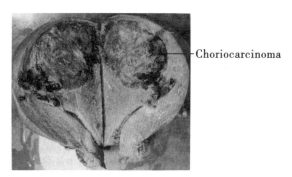

Figure 13–15　Choriocarcinoma. It presents as a bulky hemorrhagic mass invading the uterine wall

Histologically, it does not produce chorionic villi and consists entirely of proliferating syncytiotropho-blasts and cytotrophoblasts(Figure 13–16). In contrast to the case with hydatidiform moles and invasive moles, chorionic villi are not formed; instead, the tumor is purely epithelial, composed of anaplastic cuboidal cytotrophoblast and syncytiotrophoblast.

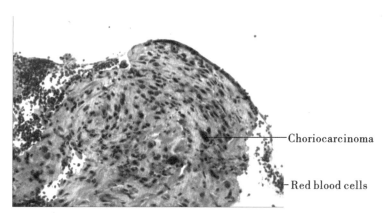

Figure 13 – 16　Choriocarcinoma (200 ×, hematoxylin and eosin stain). Photomicrograph illustrates both neoplastic cytotrophoblast and syncytiotrophoblast

13.3.3.2　Metastasis

Choriocarcinoma easily invades and destroies blood vessels, therefore, in addition to local infiltration, metastasis through vascular stream is the most common way. Metastatic organs which are most common are the lung and vagina wall, in descending order of frequency, are the brain, liver, spleen, kidney and intestine. In a few cases, the metastases can be subsided after primary resection.

13.3.3.3　Clinical Features

Uterine choriocarcinoma usually manifests as irregular vaginal spotting of a bloody, brown fluid. This discharge may appear in the course of an apparently normal pregnancy, after a miscarriage, or after curettage. By the time most choriocarcinomas are discovered, there is usually widespread dissemination via the blood, most often to the lungs, vagina, brain, liver and kidneys. Lymphatic invasion is uncommon.

The treatment of gestational choriocarcinoma depends on the stage of the tumor and usually consists of evacuation of the contents of the uterus and chemotherapy. Almost 100% of affected patients can be cured, even those with metastases at distant sites such as the lungs. Many of the cured patients have had normal subsequent pregnancies and deliveries.

13.3.4   Placental Site Trophoblastic Tumor

Placental site trophoblastic tumors (PSTT) comprise less than 2% of gestational trophoblastic neoplasm. These tumors are derived from the placental site or intermediate trophoblast. These uncommon diploid tumors, often 46 XX in karyotype, typically arise a few months after pregnancy (half of the cases). Besides normal pregnancy, it may also follow a spontaneous abortion or hydatidiform mole.

13.3.4.1   Morphology

In normal pregnancy, extavillous trophoblasts are found in nonvillous sites such as the implantation site, in islands of cells within the placental parenchyma, and in the placental membranes. Normal extravillous trophoblasts are polygonal mononuclear cells that have abundant cytoplasm and produce human placental lactogen. Histologically, PSTT is composed of malignant trophoblastic cells diffusely infiltrating the endomyometrium.

13.3.4.2   Clinical Features

An indolent clinical course is typical, with a generally favorable outcome if the tumor is confined to the endomyometrium. PSTT presents as a uterine mass, accompanies by either abnormal uterine bleeding or amenorrhea. Because intermediate trophoblasts do not produce HCG in large amounts, HCG concentrations are only slightly elevated. Of note, PSTTs are not as sensitive to chemotherapy as other trophoblastic tumors, and the prognosis is poor when spread has occurred beyond the uterus. Patients with localized disease have an excellent prognosis, but about 10% to 15% of women die of disseminated disease.

13.4   Tumors of the Ovary

Tumors of the ovary represent about 30% of all cancers of the female genital system. Age-adjusted incidence rates are highest in the economically advanced countries where they are almost as common as cancers of the corpus uteri and invasive cancer of the cervix. Carcinomas of surface epithelial-stromal origin account for 90% of these cancers in North America and Western Europe. In some Asian countries, including Japan, germ cell tumours account for a significant proportion (20%) of ovarian malignancies. High parity and the use of oral contraceptives are consistently associated with a reduced risk of developing surface epithelial-stromal tumours while long-term estrogen replacement therapy appears to increase the risk in postmenopausal women.

13.4.1   Surface Epithelial-stromal Tumors

13.4.1.1   Definition

Surface epithelial-stromal tumors are the most common neoplasms of the ovary. They originate from the ovarian surface epithelium or its derivatives and occur in women of reproductive age and beyond. They are histologically composed of one or more distinctive types of epithelium, admixed with a variable amount of stroma. Their biological behaviour varies with histological type.

13.4.1.2 Epidemiology

The age-adjusted incidence rates vary from less than 2 new cases per 100,000 women in Southeast Asia and Africa to over 15 cases in Northern and Eastern Europe. The economically advanced countries of North America, Europe, Australia, New Zealand and temperate South America show the highest rates. In the United States more women die from ovarian cancer today than from all other pelvic gynaecological cancer sites combined. Incidence rates have been either stable or have shown slow increase in most western countries, whereas they have risen steadily in parts of Eastern Asia.

13.4.1.3 Etiology

Two factors consistently associated with a reduced risk of the disease are high parity and the use of oral contraceptives. Three recent studies have shown an increased risk of ovarian cancer in postmenopausal women treated with high-dose estrogen replacement therapy for 10 years or greater. Very little is known of the aetiology of non-familial cases. The protective effects of pregnancies and of oral contraception suggest a direct role for ovulation in causing the disease, but no convincing mechanism linking the risk factors with malignant transformation has been proposed. Several dietary factors have been related to ovarian cancer. There is emerging evidence that the Western lifestyle, in particular, obesity, is associated with an increased risk.

13.4.1.4 Clinical Features

(1) Signs and Symptoms

Women with ovarian cancer have a poor prognosis. The mean 5-year survival rate in Europe is 32%. This unfavorable outcome is largely ascribed to a lack of early warning symptoms and a lack of diagnostic tests that allow early detection. As a result, approximately 70% of patients present when this cancer is in an advanced stage, i. e. it has metastasized to the upper abdomen or beyond the abdominal cavity. It is now recognized that the overwhelming majority of women diagnosed with ovarian cancer actually have symptoms, but they are subtle and easily confused with those of various benign entities, particularly those related to the gastrointestinal tract. Physical signs associated with early stage ovarian cancer may be limited to palpation by pelvic examination of a mobile, but somewhat irregular, pelvic mass(stage Ⅰ). As the disease spreads into the pelvic cavity, nodules may be found in the cul-de-sac, particularly on bimanual rectovaginal examination(stage Ⅱ). Ascites may occur even when the malignancy is limited to one or both ovaries(stage IC). As the disease involves the upper abdomen, ascites may be evident. A physical examination of the abdomen may demonstrate flank bulging and fluid waves associated with the ascites. Metastatic disease is commonly found in the omentum, such that the latter may be readily identified in the presence of advanced stage(stage Ⅲ) ovarian cancer as a ballottable or palpable mass in the mid-abdomen, usually superior to the umbilicus and above the palpable pelvic mass. Finally, the disease may spread through lymphatics to either the inguinal or left supraclavicular lymph nodes, which may be readily palpable. It may advance into the pleural cavity as a malignant effusion, usually on the right side or bilateral, in which the lung bases exhibit dullness to percussion and decreased breath sounds and egophony with auscultation(stage Ⅳ). Advanced intra-abdominal ovarian carcinomatosis may also present with signs of intestinal obstruction including nausea, vomiting and abdominal pain.

(2) Imaging

Due to its wide availability, ultrasound(US) is the imaging method of choice to assess an ovarian lesion and to determine the presence of solid and cystic elements. The distinction between benign, borderline and malignant tumours is generally not possible by US, either alone or in combination with magnetic resonance imaging(MRI)or computed tomography(CT). None of these methods has a clearly established role in preoperative tumour staging. Surgical exploration remains the standard approach for staging.

(3)Tumor Spread and Staging

About 70% –75% of patients with ovarian cancer have tumour spread beyond the pelvis at the time of diagnosis. Ovarian cancers spread mainly by local extension, by intra-abdominal dissemination and by lymphatic dissemination, but rarely also through the blood stream. The International Federation of Gynecology and Obstetrics(FIGO)Committee on Gynecologic Oncology is responsible for the staging system that is used internationally today. The p TNM-system is based on the postoperative pathological staging for histological control and confirmation of the disease.

(4)Histogenesis

The likely origin of ovarian surface epithelial-stromal tumours is the mesothelial surface lining of the ovaries and/or invaginations of this lining into the superficial ovarian cortex that form inclusion cysts.

(5)Genetic Susceptibility

Familial clustering Numerous epidemiological investigations of ovarian cancer have attempted to quantify the risks associated with a positive family history. Whereas ovarian cancer has not been as extensively studied as breast cancer, several studies point to familial clustering. The relative risk of ovarian cancer for first degree relatives varies from 13. 6 to 25. 5, the latter if both mother and sister are affected.

BRCA1/2 A number of specific genes have been identified as playing a role. The most important of these, BRCA1 and BRCA2, are discussed in chapter 8. In contrast to breast cancer in which only a minority of the familial clustering could be explained by known major susceptibility loci such as BRCA1 and BRCA2, it is likely that the majority of the familial risk of ovarian cancer is explained by BRCA1 and to a lesser extent BRCA2, MLH1 and MSH2. Using statistical modelling and the results from BRCA1 and BRCA2 mutation testing in 112 families with at least two cases of ovarian cancer(allowing for insensitivity of the mutation detection assay), BRCA1 and BRCA2 accounted for nearly all of the non-chance familial aggregation.

HNPCC Ovarian cancer is a minor feature of the hereditary nonpolyposis colon cancer syndrome caused by mutations in genes associated with DNA base mismatch repair, the most frequent of which are MLH1 and MSH2.

13.4.2   Association with Endometrial Cancer

Several studies provide evidence of associations between ovarian and other cancers, particularly endometrial cancer. The relative risk of developing endometrial cancer is about 13. 6 among mothers and sisters of ovarian cancer cases, although in both studies the risk fell just short of statistical significance.

13.5   Prostatic Diseases

The prostate is a pear-shaped glandular organ that weighs up to 20g in the normal adult male and that depends for its differentiation and subsequent growth on androgenic hormones synthesized in the testis. It can be divided into peripheral, central, transitional, and periurethral gland regions, the most important of which are the peripheral and transition zones(Figure 13 –17). The types of proliferative lesions are different in each region. The periurethral regions are the exclusive sites of origin of benign prostatic hyperplasia, whereas the peripheral zone is most susceptible to prostatitis and carcinoma. The normal prostate glands has two cell layers, a flat basal cell layer and an overlying columnar secretory cell layer. Surrounding prostatic stroma contains a mixture of smooth muscle and fibrous tissue.

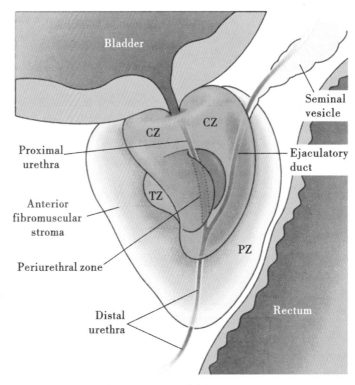

Figure 13-17 **Adult prostate**

The normal prostate contains several distinct regions, including a central zone(CZ), a peripheral zone(PZ), a transitional zone(TZ), and a periurethral zone. Most carcinomas arise from the peripheral glands of the organ and often are palpable during digital examination of the rectum. Nodular hyperplasia, by contrast, arises from more centrally situated glands and is more likely than carcinoma to produce urinary obstruction early in its course

13.5.1 Benign Prostatic Hyperplasia(Nodular Hyperplasia)

Benign prostatic hyperplasia(BPH) is an extremely common abnormality that, when extensive, results in varying degrees of urinary obstruction, sometimes requiring surgical intervention. The term nodular hyperplasia, as proposed by Moore in his classic study, is a more exact designation. The disease is characterized by a nodular enlargement of the gland caused by hyperplasia of both glandular and stromal components. It results in an increase in the weight of the organ well beyond the 20 g regarded as normal for adult individuals. The clinical incidence of this disease is only 8% during the fourth decade, but it reaches 50% in the fifth decade and 75% in the eighth decade. It is present in a significant number of men by the age of 40, and its frequency rises progressively with age. No predisposing or protecting factors(other than castration) have been identified. It has been established that excessive androgen-dependent growth of stromal and glandular elements has a central role. BPH does not occur in males castrated before the onset of puberty or in men with genetic diseases that block androgen activity. Dihydrotestosterone(DHT), the ultimate mediator of prostatic growth, is synthesized in the prostate from circulating testosterone by the action of the enzyme 5α-reductase, type 2. DHT binds to nuclear androgen receptors, which regulate the expression of genes that support the growth and survival of prostatic epithelium and stromal cells. Although testosterone can also bind to androgen receptors and stimulate growth, DHT is 10 times more potent. Clinical symptoms of lower urinary tract obstruction caused by prostatic enlargement may also be exacerbated by contraction of prostatic smooth muscle mediated by α1-adrenergic receptors.

13.5.1.1　Morphology

BPH virtually always occurs in the inner, transitional zone of the prostate. At autopsy the average weight of a prostate gland affected by nodular hyperplasia is 33 g ± 16 g. Specimens obtained surgically weigh 100 g on average, but on rare occasions weights of over 800 g have been recorded. Grossly, variously sized nodules with a gray to yellow color and a granular appearance are seen projecting above the cut surface(Figure 13-18).

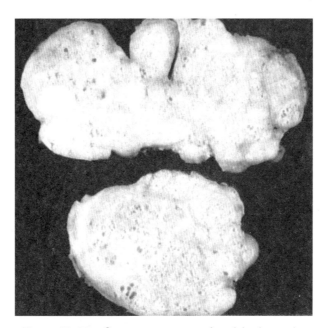

Figure 13-18　Gross appearance of nodular hyperplasia in material obtained from uprapubic prostatectomy. Note the multinodular appearance and the admixture of solid and microcystic areas

The nodules may appear solid or contain cystic spaces, the latter corresponding to dilated glandular elements. The urethra is usually compressed by the hyperplastic nodules, often to a narrow slit. In some cases, hyperplastic glandular and stromal elements lying just under the epithelium of the proximal prostatic urethra may project into the bladder lumen as a pedunculated mass, producing a ball-valve type of urethral obstruction. In only about 5% will a focal lesion of nodular hyperplasia be found in the peripheral zone of the organ.

Microscopically, the earliest change is a stromal proliferation bout small sinusoidal spaces in the periurethral regions and, to a lesser degree, in the periductal and intralobular areas(Figure 13-19). The hyperplastic nodules are composed of variable proportions of proliferating glandular elements and fibromuscular stroma. These proportions are somewhat different in patients with symptomatic and those with asymptomatic nodular hyperplasia. The glands are dilated or even cystic and often contain in spissated, proteinaceous secretory material known as corpora amylacea, which is sometimes calcified. The epithelium ranges from flat to columnar, sometimes facing each other in the same gland('functional polarization'); the cytoplasm is pale, and the nuclei are regular and centrally located(Figure 13-20). The nucleoli are inconspicuous. Papillary infoldings are common. A continuous basal cell layer is seen immediately above a well-developed basement membrane. Small clusters of lymphocytes are common in the interstitium and around the ducts. They are probably the result rather than the cause of the hyperplasia; a diagnosis of chronic prostatitis is not warranted because of their mere presence.

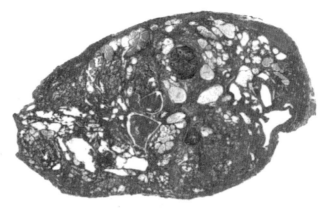

Figure 13 – 19   Whole mount of nodular hyperplasia of prostate, showing nodular configuration and cystic changes

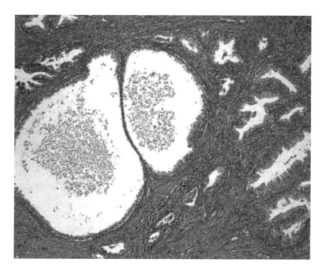

Figure 13 – 20   Nodular hyperplasia of prostate, with cystic dilation of the glands. Characteristically, the epithelium is tall on one side and flattened on the other

13.5.1.2 Clinical Features

Clinical manifestations of prostatic hyperplasia occur in only about 10% of men with pathologic evidence of BPH. Because BPH preferentially involves the inner portions of the prostate, the most common manifestations are related to lower urinary tract obstruction, often in the form of difficulty in starting the stream of urine(hesitancy)and intermittent interruption of the urinary stream while voiding. These symptoms frequently are accompanied by urinary urgency, frequency, and nocturia, all indicative of bladder irritation. Similar symptoms also may arise from urethral stricture or as a consequence of impaired bladder detrusor muscle contractility in both men and women. The presence of residual urine in the bladder due to chronic obstruction increases the risk of urinary tract infections. In some affected men, BPH leads to complete urinary obstruction, with resultant painful distention of the bladder and, in the absence of appropriate treatment, hydronephrosis.

The conventional treatment for nodular hyperplasia is surgical. The involved area may be excised by various techniques, such as transurethral resection (TUR), suprapubic prostatectomy, and laser enucleation. It should be realized that these procedures remove only the newly formed nodules. The compressed peripheral portions of the gland remain; these expand by stromal growth to surround the prostatic urethra and may be the source of recurrent hyperplasia. Not surprisingly, the chance of a patient undergoing a second operation for this disorder is substantially higher after a TUR than an open prostatectomy. Adenocarcinoma can also develop in the residual gland many years after surgery. Medical alternatives to surgery include various medications aimed at blocking the actions of androgens by preventing their secretion or their conversion to their tissue active form or at relaxing the stromal muscle cells. Among these, the drug most widely used is finasteride, which works by inhibiting $5-\alpha$ reductase, the enzyme that converts testosterone to the potent androgen dihydrotestosterone. The morphologic changes induced by this compound in the prostate are relatively minor and nonspecific. They include focal atrophy, increase in the stromal-epithelial ratio, squamous metaplasia, and transitional metaplasia.

13.5.2 Prostatitis

Prostatitis is divided into four categories: ①acute bacterial prostatitis (2% to 5% of cases), caused by the same organisms associated with other acute urinary tract infections; ②*chronic bacterial prostatitis* (2% to 5% of cases), also caused by common uropathogens; ③*chronic nonbacterial prostatitis*, or *chronic pelvic pain syndrome* (90% to 95% of cases), in which no uropathogen is identified despite the presence of local symptoms; ④*asymptomatic inflammatory prostatitis* (incidence unknown), associated with incidental identification of leukocytes in prostatic secretions without uropathogens. The prostate is usually not biopsied in men with symptoms of acute or chronic prostatitis, since the findings are usually non-specific and are not helpful in managing patients. The exception is in patients with granulomatous prostatitis, in which a specific etiology may be established. In the United States, the most common cause is instillation of bacilli Calmette-Guérin (BCG) within the bladder for treatment of superficial bladder cancer. BCG is an attenuated tuberculosis strain that produces a histologic picture in the prostate indistinguishable from tuberculosis. Disseminated prostatic tuberculosis is rare in the Western world. Fungal granulomatous prostatitis is typically seen only in immunocompromised hosts. Nonspecific granulomatous prostatitis is relatively common and represents are action to secretions from ruptured prostatic ducts and acini. Postsurgical prostatic granulomas also may be seen.

Clinical Features

Clinically, acute bacterial prostatitis is associated with fever, chills, and dysuria; it may be complicated by sepsis. On rectal examination, the prostate is exquisitely tender and boggy. Chronic bacterial prostatitis usually is associated with recurrent urinary tract infections bracketed by asymptomatic periods. Presenting manifestations may include low back pain, dysuria, and perineal and suprapubic discomfort. Both acute and chronic bacterial prostatitis are treated with antibiotics. The diagnosis of chronic nonbacterial prostatitis (chronic pelvic pain syndrome) is difficult. It requires completion of the NIH Chronic Prostatitis Symptom Index survey by the patient, digital rectal examination, urinalysis, and sequential collection of urine and prostatic fluid specimens, before, during, and after prostatic massage. This technique of collecting samples prevents contamination from the bladder and urethra and is issued to document prostatic inflammation (by presence of leukocytes) in the absence of infection. There are no proven therapies for chronic pelvic pain syndrome.

13.5.3 Infarct

Infarct of the prostate occurs predominantly in large prostates affected by nodular hyperplasia. Its reported incidence is probably related to the thoroughness of the microscopic examination. It has been traditionally reported in TUR specimens, but it can also be recognized in prostatic needle biopsies. The size and number of the infarcts are directly related to the degree of prostatic hyperplasia. True infarcts occurring on a vascular basis should be distinguished from necrotic changes involving a gland or group of glands but sparing the stroma, a change sometimes seen in nodular hyperplasia.

The mechanism of infarct is unknown but may be related to the presence of prostatic infection or trauma resulting from an indwelling catheter, cystitis, or prostatitis, all of which may result in thrombosis of the intraprostatic portion of the urethral arteries.

Grossly, prostatic infarcts vary in size from a few millimeters up to 5 cm. They are speckled, grayish yellow, and often contain streaks of blood. The peripheral margins are usually sharp and hemorrhagic and may impinge on the urethra (Figure 13–21). Microscopically, the infarcts are of anemic type, with sharply outlined areas of coagulative necrosis involving glands and stroma. Prominent squamous metaplasia may develop in the ducts at the periphery of the infarct, a change that should not be confused with squamous cell carcinoma (Figure 13–22). This metaplastic change is confined to the expanded ducts, keratinizes only rarely, and does not extend to the surrounding prostatic tissue. It should be remembered that true squamous cell carcinomas of the prostate are exceptionally rare.

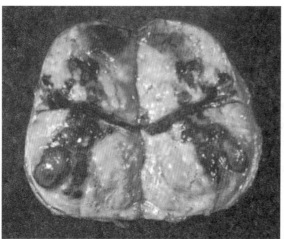 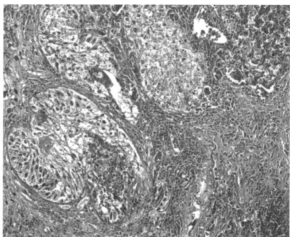

Figure 13–21　**Gross appearance of infarct of prostate. The lesion has a bright red color and bulges on the cut surface. Nodular hyperplasia is also present**

Figure 13–22　**Prominent metaplastic changes at the edge of a prostatic infarct. These are sometimes overdiagnosed as carcinoma**

Most prostatic infarcts are clinically silent. Occasionally, they cause acute urinary retention because of the accompanying edema. Since they are often adjacent to the urethra, gross hematuria can also occur. Diffuse oozing of blood from the overlying mucosa maybe seen cystoscopically.

13.5.4　Calculi

Prostatic calculi are seen in about 7% of prostates with nodular hyperplasia. They should be distinguished from those found in the prostatic urethra, which may have their origin in the bladder, ureter, or renal pelvis.

The corpora amylacea seen in glands with nodular hyperplasia may act as the nucleus for stone formation as a result of improper drainage, infection of the acini, and calcium deposition. Blood clots, epithelial detritus, and bacteria are also present in the stone nucleus. The main inorganic elements are phosphated salts(calcium,magnesium,amino magnesium,potassium),calcium carbonate,and calcium oxalate.

Because of their extreme hardness,large prostatic calculi may be erroneously diagnosed as carcinoma on palpation. They are radiopaque and easily detectable in plain X-rays. They are not associated with an increased risk for the development of prostatic carcinoma. If they are extremely large and numerous,a prostatectomy may be required.

13.5.5   Carcinoma of the Prostate

Adenocarcinoma of the prostate occurs mainly in men older than 50 years of age. It is the most common internal malignancy among men,accounting for 25% of cancer in men in the United States in 2009 and is responsible for 10% of cancer deaths in this population. Prostate cancer is the leading cause of new cancer in men and is second only to lung cancer as a leading cause of cancer-related deaths in men. Rates among black males are one and a half those of white males. The age-adjusted incidence is on the increase in most countries. Hormonal factors play a role in the development of prostatic carcinoma,a fact that has been dramatically highlighted. The disease does not occur in eunuchs castrated before puberty,and its incidence is low in patients with hyperestrogenism resulting from liver cirrhosis. It has been estimated that 5%–10% of prostatic carcinomas have a genetic link. If a man's brother or father had prostatic carcinoma,his own risk of developing the disease is two to three times greater than average. There is no demonstrable correlation with diet,venereal disease,sexual habits,smoking, or occupational exposure. There is no convincing evidence that patients with nodular hyperplasia(or those who have had a transurethral resection for it)are at an increased risk for the development of prostatic carcinoma,although the two conditions often coexist. Conversely,there is agreement as to the fact that high-grade prostatic intraepithelial neoplasia(PIN)is a well-documented precursor of prostatic adenocarcinoma.

Almost 75% of the men diagnosed with prostatic cancer are aged 65 or older,but the tumors can be seen in younger adults and even in children and adolescents. Their frequency increases with age,a fact well substantiated by careful observations at autopsy. The frequency with which incidental carcinoma is found at post mortem examination varies between 15% and 70% and is directly related to the age of the patient and the thoroughness of the sampling. Similar figures have been obtained from the examination of cystoprostatectomy specimens performed for bladder carcinoma:in one such series,incidental prostatic adenocarcinoma was found in 42% of the specimens.

13.5.5.1   Pathogenesis

Clinical and experimental observations suggest that androgens,heredity,environmental factors,and acquired somatic mutations have roles in the pathogenesis of prostate cancer.

1)Androgens are of central importance. Cancer of the prostate does not develop in males castrated before puberty,indicating that androgens somehow provide the "soil",the cellular context,within which prostate cancer develops. This dependence on androgens extends to established cancers,which often regress for a time in response to surgical or chemical castration. Notably,tumors resistant to anti-androgen therapy often acquire mutations that permit androgen receptors to activate the expression of their target genes even in the absence of the hormones. Thus,tumors that recur in the face of anti-androgen therapies still depend on gene products regulated by androgen receptors for their growth and survival. However,while prostate cancer,like normal prostate,is dependent on androgens for its survival,there is no evidence that androgens initiate carcinogenesis.

2)Heredity also contributes,as there is an increased risk among first-degree relatives of patients with prostate cancer. Incidence of prostatic cancer is uncommon in Asians and highest among blacks and is also high in Scandinavian countries. Genome-wide association studies have identified a number of genetic variants that are associated with increased risk, including a variant near the MYC oncogene on chromosome 8q24 that appears to account for some of the increased incidence of prostate cancer in males of African descent. Similarly, in white American men, the development of prostate cancer has been linked to a susceptibility locus on chromosome 1q24–q25.

3) Environment also plays a role, as evidenced by the fact that in Japanese immigrants to the United States the incidence of the disease rises(although not to the level seen in native-born Americans). Also, as the diet in Asia becomes more westernized, the incidence of clinical prostate cancer in this region of the world appears to be increasing. However, the relationship between specific dietary components and prostate cancer risk is unclear.

4) Acquired somatic mutations, as in other cancers, are the actual drivers of cellular transformation. One important class of somatic mutations is gene rearrangements that create fusion genes consisting of the androgen-regulated promoter of the TMPRSS2 gene and the coding sequence of ETS family transcription factors(the most common being ERG). TMPRSS2–ETS fusion genes occur in approximately 40% to 50% of prostate cancers; it is possible that unregulated increased expression of ETS transcription factors interfere with prostatic epithelial cell differentiation. Other mutations commonly lead to activation of the oncogenic PI3K/AKT signaling pathway; of these, the most common are mutations that inactivate the tumor suppressor gene PTEN, which acts as a brake on PI3K activity.

13.5.5.2　Morphology

Most carcinomas detected clinically are not visible grossly. More advanced lesions appear as firm, gray-white lesions with ill-defined margins that infiltrate the adjacent gland(Figure 13–23).

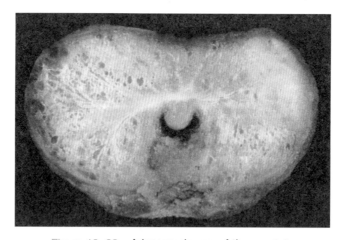

Figure 13–23　**Adenocarcinoma of the prostate**

Carcinomatous tissue is seen on the posterior aspect(lower left). Note the solid whiter tissue of cancer, in contrast with the spongy appearance of the benign peripheral zone on the contralateral side

On histologic examination, most lesions are moderately differentiated adenocarcinomas that produce well-defined glands. The glands typically are smaller than benign glands and are lined by a single uniform layer of cuboidal or low columnar epithelium, lacking the basal cell layer seen in benign glands. In further contrast with benign glands, malignant glands are crowded together and characteristically lack branching and papillary infolding. The cytoplasm of the tumor cells ranges from pale-clear(as in benign glands) to a distinctive amphophilic(dark purple) appearance. Nuclei are enlarged and often contain one or more prominent nucleoli(Figure 13-24). Some variation in nuclear size and shape is usual, but in general, pleomorphism is not marked. Mitotic figures are uncommon. With increasing grade, irregular or ragged glandular structures, cribriform glands, sheets of cells, or infiltrating individual cells are present. In approximately 80% of cases, prostatic tissue removed for carcinoma also harbors presumptive precursor lesions, referred to as high-grade prostatic intraepithelial neoplasia(HGPIN).

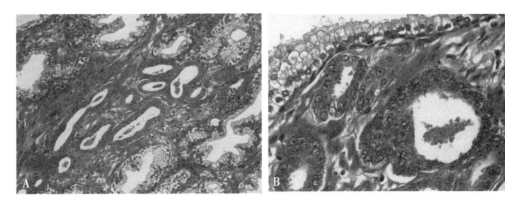

Figure 13-24   Adenocarcinoma of the prostate demonstrating small glands crowded in between larger benign glands(A). B, Higher magnification shows several small malignant glands with enlarged nuclei, prominent nucleoli, and dark cytoplasm, as compared with the larger, benign gland

Prostate cancer is graded by the Gleason system, created in 1967 and updated in 2005. According to this system, prostate cancers are stratified into five grades on the basis of glandular patterns of differentiation. Grade 1 represents the most well-differentiated tumors and grade 5 tumors show no glandular differentiation. Since most tumors contain more than one pattern, a primary grade is assigned to the dominant pattern and a secondary grade to the next most frequent pattern. The two numerical grades are then added to obtain a combined Gleason score. Tumors with only one pattern are treated as if their primary and secondary grades are the same, and, hence, the number is doubled. Thus the most well-differentiated tumors have a Gleason score of 2(1+1) and the most poorly-differentiated tumors merit a score of 10(5+5).

13.5.5.3   Clinical Features

Skillful rectal examination remains a practical and efficient method for the detection of prostatic carcinoma; however, pathologic confirmation is always necessary because early carcinomas cannot be distinguished with assurance from foci of nodular hyperplasia, granulomatous prostatitis, tuberculosis, infarct, or lithiasis. Transrectal ultrasonography can detect carcinomas(which appear as hypoechoic lesions) as small as 5 mm in diameter; however, it will miss up to 30% of the prostatic tumors that are isoechoic and has not proved an efficient tool for screening.

PSA is secreted by all but the most undifferentiated prostatic tumors. Gram for gram, the average prostatic carcinoma produces 10 times or more the amount of PSA produced by normal tissue, and this is reflected in the circulatory levels of this marker. Serum determination of PSA has all but replaced the time-honored determination of PAP. The test has a high sensitivity and specificity, is rapid and inexpensive, and is minimally invasive. Mild serum elevations of PSA can be seen with nodular hyperplasia, but levels above 4 call for serial determination, with the performance of a biopsy if they continue to rise. Almost half of patients with prostatic carcinomas have levels over 10 mg/ml. Elevations of serum PSA also occur in prostatitis, prostatic infarct, and major trauma to the prostate, such as needle biopsy or TUR, but these elevations should be transitory and resolve with proper treatment.

The combination of digital rectal examination, transrectal ultrasonography, and serum PSA represents a powerful diagnostic triad for the detection of early prostatic carcinoma. It is not clear whether measurement of the PSA density(PSA level as a function of prostatic volume)will provide a more specific test for carcinoma.

13.6   Tumors of Testicles and Penis

13.6.1   Testicular Neoplasms

Testicular neoplasms occur in roughly 6 per 100,000 males. In the 15–to 34–year-old age group,when these neoplasms peak in incidence,they are the most common tumors of men. Tumors of the testis are a heterogeneous group of neoplasms that include germ cell tumors and sex cord-stromal tumors. In postpubertal males,95% of testicular tumors arise from germ cells,and all are malignant. By contrast,neoplasms derived from Sertoli or Leydig cells(sex cord-stromal tumors)are uncommon and usually benign. The focus of the remainder of this discussion is on testicular germ cell tumors.

The cause of testicular neoplasms remains unknown. Testicular tumors are more common in whites than in blacks,and the incidence has increased in white populations over recent decades. As noted previously, cryptorchidism is associated with a three-to five-fold increase in the risk of cancer in the undescended testis,as well as an increased risk of cancer in the contralateral descended testis. A history of cryptorchidism is present in approximately 10% of cases of testicular cancer. Intersex syndromes,including androgen insensitivity syndrome and gonadal dysgenesis,also are associated with an increased frequency of testicular cancer. Family history is important,because brothers of males with germ cell tumors have an 8–to 10–fold increased risk over that of the population at large,presumably owing to inherited risk factors. The development of cancer in one testis is associated with a markedly increased risk of neoplasia in the contralateral testis. An isochromosome of the short arm of chromosome 12,I(12p),is found in virtually all germ cell tumors,regardless of their histologic type. The gene(s)that are dysregulated by this chromosomal abnormality,as well as the other mutations that contribute to the molecular pathogenesis of germ cell tumors,are an area of ongoing research.

Most testicular tumors in postpubertal males arise from the in situ lesion intratubular germ cell neoplasia. This lesionis present in conditions associated with a high risk of developing germ cell tumors(e. g. , cryptorchidism,dysgeneticgonads). These in situ lesions can be found in grossly "normal" testicular tissue adjacent to germ cell tumors in virtually all cases.

Testicular germ cell tumors are sub-classified into seminomas and nonseminomatous germ cell tumors. Seminomas,sometimes referred to as "classic" seminomas to distinguish them from the less common spermatocytic seminoma(discussed further on),account for about 50% of testicular germ cell neoplasms. They are histologically identical to ovarian dysgerminomas and to germinomas occurring in the central nervous system and other extragonadal sites.

13.6.1.1   Morphology

The histologic appearances of germ cell tumors may be pure(i. e. ,composed of a single histologic type)or mixed(seen in 40% of cases). Seminomas are soft,well-demarcated,gray-white tumors that bulge from the cut surface of the affected testis(Figure 13–25). Large tumors may contain foci of coagulation necrosis,usually without hemorrhage. Microscopically,seminomas are composed of large,uniform cells with distinct cell borders, clear, glycogen-rich cytoplasm, and round nuclei with conspicuous nucleoli (Figure 13–26). The cells often are arrayed in small lobules with intervening fibrous septa. A lymphocytic infiltrate usually is present and may, on occasion, overshadow the neoplastic cells. Seminomas may also be accompanied by an ill-defined granulomatous reaction. In approximately 15% of cases, syncytiotrophoblasts are present that are the source of the minimally elevated serum hCG concentrations encountered in some males with pure seminoma. Their presence has no bearing on prognosis.

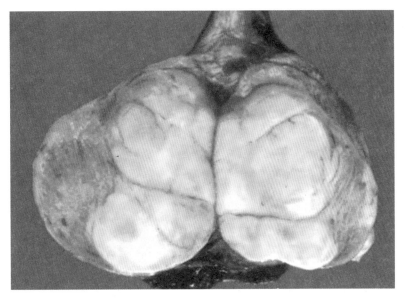

Figure 13 – 25   Seminoma of the test is appearing as a well-circumscribed, pale, fleshy, homogeneous mass

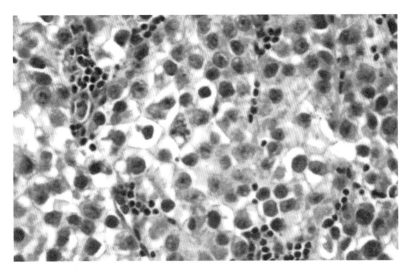

Figure 13–26   Seminoma of the testis. Microscopic examination reveals large cells with distinct cell borders, pale nuclei, prominent nucleoli, and a sparse lymphocytic infiltrate

Although related by name to seminoma, spermatocytic seminoma is a distinct clinical and histologic entity. This is an uncommon tumor. It occurs in much older individuals than other testicular tumors; affected patients generally are older than 65 years of age. In contrast with classic seminomas, spermatocytic seminomas lack lymphocytic infiltrates, granulomas, and syncytiotrophoblasts; are not admixed with other germ cell tumor histologies; are not associated with intratubular germ cell neoplasia; and do not metastasize. The tumor usually comprises polygonal cells of variable size that are arranged in nodules or sheets.

Embryonal carcinomas are ill-defined, invasive masses containing foci of hemorrhage and necrosis

(Figure 13–27). The primary lesions may be small, even in patients with systemic metastases. The tumor cells are large and primitive looking, with basophilic cytoplasm, indistinct cell borders, and large nuclei with prominent nucleoli. The neoplastic cells may be arrayed in undifferentiated, solid sheets or may contain primitive glandular structures and irregular papillae (Figure 13–28). In most cases, cells characteristic of other germ cell tumors (e. g. , yolk sac tumor, teratoma, choriocarcinoma) are admixed with the embryonal areas. Pure embryonal carcinomas account for only 2% to 3% of all testicular germ cell tumors.

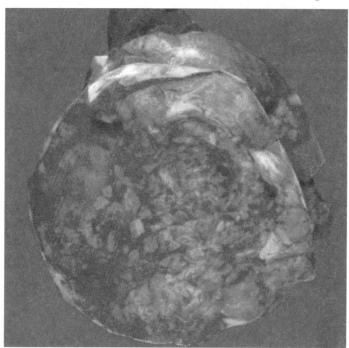

Figure 13–27　Embryonal carcinoma. In contrast with the seminoma illustrated in Figure 13–25, this tumor is a hemorrhagic mass

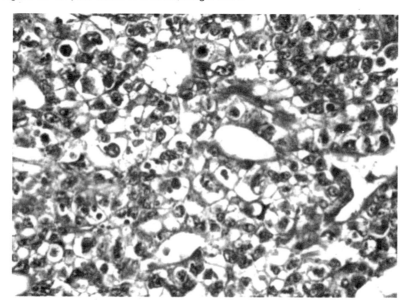

Figure 13–28　Embryonal carcinoma. Note the sheets of undifferentiated cells and primitive gland-like structures. The nuclei are large and hyperchromatic

Yolk sac tumors are the most common primary testicular neoplasm in children younger than 3 years of age;in this age group it has a very good prognosis. In adults,yolk sac tumors most often are seen admixed with embryonal carcinoma. On gross inspection,these tumors often are large and may be well demarcated. Histologic examination discloses low cuboidal to columnar epithelial cells forming microcysts,lacelike(reticular)patterns,sheets,glands,and papillae(Figure 13–29). A distinctive feature is the presence of structures resembling primitive glomeruli, the so-called Schiller-Duvall bodies. Tumors often have eosinophilic hyaline globules in which α1–antitrypsin and alpha fetoprotein(AFP)can be demonstrated by immunohistochemical techniques. As mentioned later,AFP can also be detected in the serum.

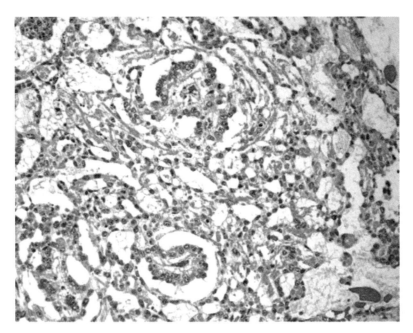

Figure 13–29   Yolk sac tumor demonstrating areas of loosely textured, microcystic tissue and papillary structures resembling a developing glomerulus(Schiller-Duval bodies)

Choriocarcinomas are tumors in which the pluripotential neoplastic germ cells differentiate along trophoblastic lines. Grossly, the primary tumors often are small,nonpalpable lesions,even those with extensive systemic metastases. Microscopic examination reveals that choriocarcinomas are composed of sheets of small cuboidal cells irregularly intermingled with or capped by large,eosinophilic syncytial cells containing multiple dark,pleomorphic nuclei;these represent cytotrophoblastic and syncytiotrophoblastic differentiation,respectively(Figure 13–30). HCG within syncytiotrophoblasts can be identified by immunohistochemical staining and is elevated in the serum.

Teratomas are tumors in which the neoplastic germ cells differentiate along somatic cell lines. These tumors form firm masses that on cut surface often contain cysts and recognizable areas of cartilage. They may occur at any age from infancy to adult life. Pure forms of teratoma are fairly common in infants and children,being second in frequency only to yolk sac tumors. In adults,pure teratomas are rare,constituting 2% to 3% of germ cell tumors,and as with embryonal carcinomas,most are seen in combination with other histologic types. Teratomas are composed of a heterogeneous,helterskelter collection of differentiated cells or organoid structures,such as neural tissue,muscle bundles,islands of cartilage,clusters of squamous epithelium,structures reminiscent of thyroid gland,bronchial epithelium,and bits of intestinal wall or brain substance,all embedded in a fibrous or myxoid stroma(Figure 13–31). Elements may be mature(resembling various tissues within the adult)or immature(sharing histologic features with fetal or embryonal tissues). In prepubertal males, teratomas are typically benign, whereas teratomas in postpubertal males are malignant, being capable of metastasis regardless of whether they are composed of mature or immature elements.

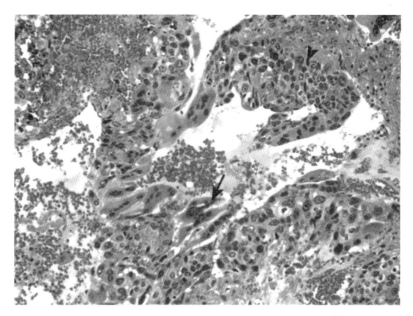

Figure 13–30 **Choriocarcinoma**

Both cytotrophoblastic cells with central nuclei (arrowhead, upper right) and syncytiotrophoblastic cells with multiple dark nuclei embedded in eosinophilic cytoplasm (arrow, middle) are present. Hemorrhage and necrosis are prominent

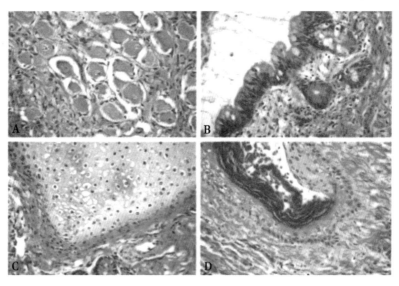

Figure 13–31 **Teratoma**

Testicular teratomas contain mature cells from endodermal, mesodermal, and ectodermal lines. A-D, Four different fields from the same tumor specimen contain neural (ectodermal) (A), glandular (endodermal) (B), cartilaginous (mesodermal) (C), and squamous epithelial (D) elements

Dermoid cysts and epidermoid cysts, common in the ovary, are rare in the testis. These tumors should not be considered teratomas since they are uniformly benign regardless of the patient's age.

Rarely, non-germ cell tumors may arise in teratoma-a phenomenon referred to as "teratoma with malignant transformation." These neoplasms may take the form of a focus of squamous cell carcinoma, mucin-secreting adenocarcinoma, or sarcoma. The importance of non-germ cell malignancies arising in a teratoma is that when the non-germ cell component spreads outside of the testis it does not respond to chemotherapy; thus, the only hope for cure resides in the local resectability of the metastases.

13.6.1.2   Clinical Features

Patients with testicular germ cell neoplasms present most frequently with a painless testicular mass that (unlike enlargements caused by hydroceles) is non-translucent. Biopsy of a testicular neoplasm is associated with a risk of tumor spillage, which would necessitate excision of the scrotal skin in addition to orchiectomy. Consequently, the standard management of a solid testicular mass is radical orchiectomy, based on the presumption of malignancy. Some tumors, especially nonseminomatous germ cell neoplasms, may have metastasized widely by the time of diagnosis in the absence of a palpable testicular lesion.

Seminomas and nonseminomatous tumors differ in their behavior and clinical course. Seminomas often remain confined to the testis for long intervals and may reach considerable size before diagnosis. Metastases most commonly are encountered in the iliac and paraaortic lymph nodes, particularly in the upper lumbar region. Hematogenous metastases occur late in the course of the disease. By contrast, nonseminomatous germ cell neoplasms tend to metastasize earlier, by lymphatic as well as hematogenous routes. Hematogenous metastases are most common in the liver and lungs. Metastatic lesions may be identical to the primary testicular tumor or may contain elements of other germ cell tumors.

Assay of tumor markers secreted by germ cell tumors is important in two ways; these markers are helpful diagnostically, but have an even more valuable role in following the response of tumors to therapy after the diagnosis is established. Human chorionic gonadotropin(HCG) is always elevated in patients with choriocarcinoma and, as noted, can be minimally elevated in persons with other germ cell tumors containing syncytiotrophoblastic cells without cytotrophoblasts. Increased alpha fetoprotein(AFP) in the setting of a testicular neoplasm indicates a yolk sac tumor component. The levels of lactate dehydrogenase (LDH) correlate with the tumor burden.

The treatment of testicular germ cell neoplasms is a remarkable cancer therapy success story. In fact, after being treated for widely metastatic testicular cancer, Lance Armstrong won the grueling Tour de France bicycle race a record seven times! Seminoma, which is extremely radiosensitive and tends to remain localized for long periods, has the best prognosis. More than 95% of patients with early-stage disease can be cured. Among nonseminomatous germ cell tumors, the histologic subtype does not influence the prognosis significantly, and hence these are treated as a group. Approximately 90% of the patients achieve complete remission with aggressive chemotherapy, and most are cured. Pure choriocarcinoma carries a dismal prognosis. However, when it is a minor component of a mixed germ cell tumor, the prognosis is not so adversely affected. With all testicular tumors, recurrences, typically in the form of distant metastases, usually occur within the first 2 years after treatment.

13.6.2   Penile Neoplasms

More than 95% of penile neoplasms arise on squamous epithelium. In developing countries, however, penile carcinoma occurs at much higher rates. Most cases occur in uncircumcised patients older than 40 years of age. Several factors have been implicated in the pathogenesis of squamous cell carcinoma of the penis, including poor hygiene(with resultant exposure to potential carcinogens in smegma), smoking, and infection with human papillomavirus(HPV), particularly types 16 and 18.

Squamous cell carcinoma in situ of the penis(Bowen disease) occurs in older uncircumcised males and appears grossly as a solitary plaque on the shaft of the penis. Histologic examination reveals morphologically malignant cells throughout the epidermis with no invasion of the underlying stroma(Figure 13-32). It gives rise to infiltrating squamous cell carcinoma in approximately 10% of patients.

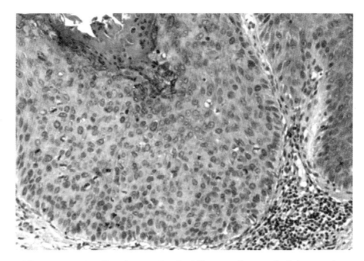

Figure 13-32　Carcinoma in situ(Bowen disease) of the penis. The epithelium above the intact basement membrane shows delayed maturation and disorganization(left). Higher magnification(right) shows several mitotic figures, some above the basal layer, a dyskeratotic cell, and nuclear pleomorphism

Invasive squamous cell carcinoma of the penis appears as a gray, crusted, popular lesion, most commonly on the glans penis or prepuce. In many cases, infiltration of the underlying connective tissue produces an indurated, ulcerated lesion with irregular margins(Figure 13-33). Histologically, it is a typical keratinizing squamous cell carcinoma. The prognosis is related to the stage of the tumor. With localized lesions, the 5-year survival rate is 66%, whereas metastasis to inguinal lymph nodes carries a grim 27% 5-year survival rate. Verrucous carcinoma is a variant of squamous cell carcinoma characterized by a papillary architecture, virtually no cytologic atypia, and rounded, pushing deep margins. Verrucous carcinomas are locally invasive but do not metastasize.

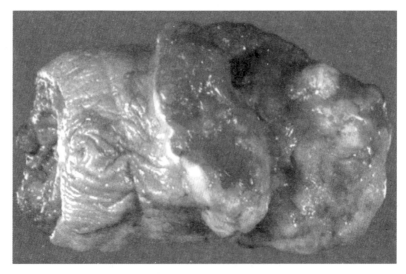

Figure 13-33　Carcinoma of the penis. The glans penis is deformed by an ulcerated, infiltrative

13.7 Breast Disease

13.7.1 Proliferative Change

Lesions of the female breast are much more common than lesions of the male breast and usually take the form of palpable, sometimes painful nodules or masses. Breast cancer is the most common cancer in women(excluding neoplasia of the skin) and is second only to lung cancer as a cause of cancer-related death.

13.7.1.1 Fibrocystic Change of the Breast

The designation fibrocystic is a kind of non-neoplastic lesions, which is characterized by distal catheter and expansion of acinus, interstitial fibrous tissue and epithelial hyperplasia. Fibrocystic changes are the most common breast abnormality seen in premenopausal women. The changes tend to arise between age 25 – 45 and are most likely a consequence of the cyclic breast changes that occur normally in the menstrual cycle. The incidence is related to ovarian endocrine disorders (Especially progesterone and estrogen.). But still now, we have no idea about the exactly pathogenesis.

Morphology

1) Nonproliferative Changes: (Cysts and Fibrosis) These cysts are interlaced with proliferative interstitial fibers, creating a variegated appearance. Under the microscope, cysts are covered with columnar epithelium, cuboidal epithelium or without epithelium covering. Fibrosis in interstitium will develop further after the cysts rupture. Metaplasia apocrine often occur in cyst epithelium (big cell size and eosinophilic cytoplasm), which is similar to large sweat gland epithelium in morphology. A single, large cyst may form within one breast, but changes usually are multifocal and often bilateral. The involved areas appear as ill-defined, diffusely increased densities and discrete nodularities on mammography. The cysts range from less than 1 cm and up to 5 cm in diameter. Unopened, they are brown to blue(blue dome cysts) and are filled with watery, turbid fluid. The secretions within the cysts may calcify, producing microcalcifications on mammograms. Histologic examination reveals an epithelial lining that in larger cysts may be flattened or even totally atrophic (Figure 13-34). Frequently, the lining cells are large and polygonal with abundant granular, eosinophilic cytoplasm and small, round, deeply chromatic nuclei. Such morphology is called apocrine metaplasia and virtually always is benign. The stroma surrounding all types of cysts usually consists of compressed fibrous tissue that has lost the delicate, myxomatous appearance of normal breast stroma. A stromal lymphocytic infiltrate is common in this and all other variants of fibrocystic changes.

2) Proliferative Changes: (Epithelial Hyperplasia) the terms epithelial hyperplasia and proliferative fibrocystic change encompass a range of proliferative lesions within the ductules, the terminal ducts, and sometimes the lobules of the breast. Some of the epithelial hyperplasia are mild and orderly, and carry little risk of carcinoma, but at the other end of the spectrum are the more florid atypical hyperplasia that carry a significantly greater risk, commensurate with the severity and typicality of the changes. The epithelial hyperplasia are often accompanied by other histologic variants of fibrocystic change. Proliferative fibrocystic changes are often accompanied by terminal ducts and epithelial hyperplasia. According to the different degree of hyperplasia: ①Mild hyperplasia; ②Flourishing hyperplasia; ③Heterogeneous hyperplasia; ④Carcinoma in situ.

The gross appearance of epithelial hyperplasia is not distinctive and is dominated by coexisting fibrous or cystic changes. Histologic examination shows an almost infinite spectrum of proliferative alterations. The ducts, ductules, or lobules may be filled with orderly cuboidal cells within which small gland patterns(called fenestrations) can be discerned. Sometimes, the proliferating epithelium projects as multiple small papillary excrescences into the ductal lumen(ductal papillomatosis). The degree of hyperplasia, judged in part by the number of layers of intraductal epithelium, can be mild, moderate, or marked. Occasionally, hyperplasia produces microcalcifications on mammography, raising concern for cancer. In some instances the hyperplastic cells have features bearing some resemblance to ductal carcinoma in situ(described later). Such hyperplasia is called atypical ductal hyperplasia. Atypical lobular hyperplasia is used to describe hyperplasias that exhibit changes that approach but do not meet diagnostic criteria for lobular carcinoma in situ. Both atypical ductal and lobular hyperplasia are associated with an increased risk of invasive carcinoma.

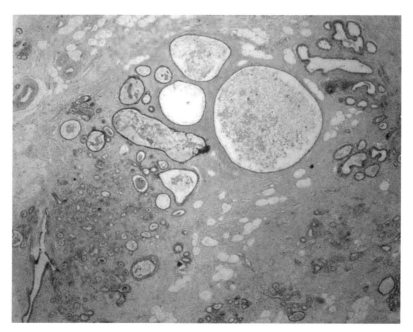

Figure 13–34   non-hyperplastic fibrocystic changes

13.7.1.2   Sclerosing Adenosis

This variant is less common than cysts and hyperplasia, but it is significant because its clinical and morphologic features may be deceptively similar to those of carcinoma. These lesions contain marked intralobular fibrosis and proliferation of small ductules and acing.

Grossly, the lesion has a hard, rubbery consistency, similar to that of breast cancer. Histologically, sclerosing adenosis is characterized by proliferation of lining epithelial cells and myoepithelial cells in small ducts and ductules, yielding masses of small gland patterns within a fibrous stroma. Aggregated glands or proliferating ductules may be virtually back to back, with single or multiple layers of cells in contact with one another(adenosis). Marked stromal fibrosis, which may compress and distort the proliferating epithelium, is always associated with the adenosis; hence, the designation sclerosing adenosis. This overgrowth of fibrous tissue may completely compress the lumina of the acini and ducts, so that they appear as solid cords of cells. This pattern may then be difficult to distinguish histologically from an invasive scirrhous carcinoma. The presence of double layers of epithelium and the identification of myoepithelial elements are helpful in suggesting a benign diagnosis.

13.7.2   Fibroadenoma

Fibroadenoma is by far the most common benign neoplasm of the female breast. Fibroadenomas usually appear in young women. The peak incidence is in the third decade of life.

13.7.2.1   Morphology

The fibroadenoma occurs as a discrete, usually solitary, freely movable nodule, 1–10 cm in diameter. Rarely, multiple tumors are encountered and, equally rarely, they may exceed 10 cm in diameter (giant fibroadenoma). Whatever their size, they are usually easily "shelled out." Grossly, all are firm, with a uniform tan-white color on cut section, punctuated by softer yellow-pink specks representing the glandular areas. Histologically there is a loose fibroblastic stroma containing ductlike, epithelium-lined spaces of various forms and sizes. These ductlike or glandular spaces are lined with single or multiple layers of cells that are regular and have a well-defined, intact basement membrane. Although in some lesions the ductal spaces are open, round to oval, and fairly regular (pericanalicular fibroadenoma), others are compressed by extensive proliferation of the stroma, so that on cross-section they appear as slits or irregular, star-shaped structures (intracanalicular fibroadenoma) (Figure 13–35).

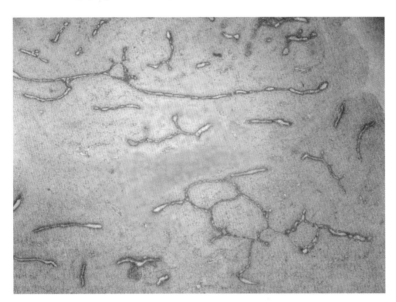

Figure 13–35   **Fibroadenoma with intracanalicular pattern**

13.7.2.2   Clinical Features

Clinically, fibroadenomas usually present as solitary, discrete, movable masses. They may enlarge late in the menstrual cycle and during pregnancy. After menopause they may regress and calcify. Cytogenetic studies reveal that the stromal cells are monoclonal and so represent the neoplastic element of these tumors. The basis of ductal proliferation is not clear; perhaps the neoplastic stromal cells secrete growth factors that induce proliferation of epithelial cells.

13.7.3   Breast Cancer

13.7.3.1   Etiology

Breast cancer makes this scourge second only to lung cancer as a cause of cancer death in women. It is uncommon in women younger than age 30. Thereafter, the risk steadily increases throughout life, but after menopause the upward slope of the curve almost plateaus. About 5% to 10% of breast cancers are related to specific inherited mutations. About half of women with hereditary breast cancer have mutations in gene BRCA1(on chromosome 17q21.3), and an additional one-third have mutations in BRCA2(on chromosome 13q12-13). Women are more likely to carry a breast cancer susceptibility gene if they develop breast cancer before menopause, have bilateral cancer, have other associated cancers(e. g. , ovarian cancer), have a significant family history or belong to certain ethnic groups.

Prolonged exposure to exogenous estrogens, oral contraceptives and Ionizing radiation to the chest increases the risk of breast cancer. Many others less well-established risk factors, such as obesity, alcohol consumption, and a diet high in fat, have been implicated in the development of breast cancer on the basis of population studies. Obesity is a recognized risk factor in postmenopausal women.

13.7.3.2　Morphology

(1)Noninvasive(in Situ)Carcinoma

There are two types of noninvasive breast carcinoma: DCIS and LCIS. Morphologic studies have shown that both usually arise from the terminal duct lobular unit. DCIS tends to fill, distort, and unfold involved lobules and thus appears into involve ductlike spaces. In contrast, LCIS usually expands but does not alter the underlying lobular architecture. Both are confined by a basement membrane and do not invade into stroma or lymphovascular channels. Non-invasive carcinoma has a tendency to develop to infiltrate cancer, WHO in 2012 included it in the precancerous lesion category.

1)DCIS(Ductal carcinoma in situ) DCIS has a wide variety of histologic appearances. Architectural patterns are often mixed and include solid, comedo, cribriform, papillary, micropapillary, and clinging types. DCIS is generally divided into three nuclear grades: low, intermediate and high.

DCIS of low nuclear grade is composed of small, monomorphic cells, growing in arcades, micropapillae, cribriform or solid patterns. The nuclear is of uniform size and have a regular chromatin pattern with inconspicuous nucleolus, mitotic figures are rare. DCIS of intermediate nuclear grade is composed of cells that show mid to moderate variability in size, shape and placement, variably coarse chromatin, and variably prominent nuclear. DCIS of high nucleolus grade is composed of high atypical cells most often proliferating in solid, cribriform or micropapillary patterns.

Nuclei are pleomorphic, poorly polarized, with irregular contours and distribution, coarse, clumped chromatin and prominent nuclear. Mitotic figures are usually common. Comedo necrosis is frequently present (Figure 13-36).

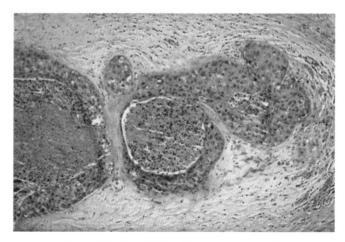

Figure 13-36　**DCIS with comedo necrosis**

Comedo：The comedo subtype is distinctive and is characterized by cells with high-grade nuclei distending spaces with extensive central necrosis. The name derives from the toothpaste-like necrotic tissue that can be extruded from transected ducts with gentle pressure. At least one-third of women with small areas of untreated low-nuclear-grade DCIS will eventually develop invasive carcinoma. Under the microscope, cell size increasing, cytoplasmic acid, differentiation, and different cell size, conspicuous can been fourd nucleoli, accompanied by nuclear fission. The cancer cells arrange insolid sheet, with necrosis in the center and calcification in necrotic areas. Interstitial fibrous tissue hyperplasia and chronic inflammatory infiltration are observed around the ducts.

　　2）LCIS（Lobular carcinoma in situ）. LCIS does not form masses and is only rarely associated with calcifications. Approximately one-third of women with LCIS will eventually develop invasive carcinoma. Subsequent invasive carcinomas arise in either breast at significant frequency. About one-third of these cancers will be of lobular type（as compared with −10% of cancers in women who develop de novo lobular carcinoma）, but most are of no special type. LCIS is both a marker of increased risk of developing breast cancer in either breast and a direct precursor of some cancers. The cancer cells are present in the distended ducts and ducts of the distal mammary glands. There is no cancer cell necrosis, interstitial inflammatory response and fibrous tissue hyperplasia. The incidence of invasive carcinoma is similar to that in ductal carcinoma in situ.

　　（2）Invasive Carcinoma

Invasive carcinoma includes invasive carcinoma of no special type（invasive ductal carcinoma）and invasive carcinoma of special type（inflammatory carcinoma、invasive lobular carcinoma、carcinoma with medullary features、mucinous carcinoma、metaplastic carcinoma、tubular carcinomas et al）. The microscopic appearance is quite heterogeneous, ranging from tumors with well-developed tubule formation and low-grade nuclei to tumors consisting of sheets of anaplastic cells. The tumor margins are usually irregular but are occasionally pushing and circumscribed. Invasion of lymphovascular spaces or along nerves may be seen. Advanced cancers may cause dimpling of the skin, retraction of the nipple, or fixation to the chest wall.

　　1）Invasive carcinoma of no special type

Invasive ductal carcinoma is a term used for all carcinomas that cannot be subclassified into one of the specialized types described below and does not indicate that this tumor specifically arises from the ductal system. Carcinomas of "no special type" or "not otherwise specified" are synonyms for ductal carcinomas. The majority（70% to 80%）of cancers fall into this group. This type of cancer is usually associated with DCIS, but rarely LCIS is present. Most ductal carcinomas produce a desmoplastic response, which replaces normal breast fat（resulting in a mammographic density）and forms a hard, palpable mass. About two-thirds express estrogen or progestagen receptors, and about one-third overexpress HER2/NEU.

　　2）Invasive carcinoma of special type. ①Inflammatory carcinoma：Inflammatory carcinoma is defined by the clinical presentation of an enlarged, swollen, erythematous breast, usually without a palpable mass. The underlying carcinoma is generally poorly differentiated and diffusely invades the breast parenchyma. The blockage of numerous dermal lymphatic spaces by carcinoma results in the clinical appearance. True inflammation is minimal or absent. Most of these tumors have distant metastases, and the prognosis is extremely poor. ②Invasive lobular carcinoma：Invasive lobular carcinoma consists of cells morphologically identical to the cells of LCIS. The cells invade individually into stroma and are often aligned in strands or chains. Occasionally they surround cancerous or normal-appearing acini or ducts, creating a so-called bull's-eye pattern. Lobular carcinomas, more frequently than ductal carcinomas, metastasize to cerebrospinal fluid, serosal surfaces, gastrointestinal tract, ovary and uterus, and bone marrow. Lobular carcinomas are also more frequently multicentric and bilateral（10% −20%）. These tumors comprise fewer than 20% of all breast carcinomas.

③Carcinoma with medullary features: Medullary carcinoma consists of sheets of large anaplastic cells with pushing, well-circumscribed borders. Clinically, they can be mistaken for fibroadenomas. There is invariably a pronounced lymphoplasmacytic infiltrate. DCIS is usually absent or minimal. Medullary carcinomas, or medullary-like carcinomas, occur with increased frequency in women with BRCA1 mutations, although most women with medullary carcinoma are not carriers. ④Mucinous carcinoma: Colloid (mucinous) carcinoma is also a rare subtype. The tumor cells produce abundant quantities of extracellular mucin that dissects into the surrounding stroma. Like medullary carcinomas, they often present as well-circumscribed masses and can be mistaken for fibroadenomas. Grossly the tumors are usually soft and gelatinous. ⑤Tubular carcinomas: Microscopically, the carcinomas consist of well-formed tubules with low-grade nuclei. Lymph node metastases are rare, and prognosis is excellent.

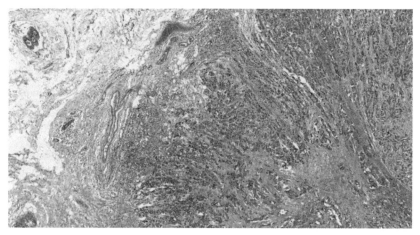

Figure 13-37　Invasive carcinoma of no special type, tumors with strip shape infiltrated into the interstitium

13. 7. 3. 3　Spreading

Spread eventually occurs through direct spreading, lymphatic and hematogenous channels.

(1) Direct Spreading

The cancer cells can infiltrate in the corresponding breast lobules, the fatty tissue surrounding the catheter, and even the pectoralis major and chest wall.

(2) Lymphatic Metastasis

Lymph node metastases are present in about 40% of cancers presenting as palpable masses. Outer quadrant and centrally located lesions typically spread first to the axillary nodes. Those in the inner quadrants often involve the lymph node along the internal mammary arteries. The supraclavicular nodes are sometimes the primary site of spread, but they may become involved only after the axillary and internal mammary nodes are affected. More distant dissemination eventually ensues, with metastatic involvement of almost any organ or tissue in the body.

(3) Hematogenous Channels

Advanced breast cancer can be transferred to the lungs, bone, liver, adrenal gland and brain (uncommon), spleen and pituitary.

13. 7. 3. 4　Prognosis

The prognosis of breast carcinoma is related with several factors as following:

1) The size of the primary carcinoma. Invasive carcinomas smaller than 1cm have an excellent progno-

sis in the absence of lymph node metastases and may not require systemic therapy.

2) The grade of the carcinoma. The most common grading system for breast cancer evaluates tubule formation, nuclear grade, and mitotic rate to divide carcinomas into three groups. Well-differentiated carcinomas have a significantly better prognosis as compared with poorly differentiated carcino-mas. Moderately differentiated carcinomas ini-tially have a better prognosis, but survival at 20 years approaches that of poorly differentiated carcinomas.

3) The histologic type of carcinoma. All specialized types of breast carcinoma(tubular, medullary, cribriform, adenoid cystic, and mucinous) have a somewhat better prognosis than carcinomas of no special type ("ductal carcinomas").

4) The presence or absence of estrogen or progesterone receptors. The presence of hormone receptors confers a slightly better prognosis.

5) The proliferative rate of the cancer. Proliferation can be measured by mitotic counts, flow cytometry, or immunohistochemical markers for cell cycle proteins. Mitotic counts are included as part of the grading system. The optimal method for evaluating proliferation has not been determined. High proliferative rates are associated with a poorer prognosis.

6) Aneuploidy. Carcinomas with an abnormal DNA content(aneuploidy) have a slightly worse prognosis as compared with carcinomas with a DNA content similar to normal cells.

7) Amplification of HER2/NEU. Amplification of this membrane-bound protein is almost always caused by amplification of the gene. Therefore, overexpression can be determined by immunohistochemistry(which detects the protein in tissue sections) or by fluorescence in situ hybridization(which detects the number of gene copies). Overexpression is associated with a poorer prognosis.

13.7.4   Male Breast

As in females, male breasts are subject to hormonal influences, but they are considerably less sensitive than are female breasts. Nonetheless, enlargement of the male breast, or gynecomastia, may occur in response to absolute or relative estrogen excesses. Gynecomastia, then, is the male analogue of fibrocystic change in the female. The most important cause of such hyperestrinism in the male is cirrhosis of the liver, with consequent inability of the liver to metabolize estrogens. Other causes include Klinefelter syndrome, estrogen-secreting tumors, estrogen therapy, and, occasionally, digitalis therapy. Physiologic gynecomastia often occurs in puberty and in extreme old age. The morphologic features of gynecomastia are similar to those of intraductal hyperplasia. Grossly, a button-like, subareolar swelling develops, usually in both breasts but occasionally in only one.

Carcinoma:This is a rare occurrence, with a frequency ratio to breast cancer in the female of 1 : 125. It occurs in advanced age. Because of the scant amount of breast substance in the male, the tumor rapidly infiltrates the overlying skin and underlying thoracic wall. Both morphologically and biologically, these tumors resemble invasive carcinomas in the female. Unfortunately, almost half have spread to regional nodes and more distant sites by the time they are discovered.

Chapter 14

Endocrine System Diseases

◆ Introduction

The endocrine system contains a highly integrated and widely distributed group of organs, including endocrinic glands and endocrinic cells. Anatomically, the endocrine system consists of 6 distinct organs: pituitary, adrenals, thyroid, parathyroids, gonads, and pancreatic islets. The cells of this system elaborate polypeptide hormones; owing to these biochemical properties, it has also been called as APUD cell system(acronym for Amine Precursor Uptake and Decarboxylation properties).

Combined with the nerve system, the endocrine system orchestrates a state of metabolic equilibrium, or homeostasis of the body. The endocrine system diseases share some common features, such as

(1)Cell shape change is concordant with function change.

(2)Local lesion causes general impacts(metabolic imbalance).

(3)The categories of diseases include inflammation, tumor, and hyperplasia, hypertrophy and atrophy. Inflammation and tumor can be seen in any system. Hyperplasia, hypertrophy and atrophy, as the pure morphology in a disease, are the features of endocrine system diseases. We have known in the chapter of cellular and tissue adaptation and injury, hyperplasia and hypertrophy happen because of either over workload or over hormone stimulation. Endocrine organs often receive hormone stimulation and it easily induces the hyperplasia and hypertrophy.

(4)Sometimes it is difficult to judge the hyperplasia and adenoma.

(5)Cellular atypia can be seen in both benign and malignant tumor. The cellular atypia is not the criteria to differentiate both.

14.1 Pituitary Gland

The pituitary is a small bean-shaped organ. It is located at the base of the brain, where it lies nestled within the confines of the sella turcica in close proximity to the optic chiasm and the cavernous sinuses. The pituitary is composed of two distinct components: the anterior lobe(Adenohypophysis) and the posterior lobe (Neurohypophysis). Pituitary is an important endocrine organ which secretes different hormones to conduct other subordinate endocrine organ's function.

Most endocrine cells are in the anterior pituitary. The adenohypophysis(anterior pituitary) releases six hormones that are in turn under the control of various stimulatory and inhibitory hypothalamic releasing factors: TSH, thyroid-stimulating hormone (thyrotropin); PRL, prolactin; ACTH, adrenocorticotrophic hormone (corticotropin); GH, growth hormone (somatotropin); FSH, follicle-stimulating hormone; LH, luteinizing hormone.

The hormones in the posterior pituitary are synthesized within the hypothalamus and then transmitted down the nerve axons in the pituitary stalk to the post lobe, include antidiuretic hormone(ADH) and oxytocin.

14.1.1 Hyperpituitarism and Pituitary Adenoma

Hyperpituitarism arises from excessive secretion of trophic hormones. It most often results from an anterior pituitary adenoma. Other, less common causes include hyperplasia and carcinomas of the anterior pituitary, secretion of hormones by some extra-pituitary tumors, and certain hypothalamic disorders.

14.1.1.1 Pituitary Giantism and Acromegaly(Over Production of GH)

Overproduction of GH in children and adolescents, whose epiphyses have not yet fused, causes excessive growth in the length of bones, and the subject becomes too tall. This condition is called pituitary giantism. Some associated coarsening of the facial features usually occurs in response to the effect of GH on the structure of the facial bones.

In adults, excessive GH causes acromegaly. Because the epiphyses have fused, there can be no growth in height, but the GH produces thickening and coarsening of bones and generalized enlargement of viscera. Affected individuals have coarse facial features, large prominent jaws, and large spade-like hands, but they are no taller than normal.

14.1.1.2 Over Production of Prolactin

In a non-pregnant woman, excessive secretion of prolactin may cause spontaneous secretion of milk from the breasts(galactorrhea) and cessation of menstrual periods(amenorrhea). Galactorrhea results from the effect of the hormone on breast tissue. Amenorrhea occurs because high level of prolactin also inhibits secretion of pituitary gonadotropins FSH and LH, which in turn leads to cessation of ovulation and menstrual cycles.

14.1.1.3 Pituitary Adenoma

Pituitary adenomas are benign neoplasms of anterior lobe of the pituitary and are often associated with the excessive secretion of pituitary hormones and symptoms of corresponding hyperfunction. Clinically diagnosed pituitary adenomas are responsible for about 10% of intracranial neoplasms; they are discovered incidentally in up to 25% of routine autopsies.

(1) Morphology

Gross view: Pituitary adenomas can be macroadenomas(>1 cm in diameter) or microadenomas(<1 cm in diameter), and clinically, they can be functional or silent. Silent and hormone-negative adenomas are likely to come to clinical attention at a later stage than those associated with endocrine abnormalities and are therefore more likely to be macroadenomas. The usual pituitary adenoma is a well-circumscribed, soft lump that may, in the case of smaller tumors, be confined by the sella turcica. Larger lesions typically extend superiorly through the sellar diaphragm into the suprasellar region, where they often compress the optic chiasm and adjacent structures. Foci of hemorrhage and/or necrosis are common in larger adenomas.

Microscopical view: In normal anterior pituitary lobe, there are at least 3 kinds of different staining cells cross distribution: acidophilic, basophilic, or chromophobic, depending on the type and amount of secretory product within the cell. But Pituitary adenomas usually are composed of relatively uniform cells. The cells are polygonal with or without mild nuclear atypia and arrayed in sheets, cords, or papillae with abundant capillaries. Supporting connective tissue, or reticulin, is sparse. This cellular monomorphism and the absence of a significant reticulin network are key morphological changes of pituitary adenomas.

Different cell proliferation will cause different clinical symptoms. But the functional status of the adenoma cannot be reliably predicted from its histologic appearance because of same staining cells secreting different hormones. The functional status can be judged only depending on the immnochemical staining, using 6 antibodies against 6 hormones respectively.

From the table 14-1, we can see that the 3 types of hormone cells show acidophilic, and 3 show basophilic. IHC reveals that prolactin cell adenoma is the most common type, followed by null cell adenoma. Null cell is not chromophobe cell. It is negative against any antibodies of 6 hormones. Then adrenocorticotropic hormone cell adenoma and gonadotroph cell adenoma. Growth hormone cell adenoma and mixed growth/prolactin cell adenoma are not so popular, but they cause significant symptoms.

Table 14-1　Pituitary Adenoma detected by IHC

Cell origin of adenoma	Frequency(%)	Cell type
Prolactin cell	20-30	acidophilic
Growth hormone cell	5	acidophilic
Mixed growth/prolactin cell	5	acidophilic
Adrenocorticotropic hormone cell	10-15	basophilic
Gonadotroph cell	10-15	basophilic
Null cell	20	
Thyroid-stimulating hormone cell	1	basophilic
Other hormonal adenoma	15	

(2) Clinical Symptoms

Systemic symptoms: Relative endocrinic dysfunction will be different in different cell type's adenoma. Increased prolactin will cause amenorrhea, galactorrhea, low libido and infertility. The corticotroph cell adenoma will cause the hypercortisolism. The gonadotroph cell adenoma will cause low libido. The excessive growth hormone will cause different symptoms in children and teenage and adult. It cause gigantism in children and teenage and acromegaly in adults. No doubt the thyroid-stimulating hormone cell adenoma cause hyperthyroidism. Sometimes, both silent and hormone-negative pituitary adenomas may cause hypopituitarism as they encroach on and destroy adjacent anterior pituitary parenchyma.

Local symptoms: As the adenomas expand, they frequently erode the sella turcica and anterior clinoid processes. It also can induce bitemporal hemianopsia because of optic chiasma being compressed.

14.1.2　Hypopituitarism

It means hypofunction of anterior pituitary. It may occur with loss or absence of 75% or more of the anterior pituitary parenchyma frequently caused by nonsecretory pituitary adenomas, ischemic necrosis of anterior pituitary, or ablation of the pituitary by surgery or radiation. In this condition, the anterior lobe fails to secret enough hormones. Then the functions of the thyroid gland, adrenal gland, and gonads are impaired because trophic hormone stimulation is lost. *Sheehan syndrome*, or postpartum necrosis of the anterior pituitary, which is the most common form of clinically significant ischemic necrosis of the anterior pituitary. In pregnancy period, the anterior pituitary usually enlarges because of prolactin cell hypertrophy and hyperplasia. But the blood supply for enlarged anterior pituitary does not increase. That makes the enlarged anterior pituitary to be very vulnerable to ischemia. When heavy hemorrhage or shock occurs, necrosis of anterior pituitary will happen in turn.

14.1.3   Hypothalamus and Posterior Pituitary Disorders

The hypothalamic neurons produce two peptides: antidiuretic hormone (ADH) and oxytocin. They are stored in axon terminals in the neurohypophysis and released into the circulation in response to appropriate stimuli. Oxytocin stimulates the contraction of smooth muscle in the pregnant uterus and those surrounding the lactiferous ducts of the mammary glands. Abnormal oxytocin synthesis and release have not been associated with significant clinical abnormalities. The clinically important posterior pituitary syndromes involve ADH production. Diabetes Insipidus is a rare disease characterized by failure of the posterior lobe of the pituitary gland to secrete ADH. Because lack of ADH, the affected person is unable to absorb water from the renal collecting tubules and excretes a large volume of extremely dilute urine. Serum sodium and osmolality are increased as a result of excessive renal loss of free water. Large amounts of water must be consumed to compensate for the excessive water loss in the urine and to prevent dehydration.

14.2   Thyroid Gland

The thyroid gland consists of two lateral lobes connected by a narrow isthmus. It is located in the overlying of the upper part of the trachea and is regulated by pituitary thyroid-stimulating hormone (TSH). The four parathyroid glands are located on its posterior surface.

Histologically, the thyroid gland is composed of multiple minute spherical vesicles called thyroid follicles. Each follicle consists of a central mass of eosinophilic protein material called colloid, surrounded by a layer of cuboid epithelial cells called follicle cells. Parafollicular cells exist between follicles, they have clear cytoplasm, so are called "C" cells.

Under the influence of TSH, the follicular cells synthesize two hormones called triiodothyronine (T3) and thyroxin (T4), which regulate the body's metabolic process and are also required for the normal development of the nervous system. The term thyroid hormone is a general term referring to both of the T3 and T4.

The figure (Figure 14-1) shows the cuboid cells of thyroid follicle under high power of microscope. The pink mass in follicle is colloid which is the secretion of follicle cell—thyroglobulin.

If many TSH molecules bind to the follicle cell, the cell will synthesize more thyroxine. It will hypertrophy to high columnar shape to match overload work. On the other hand, if TSH reduces, the follilcle cells will withdraw to low cuboid and work few. So the morphology of follicle cells is helpful for us to judge the function of thyroid (Figure 14-2).

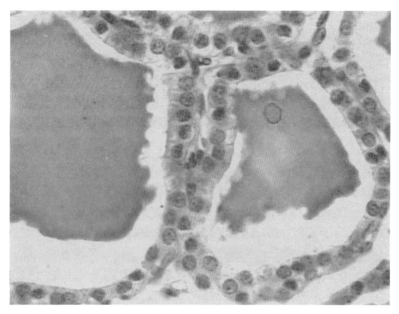

Figure 14-1 **Thyroid follicle**

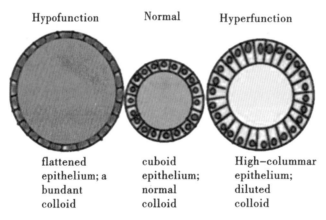

Figure 14-2   Morphology and function of thyroid

14.2.1 Goiter

An enlargement of the thyroid gland is called goiter. The gland maybe uniformly enlarged, called a diffuse goiter, or multiple nodules of proliferating thyroid tissue may form a nodular goiter. A goiter that does not secrete excess thyroid hormone is called a nontoxic goiter. On the other hand, an enlarged gland that produces an excessive amount of hormone and causes symptoms of hyperthyroidism is called a toxic goiter.

14.2.1.1 Nontoxic Goiter

Nontoxic goiter refers to simple thyroid enlarged without thyroidism in majority cases.

(1) Etiology and Pathogenesis

Three major factors predispose to the development of nontoxic goiter:

1) Iodine deficiency: If iodine is deficient in the diet, not enough iodine will be available to produce adequate thyroid hormone for the needs of the individual. The low level of thyroid hormone leads to a compensatory increase in TSH produced by pituitary. Hypertrophy and hyperplasia and goitrous enlargement will

occur in turn in response to TSH stimulation. And it is an attempt to extract the meager amount of iodine from the blood more efficiently to make enough hormones.

Deficiency of enzymes required for synthesis of the thyroid hormone or ingestion of substances that interfere with the function of these enzymes

The enzyme-deficient gland is unable to produce sufficient hormone without enlarging. It is the cause of the familial or heritage goiter. The ingestion of substances that interfere with thyroid hormone synthesis at some level, such as calcium and some "natural" food(cabbage, cauliflower and turnips)has been documented to be goitrogenic. Over calcium induces intestine to decrease the absorption of iodine and cyanide, some vegetables interfere with the iodine aggregation toward thyroid.

2)Increased hormone requirements：In some individuals, the thyroid gland may be able to produce adequate hormone under normal circumstances but may be unable to increase its output in response to increased requirement without enlarging, such as in puberty, during pregnancy and under conditions of stress.

3)Excessive intake of iodine：Excessive iodine occupies most of the functional groups of peroxidase. Then tyrosine oxidation will be interfered and organic process of iodine will be blocked. As a result, inadequate thyroid hormone leads to a compensatory enlargement of thyroid gland.

(2)Morphology

Compensatory increase in TSH produced by pituitary induces recurrent and persistent hyperplasia and hypertrophy of thyroid gland. The process can be divided into three stages.

Stage of hyperplasia(Diffuse hyperplastic goiter)：Under microscope, follicles hypertrophy and hyperplasia with few colloid can be observed. The follicles are lined by crowded columnar cells and the small blood vessels between follicles are hyperemic. In gross, the thyroid gland is diffusely and symmetrically enlarged with smooth surface and soft texture.

Stage of stored colloid(Diffuse colloid goiter)：Long-term iodine deficiency can cause large colloid storage. But the change is not uniform throughout the gland. Some follicles are distended with mass colloid, whereas others remain small. The follicular epithelium is flattened and cubical, and colloid is abundant during periods of involution(Figure 14-3, Figure 14-4). In gross, the cut surface of thyroid is usually brown, somewhat glassy, and translucent.

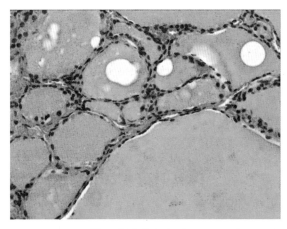
Figure 14-3   **Thyroid follicle in the stage of stored colloid**

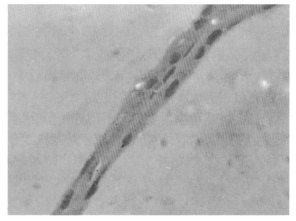
Figure 14-4   **flattened follicular epithelium and abundant colloid**

Stage of nodules(Multinodular goiter)：With time, recurrent hyperplasia and involution combine to produce an irregular enlargement of the thyroid, termed multinodular goiter. In gross, irregular nodules containing variable amounts of brown gelatinous colloid are present on cut section (Figure 14 – 5). Regressive change occurs frequently, particularly in older lesions, such as hemorrhage, fibrosis and cystic dilatation. The microscopic appearance includes some colloid-rich follicles lining by inactive epithelium, hypertrophy and hyperplasia of some follicles, and fibers hyperplasia and separating the follicles to form nodules (Figure 14–6).

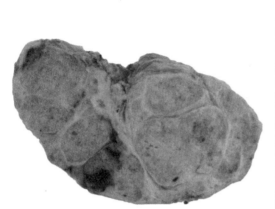

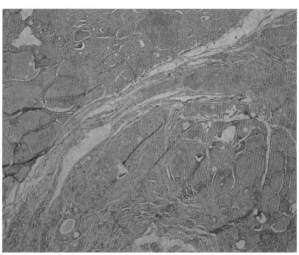

Figure 14–5   **Multinodular goiter in gross**   Figure 14 – 6   **Multinodular goiter in microscopic appearance**

14.2.1.2   Toxic goiter

Toxic goiter refers to a group of goiters with thyrotoxicosis. Thyrotoxicosis is a hypermetabolic state caused by excessive levels of thyroid hormone regardless of cause. The syndrome of thyrotoxicosis is manifested by nervousness, palpitation, rapid pulse, fatigability, muscular weakness, weight loss with good appetite, diarrhea, heat intolerance, warm skin, excessive perspiration, emotional liability, menstrual changes, a fine tremor of hand, eye change, and variable enlargement of thyroid gland. In individuals with ophthalmopathy, the tissues of the orbit are edematous, because of the presence of hydrophilic glycosaminoglycans. In addition, there is infiltration by lymphocytes, mostly T cells. Orbital muscles are edematous initially but may undergo fibrosis late in the course of the disease. The disease has a peak incidence from the ages of 20 to 40, with female being affected more commonly than male.

(1) Etiology and Pathogenesis

Thyrotoxicosis can be caused by different disorders, which include: Graves disease, hyperfunctional thyroid adenoma, goiter with hyperthyroidism, some types of thyroiditis, Increased TSH from pituitary adenoma or TRH from thalamus. Graves disease is the most common cause of toxic goiter, which is autoimmune disease induced by autoantibodies to the TSH receptor. The autoantibodies to the TSH receptor are detectable in almost all patients with Graves disease. Several autoantibodies mimic the action of TSH, resulting in the stimulation of thyroid epithelial cell activity. What propels B cells to make autoantibodies is not clear. CD4$^+$ helper T cells are highly suspected to be starter, many of which are found within the thyroid. Genetic factors are also important in the causation of Graves disease. There is a genetic susceptibility to Graves disease associated with the presence of certain HLA haplotypes, specifically HLA-B8 and-DR3, and allelic variants (polymorphisms) in genes encoding the inhibitory T-cell receptor CTLA-4 and the tyrosine phosphatase PTPN22.

(2) Morphology

In the typical case of Graves disease, the thyroid gland is diffusely enlarged because of the presence of diffuse hypertrophy and hyperplasia of thyroid follicular epithelial cells. The gland is usually smooth and soft, and its capsule is intact(Figure 14–7). Microscopically, the follicular epithelial cells in untreated cases are tall, columnar, and more crowded than usual. This crowding often results in the formation of small papillae, which project into the follicular lumen(Figure 14–8). Such papillae lack fibrovascular cores, in contrast to those of papillary carcinoma. The colloid is typically pale with prominent peripheral scalloping indicating high turnover. Stroma may show lymphoid infiltrate(Figure 14–9), sometimes with germinal center formation. Stroma fibrosis occurs later. Radiotherapy can induce atypical changes in the follicular epithelium.

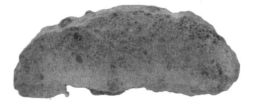

Figure 14–7   Diffusely enlarged thyroid

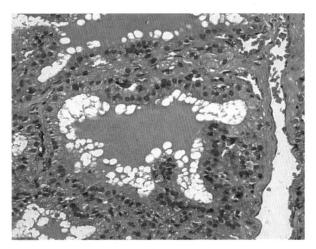

Figure 14–8   Small papillae and peripheral scalloping

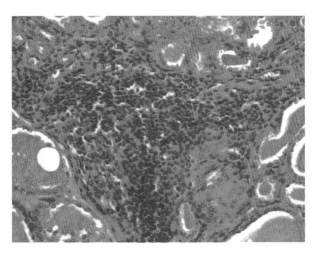

Figure 14–9   Lymphoid infiltration

Changes in extra-thyroidal tissues include generalized lymphoid hyperplasia. In individuals with ophthalmopathy, the tissues of the orbit are edematous, because of the presence of hydrophilic glycosaminoglycans. In addition, there is infiltration by lymphocytes, mostly T cells. Orbital muscles are edematous initially but may undergo fibrosis late in the course of the disease.

14.2.2　Hypothyroidism

Hypothyroidism is a low metabolism syndrome caused by sero-thyroxin level declined by either structure or functional reason. Hypothyroidism can be divided into primary and secondary categories, depending on whether the hypothyroidism arises from an intrinsic abnormality in the thyroid or results from hypothalamic or pituitary disease. The common cause of primary hypothyroidism is caused because majority gland destroyed by thyroid surgery, radiation, some drugs, some infiltrative disorders or thyroiditis. Secondary hypothyroidism is caused by TSH deficiency resulting from any of the causes of hypopituitarism, including a pituitary tumor, postpartum pituitary necrosis, or trauma. Sometimes hypothyroidism also can be caused by TRH deficiency because of hypothalamus disorders.

14.2.2.1　Myxedeyma

Hypothyroidism in older children or adults is sometimes called myxedema. It is manifested by a general slowing of the body's metabolic processes. Frequently, there are localized accumulations of mucinous material in the skin, from which the disease received its name. Manifestations of myxedema include generalized apathy and mental sluggishness that in the early stages of disease may mimic depression. Individuals with myxedema are listless, cold intolerant, and often obese. Mucopolysaccharide-rich edema accumulates in skin, subcutaneous tissue, and a number of visceral sites, with resultant broadening and coarsening of facial features, enlargement of the tongue, and deepening of the voice. Bowel motility is decreased, resulting in constipation. Pericardial effusions are common; in later stages the heart is enlarged, and heart failure may supervene.

14.2.2.2　Cretinism

It refers to hypothyroidism developing in infancy or early childhood. This disorder is common in areas of the world where dietary iodine deficiency is endemic. Clinical features of cretinism include impaired development of skeletal system and central nervous system. The severity of the mental impairment in cretinism seems to be directly influenced by the time at which thyroid deficiency occurs in utero.

14.2.3　Thyroiditis

Thyroiditis is a group of disorders characterized by some form of thyroid inflammation. These diseases include conditions that result in acute illness with severe thyroid pain and disorders in which there is relatively little inflammation and the illness is manifested primarily by thyroid dysfunction. This section focuses on the more common and clinically significant types of thyroiditis:①subacute thyroiditis;②Hashimoto thyroiditis(or chronic lymphocytic thyroiditis) ;③Riedel's thyroiditis.

14.2.3.1　Subacute Thyroiditis

Subacute thyroiditis, also known as granulomatous thyroiditis or De Quervain's thyroiditis is much less common than Hashimoto disease. It clinically presents with sore throat, marked tenderness in thyroid area, fever and malaise. De Quervain's thyroiditis most commonly affects middle-aged women. Subacute thyroiditis is believed to be caused by a *viral infection* or a postviral inflammatory process. The majority of patients have a history of an upper respiratory infection just before the onset of thyroiditis. In contrast to autoimmune thyroid disease, the immune response is not self-perpetuating, so the process is limited.

Morphology:The gland is firm, with an intact capsule, and may be unilaterally or bilaterally enlarged.

Histologically, there is disruption of thyroid follicles, with extravasation of colloid leading to foreign-body giant cell granulomas and chronic inflammatory cells infiltration (Figure 14 – 10). Granuloma are indistinct and usually noncaseating and surrounded by follicles. Some giant cell can contain ingested colloid materials. Healing occurs by resolution of inflammation and fibrosis.

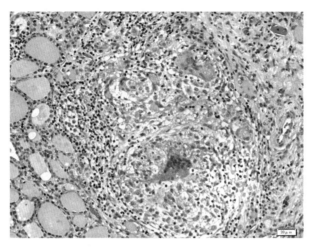

Figure 14–10   **Foreign-body giant cell granulomas**

14.2.3.2   Chronic Lymphocytic(Hashimoto) Thyroiditis

Hashimoto thyroiditis is the most common cause of hypothyroidism in areas of the world where iodine levels are sufficient. It is an immune-mediated inflammatory disease, also called autoimmune thyroiditis. This disorder is most common between 45 and 65 years of age and is more common in women than in men, with a female predominance of 10 : 1 to 20 : 1. Although it is primarily a disease of older women, it can occur in children and is a major cause of nonendemic goiter in children.

Grossly, the thyroid is usually diffusely and symmetrically enlarged, although more localized enlargement may be seen in some cases. The capsule is intact, and the gland is well demarcated from adjacent structures. The cut surface is pale, gray-tan, firm, and somewhat friable. Microscopic examination reveals marked lymphocytic infiltration of the thyroid parenchyma with well-developed germinal center formation (Figure 14–11). The follicles are small and atrophic and show marked oncocytic change of follicular epithelium cells distinguished by the presence of abundant eosinophilic, granular cytoplasm and enlarged,

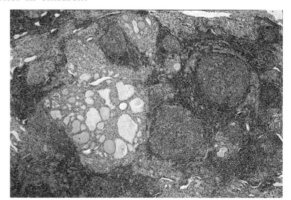

Figure 14–11   **Marked lymphocytic infiltration and atrophic follicles**

hyperchromatic nuclei, termed Hürthle, or oxyphil cells. Ultrastructurally the Hürthle cells are characterized by numerous prominent mitochondria. Interstitial connective tissue is increased and usually abundant, except for fibrosing variant. Unlike in Reidel's thyroiditis, the fibrosis does not extend beyond the capsule of the gland.

14.2.3.3   Riedel's Thyroiditis

It is also called fibrous thyroiditis, chronic woody thyroiditis, or invasive thyroiditis. Riedel thyroiditis is a rare disorder of unknown etiology and more common in older age women. It is characterized by extensive fibrosis involving the thyroid and contiguous neck structures. The presence of a hard and fixed thyroid mass clinically simulates a thyroid neoplasm. It may be associated with idiopathic fibrosis in other sites in the body, such as the retroperitoneum.

Grossly, only part of thyroid gland is involved by a hard, stone-like fibrotic process. The cut surface show solid, fibrotic tissue that often extend beyond the thyroid capsule into perithyroid tissue. In histology, thyroid parenchyma is replaced by extensive fibrosis, frequent hyalinization, admixed with focal chronic inflammation cells. Important feature is presence of chronic inflammation of venous walls within areas of fibrosis and no giant cell is present.

14.2.4 Neoplasm of Thyroid Gland

The thyroid gland gives rise to a variety of neoplasms, ranging from circumscribed, benign adenomas to highly aggressive, anaplastic carcinomas. Fortunately, the overwhelming majority of solitary nodules of the thyroid prove to be benign lesions, either follicular adenomas or localized, non-neoplastic conditions (e. g. , nodular hyperplasia, simple cysts, or foci of thyroiditis). In the following sections, we will consider the major thyroid neoplasms, including adenomas and carcinomas of various types.

14.2.4.1 Adenoma

Adenomas of the thyroid are benign neoplasms derived from follicular epithelium. As in the case of all thyroid neoplasms, follicular adenomas are usually solitary. Clinically and morphologically, they may be difficult to distinguish, between either hyperplastic nodules or, on the other hand, from the less common follicular carcinomas. Although the vast majority of adenomas are nonfunctional, a small proportion produces thyroid hormones ("toxic adenomas") and causes clinically apparent thyrotoxicosis.

(1) Morphology

The typical thyroid adenoma is a solitary round to oval tumor with a complete fibrous capsule, which compress the adjacent non-neoplastic thyroid. On the cut surface, it shows a firm, homogeneous, grey-white or brown mass (Figure 14-12). These features are important in making the distinction from multinodular goiters, which contain multiple nodules on their cut surface (even though the patient may present clinically with a solitary dominant nodule), they donet demonstrate compression of the adjacent thyroid parenchyma, and lack a well-formed capsule (Table 14-2).

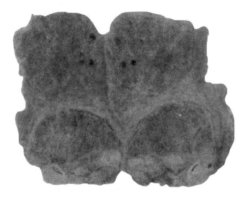

Figure 14 – 12   Thyroid adenoma with a complete fibrous capsule

Table 14-2　Discrimination of thyroid adenoma and nodular goiter

parameters	thyroid adenoma	nodular goiter
Nodular	single	multiple
capsule	intact	Not intact
glands in capsule	concordant	Not concordant
glands in and out of capsule	different	same
Compressed gland near the outside of capsule	yes	no

　　Microscopically, the constituent cells are arranged in uniform follicles (Figure 14-13). The follicular growth pattern within the adenoma is usually quite distinct from the surrounding non-neoplastic gland, and this is another distinguishing feature from multinodular goiters, in which nodular and uninvolved thyroid parenchyma demonstrate comparable growth patterns. The neoplastic cells are uniform, with well-defined cell borders. Similar to endocrine tumors at other anatomic sites, even benign follicular adenomas may, on occasion, exhibit focal nuclear pleomorphism, atypia, and prominent nucleoli (endocrine atypia); by itself this does not constitute a feature of malignancy. The hallmark of all follicular adenomas is the presence of an intact well-formed capsule encircling the tumor. Careful evaluation of the integrity of the capsule is therefore critical in the distinction of follicular adenomas from follicular carcinomas, which demonstrate capsular and/or vascular invasion (see below). Thyroid adenoma can have different patterns (subtypes): Simple adenoma exhibits mature follicles with a normal amount of colloid. Colloid adenoma is similar to simple adenoma, except the follicles are larger and containing more colloid. Embryonal adenoma is distinguished by a trabecular pattern in which poorly formed follicles contain little or no colloid. Fetal adenoma is similar to embryonal adenoma but tend to be arranged in microfollicles containing little colloid. Hürthle cell adenoma, the neoplastic cells acquire brightly eosinophilic granular cytoplasm (oxyphil or Hürthle cell change). Histologic subtypes have no clinical importance.

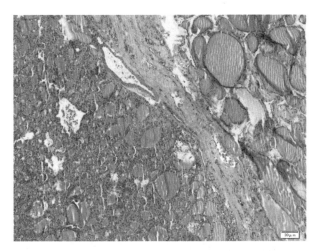

Figure 14-13　Uniform follicles in thyroid adenoma on the left side

(2) Clinical Features

Most adenomas of the thyroid present as painless nodules, often discovered during a routine physical examination. Larger masses may produce local symptoms such as difficulty in swallowing. Additional techniques used in the preoperative evaluation of suspected adenomas are ultrasonography and fine-needle aspiration biopsy. Because of the need for evaluating capsular integrity, the definitive diagnosis of thyroid adenoma can only be made after careful histologic examination of the resected specimen. Suspected adenomas of the thyroid are therefore removed surgically to exclude malignancy. Thyroid adenomas have an excellent prognosis and do not recur or metastasize.

14.2.4.2　Carcinoma

The major subtypes of thyroid carcinoma and their relative frequencies are as follows：

Papillary carcinoma(75% to 85% of cases)；Follicular carcinoma(10% to 20% of cases)；Medullary carcinoma(5% of cases)；Anaplastic carcinoma(<5% of cases)

Most thyroid carcinomas are derived from the follicular epithelium, except for medullary carcinomas; the latter are derived from the parafollicular, or C cells. Because of the unique clinical and biologic features associated with each variant of thyroid carcinoma, these subtypes will be described separately.

(1)Papillary Carcinoma

Papillary carcinomas represent the most common form of thyroid cancer. They may occur at any age, and they account for the vast majority of thyroid carcinomas associated with previous exposure to ionizing radiation.

1)Morphology：Papillary carcinomas may present as solitary or multifocal lesions that are well circumscribed and even encapsulated. The lesions may contain areas of fibrosis and calcification and are often cystic. The tumors have white-grey, firm, granular cut surface, and may have small papillary structures. Papillary carcinoma can be diagnosed only after microscopic examination. A papillary architecture, complex branching true papillae (contain fibro-vascular stalks) , usually accompanied with formation of psammoma body, is present in many cases(Figure 14–14). As currently used, the diagnosis of papillary carcinoma is based on nuclear features even in the absence of a papillary architecture. The nuclei of papillary carcinoma cells are large, oval, or irregular, contain very finely dispersed chromatin, which imparts an optically clear appearance (Figure 14 – 15) , giving rise to the designation " ground-glass " , with crowding/overlapping, nuclear grooves, or nuclear pseudoinclusions. Although some tumors are composed predominantly or exclusively of follicles, these follicular variants still behave biologically as papillary carcinomas if they have the nuclear features described.

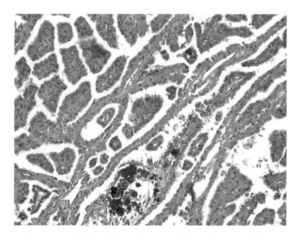

Figure 14–14　Complex branching true papillae

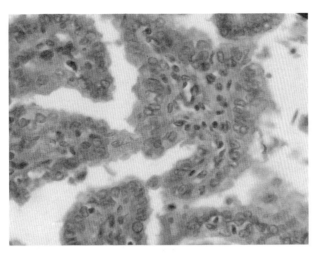

Figure 14-15   **Ground-glass nuclei**

2) Clinical Features: Papillary carcinomas present most often as a painless mass in the neck, either within the thyroid or as metastasis in a cervical lymph node. But regional lymph node metastasis typically does not adversely affect long-term prognosis. In a minority of patients, hematogenous metastases are present at the time of diagnosis, most commonly to the lung. In general, the prognosis is less favorable among elderly persons and in patients with invasion of extra-thyroidal tissues or distant metastases.

(2) Follicular Carcinoma

Follicular carcinoma is defined as a malignant epithelial tumor with follicular cell differentiation and no features of the other distinctive types of thyroid malignancy. It is the second most common form of thyroid cancer. They usually present at an older age than papillary carcinomas.

1) Morphology: Grossly, it is similar to follicular adenoma that may be impossible to distinguish from follicular adenomas on gross examination. This distinction requires extensive histologic sampling of the tumor-capsule-thyroid interface, to exclude capsular (Figure 14 – 16) and/or vascular invasion (Figure 14-17). Extensive invasion of adjacent thyroid parenchyma or nerves makes the diagnosis of carcinoma obvious in some cases(Figure 14-18). Microscopically, most follicular carcinomas are composed of fairly uniform cells forming small follicles, reminiscent of normal thyroid.

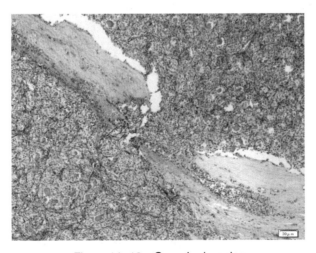

Figure 14-16   **Capsular invasion**

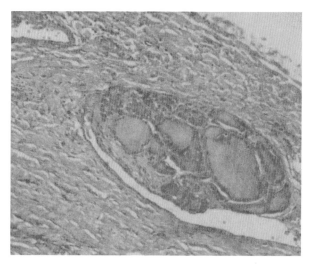

Figure 14-17　vascular invasion

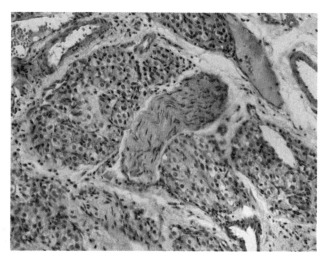

Figure 14-18　Extensive invasion of nerves

2) Clinical features: Follicular carcinomas present most frequently as solitary "cold" thyroid nodules. These neoplasms tend to metastasize through the bloodstream to the lungs, bone, and liver. Regional nodal metastases are uncommon, in contrast to papillary carcinomas.

3) Medullary carcinoma: Medullary carcinoma is a malignant neuroendocrine neoplasm composed of cells with C-cell differentiation, characterized by not containing thyroglobulin (TG) (Figure 14-19) but calcitonin. Medullary carcinomas may arise as a solitary nodule or may present as multiple lesions involving both lobes of the thyroid. Larger lesions often contain areas of necrosis and hemorrhage and may extend through the capsule of the thyroid. Microscopically, medullary carcinomas are composed of polygonal to spindle-shaped cells, which may form nests, trabeculae, and even follicles (Figure 14-20). Acellular amyloid deposits, derived from altered calcitonin molecules, are present in the adjacent stroma in many cases and are a distinctive feature of these tumors. Calcitonin is readily demonstrable both within the cytoplasm of the tumor cells and in the stromal amyloid by immunohistochemical methods (Figure 14-21).

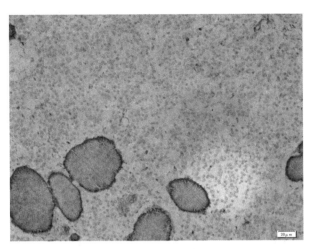

Figure 14-19   TG(-)in medullary carcinoma

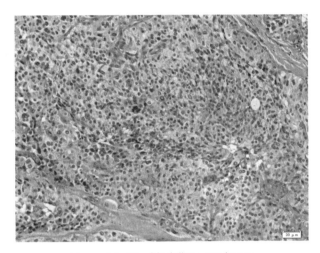

Figure 14-20   Medullary carcinoma

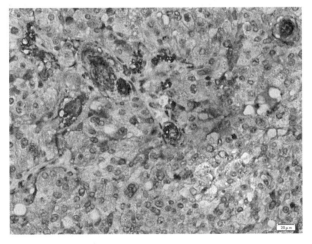

Figure 14-21   Calcitonin(+)in medullary carcinoma

4) Anaplastic carcinoma: Anaplastic carcinomas of the thyroid are among the most aggressive human neoplasms, with a near-uniform mortality rate, which is totally or partially undifferentiated. Individuals with

anaplastic carcinoma are older than those with other types of thyroid cancer, with a mean age of 65 years. Anaplastic carcinomas present as bulky masses that typically grow rapidly beyond the thyroid capsule into adjacent neck structures. Microscopically, these neoplasms are composed of highly anaplastic cells, which may take on several histologic patterns, including ①large, pleomorphic giant cells; ②spindle cells with a sarcomatous appearance; ③mixed spindle and giant-cell lesions; ④small cells, resembling those seen in small-cell carcinomas at other sites. It is unlikely that a true small-cell carcinoma exists in the thyroid, and most of the "anaplastic small-cell" tumors ultimately proved to be medullary carcinomas or malignant lymphomas. Foci of papillary or follicular differentiation may be present in some tumors, suggesting origin from a better differentiated carcinoma.

14.3 Adrenal Gland

The adrenal glands are paired endocrine organs, located above the kidney. Each adrenal consists of two separate endocrine glands, the cortex and the medulla, which differ in their development, structure, and function. This section deals firstly with disorders of the adrenal cortex, and then of the medulla.

14.3.1 The Adrenal Cortex

The cortex consists of three layers of distinct cell types. Beneath the capsule of the adrenal is the narrow layer of zona glomerulosa. An equally narrow zona reticularis abuts the medulla. Intervening is the broad zona fasciculata, which makes up about 75% of the total cortex. The adrenal cortex synthesizes three different types of steroids: ①glucocorticoids (principally cortisol), which are synthesized primarily in the zona fasciculata with a small contribution from the zona reticularis; ②mineralocorticoids, the most important being aldosterone, which is generated in the zona glomerulosa; ③sex steroids (estrogens and androgens), which are produced largely in the zona reticularis. Diseases of the adrenal cortex can be conveniently divided into those associated with cortical hyperfunction and those characterized by cortical hypofunction.

14.3.1.1 Adrenocortical Hyperfunction(Hyperadrenalism)

Just as there are three basic types of corticosteroids elaborated by the adrenal cortex (glucocorticoids, mineralocorticoids, and sex steroids), so there are three distinctive hyperadrenal clinical syndromes: ①cushing syndrome, characterized by an excess of cortisol; ②hyperaldosteronism; ③adrenogenital or virilizing syndromes, caused by an excess of androgens. The clinical features of some of these syndromes overlap somewhat because of the overlapping functions of some of the adrenal steroids.

(1)Cushing syndrome

This disorder is caused by any condition that produces an elevation in glucocorticoid levels. The glucocorticoids excess causes disturbances of carbohydrate, protein, and fat metabolism. The blood glucose rises. Protein synthesis is impaired and body proteins are broken down, which leads to loss of muscle fibers and muscle weakness. Bones become weaker and more susceptible to fracture as the protein breakdown leads to loss of the connective tissue framework of the bones. The amount and distribution of body fat is altered. Fat tends to accumulate on the trunk, while the extremities appear thin and wasted because of muscle atrophy. The skin becomes thin and bruises easily. Stretch marks(striae)often appear in the skin as fat deposits accumulate in the subcutaneous tissues of the trunk. The face appears full and rounded, which is sometimes called a "moon face". Salt and water are retained because of the increased output of mineralocorticoids, leading to an increase in blood volume and a rise in blood pressure.

Four distinct conditions may give rise to this syndrome:

An ACTH-producing tumor of the pituitary, which stimulates the adrenal gland to enlarge and produce excess hormone. The most common cause of a corticosteroid excess is a small ACTH secreting pituitary adenoma, and this condition is called Cushing's disease, accounts for more than half of the cases of spontaneous, endogenous Cushing syndrome.

A corticosteroid-hormone-producing tumor of the adrenal cortex.

Administration of large amounts of corticosteroid hormone to treat diseases that respond to the hormone, as may be required to help suppress the immune response in recipients of organ transplants or patients with autoimmune diseases, or to help induce remission in patients with leukemia.

A malignant tumor, such as a small cell lung carcinoma, that produces ACTH or a similar protein that resembles the "real" hormone.

The morphology of the adrenal glands depends on the cause of the hypercortisolism. The adrenals have one of the following abnormalities: ①cortical atrophy; ②diffuse hyperplasia; ③nodular hyperplasia; ④an adenoma, rarely a carcinoma.

(2)Overproduction of Aldosterone

Aldosterone promotes absorption of salt and water by the kidneys in exchange for potassium which is excreted, and its secretion is regulated primarily by the rennin-angiotension-aldosterone. In roughly 80% of cases, primary hyperaldosteronism is caused by an aldosterone-secreting adenoma in one adrenal gland, a condition referred to as Conn syndrome. The clinical manifestations of primary hyperaldosteronism are those of hypertension and hypokalemia. The aldosterone excess produced by the tumor promotes excessive absorption of sodium and excessive excretion of potassium by the kidneys. Since water is absorbed along with the sodium, the blood volume increases along with the sodium concentration and the blood pressure also rises along with the blood volume. The excessive hormone-induced excretion of potassium lowers blood potassium, which impairs neuromuscular function and leads to muscle weakness. The high aldosterone output exerts a negative feedback effect on rennin production by the kidneys, and plasma rennin falls.

(3)Overproduction of Adrenal Sex Hormones

Adrenal gland dysfunction associated with abnormal production of sex hormone is uncommon. This may result from congenital hyperplasia of the adrenal gland or from an adrenal sex-hormone-producing tumor. Adrenal tumors that elaborate sex hormones are rare. When such a tumor develops, however, either androgen or estrogen may be produced. The clinical features depend on the age of the individual when the tumor becomes manifested and on the sex of affected person. In a child, the tumor produces precocious puberty, and the character of the sexual development depends on the type of hormone elaborated. In adults, an estrogen-producing neoplasm elicits no hormonal symptoms in women but induces feminization in men. An antrogen-secreting tumor masculinizes a woman but causes no hormonal symptoms in a man.

14.3.1.2 Adrenal Insufficiency

Adrenocortical insufficiency, or hypofunction, may be caused by either primary adrenal disease(primary hypoadrenalism) or decreased stimulation of the adrenals resulting from a deficiency of ACTH(secondary hypoadrenalism). The patterns of adrenocortical insufficiency can be considered under the following headings: ①primary acute adrenocortical insufficiency(adrenal crisis); ②primary chronic adrenocortical insufficiency(Addison disease); ③secondary adrenocortical insufficiency.

(1)Acute Adrenocortical Insufficiency

Acute adrenocortical insufficiency occurs most commonly in the clinical settings listed below:

Individuals with chronic adrenocortical insufficiency may develop an acute crisis after any stress that taxes their limited physiologic reserves.

In patients maintained on exogenous corticosteroids, rapid withdrawal of steroids or failure to increase steroid doses in response to an acute stress may precipitate a similar adrenal crisis, because of the inability of the atrophic adrenals to produce glucocorticoid hormones.

Massive adrenal hemorrhage may destroy the adrenal cortex sufficiently to cause acute adrenocortical insufficiency. This condition may occur in patients maintained on anticoagulant therapy, in postoperative patients who develop disseminated intravascular coagulation, during pregnancy, and in patients suffering from overwhelming sepsis(Waterhouse-Friderichsen syndrome). The pathogenesis of the Waterhouse-Friderichsen syndrome remains unclear, but it probably involves endotoxin-induced vascular injury with associated disseminated intravascular coagulation.

(2)Chronic Adrenocortical Insufficiency(Addison Disease)

Addison disease, or chronic adrenocortical insufficiency, is an uncommon disorder resulting from progressive destruction of the adrenal cortex. In most cases, the disease results from more than 90% of all cases and are attributable to one of four disorders; autoimmune adrenalitis, tuberculosis, the acquired immune deficiency syndrome(AIDS)or metastatic cancers.

In general, clinical manifestations of adrenocortical insufficiency do not appear until at least 90% of the adrenal cortex has been compromised. The initial manifestations often include progressive weakness and easy fatigability, which may be dismissed as nonspecific complaints. Gastrointestinal disturbances are common and include anorexia, nausea, vomiting, weight loss, and diarrhea. In individuals with primary adrenal disease, increased levels of ACTH precursor hormone stimulate melanocytes, with resultant *hyperpigmentation* of the skin and mucosal surfaces. The face, axillae, nipples, areolae, and perineum are particularly common sites of hyperpigmentation. By contrast, hyperpigmentation is not seen in individuals with secondary adrenocortical insufficiency. Decreased mineralocorticoid(aldosterone)activity in patients with primary adrenal insufficiency results in potassium retention and sodium loss, with consequent hyperkalemia, hyponatremia, volume depletion, and hypotension; in contrast, secondary hypoadrenalism is characterized by deficient cortisol and androgen output but normal or near-normal aldosterone synthesis. Hypoglycemia may occasionally occur as a result of glucocorticoid deficiency and impaired gluconeogenesis. Stresses such as infections, trauma, or surgical procedures in such patients may precipitate an acute adrenal crisis, manifested by intractable vomiting, abdominal pain, hypotension, coma, and vascular collapse. Death follows rapidly unless corticosteroids are replaced immediately.

14.3.1.3 Adrenocortical Neoplasms

(1)Adrenocortical Adenomas

Adrenocortical adenomas were described in the earlier discussions of Cushing syndrome and hyperaldosteronism. Most cortical adenomas do not cause hyperfunction and are usually encountered as incidental findings at the time of autopsy or during abdominal imaging for an unrelated cause. In fact, the half-facetious appellation of "adrenal incidentaloma" has crept into the medical lexicon to describe these incidentally discovered tumors. On cut surface, adenomas are usually yellow to yellow-brown, owing to the presence of lipid within the neoplastic cells(Figure 14-22). As a general rule they are small, averaging 1 to 2 cm in diameter. Microscopically, adenomas are composed of cells similar to those populating the normal adrenal cortex. The nuclei tend to be small, although some degree of pleomorphism may be encountered even in benign lesions("endocrine atypia"). The cytoplasm of the neoplastic cells ranges from eosinophilic to vacuolated (Figure 14-23), depending on their lipid content; mitotic activity is generally inconspicuous.

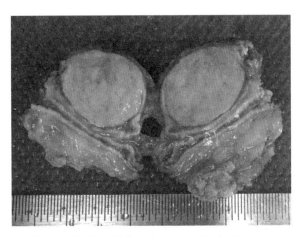

Figure 14-22　Yellow adrenocortical adenoma

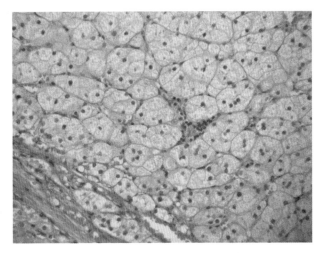

Figure 14-23　Vacuolated cytoplasm

(2) Adrenocortical Carcinomas

Adrenocortical carcinomas are rare neoplasms that may occur at any age, including in childhood. In most cases, adrenocortical carcinomas are large, invasive lesions that efface the native adrenal gland. On cut surface, adrenocortical carcinomas are typically variegated, poorly demarcated lesions containing areas of necrosis, hemorrhage, and cystic change. Microscopically, adrenocortical carcinomas may be composed of well-differentiated cells resembling those seen in cortical adenomas or bizarre, pleomorphic cells, which may be difficult to distinguish from those of an undifferentiated carcinoma metastatic to the adrenal. Adrenal cancers have a strong tendency to invade the adrenal vein, vena cava, and lymphatics. Metastases to regional and periaortic nodes are common, as are distant hematogenous spread to the lungs and other viscera. Bone metastases are unusual. The median patient survival is about 2 years.

14.3.2　Adrenal Medulla

The adrenal medulla is composed of chromaffin cells, which synthesize and secrete catecholamines, mainly epinephrine. The most important diseases of the adrenal medulla are neoplasms, which include both neuronal neoplasms(including neuroblastomas and more mature ganglion cell tumors) and neoplasms composed of chromaffin cells(pheochromocytomas).

Pheochromocytomas

Pheochromocytomas are neoplasms composed of chromaffin cells, which, like their non-neoplastic counterparts, synthesize and release catecholamines and in some cases, other peptide hormones. These tumors are of special importance because, although uncommon, they (like aldosterone-secreting adenomas) give rise to a surgically correctable form of hypertension.

(1) Morphology

Pheochromocytomas range from small, circumscribed lesions confined to the adrenal to large, hemorrhagic masses weighing several kilograms. On cut surface, smaller pheochromocytomas are yellow-tan, well-defined lesions that compress the adjacent adrenal. Larger lesions tend to be hemorrhagic, necrotic, and cystic and typically efface the adrenal gland. Microscopically, pheochromocytomas are composed of polygonal to spindle-shaped chromaffin cells and their supporting cells, compartmentalized into small nests by a rich vascular network (Figure 14-24). The cytoplasm of the neoplastic cells often is basophilous and has a finely granular appearance (Figure 14-24), highlighted by a variety of silver stains, because of the presence of granules containing catecholamines. Chromogranin is always positive within the cytoplasm of the tumor cells (Figure 14-25). Both capsular and vascular invasion may be encountered in benign lesions, and the presence of mitotic figures does not imply malignancy. Therefore, the definitive diagnosis of malignancy in pheochromocytomas is based exclusively on the presence of metastases. These may involve regional lymph nodes as well as more distant sites, including liver, lung, and bone.

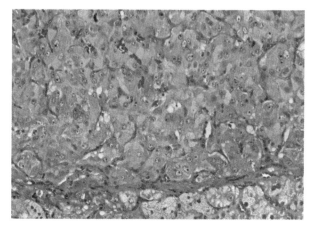

Figure 14-24   Polygonal chromaffin cells

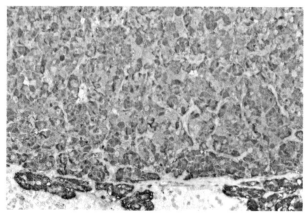

Figure 14-25   Chromogranin (+)

(2) Clinical Features

The dominant clinical manifestation of pheochromocytoma is hypertension. Classically, this is described as an abrupt, precipitous elevation in blood pressure, associated with tachycardia, palpitations, headache, sweating, tremor, and a sense of apprehension. Such episodes may also be associated with pain in the abdomen or chest, nausea, and vomiting. In practice, isolated, paroxysmal episodes of hypertension occur in fewer than half of individuals with pheochromocytoma. In about two-thirds of patients the hypertension occurs in the form of a chronic, sustained elevation in blood pressure, although an element of labile hypertension is often present as well. Whether sustained or episodic, the hypertension is associated with an increased risk of myocardial ischemia, heart failure, renal injury, and cerebrovascular accidents. In some cases, pheochromocytomas secrete other hormones such as ACTH and somatostatin and may therefore be associated with clinical features related to the secretion of these and other peptide hormones. The laboratory diagnosis of pheochromocytoma is based on demonstration of increased urinary excretion of free catecholamines and their metabolites, such as vanillylmandelic acid and metanephrines. Isolated benign pheochromocytomas are treated with surgical excision, after preoperative and intraoperative medication of patients with adrenergic-blocking agents. Multifocal lesions may require long-term medical treatment for hypertension.

14.4 Endocrine Pancreas

The endocrine pancreas consists of about 1 million microscopic clusters of cells, the islets of Langerhans, which contain 4 major cell types-β, α, δ, and PP (pancreatic polypeptide) cells. The cells can be differentiated morphologically by their staining properties, by the ultrastructural structure of their granules, and by their hormone content. The β cell produces insulin, which is the most potent anabolic hormone known, with multiple synthetic and growth-promoting effects; the α cell secretes glucagon, inducing hyperglycemia by its glycogenolytic activity in the liver; δ cells contain somatostatin, which suppresses both insulin and glucagon release; and PP cells contain a unique pancreatic polypeptide (vasoactive intestinal peptide, VIP) that exerts several gastrointestinal effects, such as stimulation of secretion of gastric and intestinal enzymes and inhibition of intestinal motility.

14.4.1 Diabetes Mellitus

Diabetes mellitus is not a single disease entity but rather a group of metabolic disorders sharing the common underlying feature of hyperglycemia. Hyperglycemia in diabetes results from defects in insulin secretion, insulin action, or, most commonly, both. The chronic hyperglycemia and attendant metabolic dysregulation of diabetes mellitus may be associated with secondary damage in multiple organ systems, especially the kidneys, eyes, nerves, and blood vessels.

14.4.1.1 Classification

The vast majority of cases of diabetes fall into one of two broad classes, depending on whether the diabetes results primarily from insulin deficiency or from inadequate response to insulin. Type 1 diabetes is characterized by an absolute deficiency of insulin secretion caused by pancreatic β-cell destruction, usually resulting from an autoimmune attack. Type 1 diabetes accounts for approximately 10% of all cases. Type 2 diabetes is caused by a combination of peripheral resistance to insulin action and an inadequate compensatory response of insulin secretion by the pancreatic β cells ("relative insulin deficiency"). Approximately 80% to 90% of patients have type 2 diabetes.

(1) Pathogenesis of Type 1 Diabetes Mellitus

Type 1 diabetes is an autoimmune disease in which islet destruction is caused primarily by T lymphocytes reacting against as yet poorly defined β-cell antigens, resulting in a reduction in β-cell mass. Type 1 diabetes most commonly develops in childhood, becomes manifest at puberty, and is progressive with age. Most individuals with type 1 diabetes depend on exogenous insulin supplementation for survival, and without insulin, they develop serious metabolic complications such as acute ketoacidosis and coma. Although the clinical onset of type 1 diabetes is abrupt, this disease in fact results from a chronic autoimmune attack on β cells that usually starts many years before the disease becomes evident. The classic manifestations of the disease (hyperglycemia and ketosis) occur late in its course, after more than 90% of the β cells have been destroyed.

(2) Pathogenesis of Type 2 Diabetes Mellitus

The pathogenesis of type 2 diabetes remains enigmatic. Environmental influences, such as a sedentary life style and dietary habits, clearly have a role, as will become evident when obesity is considered. Nevertheless, genetic factors are even more important than in type 1 diabetes, with linkage demonstrable to multiple "diabetogenic" genes. The two metabolic defects that characterize type 2 diabetes are ①a decreased ability of peripheral tissues to respond to insulin (insulin resistance) and ②β-cell dysfunction that is manifested as inadequate insulin secretion in the face of insulin resistance and hyperglycemia. In most cases, insulin resistance is the primary event and is followed by increasing degrees of β-cell dysfunction.

Insulin resistance is defined as resistance to the effects of insulin on glucose uptake, metabolism, or storage. Insulin resistance is a characteristic feature of most individuals with type 2 diabetes and is an almost universal finding in diabetic individuals who are obese.

14.4.1.2 Morphology of Diabetes and Its Late Complications

Pathologic findings in the pancreas are variable and not necessarily dramatic. The important morphologic changes are related to the many late systemic complications of diabetes. In individuals with tight control of diabetes the onset may be delayed. In most patients, however, morphologic changes are likely to be found in arteries (macrovascular disease), basement membranes of small vessels (microangiopathy), kidneys (diabetic nephropathy), retina (retinopathy), nerves (neuropathy), and other tissues. These changes are seen in both type 1 and type 2 diabetes.

(1) Pancreas

Lesions in the pancreas are inconstant and rarely of diagnostic value. Distinctive changes are more commonly associated with type 1 than with type 2 diabetes.

Reduction in the number and size of islets is most often seen in type 1 diabetes, particularly with rapidly advancing disease. Eosinophilic infiltrates may also be found, particularly in diabetic infants who fail to survive the immediate postnatal period.

In type 2 diabetes, there may be a subtle reduction in islet cell mass, demonstrated only by special morphometric studies. Amyloid replacement of islets in long-standing type 2 diabetes appears as deposition of pink, amorphous material beginning in and around capillaries and between cells. At advanced stages the islets may be virtually obliterated; fibrosis may also be observed. This change is often seen in long-standing cases of type 2 diabetes.

(2) Macrovascular Disease

Diabetes exacts a heavy toll on the vascular system. The hallmark of diabetic macrovascular disease is accelerated atherosclerosis affecting the aorta and large and medium-sized arteries. Except for its greater severity and earlier age of onset, atherosclerosis in diabetics is indistinguishable from that in nondiabetics. Hyaline arteriolosclerosis, the vascular lesion associated with hypertension, is both more prevalent and more severe in diabetics than in nondiabetics, but it is not specific for diabetes and may be seen in elderly nondiabetics without hypertension.

(3) Microangiopathy

One of the most consistent morphologic features of diabetes is diffuse thickening of basement membranes. The thickening is most evident in the capillaries of the skin, skeletal muscle, retina, renal glomeruli, and renal medulla. However, it may also be seen in such nonvascular structures as renal tubules, the Bowman capsule, peripheral nerves, and placenta.

(4) Diabetic Nephropathy

The kidneys are prime targets of diabetes. Three lesions are encountered: ①glomerular lesions; ②renal vascular lesions, principally arteriolosclerosis; ③pyelonephritis, including necrotizing papillitis.

The most important glomerular lesions are capillary basement membrane thickening; diffuse mesangial sclerosis, and nodular glomerulosclerosis(Figure 14−26). The glomerular capillary basement membranes are thickened throughout their entire length. Diffuse mesangial sclerosis consists of a diffuse increase in mesangial matrix along with mesangial cell proliferation and is always associated with basement membrane thickening. When glomerulosclerosis becomes marked, patients manifest the nephrotic syndrome, characterized by proteinuria, hypoalbuminemia, and edema. Nodular glomerulosclerosis describes a glomerular lesion made distinctive by ball-like deposits of a laminated matrix situated in the periphery of the glomerulus. These nodules are PAS positive and usually contain trapped mesangial cells(Figure 14−27). This distinctive change has been called the Kimmelstiel-Wilson lesion, after the pathologists who described it.

Pyelonephritis is an acute or chronic inflammation of the kidneys that usually begins in the interstitial tissue and then spreads to affect the tubules. Both the acute and chronic forms of this disease occur in nondiabetics as well as in diabetics but are more common in diabetics than in the general population, and once affected, diabetics tend to have more severe involvement. One special pattern of acute pyelonephritis, necrotizing papillitis(or papillary necrosis) , is much more prevalent in diabetics than in nondiabetics.

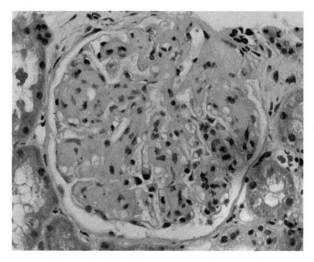

Figure 14−26 Diffuse mesangial sclerosis

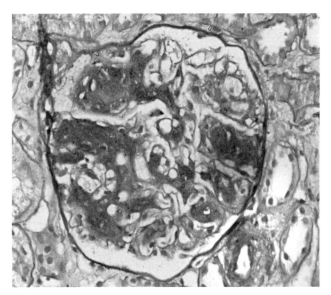

Figure 14-27   **PAS staining positive**

(5) Ocular Complications of Diabetes

, Visual impairment, sometimes even total blindness, is one of the more feared consequences of long-standing diabetes. The ocular involvement may take the form of retinopathy, cataract formation, or glaucoma. Retinopathy, the most common pattern, consists of a constellation of changes that together are considered by many ophthalmologists to be virtually diagnostic of the disease. The lesion in the retina takes two forms: non-proliferative(background) retinopaty and proliferative retinopathy. Nonproliferative retinopathy includes intraretinal or preretinal hemorrhages, retinal exudates, microaneurysms, venous dilations, edema, and, most importantly, thickening of the retinal capillaries(micro-angiopathy). The so-called proliferative retinopathy is a process of neovascularization and fibrosis. This lesion leads to serious consequences, including blindness, especially if it involves the macula. Vitreous hemorrhages can result from rupture of newly formed capillaries; the resultant organization of the hemorrhage can pull the retina off its substratum(retinal detachment).

(6) Diabetic Neuropathy

The central and peripheral nervous systems are not spared by diabetes. The most frequent pattern of involvement is a peripheral, symmetric neuropathy of the lower extremities that affects both motor and sensory function but particularly the latter. Other forms include peripheral neuropathy, which produces disturbances in bowel and bladder function and sometimes sexual impotence, and diabetic mononeuropathy, which may manifest as sudden footdrop, wristdrop, or isolated cranial nerve palsies. The neurologic changes may be caused by microangiopathy and increased permeability of the capillaries that supply the nerves as well as direct axonal damage due to alterations in sorbitolmetabolism(as discussed).

14.4.2   Islet Cell Tumor

Pancreatic endocrine neoplasms, also known as "islet cell tumors", are rare in comparison with tumors of the exocrine pancreas, accounting for only 2% of all pancreatic neoplasms. They are most common in adults, may be single or multiple, and benign or malignant, the latter metastasizing to lymph nodes and liver. Pancreatic endocrine neoplasms have a propensity to produce pancreatic hormones, but some may be totally nonfunctional.

14.4.2.1 Insulinomas

β-cell tumors(insulinomas) are the most common of pancreatic endocrine neoplasms and may be responsible for the elaboration of sufficient insulin to induce clinically significant hypoglycemia. Insulinomas are most often found within the pancreas and are generally benign. Most are solitary lesions, although multiple tumors or tumors ectopic to the pancreas may be encountered. Solitary tumors are usually small(often < 2 cm in diameter) and are encapsulated, pale to red-brown nodules located anywhere in the pancreas. Histologically, these benign tumors look remarkably like giant islets, with preservation of the regular cords of monotonous cells and their orientation to the vasculature. Not even the malignant lesions present much evidence of anaplasia, and they may be deceptively encapsulated. By immunocytochemistry, insulin can be localized in the tumor cells.

While as many as 80% of islet cell tumors may demonstrate excessive insulin secretion, hypoglycemia is mild in all but 20%, and many cases never become clinically symptomatic. The critical laboratory findings in insulinomas are high circulating levels of insulin and a high insulin-to-glucose ratio.

14.4.2.2 Gastrinomas

Marked hypersecretion of gastrin usually has its origin in gastrin-producing tumors (gastrinomas), which are just as likely to arise in the duodenum and peripancreatic soft tissues as in the pancreas(so-called "gastrinoma triangle").

Gastrinomas may arise in the pancreas, the peripancreatic region, or the wall of the duodenum. Over half of gastrin-producing tumors are locally invasive or have already metastasized at the time of diagnosis. In approximately 25% of patients, gastrinomas arise in conjunction with other endocrine tumors, thus conforming to the MEN-1 syndrome(see below); MEN-1−associated gastrinomas are frequently multifocal, while sporadic gastrinomas are usually single. As with insulin-secreting tumors of the pancreas, gastrin-producing tumors are histologically bland and rarely exhibit marked anaplasia.

14.5 Neuroendocrine Tumors of Diffuse Neuroendocrine System (DNES NET)

14.5.1 Diffuse Neuroendocrine System

The neuroendocrine system exists in two phenotypes, either as discreet organoid aggregates(pituitary, adrenal, parathyroid) or as disseminated, nonuniform distribution of cells. This latter group has been assigned the term diffuse neuroendocrine system(DNES). DNES cells are a group of small cells that are individually dispersed among the whole body are known collectively by several names: Argentaffin and argyrophilic cells-because they stain with silver stains; APUD cells-because some of them can take up the precursors of amines and decarboxylate them; or Enteroendocrine cells-because they secrete hormone-like substances and are located in the epithelium of the enteric(alimentary) canal. Some of these cells are individually designated according to the substance that they produce. Generally, a single type of DNES cell secretes only one hormone, although occasional cell types may secrete two different hormones. Cells of the DNES have been localized not only in the digestive tract but also in the respiratory system and in the endocrine pancreas. Additionally, some of the secretory products synthesized and released by these DNES cells are identical with neurosecretions localized in the CNS. The significance of their diverse location and the substances they produce is only incompletely understood.

14.5.2   Neuroendocrine Tumors,NETs

Neuroendocrine tumors originate from diffuse neuroendocrine cells. Tumors express neuroendocrine markers and exhibit other neuroendocrine characteristics. Neuroendocrine tumor is a group of heterogeneous tumors. From pathological morphology to biological behavior, there are great differences between different tumors. Neuroendocrine neoplasms/tumors(NET) once considered "rare" have been steadily increasing in incidence and prevalence over the past 3 decades. DNES NETs occur most frequently in the lung and gastro-entero-pancreatic(GEP) regions. NETs currently represent 2% of all cancers and GEP-NETs represent the second most prevalent gastrointestinal neoplasm after colorectal cancer.

The clinical manifestations of this relatively uncommon disease are protean and nonspecific, thereby leading to alternative diagnoses and the average lag between first symptoms and diagnosis of NET of about 7 years. It is therefore understandable that 60% –80% have metastases at presentation, with the liver being the most common distant metastatic site. There is another important consequence of metastases, the "carcinoid syndrome"(diarrhea, abdominal pain, sweating, flushing, bronchospasm, tachycardia, and fibrotic heart disease). According to cell sources, tumor is divided into two types: nerve type and epithelial type. pheochromocytoma and paraganglioma are nerve type. And some NETs originating from gastrointestinal tract or pancreas belong to the epithelial type.

14.5.3   Gastroenteropancreatic Neuroendocrine Tumors

The World Health Organization(WHO) classification system(2010) in neuroendocrine tumors(NET-G1, NET-G2) and neuroendocrine carcinoma(NEC-G3) is informative(Table 14−3 for the clinical management of neuroendocrine intestinal and lung tumors(carcinoids). Tumors should be classified according to the recent WHO 2010 classification, which has been based on the recently validated concept that all NETs have malignant potential. Grading is based on morphologic criteria seen on light microscopy with conventional staining(mitoses and necrosis) and proliferative activity performed via immunohistochemistry(Ki-67).

Table 14−3   **WHO 2010 grading system**

Grade	Mitotic count	Ki-67 Index	ENETS/WHO
Low(G1)	<2/10 HPF	<3%	NET Grade 1
Intermediate(G2)	2–20/10 HPF	3% –20%	NET Grade 2
High(G3)	>20/10 HPF	>20%	NET Grade 3

Chapter 15

Diseases of Nervous System

> *Introduction*

The nervous system is an enormously complex tissue serving the organism as a processing center linking information between the outside world and the body. The disease of the nervous system has its special characteristics:

(1) The same lesions may occur at different sites and have different clinical manifestations and consequences.

(2) Raised intracranial pressure, cerebral edema, and hydrocephalus are the most common and important complications of central nervous diseases.

(3) Pathogens including bacteria, virus, parasites, rickettsia, helix etc, all can infect the brain, but bacteria, virus infections are more common.

(4) Tumors of the nervous system may arise from the cells of the coverings, from cells intrinsic to the brain, or other cell populations within the skull, or they may spread from elsewhere in the body.

(5) Even low-grade or benign tumors can have a poor clinical outcome depending on where in the brain they occur.

15.1 The Principal Pathologic Changes of the Nervous System Diseases

The nervous system is composed of neuronglial cell (astrocyte, oligodendrocyte, and ependyma), blood vessel, and microglia. It is estimated that more than half of the human genes possess the nervous system specificity.

15.1.1 The Principal Pathologic Changes of the Neuron and Nerve Fiber

Neuron is the principal functional unit of the central nervous system. It is often regarded as one of the most complex or arcane cells in the body organ systems, which may have the following lesions when ischemic anoxia, infection and toxicosis occur in the brain.

15.1.1.1 The Principal Pathologic Changes of the Neuron

(1) Acute Neuronal Injury

There are several well-characterized forms of pathologic reaction of neurons. Coagulation necrosis is the most common feature and occurs in association with acute hypoxia-ischemia injury, infection and toxicosis. Neuronal necrosis is characterized by a loss of cytoplasmic ribonucleoproteins and denaturation of cytoskeletal proteins, resulting in the development of intense cytoplasmic eosinophilia ("red neuron") in hematoxylin and eosin (H & E)-stained sections. In addition, the Nissl body in cytoplasm disappears. Coagulation necrosis is also accompanied by nuclear changes identical to those seen in other organs, including condensation of nuclear material (pyknosis) and loss of nuclear staining (karyolysis). Lastly, the outline or trace of a residual cell is called ghost cell.

(2) Simple Neuronal Atrophy

In fact, simple neuronal atrophy describes a process from neuronal degeneration to neuronal death, which is characterized by condensation of nuclear material (pyknosis) and loss of nuclear staining (karyolysis). In contrast to red neuron, however, the Nissl body in cytoplasm do not disappear. Simple neuronal atrophy often occurs in neurodegenerative disorders, such as multisystem atrophy and Amyotrophic lateral sclerosis (ALS). Loss of atrophic neuron is invisible in the early period and glial cell proliferation appears in later stage.

(3) Central Chromatolysis

Central chromatolysis, a common reaction to viral infection, hypoxia-ischemia, Vitamin B deficiency and axonal injury, is characterized by dispersion of the Nissl substance from the center to the periphery of the cell, perikaryon enlargement, peripheral displacement of the nucleus and enlargement of the nucleolus.

(4) Inclusion Body Formation

Inclusion bodies in the cytoplasm or nucleus of the neuron may be seen in some viral infections and degenerative diseases. Usually, the form and size of inclusion bodies and coloring are also different in different diseases, for example, Lewy corpuscle may occur in the cytoplasm of the substantia nigra neurons of the Parkinson patients, while tehe inclusion bodies can occur simultaneously in the nucleus and cytoplasm of cytomegalovirus infection.

(5) Neurofibrillary Degeneration

Neurofibrillary degeneration, also known as neurofibrillary tangles, is known such a phenomenon in which thickening neurofibrils condense around the nucleus and are tangled, which can be observed by the silver staining.

15.1.1.2 The Principal Pathologic Changes of the Nerve Fiber

(1) Axonal Injury and Axonal Reaction

Axonal reaction occurs when the central nervous axons or peripheral nerve axons are cut or seriously damaged. This process is associated with swelling and disintegration of axon, disintegration of myelin sheath, and cell proliferation reaction (phagocytes phagocytose disintegration product). Degenerative changes in an injured axon occur over the course of time, involving the distal regions of the axon.

(2) Demyelination

Demyelination is caused by degeneration of Schwann or injury of myelin. It refers to separation, swelling, fracture and disintegration of the myelin lamina. The remyelination ability of the myelin sheath is limited in the central nerve system.

15.1.2　The Principal Pathologic Changes of the Neuroglia

Neuroglia is composed of astrocyte, oligodendrocyte, and ependymal cell.

15.1.2.1　The Principal Pathologic Changes of Astrocyte

Astrocytes are major supporting cells in the brain. The most common reactive changes include swelling, reactive astrogliosis and inclusion body formation etc.

(1) Cellular Swelling

Cellular swelling, or swelling of the astrocyte cytoplasm, occurs in acute injury, such as hypoxia, hypoglycemia, and toxic injuries.

(2) Reactive Astrogliosis

Reactive astrogliosis is a kind of reparative reaction, somewhat analogous to a fibrous scar occurring elsewhere in the body. In contrast to fibroblasts, however, astrocytes do not produce collagen. The glial scar, accordingly, is made up predominantly of cytoplasmic processes, with little or no extracellular protein.

(3) Corpora Amylacea

In H&E-stained sections, corpora amylacea, are spherical, faintly basophilic, concentrically lamellated structures and located wherever there are astrocytic foot processes, especially in the subependymal, subpial and perivascular zones.

(4) Rosenthal Fibers

Rosenthal fibers are round, elongated, brightly eosinophilic body in astrocytic cytoplasm. Due to a mutation in the gene for GFAP, in the certain disease(e. g. Alexander disease), abundant Rosenthal fibers are found in periventricular, perivascular, and subpial locations.

15.1.2.2　The Principal Pathologic Changes of Oligodendrocyte

Satellitosis is characterized by five or more than five oligodendrocytes surrounding one degenative neuron cell, which may be related to neurotrophy.

15.1.2.3　The Principal Pathologic Changes of Microglia

Despite their name, it is now generally accepted that microglia are mesoderm-derived cells whose primary function is to serve as a fixed macrophage system in many inflammatory conditions. In the CNS, microglia cells can be activated due to injury.

(1) Neuronophagia

It refers to microglia cells aggregating around cell bodies of dying neurons and engulfing injured neurons. In addition to resident microglia, blood-derived macrophages are the principal phagocytic cells present in inflammatory foci. For example, in Japanese encephalitis, neuronophagia appears as a reaction to necrotic neurons.

(2) Microglial Nodule

Microglia cells aggregate in compact clusters to form microglial nodules due to central nervous system infections(especialy viral infections).

(3) Gitter Cell

Activated microglia cells may accumulate abundant intracellular lipid to form cells with foamy cytoplasm, which is termed gitter cells.

15.1.2.4　The Principal Pathologic Changes of Ependymal Cell

Ependymal cells line the inside of the ventricular system. Loss or disruption of ependymal cells is often associated with a local proliferation of subependymal astrocytes to produce small irregularities on the ventricular surfaces, which is termed ependymal granulations. Viral inclusions may be seen within ependymal cells due to certain viral infections, particularly cytomegalovirus(CMV).

15.2 Common Complications of the Central Nervous Diseases

Raised Intracranial Pressure, Cerebral Edema, and Hydrocephalus are the most common and important complications of central nervous diseases.

15.2.1 Raised Intracranial Pressure and Herniation

Raised intracranial pressure means CSF pressure above 2 kPa(normal value is 0.6-1.8 kPa)with the patient recumbent. Most cases are associated with the hydrocephalus, which is caused by tumor, inflammation(e.g. meningocephalitis and abscess), aemorrhage, intracranial hematoma, and cerebrospinal fluid circulation disorder. The increase of intracranial pressure can be divided into three periods: Compensatory stage, Decompensation stage and Vasomotor paralysis. Sometimes, brain displacement and encephalocoele deformation, caused by raised intracranial pressure, lead to part of the brain tissue embed in mediastinum cerebri, tentorium cerebelli or foramina magnum, then a herniation of the brain occurs.

1)Subfalcine(cingulate)herniation occurs when midline of the brain moves to the opposite caused by the occupying lesions of unilateral cerebral hemisphere(especially occurring in the frontal lobe, parietal lobe and temporal lobe), the cingulate gyrus of the same side displaces under the free margin of falx cerebri. Then the herniated cingulate gyrus is compressed, and as a result, bleeding and necrosis may occur in compressed brain tissue. The branches of the anterior cerebral artery may also be compressed, resulting in cerebral infarction of the territory supplied by that vessel.

2)Transtentorial(uncinate, mesial temporal)herniation occurs when the medial aspect of the temporal lobe is compressed against the free margin of the tentorium cerebelli. Then bad consequences come up: Firstly, the ipsilateral oculomotor nerve is compressed, resulting in transiently pupillary contraction, then pupillary dilation and impairment of ocular movements on the side of the lesion. Secondly, progression of transtentorial herniation is often accompanied by hemorrhagic lesions in the midbrain and pons, termed secondary brainstem, or Duret hemorrhages. These linear or flame-shaped lesions usually occur in the midline and paramedian regions due to tearing of penetrating veins and arteries supplying the upper brainstem. Thirdly, when the lateral shift of mesencephalon occurs, the contralateral cerebral peduncle displaces under the free margin of tentorium cerebelli, resulting in the compression of contralateral cerebral peduncle; the changes in the peduncle in this setting are known as Kernohan's notch. Lastly, the posterior cerebral artery may also be compressed, resulting in hemorrhagic infarction of the territory supplied by that vessel(such as ipsilateral occipital lobe calcarine fissure).

3)Tonsillar herniation refers to displacement of the cerebellar tonsils and medulla oblongata through the foramen magnum. This pattern of herniation is life-threatening because it causes brainstem compression and compromises vital respiratory and cardiac centers in the medulla oblongata.

15.2.2 Cerebral Edema

Cerebral edema or, more precisely, brain parenchymal edema refers to excessive accumulation of liquid in brain tissue, which is associated with a number of pathologic processes, such as hypoxia, trauma, infarct, inflammation, tumor and toxicosis. Two principal types are recognized:

1) Vasogenic edema is the most common type, which occurs when the integrity of normal blood-brain barrier is disrupted and fluids escape from the intravascular compartment predominantly into the intercellular spaces of the brain.

2) Cytotoxic edema refers to a retention of water and sodium in cytoplasm, which might be caused by generalized hypoxic-ischemic or intoxications.

In most cases, brain edema is both vasogenic and cytotoxic. On macroscopic examination, the edematous brain is heavier than normal and often appears obvious white matter edema, the gyri are flattened, the intervening sulci are narrowed, and the ventricular cavities are compressed. If the brain edema is severe, a herniation of the brain may occur. On microscopic examination, when vasogenic edema occurs, we can see the brain tissue was loosen, large amount of liquid accumulate in the widened spaces between cells and perivascular. In contrast, when cytotoxic edema occurs, we can see large amount of liquid accumulate in neurons, glial cells and vascular endothelial cells, which causes the enlargement of cell volume, hypochromatic cytoplasm.

15.2.3   Hydrocephalus

The term hydrocephalus refers to an increased volume of CSF within the ventricular system, which is always accompanied with continuous dilatation of the ventricle. Most cases occur as a consequence of obstruction to the free flow of CSF (the pattern is called noncommunicating hydrocephalus), increased production of CSF or decreased absorption (the pattern is called communicating hydrocephalus). Communicating hydrocephalus always occur in patients with cerebral cysticercosis, tumors, congenital malformation, inflammation, trauma or subarachnoid hemorrhage, etc. However, noncommunicating hydrocephalus may occur in patients with papillary tumor of the choroids plexus or chronic arachnoiditis, etc.

The pathological changes of hydrocephalus vary with different lesion sites and degree of lesion. For example, when mild hydrocephalus occurs, we can see mild ventricular dilatation and mild ventricular atrophy, however, high ventricular dilatation and severe compression of brain tissue might be seen when severe hydrocephalus occurs.

15.3   Infections of the Central Nervous System (CNS)

Bacterial, virus, rickettsia, leptospira, fungus or parasite, all can cause infections of the central nervous system (CNS). In addition, HIV can cause opportunistic infection (toxoplasmosis, cytomegalovirus infection), or central nervous system lymphoma.

There are four principal routes by which infectious microbes enter the nervous system.

1) Hematogenous spread: It is the most common means of entry; infectious agents ordinarily enter through the arterial circulation, e. g when the patient contracts sepsis, it is possible that the infective embolus entered through the arterial circulation, then came to the central nervous system.

2) Local extension: It occurs secondary to an open fracture of skull, most often the mastoiditis; an infected tooth; or tympanitis, nasosinusitis, bone erosion, and propagation of the infection into the CNS.

3) Direct implantation: It is almost invariably traumatic; rarely, it is iatrogenic (such as Lumbar puncture).

4) Through the peripheral nervous system: a few pathogens, especially certain viruses (such as rabies

virus)invade peripheral nerve to cause the damage to nervous tissue,and herpes zoster can cause infection along the olfactory nerve,the trigeminal nerve invades the central nervous system.

15.3.1 Bacterial Disease

The most common intracranial bacterial diseases are meningitis and brain abscess.

15.3.1.1 Meningitis

Meningitis includes pachymeningitis and leptomeningitis. As a result of the advent and clinical application of various antibiotics,the incidence of the pachymeningitis secondary to cranium infection is greatly reduced. So,meningitis is usually referred to as leptomeningitis including infection of the pia mater,arachnoidea and cerebrospinal fluid. Based on CSF inflammatory exudate examination and clinical evolution, meningitis is broadly classified into purulent meningitis(usually bacterial meningitis),lymphocytic meningitis(usually viral meningitis),and chronic meningitis(usually tuberculous,spirochetal,cryptococcal or fungus).

Epidemic cerebrospinalmeningitis is acute suppurative inflammation in cerebral spinal cord membrane, which is usually caused by meningococcal infection. It is usually sporadic. Sometimes it can be popular in winter and spring. Most of the patients are children and adolescents. Patients typically show systemic signs of infection superimposed on clinical evidence of meningeal irritation and neurologic impairment,including fervescence,headache,vomit,skin petechia,irritability,clouding of consciousness,and neck stiffness. Toxic shock can occur in severe cases,untreated,pyogenic meningitis can be fatal.

(1)Etiology and Pathogenesis

Meningococcus possess capsule,which can resist leukocyte phagocytosis. In most cases,bacteria in a partial secretory of the nasopharynx of a patient or a carrier can invade the body of other people by the way of droplet propagation. However,only few people can suffer from bacteremia or septicemia,and even meningitis.

(2)Pathological Changes

According to the progress of the disease,the patients experience three periods:

1)Upper respiratory tract infection:After 2-4 days of the bacteria propagation in the nasopharyngeal mucosa,patients show symptoms of upper respiratory tract infection. The major pathological changes include mucous congestion and edema,a small amount of neutrophil infiltration and Increase of secretion. Unfortunately,some patients enter the next stage-septicemia.

2)Septicemia:In this stage,blood culture can be positive,and mucocutaneous petechia or ecchymoses can be seen in most of the patients. High fever,headache,vomitting and increased neutrophils in peripheral blood can occur in patients because of the effect of endotoxin.

3)Meningitis stage:The characteristic lesion of this stage is suppurative inflammation of the cerebral spinal cord membrane. On gross appearance(Figure 15-1,Figure 15-2),hyperemia of cerebrospinal meningeal vessels and yellow purulent exudates within the leptomeninges over the surface of the brain are evident. In severely affected areas,exudation are densest in subarachnoid space,covering the sulci and gyri;in less severe areas,tracts of pus can be followed along blood vessels on the surface of the brain. Due to the obstruction of exudation,cerebrospinal fluid circulation disorder can occur and cause different degrees of ventricular dilatation. On microscopic examination,arachnoid angiectasia is obvious(Figure 15-3),and a large number of neutrophils infiltrate in subarachnoid space(Figure 15-3). In untreated meningitis,Gram stain reveals varying numbers of the causative organism,although they are frequently not demonstrable in treated cases. Generally,the parenchyma of the brain is not involved.

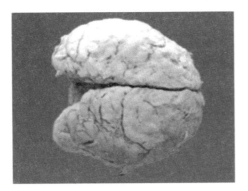

Figure 15－1　**Epidemic cerebrospinal meningitis**

　　Hyperemia of cerebrospinal meningeal vessels and yellow purulent exudates within the leptomeninges over the surface of the brain are evident. The exudates are densest in subarachnoid space, covering the sulci and gyri

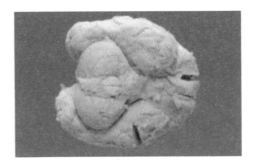

Figure 15－2　**Epidemic cerebrospinal meningitis**

　　A thick layer of suppurative exudate covers the brain stem and cerebellum and thickens the leptomeninges

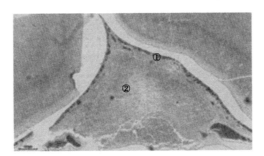

Figure 15－3　**Epidemic cerebrospinal meningitis**

　　① Arachnoid angiectasia is obvious; ② A large number of neutrophils can be seen in subarachnoid

（3）Clinical Pathological Correlation

1）Meningeal irritation: Meningeal irritation include neck stiffness and positive Kernig's sign. Neck stiffness is a protective spasm of the neck, which occurs as a result of inflammation involving the arachnoidea, pia mater and pia mater spinalis surrounding the spinal nerve root. Due to inflammation, nerve roots are pressed through the intervertebral foramen, then the patient will feel pain when the muscle in the neck or back is moving. Sometimes, infantile patients shows opisthotomus signs.

2）Symptoms of increased intracranial pressure: Symptoms of increased intracranial pressure include a severe headache, projectile vomiting, papilloedema and full bregma etc.

3）Changes of cerebrospinal fluid: CSF is cloudy or frankly purulent with raised neutrophils and protein level, but glucose content reduced markedly. Diplococcus meningitidis may be seen on a smear or can be cultured.

（4）Outcome and Complications

Most patients can recover if timely treated with extensive use of antibiotics. The current mortality rate has fallen from 70%－90% in the past to less than 5%. In very few patients, sequelae probably turn up, such as hydrocephalus, cerebral nerve damage and obstructive disease caused by arteritis of the base of the skull. Unfortunately, Some patients(children are the most common people) will develop fulminant epidemic cerebrospinal meningitis, which is fatal. According to the clinical pathological characteristics, fulminant epidemic cerebrospinal meningitis can be classified into two types:

1)Meningococcal septicemia with severe meningitis: Septic shock is the major clinical manifestation. The patient will turn up the severe clinical manifestation such as the skin and mucous membrane extensive bleeding point and ecchymosis, as well as peripheral circulatory failure, which were considered as the Waterhouse-Friderichsen syndrome. In the past few years, Waterhouse-Friderichsen syndrome was considered to result from meningitis-associated septicemia with hemorrhagic infarction of the adrenal glands and cutaneous petechiae, however, now it is considered as the result of toxic shock and DIC.

2)Fulminant meningoencephalitis: In fulminant meningitis, inflammatory cells infiltrate the walls of the leptomeningeal veins and potentially extend to substance of the brain(focal cerebritis). It can be fatal if not treated timely.

15.3.1.2 Brain Abscess

Brain abscesses are mainly caused by streptococci and staphylococci. Different infection pathways result in different positions and number of abscesses. It is caused by hematogenous spread(usually multiple foci, distributed in the various parts of the brain), or direct implantation of organisms, local extension from adjacent foci(usually single lesion).

The pathological changes of the brain abscesses are similar to the abscesses in the extracranial organs. On macroscopic examination, acute abscesses are discrete lesions with central liquefactive necrosis(Figure 15-4), however, in chronic abscesses, there is exuberant granulation tissue with neovascularization around the necrosis, a surrounding fibrous capsule, and edema. Outside the fibrous capsule is a zone of reactive gliosis with numerous gemistocytic astrocytes.

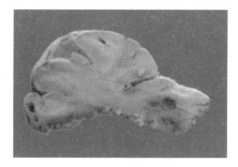

Figure 15-4 **Brain abscess**

15.3.2 Viral Disease

Viral encephalitis is due to infection of the brain by viruses, such as Herpes virus(DNA viruses, including herpes simplex virus, herpes zoster virus, EB virus and cytomegalovirus etc.), arbovirus(RNA viruses, including Japanese encephalitis virus, forest encephalitis virus etc.), enteric virusa(small RNA virus, such as poliovirus, Coxsackie virus, ECHO virus etc.), rabies virus and HIV etc.

Epidemic encephalitis B is an acute infectious disease caused by Japanese encephalitis virus. It is generally spread by mosquitoes. Pigs serve as a reservoir for the virus. It is popular in late summer and early autumn. Patients develop generalized symptoms, such as ardent fever, somnolence, twitch and coma etc. Approximately 50% -70% of the patients are children(especially under 10 years old).

15.3.2.1 Etiology and Pathogenesis

Patients with encephalitis B and host(livestock, fowl)act as reservoirs. Culex, aedes and anopheles act as the carriers of disease. Culex tritaeniorhynchus is the main vector of the disease in China. Immune defense and blood-brain barrier play an important role in the occurrence of disease.

15.3.2.2 Pathological Changes

Epidemic encephalitis B is mainly with lesions of brain parenchyma inflammation, which is most severe in the cerebral cortex, basal ganglia and thalamus. On gross appearance, leptomeningeal hyperemia and edema, widened gyri and narrowed sulc. In severe cases, petechial hemorrhage and semitransparent softening of the brain can be seen. On microscopic examination, the most characteristic histologic features of epidemic encephalitis B are perivascular and parenchymal mononuclear cell infiltration(lymphocytes, plasma cells, and macrophages)(Figure 15-5), degeneration and necrosis of nerve cell(satellitosis and neuronophagia) (Figure 15-6), glial cell reactions(including the formation of microglial nodules), and softening of the brain(Figure 15-7).

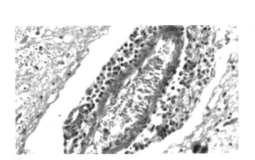

Figure 15-5　Epidemic encephalitis B. Perivascular mononuclear cell infiltration

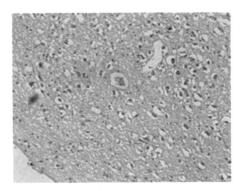

Figure 15-6　Neuronophagia

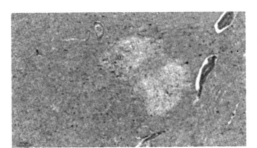

Figure 15-7　Epidemic encephalitis B. Softening of the brain

15.3.2.3 Clinical Pathological Correlation

Owing to the extensive involvement of the nerve cell and inflammatory damage of the cerebral parenchyma, most patients present with neurologic symptoms, such as somnolence or coma. Severe disease is characterized by upper motor neuron damaged symptoms, for example, muscle tone enhancement, tendon hyperreflexia, twitch and spasm, etc. Some patients can present as headache or vomit. Severe intracranial hypertension can cause hernia cerebri, which is fatal.

Fortunately, if treated, most of the patients can recover. However, few patients have neurologic sequelae or even die.

15.4 Neurodegenerative Diseases

Neurodegenerative diseases are a group of chronic, progressive disorders characterized by the gradual loss of neurons in discrete areas of the central nervous system (CNS). The mechanism underlying the disease remains unknown. There are several general characteristics: Firstly, selective loss of neuron cells. The affecting neurons might be atrophic or die. At the same time, astrogliosis might be seen. Thus, patients usually have specific clinical manifestations of the affected parts. Secondly, special neuropathologic findings can be observed in different degenerative diseases, e. g. Lewy bodies, and neurofibrillary tangles. The accumulation of abnormal protein can be found, such as Aβ protein and Tau protein in Alzheimer disease, α-synuclein in Parkinson disease.

The most common clinical features of degenerative diseases are as follow:

1) The main clinical manifestation of Alzheimer disease and Pick disease, which are involved the cerebral cortex, is dementia.

2) The main clinical manifestation of Huntington disease, Parkinson disease, Progressive supranuclear palsy and Multiple system atrophy (MSA), which are involved the Basal ganglia and brainstem, is cinesipathy.

3) The main clinical manifestation of Friedriech asynergy and ataxia telangiectasia, which are involved the cerebellum and spinal cord, is asynergy.

4) The main clinical manifestation of amyotrophic lateral sclerosis and Duchenne-Aran disease, which are involved motor neuron, is amyosthenia.

15.4.1 Alzheimer Disease

Alzheimer disease (AD) refers to the cortical degenerative disease characterized by progressive dementia, which is by far the most common cause of dementia in the elderly. Most patients become symptomatic after 50 years old, and the incidence of the disease rises with aging, the prevalence roughly reaches 47% for the 85-to 89-year-old cohort. The disease usually becomes clinically apparent as progressive mental state decay including memory, intelligence, orientation, discretion, disturbance of emotion and behavior disorder. Later, the patient will be lost in profoundly stuporous state. Eventually, in 5 to 10 years, the patient often dies of secondary infection and systemic failure.

15.4.1.1 Etiology and Pathogenesis

The cause of most Alzheimer's cases is still mostly unknown. Some cases are associated with genetic factors, level of education, metal ion damage and secondary transmitter change. Most cases are sporadic and 5% –10% of the cases are familial. Studies suggest in recent years that genes on chromosome 21, 19, 14 and 1 are related with Alzheimer disease. Familial AD show the accumuliation of Aβ protein in brain plays the major role in AD, which is derived from the abnormal degradation of APP.

15.4.1.2 Morphology

On macroscopic examination, cortical atrophy and widening of the cerebral sulci are most prominent in frontal, temporal, and parietal lobes of the brain. Ventricular enlargement are common complications after severe atrophy.

The major microscopic abnormalities of Alzheimer disease are neuritic plaques, neurofibrillary tangles, granulovacuolar degeneration and Hirano bodies.

1) Neuritic plaque, also named senile plaque, is an extracellular structure. Senile plaques are focal,

spherical collections dilated in shape, and range in size from 20 to 200 μm in diameter tortuous. Essentially, they are dystrophic neurites around a central amyloid core. In H&E staining, eosinophilic clumps may be surrounded by clear halo, and irregularly argentaffin granules or filamentous substance can be observed at the periphery. Immunohistochemistry reveals that the dominant component of the plaque core is Aβ.

2) Neurofibrillary tangles, intracellular abnormalities, are bundles of filaments in the cytoplasm of the neurons. They are visible as basophilic fibrillary structures with H & E staining but are dramatically demonstrated by silver staining. Generally, neurofibrillary tangles are commonly found in cortical neurons, especially in the entorhinal cortex, as well as pyramidal cells of the hippocampus, the amygdala, the basal forebrain, and the raphe nuclei.

3) Granulovacuolar degeneration present as a small vacuole in the cytoplasm of the neurons, and argyrophilic granules can be observed in small vacuoles. It is most commonly found in great abundance in hippocampal pyramidal cells.

4) Hirano bodies are rodlike eosinophilic bodies with actin as their major component. They are found most commonly within hippocampal pyramidal cells.

15.4.2 Parkinson Disease

Parkinson disease(PD), also named paralysis agitans, is a kind of slow progressive disease charactered as a lesion of striatal substantia nigra. It often occurs in adults of 50–80 years old.

15.4.2.1 Etiology and Pathogenesis

Parkinson disease is characterized by a progressive and selective degeneration of dopaminergic neurons of the substantia nigra, but the mechanisms are not fully understood.

Epidemiologic evidence suggested that environmental exposures may increase the risk of PD. MPTP (1-methyl-4-phenyl-1,2,3,6-tetrahydropyridine) produces moderate to severe parkinsonism in humans due to selective death of substantia nigra neurons. To date, six genes

have been found to be linked to PD, and gene PARK-1 is the most important one, which is related with α-synuclein.

15.4.2.2 Morphology

The typical macroscopic findings are pallor of the substantia nigra and locus ceruleus. On microscopic examination, there is loss of the pigmented, catecholaminergic neurons in these regions. Frequently, some remaining neurons contain single or multiple, cytoplasmic, eosinophilic, round inclusions known as Lewy bodies. Ultrastructurally, Lewy bodies are composed of fine filaments, densely packed in the core but loose at the rim.

The clinical manifestations of the patient are tremor, myotonus, exercise reduction, posture and gait instability, starting and stopping difficulties, masklike face etc. In the later stage, some patients might develop dementia. The relationship between AD and PD with subsequent development of dementia remains to be clarified. The course of PD is often over 10 years, eventually, the patient usually die from secondary infection or injury of fall.

15.5 Anoxia and Cerebrovascular Disease

Cerebrovascular disease is the most prevalent neurologic disorder in terms of both morbidity and mortality.

15.5.1 Ischemic Encephalopathy

Ischemic encephalopathy refers to severe brain damage as a result of hypotension, cardiac arrest, hemorrhage, hypoglycemia and asphyxia etc.

15.5.1.1 Influence Factor

Several principal factors influence the prognosis of patients. First, sensitivity to anoxia varies with different segments of the brain, for example, gray matter is more sensitive to anoxia than white matter. Second, local vascular distribution and vascular status are related to the injury site. In addition, the subsequent brain injury depends on the degree and duration of ischemia and anoxia, and the survival time of the patients.

15.5.1.2 Morphology

The typical pathological changes are central chromatolysis, red neuron, disintegration of myelin and axon, repair of glial scar etc, which can be observed in the brain tissue of moderate hypoxic patients or the patient's survival time is over 12 hours.

15.5.2 Obstructive Cerebrovascular Disease

Cerebral infarction results from a local arrest or reduction of cerebral blood flow. Usually thrombotic or embolic obstruction cause the vascular obstruction. Cerebral infarction is usually anemic infarction. The gray matter in the infarct area is dim after a few hours of infarction, and one week later, necrotic tissue can be liquefied.

15.5.3 Brain Hemorrhage

Brain hemorrhage includes intracerebral hemorrhage, subarachnoid hemorrhage and Mixed hemorrhage.

15.6 Demyelinating Diseases

In the central nerve system, the axon is tightly wrapped in the myelin sheath, which ensures the rapid propagation of nerve impulses. Demyelinating diseases are characterized by preferential damage to myelin, with relative preservation of axons. Myelin regeneration ability in central nervous system is limited, and secondary axonal injury can cause severe results. The clinical manifestation of the disease depends on the capacity of regenerating myelin and the degree of secondary damage to axons that occurs during the disease course.

15.6.1 Multiple Sclerosis

Multiple sclerosis(MS) is the most common demyelinating disease, and women are usually affected. The clinical course of the illness evolves as relapsing and remitting episodes of neurologic deficit during variable intervals of time. Each time, the involved part that relapses may be different, resulting in different symptoms of the nervous system. Now MS is considered as an autoimmune disease, which is influenced by genetic and environmental factors.

On macroscope examination, multiple, well-circumscribed, glassy, gray-tan, irregularly shaped plaques occur in horns of the ventricle and paraventricular white matter. The plaques can also be found in the optic nerves and chiasm, brain stem ascending and descending fiber tracts, cerebellum, and spinal cord. On microscope examination, perivascular demyelinating is the major change of the disease. Monocytes and lymphocytes present as perivascular cuffings, at the outer edge of the lesion occurring in the early stage. In active plaques, ongoing myelin breakdown with abundant macrophages containing myelin sheath debris (termed foamy cells) can be seen. In quiescent plaques, the inflammatory cells infiltrating disappear, no myelin is found, and there is a hyperplasia in the number of astrocyte.

MS lesions can occur anywhere in the CNS and, as a consequence, may induce a wide range of clinical manifestations, certain patterns of neurologic symptoms and signs are commonly observed.

15.6.2　Acute Disseminated Encephalomyelitis

Acute disseminated encephalomyelitis(ADEM) is a demyelinating disease of the central nervous system that typically presents as a monophasic disorder associated with multifocal neurologic symptoms and disability. Viral infections or vaccinations thought to induce ADEM include measles virus, rubella virus, chickenpox virus, vaccinia vaccine, and hydrophobia vaccine etc. Symptoms usually begin 1-3 weeks after infection. Major symptoms include fever, headache, nausea and vomiting, confusion and coma. The disease worsen rapidly over the course of hours to days, 80% of patients recovered well and 20% of cases have a fatal outcome.

On microscopic examination, perivascular demyelinating accompanying inflammatory response can be observed, which is considered as the characteristic of ADEM. Although the lesions progress rapidly, the axons are preserved well.

15.6.3　Acute Necrotic Hemorrhagic Encephalitis

Acute necrotic hemorrhagic encephalitis is a rare, rapid progressive and fetal disease in young people and children. Most of the lesions occur in cerebral hemisphere and brain stem. The characteristics of the lesions are similar to cerebral fat embolism-brain swelling with white matter punctate hemorrhage. On microscopic examination, the disease appears as focal necrosis of small vessels with peripheral hemorrhage, perivascular demyelinating with infiltration of neutrophil, lymphocyte and macrophage, as well as cerebral edema and meningitis. In contrast to ADEM, the necrosis of the acute necrotic hemorrhagic encephalitis is more extensive.

15.7　Tumors of the Nervous System

15.7.1　Tumors of the Central Nervous System

CNS tumors inculde primary (75%) and secondary tumors (25%). The most common primary brain tumors are gliomas (50%), meningiomas (20%), pituitary adenomas (15%) and nerve sheath tumors (8%). CNS tumors have unique characteristics:

1) There is no precancerous lesion or carcinoma in situ;

2) Benign or malignant tumors all can infiltrate the brain and lead to serious clinical deficits and poor prognosis;

3) The anatomic site of the tumor can have lethal consequences irrespective of histologic classification; for example, benign meningioma can compress medulla and cause cardiac arrest;

4) The lesion can spread along the subarachnoid space, however, few tumors metastasize outside of the

CNS;

5) Different types of intracranial tumors can develop the same clinical manifestations: epilepsia, paralysis defect of field vision, high intracranial pressure.

15.7.1.1 Gliomas

Gliomas, derived from glial cells, include astrocytic tumor, oligodendroglial tumor, and ependymal tumor. Astrocytic tumor and oligodendroglial tumor grow by progressive infiltration, invasion and penetration of the surrounding tissue, however, ependymal tumor is inclined to be solid tumor.

(1) Astrocytic Tumor

Astrocytic tumor is the most common type of glioma and accounts for 30% of primary tumors. It includes various types of astrocytomas with different clinicopathological characteristics: pilocytic astrocytoma (WHO grade I), subependymal giant cell astrocytoma (WHO grade I), pleomorphic xanthoastrocytoma (WHO grade II), diffuse astrocytoma (WHO grade II), anaplastic astrocytoma (WHO grade III), glioblastoma (WHO grade IV), as well as Gliaomatosis cerebri.

Genetic alterations have been identified in astrocytoma, such as the inactivation of TP53, RB, P16INK4a and the heterozygosity loss on chromosome 10. Inactivation of TP53 is most common gene alteration in astrocytomas. PDGF-A and its receptor overexpressed. Transition from lower-grade astrocytoma to glioblastoma is associated with DCC gene disruption.

Macroscopically, tumors are gray, expand and distort the brain. Some tumors may appear well demarcated from the surrounding brain tissue, but infiltration beyond the outer margins is always present. These tumors range in size from a few centimeters to enormous lesions, which can replace the entire hemisphere. The cut surface of the tumor is either firm or soft depending on the amount of glial fiber; sometimes, gelatinous, cystic degeneration and hemorrhage may be seen.

On microscopic examination, the tumor cells vary in size and shape; different astrocytomas show different characteristics of cell density, nucleus, vascular proliferation and necrosis. Astrocytomas are GFAP-positive.

Diffuse astrocytomas account for 10% –15% of astrocytic tumors, which are characterized by well differentiation and slow growth. The onset age is 30–40 years old. It often occurs in cerebral hemispheres, frontal lobe and lobi temporalis. The most common signs and symptoms are seizures, headaches, and focal neurologic deficits related to the anatomic site of involvement. Histologically, the tumor cells are well-differentiated, have densely cellular and occasionally have nuclear pleomorphism (Figure 15-8), mitotically active cells are rare. Several different subtypes of diffuse astrocytomas are recognized, including fibrillary, protoplasmic, gemistovytic and mixed cells type, etc. Fibrillary astrocytoma is the most common subtype. Generally, the mean length of survival time after operation was 6–8 years. Diffuse astrocytomas have an intrinsic tendency to progress to more advanced grades, such as glioblastoma.

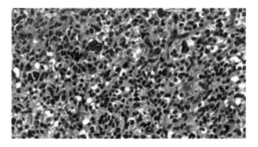

Figure 15–8 **Astrocytoma**

Anaplastic astrocytoma has a poor prognosis. The characteristics of histology are increase of tumor cell density, evident nuclear atypia, nuclear hyperchromatism, increased mitosis and vascular endothelial cell proliferation etc. In addition, naplastic astrocytoma has a tendency to progress to glioblastoma.

Glioblastoma is the most aggressive cancer that begins within the brain. It can be divided into primary and secondary categories. It often occurs in lobi temporalis, parietal lobe, frontal lobe and occipital lobe. Its histologic appearance is similar to anaplastic astrocytoma and accompanied with necrosis and vascular proliferation. However, in contrast to anaplastic astrocytoma, necrosis in glioblastoma occurs in hypercellularity areas with highly malignant cells crowding along the edges of the necrotic regions, which referred as pseudopalisading(Figure 15 – 9). Sometimes, vascular proliferation is characterized by tufts of piled-up vascular cells, When vascular cell proliferation is extreme, the tuft forms a ball-like structure, termed the glomeruloid body.

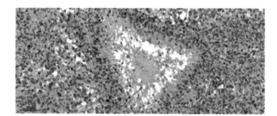

Figure 15-9   Glioblastoma(pseudopalisading)

Eventually, worse prognosis is correlated with rapid growth of the tumor. The mean length of survival time after operation is only 12 months.

WHO grade I - II tumors(Pilocytic astrocytoma, pleomorphic xanthoastrocytoma and subependymal giant cell astrocytoma) usually grow slowly, have relatively benign behavior and favorable prognosis. The tumors usually were well-circumscribed with the surrounding brain. They typically occur in children and young adults. On microscopic examination, pilocytic astrocytoma is special, which are composed of bipolar cells with long, thin "hairlike" processes; Rosenthal fibers, eosinophilic granular bodies, and microcysts are often present.

(2) Oligodendroglial Tumor

Oligodendroglial tumors include oligodendroglioma and anaplastic oligodendroglioma. Oligodendroglioma, derived from oligodendrocyte, is considered as WHO grade II . The lesions are found mostly in the cerebral hemispheres, especially in the frontal lobe. It occurs most often in 40–45 years old adults. On macroscopic examination, oligodendrogliomas are gray masses, soft, well-circumscribed but invasive growth, often with cysts, focal hemorrhage, and calcification. On microscopic examination, the tumors are composed of sheets of regular small and round cells with spherical nuclei(like normal oligodendrocytes) surrounded by a clear halo of cytoplasm. The tumor cells array dispersively, sometimes there is often formation of secondary structures, particularly with perineuronal satellitosis. In addition, it typically contains a delicate network of anastomosing capillaries, and may be accompanied by different degrees of calcification and psammoma body formation. Histochemical and immunohistochemical staining show that galactolipid, carbonic anhydrase isozyme C, CD57, MAP or MBP are all positive. The most common genetic alterations in oligodendrogliomas are loss of heterozygosity for chromosomes 1p and 19q.

Oligodendroglioma is sensitive to chemotherapy. As a result of slowly growth of the tumor, patients with oligodendroglioma have an average survival of about 10 years after operation. The most common presenting signs and symptoms are epilepsia or focal paralysis. In contrast to oligodendroglioma, anaplastic oligodendroglioma grows fast, and the mean length of survival time after operation is only 3.5 years.

(3) Ependymal Tumor

Ependymal tumors include ependymoma and anaplastic ependymoma.

Ependymoma is considered as WHO grade Ⅱ. Ependymoma arises from ependyma-lined ventricular system, including the oft-obliterated central canal of the spinal cord. It typically constitutes 2% –9% of the neuroepithelial tumors, and most often occurs in children and adolescents. On macroscopic examination, ependymomas are gray masses, well-circumscribed, globular or lobulated, often with cysts, focal hemorrhage, and calcification(similar to oligodendroglioma). On microscopic examination, ependymomas are composed of uniform cells, round to oval nuclei, as well as, with abundant cytoplasm. The most characteristic change of histology is the tumor cells, there may be formation of gland-like structures that resemble the embryologic ependymal canal, with long, delicate processes extending into a lumen(Figure 15 – 10); more frequently present are perivascular pseudorosettes in which tumor cells are arranged around vessels with an intervening zone consisting of thin ependymal processes directed toward the wall of the vessel(Figure 15–11). Anaplastic ependymomas occur with increased cell density, high mitotic rates, areas of necrosis, and less evident ependymal differentiation. Ependymomas grow slowly, and the patients can survive for 8–10 years.

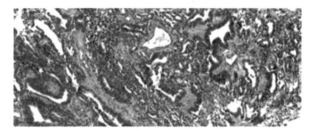

Figure 15–10　**Ependymoma**

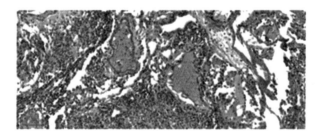

Figure 15–11　**Ependymoma**

15.7.1.2　Medulloblastoma

Medulloblastoma, the most common embryonal tumor of the central nervous system, derived from the embryonal external granular layer cells of cerebellum or subependymal stromal cells, occurs predominantly in children. It accounts for 20% of the children tumors and is considered as WHO grade Ⅱ. Up to 75% of children medulloblastoma is located in the vermis of the cerebellum and may be seen extending to the fourth ventricle. On macroscopic examination, it usually presents as a soft, greyish mass. On microscopic examination, medulloblastoma is usually extremely cellular, tumor cells are small, round or ovoid, with little cytoplasm and hyperchromatic nuclei. Sometimes, pathological mitotic figure can be seen. The Homer Wright rosettes is the typical structure of medulloblastoma, characterized as the tumor cells are arranged around the center of the argyrophilic fiber(Figure 15–12). In electron microscope, bi-directional differentiation of the tumor cells can be seen. In addition, the tumor has the potential to express neuronal(e. g, Syn and NSE)and glial(GFAP) phenotypes examined with immunohistochemical assay. The most common genetic alteration, occurring in medulloblastoma, is the isochromosome 17q and chromosome 17 trisomy. The tumor is highly malignant, and the prognosis is dismal; however, with opertation and regular adjuvant therapy, the 5 - year survival rate may be as high as 75%.

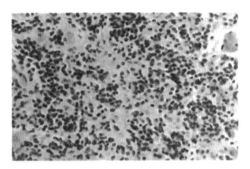

Figure 15–12 **Medulloblastoma**

15.7.1.3 Neuronal and Mixed Neuronal-glial Tumors

(1) Gangliocytoma and Gangliogima

Most of these tumors are slow growing, well differentiated and considered as WHO grade I (gangliocytoma) or WHO grade I - II (gangliogima). But the glial component of gangliogima occasionally becomes frankly anaplastic, then anaplastic ganglioglioma occurs and behaves as grade III lesions. Gangliocytomas are well-circumscribed masses with small tumor size, slightly hard in quality, grayish red cut surface, as well as focal calcification and small cysts usually found in the temporal lobe. On microscopic examination, neoplastic ganglion cells with various nuclei(mononuclear, binucleate or multinuclear) are irregularly clustered and have apparently random orientation of neurites. In addition, plasmosome and Nissl body can be seen in tumor cells, and sometimes medullated fibers and amyelinated nerve fiber will be confused among the tumor cells too. Immunohistochemical staining of the tumor tissue show GFAP is positive of glial cells as well as neuronal proteins, neurofilaments, and synaptophysin are positive of ganglion cells.

(2) Central Neurocytoma

Central neurocytoma is considered as WHO grade II. The average age of onset is 29 years old. It most often located in frontal part of the lateral ventricle, sometimes extending to lateral ventricle or the third ventricle. On microscopic examination, central neurocytomas are composed of densely uniform small cells, round nucleus and transparent cytoplasm. Pseudorosette can be seen. Synaptophysin and NeuN are positive in immunohistochemical staining.

15.7.1.4 Meningiomas

Meningiomas, accounted for 15% –26% of intracranial tumor, are the most common meningeal primary tumor that originate from the meningothelial cell of the arachnoid. They are predominantly benign tumors of adults, growing slowly, easily to be excisived, that appear to be the best prognosis in central nervous tumor and considered as WHO grade I.

On macroscopic examination, meningiomas are usually attached to the dura with expansive growth and may be found on the cerebrum convex surface. The tumors appear to be usually rounded or lobulated masses with a well-defined dural base that compress underlying brain but are easily separated from it. The surface of the mass is usually encapsulated with thin, fibrous tissue termed diolame. On the cut surface, the tumor appears to be gray, tenacious texture, sometimes gritty-textured, gross evidence of necrosis or extensive hemorrhage is almost not present. On microscopic examination, various histological types can be seen. These include syncytial, the concentric arrangement of the cells with a somewhat whorled appearance (Figure 15-12) and the whorls may undergo hyaline degeneration and become calcified with psammoma bodies (Figure 15-13); fibroblastic, with elongated cells and abundant collagen deposition between them; transitional, which share features of the syncytial and fibroblastic types. In addition, there are other rare patterns. Anaplastic(malignant) meningioma, considered as WHO grade Ⅲ, is a highly aggressive tumor that has the overall appearance of a high-grade sarcoma. Mitotic rates are often extremely high and necrosis is present. All meningiomas express vimentin, and most cases express EMA.

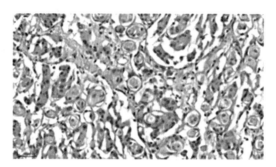

Figure 15-13 **Meningiomas**

15.7.2 Peripheral Nerve Tumors

Generally, peripheral nerve tumors are divided into two categories. One arises from neurilemmal, including Schwannoma and neurofibroma, the other is accompanied with different degrees of nerve cell differentiation, such as neuroblastoma and ganglion cell neuroma. In this section, Schwannoma and neurofibroma will be descried briefly.

(1)Schwannoma

Schwannoma(neurilemoma), arised from the neural crest-derived Schwann cell or lemmocyte, it is a benign tumor and considered as WHO grade Ⅰ. Neurilemoma is the most common tumor occurring in the canalis spinalis, it account for 25% -30% of intraspinal tumors. Within the cranial vault, the most common location of schwannomas are in the vestibular branch of the eighth nerve(so called acoustic neurinoma) and the cerebellopontine angle. While, the most common location of schwannomas in the peripheral nerve is the flexor side nerve trunk of extremities.

Gross appearance of schwannomas are round or lobulated, well-circumscribed, encapsulated masses that are attached to the nerve but can be separated from it. Tumors form hoar or luidity masses but may also have areas of cystic and hemorrhagic change. On microscopic examination, tumors show two growth patterns. In Antoni A growth pattern, cells are spindle shaped, a close parallel arrangement of which form a palisade or incomplete whirlpool, termed Verocay bodies(Figure 15-14). In Antoni B growth pattern, the tumor is less densely cellular with a loose meshwork of cells along with microcysts and myxoid changes. In most cases, two patterns of growth both can be observed in the same tumor, but only one of them will express as the main change in different areas, for example, intracranial schwannoma mainly appears to be Antoni B pattern of growth, however, Antoni A pattern of growth will appear in neurilemmoma in the spinal canal. The Schwann cell origin of these tumors is borne from their S-100 immunoreactivity. CollagenⅣ and laminin are usually cell membrane positive, too.

Clinical Features are usually associated with the location and size of tumor. Patients with small tumor can be asymptomatic, however, if the tumor is larger, paralysis or pain caused by the compression of the nerve probably occur. For example, patients with acoustic neuroma often present with hearing loss and tinnitus. Most neurilemoma can take radical operation except very few tumors attached to brain stem or spinal cord closely can not be excisived completely and relapse but they are still benign tumor.

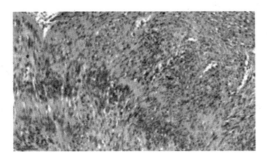

Figure 15-14   **Schwannoma**

(2) Neurofibroma

Neurofibroma, considered as WHO grade I, can be sporadic or multiple. The most common location occurs in the skin or subcutaneous tissue. Neurofibromatosis, also known as von Recklinghausen disease, is always accompanied by café-au-lait spot and axillary spots.

On macroscopic examination, the skin lesions are evident as nodules or polypoid, well-circumscribed, nonencapsulated, diffusely infiltrating into skin and subcutaneous. On the cut surface, the tumor is gray and vortexed fiber, Jelly material can be seen. However, bleeding and cystic degeneration rarely occur. The stroma of these tumors is highly collagenized and contains myxoid material. Lesions within peripheral nerves are of identical histologic appearance. On microscopic examination, the tumor is composed of Schwann cells, perineurial-like cells and fibroblasts (interweaving each other), which disperse between nerve fibers. The stroma of these tumors is highly collagenized and contains little myxoid material.

Malignant peripheral nerve sheath tumor(MPNST), which accounts for 5% of soft tissue sarcoma, most arise from peripheral neurofibroma(especially von Recklinghausen disease). MPNST is a very aggressive tumor, and considered as WHO grade II -IV. On microscopic examination, it is similar to fibroma sarcomatosum, showing more nuclear mitotic images accompanied by vascular proliferation and cell necrosis. In addition, pleomorphism of tumor cell can be seen.

MPNST most often occurs in 20-60 years old. Generally, the tumor show fast progress and poor prognosis. Five- and ten-year survival rate respectively is 34% and 23%.

15.7.3 Metastatic Tumors

Central nervous system metastatic tumors account for approximately 20% of intracranial tumors. The most common primary malignant tumor is lung cancer(accounting for about 50% of all metastases), the second is breast cancer(accounting for about 15% of all metastases), then, melanoma, kidney cancer, gastrointestinal tract malignant tumors and choriocarcinoma etc. Metastatic tumors present clinically as mass lesions and may occasionally be the first manifestation of the cancer.

The most commom metastatic route of intracranial metastatic tumors is hematogenous metastasis. The cerebrum and endocranium are frequent sites of involvement by intracranial metastatic disease, while, spinal metastasis often occurs in epidural space, pia mater spinalis and spinal cord.

On microscopic examination, the metastatic tumors are similar to the primary tumors, usually accompanied by hemorrhage, necrosis, cystis degeneration and liquefaction. The boundary between tumor and brain parenchyma is well defined as well.

Chapter 16

Infectious Disease and Deep Mycosis

16.1 Tuberculosis

16.1.1 Overview

Tuberculosis(TB)is a chronic,communicable disease caused by mycobacterium tuberculosis. Tuberculosis typically attacks the lungs but can also affect other parts of the body. It is spread through the air when people who have an active TB infection cough,sneeze,or otherwise transmit respiratory fluids through the air. Most infections are asymptomatic and latent,but about one in ten latent infections eventually progresses to active disease which,if left untreated,kills more than 50% of those who are infected.

Tuberculosis is estimated to affect 1. 7 billion individuals worldwide,with 8 to 10 million new cases and 1.7 million deaths each year. After HIV,tuberculosis is the leading infectious cause of death in the world. Infection with HIV makes people susceptible to rapidly progressive tuberculosis;over 50 million people are infected with both HIV and M. tuberculosis.

Etiology and pathogenesis:

The common human strain infects only humans. Patients with pulmonary tuberculosis who cough up bacilli in the sputum are the source of transmitted infections. Bovine tuberculosis typically involves the oropharynx or intestine because the organism is ingested in milk. The bovine strain of M. tuberculosis infects dairy,causing human infection via contaminated milk. Most infection is acquired by direct person to person transmission of airborne droplets of organisms. Tuberculosis of the lung may also occur via infection from the blood stream. Hematogenous transmission can spread infection to more distant sites,such as peripheral lymph nodes,the kidneys,the brain,and the bones. All parts of the body can be affected by the disease, though for unknown reasons it rarely affects the heart,skeletal muscles,pancreas,or thyroid.

Cell immune reaction and allergic reaction of tuberculosis(Type Ⅳ hypersensitivity)often occur simultaneously. Components of the M. tuberculosis cell wall(such as cold factor,wax D,complement,heat-shock protein,etc.)and host response(immune response and delayed hypersensitivity)contribute to its pathogenicity. The earliest phase of primary tuberculosis(<3 weeks)in the no sensitized individual is characterized by bacillary proliferation with the pulmonary alveolar macrophages and airspaces,which result into bacteremia seeding of multiple sites. The development of cell-mediated immunity occurs approximately 3 weeks after exposure. In the draining lymph nodes, processed mycobacterial antigens are presented in a major histocompatibility class II context by dendritic cell macrophages to CD4$^+$ TH1 cells, which are capable of secreting IFN-γ and activate macrophages. Activate macrophages, in turn, release a variety of mediators with important down-stream effects, including ①secretion of TNF, which is responsible for recruitment of monocytes, which in turn undergo activation and differentiation into the "epithelioid histiocytes" that characterize the granulomatous response; ②expression of the inducible nitric oxide synthase(iNOS) gene, which results in elevated nitric oxide levels at the site of infection. Nitric oxide is a powerful oxidizing agent and results in generation of reactive nitrogen intermediates and other free radicals capable of oxidative destruction of several mycobacterial constituents, from cell wall to DNA; ③generation of reactive oxygen species that can have antibacterial activity. In summary, immunity to a tubercular infection is primarily mediated by CD4$^+$ TH1 cells, which stimulate macrophages to kill bacteria. This immune response, while largely effective, comes at the cost of hypersensitivity and the accompanying tissue destruction. Reactivation of the infection or re-exposure to the bacilli in a previously sensitized host results in rapid mobilization of a defensive reaction but also increases tissue necrosis.

The clinical manifestations of the infection of TB are decided by different reactions. Three considerations are involved in the pathogenesis of TB, quantity of bacteria; virulence of pathogen; responsiveness of the body sensitivity and immune response. If TB bacteria gain entry to the bloodstream from an area of damaged tissue, they can spread throughout the body and set up many loci of infection, all appearing as tiny, white tubercles in the tissues. This severe form of TB disease, most common in young children and those with HIV, is called miliary tuberculosis. People with this disseminated TB have a high fatality rate even with treatment(about 30%). In many people, the infection waxes and wanes. Tissue destruction and necrosis are often balanced by healing and fibrosis. Affected tissue is replaced by scarring and cavities filled with caseous necrotic material. During active disease, some of these cavities are joined to the air passages bronchi and this material can be coughed up. It contains living bacteria, and so can spread the infection. Treatment with appropriate antibiotics kills bacteria and the focus allows healing to take place. Upon cure, affected areas are eventually replaced by scar tissue.

16.1.1.1 Basic Morphology of Tuberculosis

(1)Exudation

Acute inflammatory exudates are not common in tuberculosis. However, they can occur when hypersensitivity is very pronounced, such as with early infections and high bacterial virulence. Exudates appear as serous or serofibrinous inflammation. The immediate reaction causes edema, hyperemia, and neutrophilic infiltration. However, the majority of cells are mononuclear phagocytes and lymphocytes. This type of inflammation is encountered mostly in the lung, serous membranes, joints, and meninges. Mycobacterium tuberculosis can be seen in the exudation and macrophage cells. Exudation can be completely absorbed or change into necrosis or proliferation dominated lesions.

(2)Proliferation

The most characteristic lesion in tuberculosis is the granuloma with central necrosis. The morphology of this lesion depends on the balance between proliferation of the tubercle bacillus and the intensity of the host immune response(formation of the granuloma). When proliferation of the micro-organism is predominant, that will be many macrophages containing numerous bacilli; the macrophages will be loosely arranged. This is a common presentation of infection by M. avium intracellularly. When there is little proliferation of the organism and the host immune response is very strong, there are few detectable organisms and numerous well-formed granulomas with central necrosis; this is a common appearance with infection by M. tuberculosis hominis or M. bovis.

Tuberculosis granuloma is the feature of the diagnosis of the tuberculosis (Figure 16-1). It consists of aggregates of epithelioid cells, Langerhans giant cells, fibroblasts and lymphocytes. Caseous necrosis frequently is presented in the center, which shows red-stain amorphous granular substance containing tubercle bacilli. Monocytic infiltrates appear initially. They engulf bacteria and, after about 2 weeks, develop delayed hypersensitivity and epithelioid conversion. Tubercles are characterized by formation of granulomas containing compact collections of mononuclear cells called epithelioid cells, which is spindle shaped or polygonal, with abundant cytoplasm, pale eosinophilic and ambiguous realm. The epithelioid cell nucleus is round or oval, chromatin understood, even vacuolization and may have 1-2 nucleolus. These epithelioid cells arrange in concentric layers. The increase of epithelioid cell activity is conducive to the phagocytosis and killing of Mycobacterium tuberculosis. The majority of epithelioid cell can fuse together and transform into Langerhans giant cells, which are giant multinucleated giant cells (up to 300 μm in diameter) and rich in cytoplasm. The number of nuclei varies from a dozen to more than a hundred and arrange in garland or horse's hoof form or assembled together. The typical tubercles are composed of lymphocytes with epithelioid cells and Langhans'giant cells in the center. When tubercles coalesce, the center is often necrotic, replaced by eosinophilic, structureless granular material (caseous necrosis), and some lymphocytes. Granulomas with central necrosis are characteristic of tuberculosis and have diagnostic value. Fibrous scarring develops around caseous tubercles. With modern therapy, all residual evidence of previous disease may disappear except for a residual scar. Calcification commonly occurs.

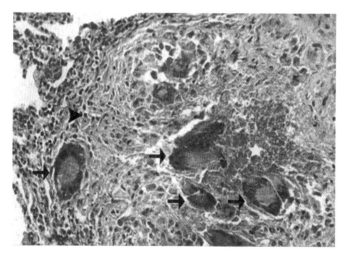

Figure 16-1   Tuberculosis granuloma. Nodule consists of collection of epitheliod cells with several Langhans' giant cells and lymphocytes. Caseous necrosis is presented in the center

Single tubercle is very small, about 0.1mm in diameter, which cannot easily be seen by naked eyes and X-ray. Three or four nodules can fuse to a large one. Grossly, the lesions often resemble well-circumscribed nodules. On cut surface, these are gray-white or yellow, homogenous or greasy. They have necrotic centers with a dry or greasy cheese-like (caseous) appearance. The centers may be liquid. Liquefaction may facilitate dissemination of TB in the body.

(3) Necrosis

The lesion of necrosis appears when there are numerous organisms or high virulence and the people are in low host immunity state or strange hypersensitivity reaction. The necrotic lesion is called caseous necrosis because it is pale yellowish or creamy-white in color, soft and friable, similar to dry cheese in gross. Microscopically, caseous necrosis showes red strained homogeneous amorphic material or some granular material with cell debris. Caseous necrosis is of equal diagnostic importance in TB. Large areas of caseous necrosis are a sign of TB progression.

These three basic pathological processes are inter-related and also can interchange according to host conditions.

16.1.1.2　Transformation of Basic Lesions

(1) Healing or Repair

1) Absorption and dissipation are main healing ways. The effusion is absorbed through lymphatics vessel. Small necrosis lesions can be absorbed and dissipate by energetic therapy. Chest X-ray shows that the lesions are dense inhomogeneous cloud shadow with unclear edge. Clinically, the patients are called on the mend and take a turn for cure.

2) Fibrosis, fibrous encapsulation and calcification of lesions are main repair ways. Tubercle with small necrosis can fibroses and be healed by organization. Large necrotic focus can be encapsulated by peripheral fibrosis tissue and the caseous center condensed to a hard calcified nodule. Chest X-ray shows the fibrotic lesion is stripe or star-like scar with clear edge and the density of calcified lesions is higher in the center. Clinically, it is called calcification induration stage.

(2) Exacerbation

1) Infiltration. When TB gets worse, the lesion appears exudation and necrosis around focus. X-ray examinations shows pachy shadow with unclear edge. Clinically, it is called infiltration and extension stage.

2) Dissolution and dissemination. Liquefied necrosis excludes mainly through natural tracts, such as branchi, urinary tract and so on. Cavity necrosis spread by branchi, lymphatics or blood stream and result in some new lesions in other sites. X-ray shows that the density of shadow is inhomogenous. The bright region and new lesions can be observed. Clinically, it is called dissolution and spread stage.

16.1.2　Pulmonary Tuberculosis

The lungs are the most commonly affected by tuberculosis than any other organs. The pattern of host response depends on whether the infection represents a primary first exposure to the organism or secondary reaction in already sensitized host. Pulmonary tuberculosis is classified into primary pulmonary tuberculosis and secondary pulmonary tuberculosis.

16.1.2.1　Primary Pulmonary Tuberculosis

Primary tuberculosis is the form of disease that develops in child who has not been previously exposed to tuberculous bacillus or immunised by BCG(Bacillus Calmette-Guérin)vaccination. So it is also called the childhood type TB, but primary lesion may also occurs in elderly persons and profoundly immunosuppressed persons who may lose their sensitivity to the tubercle bacillus and may develop primary tuberculosis more than once.

Primary tuberculosis is characterized by formation of a Primary complex(also called a Gohn complex))(Figure 16-2). Usually the involved portion of the lung is subpleural, in the midzone of the lung, with lymphatic extension to involve the hilar lymph nodes. The lesion consists of three components: primary lesion(Ghon focus); tuberculous lymphangitis; tuberculous lymphadenitis(in the hilar lymph nodes). Primary lesion is usually a 1.0-1.5 cm area of round, gray-yellow inflammatory consolidation, which locates in lower segment of the upper lobe or the upper segment of the lower lobe, close to the pleura. The center of

Ghon focus usually undergoes caseous necrosis. Tubercle bacilli can drain through lymphatic vessel to the regional hilar lymph nodes, which result in tuberculous lymphangitis and tuberculous lymphadenitis. Chest X-ray shows primary complex lesions are dumb bell-like shadow, in which the lymphangitis is in strip-like shape. Histologically, tuberculosis lesions are marked by a characteristic granulomatous inflammatory reaction that forms both caseating and noncaseating tubercles. The granulomas are usually enclosed within a fibroblastic rim punctuated by lymphocytes. Multinucleate giant cells are present in the granulomas.

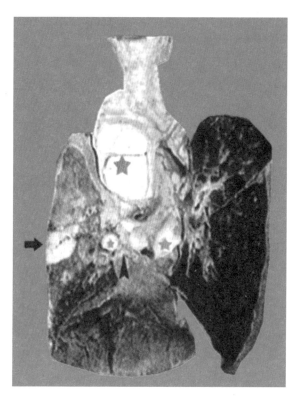

Figure 16-2 **Primary complex**

The lesion consists of three components: primary lesion
(Ghon focus); tuberculous lymphangitis; tuberculous lymphadenitis (in the hilar lymph nodes)

Primary pulmonary tuberculosis is usually asymptomatic or manifested as a mild flu-like illness. In the first few weeks, it is also lymphatic and hematogenous dissemination to other parts of the body. In 98% of cases, immunity stops disease progression and healing occurs. The lesions heal by fibrosis and may calcify, despite seeding of other organs, no lesions develop. In 2% of cases, rapidly progressive pulmonary disease causing extensive caseous consolidation of the lung, usually occurs only in malnourished or immunodeficient children.

16.1.2.2 Secondary Pulmonary Tuberculosis

This form of tuberculosis occurs in people who have immunity to tuberculosis before the infection occurs. It usually occurs in an adult as a result either of reinfection or reactivation, with the latter more common. Because of immunity, the initial reaction to the infection is much stronger and more rapid than in people with primary tuberculosis. Secondary tuberculosis tends to produce more damage to the lungs than primary tuberculosis. The subsequent course of the secondary lesions is variable. It is classified into the following types according to the pathological features and clinical course.

(1) Focal Pulmonary Tuberculosis

It is the earliest lesion of secondary pulmonary tuberculosis. The pathogenesis of focal tuberculosis is diverse, multiforme and complicated. Focal tuberculosis can be derived from the action of the primary or more often secondary period of tuberculosis. The most common site is the lung apex, one or more small focus of consolidation. The lesions are one or more small apical foci, usually a 0.5–1.0 cm in maximum diameter, well-circumscribed, grayish-white to yellow in color. Histologically, small epithelioid cell granulomas are characterized by caseous necrosis and fibrosis. Patients usually are asymptomatic. They either may heal spontaneously or with therapy, resulting in a fibro-calcific nodule, remain quiescent, or progress. Dissemination via lymphatics or the bloodstream can be prevented by hypersensitivity and cellular immunity.

(2) Infiltrative Pulmonary Tuberculosis

This is the most common type of secondary tuberculosis and usually transformes from focal pulmonary TB. It usually occurs by infection through the airways after inhaling sputum from another person with open tuberculosis. The lesions are usually located in upper part of the lungs (subclavicular or apical region). Active cellular immunity causes acute reactions with marked caseous necrosis, which cause the lesion enlargement. On chest X-ray, there are soft "woolly" infiltrates, which shows the cloud like shadow with indistinct boundary under the clavicle. When the disease develops progressively, the caseation lesions enlargement can result in irregular acute cavities. Erosion into pneumothorax evacuates the central caseous material and creates spontaneous pneumothorax or tuberculosis pyopneumothorax. Erosion into a bronchus evacuates the caseous center, creating a ragged, irregular cavity lined by caseous material that is poorly walled off by fibrous tissue. Erosion of blood vessels results in hemoptysis. Clinically, Patients can have toxic symptoms, with chronic cough and hemoptysis. With adequate treatment, the process may be arrested, although healing by fibrosis often distorts the pulmonary architecture. If healing does not occur, there may be progressive enlargement of the lesion with liquefaction necrosis, cavitation; and bronchogenic spread. The lesions can break through the pleura to cause pneumothorax or pyopneumothorax; or transform into chronic fibrocaseous tuberculosis with cavitation.

(3) Chronic Fibro-cavitative Pulmonary TB

It often result from infiltrative pulmonary tuberculosis and is a most common form of chronic pulmonary TB in an adult. This is a more severe reaction to infection than infiltrative pulmonary tuberculosis. It may affect one, many or all lobes of both lungs. The upper lobes of lung contain multiple thick-walled chronic cavities of varying size (Figure 16-3). The thickness of their walls can be more than 1 cm. Histologically, the wall of cavity is lined by a yellow-green caseous material, tuberculous granulation tissue and fibrous tissue successively. There may be coexisting bronchial disseminated many tuberculous lesions and diffuse fibrosis in the pulmonary tissues. Old and new lesions often coexist. The upper lung has more lesions and older lesions than the lower lung. In late period, the lung becomes small, indurated, with pleural extensive adhesion, the function of the lung may be severely damaged.

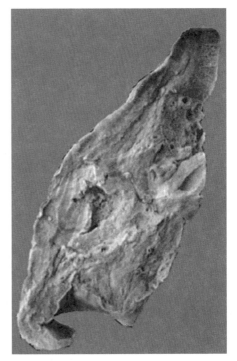

Figure 16-3   **Chronic fibro-cavitative pulmonary tuberculosis**

The upper lobe of lung contains multiple thick-walled chronic cavities of varying size. The thickness of their their walls can be more than 1 cm

Chronic fibro-cavitative pulmonary TB is called open tuberculosis because the sputum is often infective. Spreading of the infection through the infected sputum can cause tuberculosis of the larynx and intestine. Patients may have hemoptysis if the necrosis involves blood vessels. The habitus of the patient with long time proceeding of fibrous cavernous pulmonary tuberculosis is specific and is named habitus phthisicus. Pulmonary congestion and acrocyanosis are evident. In the final stage, patients will have cor pulmonale because of pulmonary hypertension.

By using of the combination of many tuberculostatic medicine and the reinforcement of patient resistance, the smaller cavity contracts and is obstructed by organization. The bigger cavity wall of granulation tissue is gradually replaced by fibrous scar tissue and covered by bronchial epithelium. Thus, although the cavities still exist, they contain no microphyte and are called openly healing.

(4) Caseous Pneumonia

Caseous pneumonia represents rapid serious progression of tuberculosis. This usually occurs in debilitated immunodeficientor highly sensitized patients. Dissemination large numbers of organisms in the focus via the bronchial tree and spreading rapidly throughout large areas of lung parenchyma and producing a diffuse bronchopneumonia or lobar exudative consolidation ("galloping consumption"). Grossly, one lobe or an entire lung may be affected(Figure 16-4). Extensive caseous necrosis is its character. According to the size of the lesion, caseous pneumonia is classified to lobular caseous pneumonia and lobar caseous pneumonia. The involved tissue is consolidated. Microscopically, there is marked cellular infiltration and necrosis. A large number of tubercle bacilli are usually present. The alveoli are filled with an exudate that contains monocytes and lymphocytes. Patients are in danger.

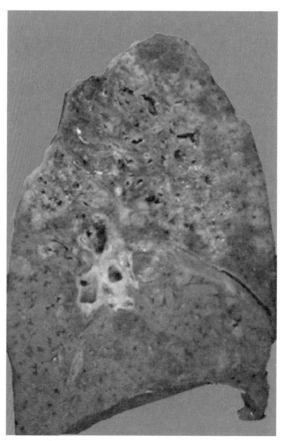

Figure 16-4 **Caseous pneumonia**

One lobe of the lung is affected

（5）Tuberculoma

The coalescence of caseous necrosis can form a large solid and spherical mass（usually 2–5 cm in diameter）（Figure 16–5）. They may be single or multiple, and commonly in the upper lobe. The lesion is usually well delineated. On chest X-ray, it is easily mistaken for a tumor. This pattern may be the result of two forms of pulmonary tuberculosis: infiltrative-pneumonic and focal. Besides this, tuberculoma form from cavernous pulmonary tuberculosis via of filling the cavity with caseous masses. Filled cavities refer to tuberculoma only conditionally, as the filling of a cavity occurs mechanically, while tuberculomas are an original phenomenon in lung tissue. The prevalence of tuberculoma among all forms of pulmonary tuberculosis is 6% – 10%. This tendency is explained by the fact that vast infiltrative pneumonic processes, under treatment and increased body resistance, become limited, condensed, lose their aggravated course. However, the process does not heal completely and precisely outlined dense formation remains. So, tuberculomas represent quiescent disease.

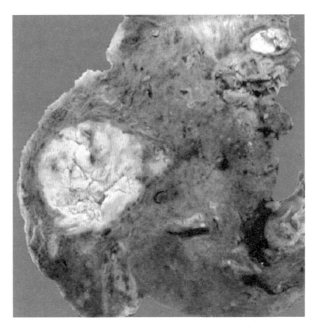

Figure 16–5   **Tuberculoma**

The coalescence of caseous necrosis form a large solid and spherical mass（usually 2–5 cm in diameter）

（6）Tuberculosis Pleuritis

According to affected feature, tuberculosis pleuritis can be divide into: moist tuberculous pleuritis（exudative tuberculous pleuritis）and dry tuberculous pleuritis（proliferative tuberculous pleuritis）.

Moist tuberculous pleuritis is an exudative inflammation dominate（serious or serofibrinous）inflammation. The course of dry serous pleurisy of tubercular etiology divided into three phases: the exudation, stabilization of the process, resorption of effusion. At exudative pleurisy essential shifts in proportions of proteins is distinguished. For definition of exudates character and etiology of pleurisy, it is extremely important the examination of pleural effusion. Serous tubercular effusion is usually transparent, yellowish in color, with densities from 1,015 up to 1,025 and contents of protein from 3% –6%. In acute phase of exudation, lymphocytes prevail in pleural effusion. （50% –60% ）; there are a small amount eosinophils, erythrocytes and mesotelial cells. With adequate therapy, effusion may be absorbed. If effusion contains much of the cellulose, it is difficult to absorb and may cause thicken and adhesion of pleura because of organization.

Dry tuberculous pleuritis(proliferative tuberculous pleuritis)is the proliferative lesion dominate inflammation. Often these lesions are at the apex of the lung, associated with granulomas, and do not involve formation of a hydrothorax. The basic clinical displays are pain in the chest, dry cough, infringement of general condition and subfebrile temperature. Localization of pain depends on place of the damage. The pain amplifies at deep breath, cough and pressing on intercostals spaces. For physical examinations of the patients, lagging of the damaged part of chest reveals at breathing and weak dull sound at percussion. Dry pleurisy can be healed by the end of treatment and have proceeds favorably. Sometimes it gets relapsing character.

16.1.2.3 Miliary Tuberculosis

Miliary pulmonary disease occurs when organisms drain through lymphatics into the lymphatic ducts, which empty into the venous return to the right side of the heart and thence into the pulmonary arteries. Individual lesions are either microscopic or small, visible(2-mm)foci of yellow-white consolidation scattered through the lung parenchyma(the word miliary is derived from the resemblance of these foci to millet seeds). Miliary lesions may expand and coalesce to yield almost total consolidation of large regions or even whole lobes of the lung. With progressive pulmonary tuberculosis, the pleural cavity is invariably involved and serous pleural effusions, tuberculous empyema, or obliterative fibrous pleuritis may develop.

(1)Acute Systemic Miliary Tuberculosis

It results from the hematogenous disseminated lesions of pulmonary Blare numbers of mycobacteria usually enter one of the pulmonary veins and via left heart, into the arterial systemic circulation and spread to the general various organs. In gross appearance, the lesions are multiple, scattered, approximate 1-2 mm in diameter size, fairly uniform size, round, gray white well demarcated nodules in the organ(Figure 16-6). Microscopically the tubercles are proliferative changes dominate, often without giant cells, but with central necrosis. Occasionally, the lesions are exudative, with necrosis in the center. Clinically, the patients have high fever, night sweats, loss of appetite, failure, hepatomegaly and splenomegaly. With adequate treatment, the prognosis is favorable. Some patients will die from tuberculous meningitis.

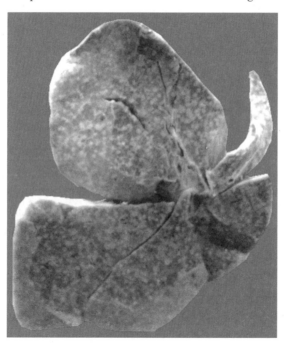

Figure 16-6　**Military tuberculosis of lung**

The lesions are multiple, scattered, approximate 1-2 mm in diameter size,
fairly uniform size, round, gray white well demarcated nodules in the lung

（2）Chronic Systemic Miliary Tuberculosis

It occurs when acute systemic miliary tuberculosis is not healed for three weeks or when tubercle bacillus invades into blood slightly and multiply for a long time. In gross appearance, the lesions are uneven in the organ. Microscopically the tubercles are often concomitant of exudation, proliferation and necrosis. The main patients are adults and the course of the disease is long.

16.1.2.4   Acute Pulmonary Military Tuberculosis

It occurs when caseous necrosis in the hilar lymphadenopathy escape into a systemic vein, either directly or by involvement of the thoracic duct, and via right heart, pulmonary artery, disseminating to the lung. The pulmonary lesions in this condition are part of acute systemic miliary tuberculosis. In gross appearance, both lungs are in congestion with dark-red in color on the cut surface and numerous grey or grey-yellow miliary nodules in size rising on surface of lung. Individual lesions are either microscopic or small.

Chronic pulmonary miliary tuberculosis.

It often occurs in adults when *tubercle bacillus* in lesions of extrapulmonary-TB drains into blood periodically. The course of disease is long and the lesions are new or old lesion, small or big together. The main pathological change is proliferation.

16.1.3   Extrapulmonary Tuberculosis

Extrapulmonary tuberculosis is usually the result of hematogenous spread of infection from the lung. It can also occur after ingestion of tubercle bacilli, e. g. , in milk. Any organ can be infected, e. g. , brain, liver, gastrointestinal tract, spleen, kidney, adrenal glands, bones and genitourinary organs.

16.1.3.1   Intestinal Tuberculosis

Intestinal tuberculosis is classified into primary intestinal tuberculosis and secondary intestinal tuberculosis. Primary intestinal tuberculosis usually occurs in children who drink contaminated Mycobacterium tuberculosis milk. It may develop into intestinal primary complex: ①a primary intestinal lesion; ②intestinal tuberculous lymphangitis; ③mesenteric tuberculous lymphadenitis. Secondary intestinal tuberculosis usually occurs in adults(21−40 years old)and most often occurs in the ileocecal region. There are two morphological forms of the disease: the ulcerative type and the hyperplastic type.

（1）Ulcerative Intestinal Tuberculosis

The organisms are trapped in mucosal lymphoid aggregates of the small and large bowel, which then undergo inflammatory enlargement with ulceration of the overlying mucosa, particularly in the ileum (85%). Grossly, irregular ring or band shaped ulcers can be seen in the mucous membrane with some caseation on the bottom, and these ulcers are perpendicular to the long axis of the ileum. On the serous membrane near these ulcers, there are many small grey-white or grey-yellow nodules with string-of-beads alignment, which are caused by tuberculosis lymphangitis. Microscopically, caseous necrosis occurs on the serous membrane surface. tuberculous granulation tissue is below the necrosis. Because of scar contraction and the adhesion with adjacent tissue, the enteric canal will become stegnotic, which is the most common complication of ulcerative intestinal tuberculosis. Perforation and hemorrhage occur from the erosion into peritoneal and vessels in the ulcer base.

（2）Proliferative Intestinal Tuberculosis

This type of disease only occurs in about 15% patients. It is characterized by formation of tuberculous granulation tissue and fibrous tissue proliferation in the intestine, which leads to the intestinal wall thickening. Usually, the clinical symptoms are intestinal cavity stenosis and obstruction. It is also characterized by formation of multiple polyps and the diagnosis should be differentiated from carcinoma.

16.1.3.2　Tuberculous Meningitis

Tuberculous meningitis occurs more often in children than adult. It is caused by bloodstream spread of Mycobacterium tuberculosis. In children, tuberculous meningitis is usually the result of bloodstream spread of primary pulmonary TB. In adults, most cases are result from tuberculosis of lung, bone, joint, urinary and genital system. Some cases are caused by rupture of tuberculoma in brain.

The base of the brain is usually the most obviously affected region. The brain surface is covered with small tubercles. Yellow gelatinous exudate accumulate in the subarachnoid space of pons, interpedunculare cistern, optic chiasm and sylvian fissure. There is only a moderate increase in cellularity of the pleiocytosis, which is made up of mononuclear cells, or a mixture of polymorphonuclear and mononuclear cells. It may also result in a well-circumscribed intraparenchymal mass (tuberculoma), which may be associated with meningitis. Meninges adhesion may obstruct the flow of cerebrospinal fluid and lead to hydrocephalus. When the inflammation is in the brain stem subarachnoid area, cranial nerve roots may be affected. The symptoms will mimic those of space-occupying lesions. Fever and headache are the cardinal features. Confusion in advanced symptom but coma bears a poor prognosis will be poor prognosis.

Confusion is a late feature and coma bears a poor prognosis.

16.1.3.3　Tuberculosis of Genitourinary System

Renal tuberculosis is usually a blood borne infection from tuberculosis of the pulmonary. The tubercle lesions often occur at the cortico-medullary junction, or in renal pyramids and papillae. With the enlargement of tubercles, the caseous necrosis coalesce into necrotic irregular cavities and result in nonfunctioning kidneys. On the cut surface, kidney shows several cavities in different sizes with coarse wall, yellowish white caseous necrosis attaches inside (Figure 16-7). Microscopically, similar to tubercles in other organs, renal tuberculous lesion is a collection of reticulo-endothelial cells, phagocytosis and giant cell formation, which is surrounded by infiltration and thin collagenous fibers. These minute tuberculosis lesions may coalesce. Necrotic material is often discharged through the ureter leaving multiple cavities within the kidney. Calcification is uncommon. The entire kidney, pelvic mucosa, ureter, and urinary bladder may become infected. Severe cases involve the entire bladder and deep layers of muscle are eventually replaced by fibrosis tissue. Due to lose of the anti-reflux mechanism, the ureteral orifice fibrosis can lead to stricture formation with hydronephrosis or scarification with vesicoureteral reflux.

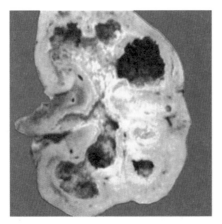

Figure 16-7　**Tuberculosis of kidney**

Several cavities in different size with coarse wall
and yellowish white caseous necrosis inside of the
kidney

The male and female genital organs are usually infected by hematogenous dissemination. In the male, infection of the seminal vesicles and prostate can also occur from the urinary tract. Common patterns of infection include: tuberculous salpingitis (infection of the fallopian tubes), tuberculous endometritis, tuberculous prostatitis and tuberculous epididymitis. Epididymis TB can result in male sterility. Females are more frequently affected. Tuberculosis of the uterus, fallopian tubes and ovaries are most common. TB of fallopian tubes is one of the causes of female sterility.

16.1.3.4 Tuberculosis of Bones and Joints

Tuberculosis of bones and joints often occur in children and teenagers by hematogenous dissemination. Early lesions often occur near the epiphyseal line (growth plates) in children before the growth plate has closed. Tuberculosis can cause destruction of cartilage and intervertebral discs with disc erosion, synovitis, and arthritis.

Bone infection complicates an estimated 1% to 3% of cases of pulmonary tuberculosis. Long bones and vertebrae are most common sites. The lesions are often solitary, but also can be multicentric, particularly in patients with an underlying immunodeficiency. The infection can cause a typical granulomatous inflammation with caseous necrosis and extensive bone destruction. The lesion usually erodes the peripheral soft tissue and results in the formation of "abscess", which is the liquefaction of necrotic material formed by the side of the bone. Because the "abscess" is not red, hot and painful, it is named "cold abscess". When abscess erodes into the skin, a sinus tract is formed. Tuberculosis of the vertebral bodies, is an important form of osteomyelitis. Infection at this site causes vertebral deformity and collapse, with secondary neurologic deficits.

Tuberculosis involves joints that matters most spine, hips, knees, feet, elbows, wrists, and shoulders, in this order of frequency, and occasionally other joints as well. The patients are young adults, or children over 6 years. Spinal tuberculosis has a tendency to spread along fascial planes (psoas abscess). Tuberculous arthritis is 'cold', which means that the skin over the infected joint is the same temperature as the normal skin. The joint is not 'hot', as it is in septic arthritis. In a synovial joint, the disease starts from the synovium and grows slowly over the cartilage; it then extends through the cartilage into the underlying bone, which decalcifies. Sometimes, cold abscesses and sinuses are formed.

16.1.3.5 Tuberculous Lymphadenitis

It is common in children and young adults. Involvement of regional lymph nodes occurs in all forms of tuberculosis. It is the result of lymphatic or hematogenous dissemination of M. tuberculosis. The cervical lymph node is the most frequent form and it also can occur in bronchial and mesenteric lymph node. Structure of lymph node is destroyed and replaced by tubercles in different sizes. The characteristic morphological element is the tuberculous granuloma. There is caseous necrosis at the center of the tubercle surrounded by epithelioid cell, Langerhans giant cell and lymphocytes. Granulomatous tubercles eventually become confluent and replace the lymphoid tissue. Lymphadenitis usually affect the localized group of nodes, with caseous necrosis and tuberculation. Enlarged and adherent lymph nodes can form a big lump (Figure 16-8).

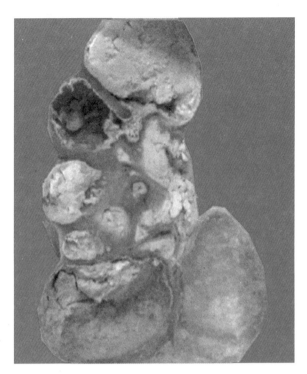

Figure 16-8　**Tuberculosis of lymph node**

Structure of lymph node is destroyed and replaced by tubercles in different size. Enlarged and adherent lymph nodes can form a big lump

16.2　Typhoid Fever

Typhoid fever is an acute infectious disease caused by salmonella typhi. It is characterized by hyperplasia of mononuclear-macrophages in the reticuloendothelium of all over the body(intestinal and the mesenteric lymph nodes, liver, spleen and bone marrow, etc.). The hallmark of clinic feature is persistent, high fever, splenomegaly, relative bradycardia, rose-colored spots on the trunk, reduction of blood neutrophils and eosinophils.

16.2.1　Etiology and Pathogenesis

Salmonella typhi is a facultative intracellular organism and infects only humans. It has Somatic antigen ("antigen"), flagellar antigen("H" antigen) and surface antigen("V1" antigen). Wildal's test is the traditional serologic test for the diagnosis of typhoid fever. It also can release endotoxin, which is the main etiological factor.

The source of infection are patients and healthy carriers. Fecal-oral transmission is the main route of infection. Flies, raw shellfish, and patients' hands are especially important vectors. The infection results from contamination of food and water with feces from a symptomatic case or a symptomatic carrier of typhoid. The ingested bacillus invades the small intestinal mucosa, where it is taken up by macrophages and transported to regional lymph nodes and multiplies in the intestinal lymphoid tissue during the ten days incubation period. Then they enter the bloodstream through the thoracic duct and are carried to the liver, bone marrow, spleen and kidneys. Ingestion by phagocytic cells causes generalized hyperplasia of the mononuclear phagocytic system. S typhi reenters the intestinal lumen by way of biliary excretion. The most prominent change is in Peyer's patches and solitary lymph follicles of the distal ileum. Healing usually begins about at the end of the third week and is complete by the fifth week in uncomplicated cases. The main mechanisms of the disease are proliferation of bacteria, coupled with an antigen-antibody hypersensitivity reaction.

16.2.2　Intestinal Morphology

The lesion of lymphoid tissue in intestine tract is usually most marked in the Peyer's patches of the distal ileum and solitary lymphoid follicles of the cecum. The whole course is divided into 4 stages and each course lasts about one week.

16.2.2.1　The Stage of Medullary Swelling

In the first week of infection there is swelling of the solitary lymphoid follicles and Peyer's patches. Peyer patches in the terminal ileum become sharply delineated, plateau-like elevations up to 8cm in diameter, with enlargement of draining mesenteric lymph nodes. The surface of the lymphoid tissue is convoluted, like the surface of the brain, thus, it is also called medullary swelling (Figure 16-9). Microscopically, Peyer's patch shows congestion and marked proliferation of macrophages. These cells have abundant pale cytoplasm with round or oval eccentric nuclei. Macrophages have increased phagocytic activity, and may contain ingested red blood cells, lymphocytes, and cellular debris. These so-called "typhoid cells" have diagnostic significance. Intermingled with the phagocytes are lymphocytes and plasma cells. Collections of these cells form typhoid nodules or granulomas. Clinically, patients have suffered from blood diseases and with staircase-like rise of typhoid cells sometimes.

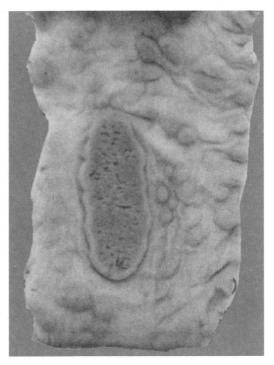

Figure 16-9　**Typhoid fever of intestine**
The stage of medullary swelling

The surface of the lymphoid tissue is convoluted, like the surface of the brain.

16.2.2.2 The Stage of Necrosis

The stage of necrosis occurs in the second week. Lymphoid tissue undergoes necrosis, forming grayish-white or grayish-green areas. Necrosis can extend deeply to the muscular propria and even the serosal coat. The development of focal necrosis can lead to softening and rupture of the lymphoid patches. Clinically, the patient has persistent high fever, bradycardia, hepatosplenomegaly, rose-coloured spots in the skin, leukocytopenia and diarrhea. The more serious complication resulting from extensive necrosis is perforation of the small vowel with usually fatal generalized peritonitis.

16.2.2.3 The Stage of Ulceration

The stage of ulceration occurs in the third week. Ulcers occur as longitudinal ulcers overlying the peyer patches in the ileum. The mucosal ulcers tend to take the shape and extent of the underlying lymphoid patches(round or oval). Necrotic mucosa sloughs off, leaving round or oval ulcers. They have slightly elevated margins. Ulcers may penetrate to the serosa and cause intestinal perforation and peritonitis. Erosion of blood vessels at the ulcer base can cause severe massive hemorrhage. Perforation and hemorrhage are both serious complications of typhoid fever. Typhoid ulcers can be differentiated from tuberculous ulcers. Tuberculous infection spreads along submucosal lymphatics to form circumferential ulcers. Ulcer healing may result in stricture. Typhoid ulcers, on the other hand, lie parallel to the long axis of the intestine, and hence healing will not cause strictures.

16.2.2.4 The Stage of Healing(the Fourth Week)

The fourth week is the stage of healing. Ulcers heal by formation of granulation tissue and re-epithelialization of the ulcer surface. Healing of these ulcerated lesions leaves a smooth scar which never shows any tendency towards stricture formation. In clinic, the patient's temperature shows a staircase-like descend to recover normally. Patients become afebrile.

But, in the antibiotic era, it is difficult to find typical four stages(swollen, necrotic, ulcerative and healing stages).

16.2.3 Changes in Other Organs

The lesions are characterized by an acute proliferative inflammation of reticuloendothelial and lymphoid tissues, e. g. bone marrow, spleen and liver. Sections of the enlarged spleen in typhoid fever show congestion and dilatation of splenic sinuses. The enlarged liver shows sinusoidal dilatation and degeneration and necrosis of liver cells. Typical granulomas can also be found in the spleen, liver, bone marrow and lymph nodes. Gallblader colonization, which may be associated with gallstones, causes a chronic carrier state.

Fever with a remittent pattern, relative bradycardia, hepatomegaly and splenomegaly, rose spots and decreased numbers of neutrophils and eosinophils are clinical characteristics of the illness. Due to endotoxaemia and bacteraemia, typhoid fever is also associated with a great variety of lesions which are widely distributed and may arise during the course of the disease. Laryngitis, bronchitis and bronchopneumonia may occur.

16.3 Bacillary Dysentery

Dysentery refers to diarrhea with abdominal cramping and tenesmus, which loose stools contain blood, pus, and mucus. Bacillary dysentery is the acute pseudomembranous inflammation caused by Shigella species.

16.3.1   Etiology and Pathogenesis

Shigella species are gram-negative bacilli. The four species of Shigella are pathogenic for humans, including Shifella sonnei, Shigella flexneri, Shigella boydii—uncommon; Shigella dysenteriae-produces a severe illness. Patients and healthy carriers are sources of infection. The routes of infection are atypical fecal-oral transmission and flies serve as an important vectors in transmission. It is transmitted by food and water contaminated by Shigella. Most of Shigella is killed by gastric acid, so few can get into small intestine. The organisms invade directly the intestinal mucosa by producing endotoxin and cause ulceration of intestinal mucosa. Endotoxin enters blood stream and results in systematic toxemia. Exotoxin, which is produced by S. dysenteriae, is the main factor that cause large-volume watery diarrhea.

16.3.2   Pathology and Clinical Features

Sigmoid colon, rectum are the most commonly affected areas. In severe conditions all the colon and the terminal ileum can be affected. The extraintestinal lesion is rare. There are three different types of bacillary dysentery: acute bacillary dysentery, chronic bacillary dysentery and toxic bacillary dysentery.

16.3.3   Acute Bacillary Dysentery

A typical disease course consists of acute catarrh inflammation, subsequent distinctive pseudomembranous inflammation and ulceration, and healing eventually.

Initial, acute catarrh inflammation is an acute inflammation with diffuse hyperemia, edema, punctuate hemorrhage, infiltrating of inflammatory cells (neutrophils) , excess mucus secretion and formation superficial erosion in the mucosa. A fibrinosuppurative exudates first patchily, then diffusely covers the mucosa and produces a dirty gray to yellow pseudomembrane. Grossly, on the surface of the mucosa of affected colon, firstly the pseudomembrane patchily distributed and then diffusely cover the mucosa and produce a dirty membranous matter(Figure 16–10). Microscopically, mucosal gland in areas of mild inflammation are preserved. In severely affected areas, there are superficial necrosis, absent glands, submucosal edema, hemorrhage, and neutrophilic infiltration. The necrotic mucosal epithelium is covered by an acute suppurative and fibrinous exudate, forming a pseudomembrane. The pseudomembrane is composed of fibrins, numerous neutrophils admixed with red cells, cell debris and bacteria. When the pseudomembrane sloughs, it leaves shallow ulcers of varying sizes. One week later, the inflammatory reaction within the intestinal mucosa builds up, the mucosa becomes soft and friable, and irregular superficial ulcerations appear(maplike ulcers). As the disease progresses, the ulcer margins are transformed into active granulation tissue. When the disease remits, this granulation tissue fills the defect, and the ulers heal by regeneration of the mucosal epithelium, sometimes with the formation of polyps.

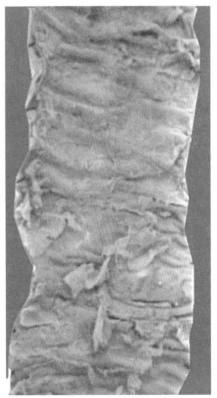

Figure 16–10   **Bacillary dysentery**

On the surface of the mucosa of affected colon, pseudomembrane patchily distributes and produces a dirty membranous matter

In clinic, patients have severe tenesmus and diarrhea with blood and pus, or blood and mucus. Because inflammation stimulates the nerve terminal of rectum and anal sphincter, patients have tenesmus and the frequency of acute defecation increases. Patients defecate mucoid loose stool, mucoid bloody perulent stool, occasionally accompanying lamellar pseudomembrane. It is usually a self-limited disease of three days to one week and rarely lasts as long as a month. Sometimes illness can transform to chronic bacillary dysentery.

16.3.4 Chronic Bacillary Dysentery

Course of bacillary dysentery has been exceeded more than 2 months. The chronic cases are characterized by repeated injury and repair, ulceration and healing, and can lead to new and old lesions coexist, chronic ulcer formation, polypoid mucosal irregularity with fibrous scarring and subsequent stenosis of the bowel.

In clinic, patients have abdominal pain, chronic diarrhea intestinal obstruction. Some patients do not any symptoms or signs, but their stool culture is persistent positive. Patients of this type will become chronic carrier and infection sources.

16.3.5 Toxic Bacillary Dysentery

The disease is usually caused by Shigella sonnei and Shigella flexneri that have low virulence and their pathogenesis is unaware. It occurs most commonly in children at the age of 2–7 years. The onset of disease is sudden. Patients have severe systemic toxic symptom and mild intestinal symptom.

Intestinal lesion is catarrh enteritis or follicular enteritis. There are severe general toxic symptoms (high fever, convulsion). Several hours later, toxic shock, coma or brain edema and respiratory failure appear rapidly.

16.4 Leprosy

Leprosy is a chronic inflammatory disease of low infectivity caused by Mycobacterium leprae. The disease mainly involves the skin and peripheral nerves. The disease spreads extensively in the world, especially in warm and wet areas.

16.4.1 Etiology and Pathogenesis

Mycobacterium leprae and Mycobacterium lepromatosis are the causative agents of leprosy. M. lepromatosis is a relatively newly identified mycobacterium isolated from a fatal case of diffuse lepromatous leprosy in 2008. An intracellular, acid-fast bacterium, M. leprae is aerobic and rod-shaped, and is surrounded by the waxy cell membrane coating characteristic of Mycobacterium species. The use of non-culture-based techniques such as molecular genetics has allowed for alternative establishment of causation. While the causative organisms up to date have been impossible to culture in vitro, it has been possible to grow them in animals. Naturally occurring infection also has been reported in non-human primates including the African chimpanzee, sooty mangabey, and cynomolgus macaque, as well as in armadillos.

Human-to-human transmission is the primary source of infection. Leprosy was previously thought to be transmitted through intact skin by direct contact. However, current evidence suggests that the bacillus is inhaled into the respiratory tract through prolonged contact with nasal secretions or open ulcers of infected people. Bacilli are taken up by macrophages and disseminated widely throughout the body. Disease results from proliferation of the micro-organisms and the host response to them. The disease has a latent period of 2–5 years. The organisms grow best at lower temperatures and are found mainly in the peripheral nerves and skin. In the skin, leprosy causes atrophy of cutaneous appendages resulting in loss of sweating, and loss of eyebrows or hair. In the peripheral nerves, nerve trunks become thick. Patients lose sensation. Limbs become disabled.

16.4.2　Morphology and Clinicopathologic

The disease is termed a chronic granulomatous disease, similar to tuberculosis, because it produces inflammatory nodules(granulomas) in the skin and nerves over time. Leprosy can be classified as three types: tuberculoid leprosy, lepromatous leprosy and borderline leprosy.

Tuberculoid leprosy accounts for 70% of cases of leprosy disease. The form occurs in patients who have strong immune responses to infection. The characteristic lesion is the result of formation of tuberculoid granulomas. Grossly, the lesions are symmetric, and localized to one or more areas of skin, especially the legs and feet. They are annular, flat and lack sensation. The cutaneous nerves are often palpably enlarged. Microscopically, the granulomatous foci consist of epithelioid cells, Langhans giant cells, and numerous lymphocytes at the periphery. They closely resemble the lesions of tuberculosis. Caseous necrosis is rare, but occurs in lesions of nerve stem, which usually affects appendages of the skin and results in hypesthesia and absent sweating. This type of leprosy is less infectious and progresses slowly. The results of treatment and prognosis are better than in other forms. The lepromin skin test is positive, reflecting the immune response. M. leprae can be detected by acid-fast stains but there are fewer organisms than in Lepromatous leprosy.

Lepromatous leprosy accounts for 20% of cases of leprosy disease. This form of the disease occurs when patients fail to develop an immune response. As a result, bacilli proliferate readily and cause more extensive disease than in the tuberculoid form. Lepromatous leprosy presents with granuloma composed of foam cells and few lymph cells. Foam cells originate from macrophage cells, many of which contain lepra bacilli, called lepra cells. Lesions surround small vessels and appendages of the skin and can progress to fuse. There is a no cell infiltration layer between epidermis and infiltrative focus, which is one of the features of lepromatous leprosy. Lepromatous leprosy involves the nose, lymph nodes, liver, spleen and testes. A distinctive deformity of the face is known as leonine face. Lesions in the nose cause collapse of the bridge of the nose or perforation of the septum. The lepromin test is negative because patients have not developed an immune response to the organism.

Borderline leprosy is also called as indeterminate leprosy and of intermediate severity. These lesions have features that resemble both tuberculoid and lepromatous forms of the disease. Skin lesions resemble tuberculoid leprosy but are more numerous and irregular; large patches may affect the whole limb, and peripheral nerve involvement with weakness and loss of sensation is common. This type is unstable and may become more like lepromatous leprosy or may undergo a reversal reaction, becoming more like the tuberculoid leprosy form. These lesions may heal or may progress to either tuberculoid or lepromatous leprosy.

16.5　Leptospirosis

Leptospirosis is caused by infection with bacteria of the genus Leptospira and affects humans as well as other animals. It is among the world's most common diseases transmitted to people from animals. It distributes worldwide, especially in tropical and subtropical areas. There is a direct correlation between the amount of rainfall and the incidence of leptospirosis, making it seasonal in temperate climates and year-round in tropical climates.

16.5.1 Etiology and Pathogenesis

Leptospirosis is transmitted by the urine of an infected animal and is contagious as long as it is still moist. Rats, mice, and moles are important primary hosts. Humans become infected through contact with water, food, or soil containing urine from these infected animals. This may happen by swallowing contaminated food or water or through skin contact. The disease is not known to be spread from person to person and cases of bacterial dissemination in convalescence are extremely rare in humans. Leptospirosis is common among water-sport enthusiasts in specific areas because prolonged immersion in water can promote the entry of the bacteria. Surfers and whitewater paddlers are at especially high risk in areas that have been shown to contain the bacteria, and can contract the disease by swallowing contaminated water, splashing contaminated water into their eyes or nose, or exposing open wounds to infected water. The pathogensis of leptospirosis is still indistinct. Leptospiral toxin is one of the etiology factors, and its specificity and function still need to research.

16.5.2 Morphology and Clinicopathologic

The genus Leptospira is thought to comprise many species, which have specific surface antigen and collective inner antigen. Different species of Leptospira have different virulence to human and involve different organs. Leptospiral infection in humans causes a range of symptoms, and some infected persons may have no symptoms at all. In clinic, the develop ment process of leptospirosis is divided into three stages: early, middle and late. This classification has great significance in guiding the clinical practice, especially the early diagnosis and treatment.

16.5.2.1 Early Stage(Septicmic Stage)

The symptoms in humans appear after a 1-3 day incubation period. Symptoms of leptospirosis include high fever, severe headache, chills, muscle aches, and vomiting, and may include jaundice, red eyes, abdominal pain, diarrhea, and rash. Initial presentation may resemble pneumonia. The first phase resolves, and the patient is briefly asymptomatic until the second phase begins.

16.5.2.2 Middle Stage(Septicmic with Tissue Damage stage)

It occurs after 4-10 day incubation period and inner organ damage is seen in this stage. This is characterized by meningitis, liver damage(causing jaundice), and renal failure. Cardiovascular problems are also possible and in severe cases commonly death occurs in this stage.

16.5.2.3 Late Stage(Convalescent Stage)

Most patients recover from illness after 2-to-3 week onset. High fever symptoms gradually subsided. Myocarditis, pericarditis, meningitis, and uveitis are also possible sequelae. Some patients have ocular and neurologic sequelae due to specific immunological reaction.

16.5.3 Pathology

The pathological changes of leptospirosis are acute systemic toxic injury and usually involves capillary, which results in distribution of circulation. It shows degeneration, necrosis, and severe functional disturbance of parenchymatous organs.

(1) Liver

The lesions can be mild and severe. Mild lesions only show slight interstitial edema and congestion of blood vessels and scattered focal necrosis under microscope. In severe cases, jaundice and hepatomegaly may occur. Under microscope, the lesion is marked by obvious liver necrosis, liver cells swelling, fatty degeneration and vacuolization, portal to neutral cell based cell infiltration. Partial necrosis of liver cells and mitotic, serous liver cells arrange in discrete disorder, which lead to biliary excretion disorder. Liver cell necrosis cause dyssynthesis of blood coagulation factor and hemorrhage can be observed in skin and mucosa wildly。

(2) Kidney

The lesion is mainly interstitial nephritis. The appearance of the renal cortex kidney may have bleeding or hemorrhage spot under the renal capsule. Microscopically, the main lesions are renal tubular epithelial cloudy swelling and necrosis especially in the distal convoluted tubule and Heinz loop. Renal tubular lumen can be filled with blood cells or transparent tube type, which causes renal tubular dilatation proximal renal tubules. In general, the glomerular lesions are not serious.

(3) Lungs

The main lesion is characterized by pulmonary hemorrhage, which is a frequent cause of death in anicteric cases. Hemorrhage can be observed on the surface of lung. tracheal, bronchial mucosa and even a large number of interstitial and intra alveolar also showed obvious edema and hemorrhage.

(4) Heart

Hemorrhage can be observed in pericardial membrane. Myocardial cells show hyalinized degeneration and focal necrosis. Interstitial edema also can be seen. Patients may have tachycardia, cardiac dysrhythmia and some other symptoms of myocarditis.

(5) Striated Muscle

Bleeding point can be seen in intercostal muscles, psoas major muscle, gastrocnemius muscle, abdominal muscle and diaphragm, the upper wall and thigh muscles. Microscopically, striated structure of muscle fibers disappears. Particles or hyaline degeneration appear in the muscle fiber cell cytoplasm. Hemorrhage, edema and inflammatory cell infiltration may occur in stroma.

(6) Nervous System

Brain parenchyma and meninges appear edemic, congestion, hemorrhage and inflammatory cell infiltration. Nerve cell degeneration can be seen in some cases. Cerebral arteritis may occur in some cases in convalescent stage, especially in children. Cerebral infarction and cerebral atrophy can be seen in subdural or subarachnoid. The main pathological changes are multiple arteritis in pavimentum cerebri and brain parenchyma damage, which result in hemiplegi and aphasia.

16.6 Rabies

Rabies is a viral disease that causes acute encephalitis in warm-blooded animals. The disease is zoonotic, meaning it can be transmitted from one species to another, such as from dogs to humans, commonly by a bite from an infected animal. For a human, rabies is almost invariably fatal if post exposure prophylaxis is not administered prior to the onset of severe symptoms. The rabies virus infects the central nervous system, ultimately causing disease in the brain and death.

16.6.1 Etiology and Pathogenesis

Rabies virus contains 5 kinds of protein, the glycoprotein(G), a nuclear protein(N), polymerase(L), phosphoprotein(NS) and membrane protein(M) etc. Glycoprotein can bind with acetylcholine binding, which leads to the affinity for neural tissue feature of rabies virus. Rabies virus invades from skin or mucosal damage site. Once within a muscle or nerve cell, the virus undergoes the replication. Then the virus invades peripheral nerve and spreads to the central nervous system along the peripheral nerve axoplasm. Virus mainly invades neurons of the brainstem and cerebellum. The rabies virus also can diffuse from the central nervous system to peripheral nerve system, especially invasion in the salivary glands of tongue taste buds, olfactory epithelium. Damage of the vagus nerve nucleus, nucleus of hypoglossal nerve and swallowing the damaged nerve nucleus, cause respiratory muscle and swallowing muscle spasm, which result in hydrophobia, dyspnea, dysphagia in clinic; sympathetic nerve stimulation cause increased saliva secretion and sweating; damage of vagus ganglion, sympathetic ganglion and the cardiac ganglia can cause cardiovascular system function disorder, and even sudden death.

16.6.2 Morphology and Clinicopathologic

The lesions are acute disseminated encephalomyelitis, especially in hippocampus of dorsal root ganglion and spinal cord on the bite site. Usually, there is no meningeal lesions. The brain parenchyma showed hyperemia, edema and bleeding. Under low microscopic, there is nonspecific degeneration and inflammatory changes, such as nerve cell vacuolization, decomposition, hyaline degeneration and chromatin perivascular infiltration of mononuclear cells.

The characteristic lesion is eosinophilic inclusion, called Negri body. Negri bodies are round or oval, dyed cherry red, uniform diameter of about 3-10 nm and most common in the hippocampus and the Meura Kenno organization the nerve cells in the cerebral cortex. They also can be found in the cone cell layer, spinal cord nerve cells, posterior horn, retinal ganglion cells layer and ganglion sympathetic ganglion. Under electron microscope, Negri bodies are the virus colony and contain baculovirus particles.

Salivary acinar cell degenerate, with the mononuclear cells infiltration. Acute degeneration shows in pancreatic acini and epithelial cells, parietal cells of the gastric mucosa, adrenal medulla cells and renal tubular epithelial cells.

Early-stage symptoms of rabies are malaise, headache and fever, progressing to acute pain, violent movements, uncontrolled excitement, depression, and hydrophobia. Finally, the patient may experience periods of mania and lethargy, eventually leading to coma. The primary cause of death is usually respiratory insufficiency. Because the mortality rate is almost 100%, positive and effective treatment of wounds and preventive vaccination are very important.

16.7　Sexually Transmitted Disease

Diseases transmitted during sexual contact are sexually transmitted diseases(STD), but none of STD is acquired solely via coitus. It also can be transmitted by the parents to the fetus or newborn way. In our country, it is called venereal disease. The classical venereal diseases include syphilis, gonorrhea, chancroid and lymphogranuloma venereum. Today venereal diseases contain more than 20 kinds of STD. The STDs are largely diseases of life-style, and their incidence is higher among patients with multiple sexual partners. As a consequence, the coexistence of many STDs is prevalent in groups with high levels of sexual activity. In China, common sexually transmitted microbial pasthogens are now Neisseria gonorrhoeae(gonorrhea), human papillomavirus(HPV)(condyloma acuminatum)and Treponema pallidum(syphilis).

16.7.1   Gonorrhea

Gonorrhoea is a sexually transmitted bacterial infection, caused by the gram-negative diplococcus Neisseria gonorrhoea. Neisseria gonorrhoeae(syn. gonococcus)causes acute suppurative inflammation of the urethra and periurethral glands, which may also extend to the prostate and epididymis. About 90% of males develop a purulent urethral discharge with pain on passing urine as a result of infection, in contrast to females in whom about 70% of gonococcal infections are asymptomatic. Gonorrhoea is a common infection, mainly occurring in 20-24 years old young adults, and has a high infectivity.

16.7.1.1   Etiology and Pathogenesis

Neisseria gonorrhoea occurs only in humans. It is morphologically identical to Neisseria meningitidis, an important cause of bacterial meningitis. Neisseria gonorrhoeae is a facultative intracellular pathogen that binds to and invades epithelial cells through the pili in the envelope of gonococcus and secreted IgA proteolystic enzyme. The polysaccharides of capsular contribute to virulence through inhibiting phagocytosis in the absence condition of antigonococcal antibody. In addition, the pathogen releases peptidoglycans and endotoxin, which induce host cell secretion of TNF-α that may cause damages of infectious epithelial cells. Patients and asymptomatic carriers are source of infection. Usually, it is transmitted by the sexual contacts in the adults, or by the indirect contact in the children. In addition, gonococcal infection may be transmitted to the fetus during delivery through the birth canal; producing neonatal ophthalmitis. Transmission by fomites such as toilet seats or towels is not likely since N. gonorrhoea cannot survive long outside the human body.

16.7.1.2   Morphology and Clinicopathologic

The primary acute infection affects the urethra and the periurethral glands in both sexes and the endocervix in the female. Because stratified squamous epithelium is resistant to invasion by N. gonorrhoea, lesions do not usually occur on the external genitalia or in the vagina. Bacteria infect columnar and transitional cells of the mucous membranes and cause an acute suppurative infection, sometimes with abscess formation, then followed by granulation tissue formation and fibrosis. N. gonorrhoea is usually seen easily within the cytoplasm of polymorphonuclear leukocytes at the sites of infection.

In males, acute gonorrhea usually causes severe urethritis with urinary frequency, urgency, and pain on urination. There is a marked purulent exudate. In female patients, acute symptoms are often less severe but chronic infection of the endometrium, fallopian tubes, ovaries, and peritoneum may cause pelvic pain and vaginal discharge. Congenital infection can cause purulent infection of the eyes and result in blindness. Neisseria gonorrhoeae may spread to the whole body by hematogenous routs, which result in a serious systemic infection. Although the disease often has the typical signs and symptoms, clinical manifestations are variant. The clinical manifestations of disseminated gonococcal infection(DGI)include simple skin damage, arthritis, tenosynovitis or septic arthritis disease spectrum. A few severe DGI can appear endocarditis or meningitis symptoms.

16.7.2   Condyloma Acuminatum

Condyloma acuminatum, also known as genital warts, caused by Human papilloma viruses(HPV), are increasing in prevalence and now probably the most commonest type of lesion seen in patients attending departments of genito-urinary medicine. HPV are a large group of more than 70 double-stranded DNA viruses that can infect squamous epithelium in the skin, mucocutaneous surfaces, and respiratory tract. In the genital tract, HPV Types 6, 11, 16, and 18 are especially common. They are spread by sexual intercourse.

16.7.2.1 Etiology and Pathogenesis

HPV is a kind of DNA virus. Human is the only host for papilloma viruses. Using molecular hybridization, more than 120 subtypes were identified. About 40 species are involved in reproductive tract infection and different types of HPV can cause the different clinical manifestations. The incubation period was from 1 to 8 months, average 3 months. The main clinical manifestations depend on the type of HPV genital epithelium after HPV infection, position and state of the body infection, especially cell immune state. Both sexually vulnerable male wrapping chalaza side, coronary ditch, female joint is most easily clinically lesions. Patients with immune function defect, especially when the cell immune function defects, such as long-term use of corticosteroids or immunosuppressants are prone to infection.

16.7.2.2 Morphology and Clinicopathologic

In the genital organs, human papilloma viruses cause genital warts (condyloma accuminata), epithelial dysplasia, and squamous carcinoma. The primary lesion is small and soft light red papules as big as needle cap or a grain of rice. Then its number and volume increase gradually, then it changes into papillomatous with cauliflower appearance, rough surface, soft texture. The characteristic lesion is hyperplastic, fleshy wart or condyloma acuminatum. This wart occurs most commonly on the glans penis and inner lining of the prepuce or in the terminal urethra. Less often, lesions develop on the shaft of the penis, the perianal region or the scrotum. Histologically, the epidermis shows papillomatous hyperplasia. Many of the epidermal cells show cytoplasmic vaculation (koilocytes), a feature indicating a viral etiology. Vacuolated cells are the characteristic of the lesion and usually located in the upper of prickle cells. The cell body is big, round hyperchromatic nuclei, perinuclear vacuolization and pale staining. Basilar cells proliferate and parabasal cells enlarge with a foamy nuclear chromatin. There is a chronic inflammatory infiltrate and extension of capillary or lymphatic vessels within the dermis. Viral DNA can be identified by in situ hybridization, PCR and in situ PCR. Viral proteins may be detected by immunohistochemistry.

Dysplasia is characterized by lack of normal maturation (differentiation) of the squamous epithelium from the basal epithelial layer towards the surface, by nuclear atypical, and by increased numbers of mitoses. Dysplasia is a precancerous lesion. It can occur at any site infected by HPV but is especially important in the vulva, vagina, and cervix. HPV Types 16 and 18 are considered to be important causes of genital epithelial dysplasia.

Carcinoma in situ and invasive squamous carcinoma result from progression of dysplasia. HPV infection is considered to be the main cause of carcinoma in the genital tract, especially carcinoma of the penis, carcinoma of the vulva, vagina, and cervix.

16.7.3 Syphilis

Syphilis is a chronic venereal infection caused by the spirochete, Treponema pallidum. It has remained an endemic infection in all parts of the world, especially in large cities. There is a strong racial disparity, with African Americans affected 30 times more often than whites.

16.7.3.1 Etiology and Pathogenesis

Treponema pallidum is a fastidious spirochete whose only natural hosts are humans. T. pallidum must be stained with silver or viewed by darkfield microscopy to be detected. It cannot be grown in culture. The usual source of infection is an active cutaneous or mucosal lesion in a sexual partner in the early (primary or secondary) stages of syphilis. The organism is transmitted from such lesions during sexual intercourse across minute breaks in the skin or mucous membranes of the uninfected partner. In cases of congenital syphilis, T. pallidum is transmitted across the placenta from mother to fetus, particularly during the early stages of maternal infection. Once introduced into the body, the organisms are rapidly disseminated to distant sites by lymphatics and the bloodstream. Systemic dissemination of organisms continues and the host mounts an immune response. Specific antibody of syphilis is produced in the sixth week after injection and has serological diagnostic value. Syphilis is classified into two types: congenital syphilis and acquired syphilis.

16.7.3.2   Pathology

Syphilis may affect nearly any organ or tissue in the body. The basic pathologic changes of syphilis are the same, irrespective of the site. The lesions of syphilis vary with the stage of disease. There are two fundamental microscopic lesions of syphilis.

1) Proliferative endarteritis and an accompanying inflammatory infiltrate rich in plasma cells. The lesion can occur in all the stage of syphilis. This lesion is characterized by concentric proliferation of endothelial and fibroblastic cells of small vessels, with a surrounding mononuclear infiltrate, known as periarteritis. Local ischemia caused by the vascular changes undoubtedly accounts for some of the local cell death and fibrosis seen in syphilis. The infiltration of plasma cells around blood vessels has diagnostic significance. Spirochetes are readily demonstrable in histologic sections of early lesions with the use of standard silver stains (e. g. , Warthin-Starry stains).

2) Gumma in late syphilis(tertiary syphilisis), another pattern of tissue injury is a form of granulomatous necrosis. Because of its rubbery texture, such a lesion is known as a gumma. It is an irregular, firm mass of necrotic tissue surrounded by resilient connective tissue, which is similar to tubercle. Histologically, the gumma is characterized by central coagulative necrosis and peripheral epithelioid cells, admixed with giant cells. The central zone of structured necrosis in the original architecture can usually be distinguished. Granulation tissue heavily infiltrated by plasma cells and lymphocytes. This focus is enclosed by a fibroblastic wall, in which the small vessels may show endarteritis and periarteritis. Healing of a gumma is by absorption of the necrotic center and by progressive fibrous proliferation, leading to scarring.

16.7.3.3   Congenital Syphilis

T. pallidum may be transmitted across the placenta from an infected mother to the fetus at any time during pregnancy. In the absence of treatment, 40% of infected infants die in utero, typically after the fourth month. In cases of congenital syphilis, the placenta is enlarged, pale, and edematous. Microscopy reveals proliferative endarteritis involving the fetal vessels, a mononuclear inflammatory reaction(villitis), and villous immaturity. According to the clinical manifestations, congenital syphilis can be devided into two types: early(prior to age 2 years) and late(after age 2 years) congenital syphilis.

1) Early congenital syphilis for stillborn infants, the most common manifestations are hepatomegaly, bone abnormalities, pancreatic fibrosis, and pneumonitis. Infantile syphilis refers to congenital syphilis in liveborn infants that is clinically manifest at birth or within the first few months of life. Affected infants present with chronic rhinitis(snuffles) and mucocutaneous lesions, similar to those seen in secondary syphilis in adults. Visceral and skeletal changes resembling those seen in stillborn infants may also be present.

2) Late congenital syphilis: It refers to cases of untreated congenital syphilis of more than 2 years' duration. Classic manifestations include the Hutchinson triad: notched central incisors, interstitial keratitis with blindness, and deafness from eighth cranial nerve injury. Other changes include a saber shin deformity caused by chronic inflammation of the periosteum of the tibia, deformed molar teeth("mulberry" molars), chronic meningitis, chorioretinitis, and gummas of the nasal bone and cartilage with a resultant "saddle-

nose" deformity.

16.7.3.4 Acquired Syphilis

Acquired syphilis may progress through three distinct phases: primary, secondary and tertiary syphilis. The lesions of syphilis vary with the stage of disease. The primary lesion, termed a chancre, appears at the point of entry between 9 and 90 days (a mean of 21 days) after the initial infection. The secondary syphilis usually occurs within 7–8 weeks after the primary chancre. Tertiary syphilis usually develops within 4–5 years of infection.

(1) Primary Syphilis

It is characterized by the presence of a chancre at the site of initial inoculation. The primary chancre in males is usually on the penis. In females, multiple chancres may be present, usually in the vagina or on the uterine cervix. The chancre begins as a small, firm papule, which fully developed is a hard, painless, indurated ulcer with regular, well-demarcated margins and a "clean," moist base. This occurs within 3 months at the site of inoculation. Regional lymph nodes are often slightly enlarged and firm, but painless. Histologically, the lesion is characterized by granulation tissue underlying the ulcer, endothelial proliferation in small blood vessels, heavy plasma-cell and lymphocytic infiltration. The ulcer can be healed by fibrosis, producing a small scar. Spirochetes may be demonstrable by a silver impregnation stain, such as the Levaditi stain. Even without therapy, the primary chancre resolves over a period of several weeks to form a subtle scar.

(2) Secondary Syphilis

The manifestations of secondary syphilis are varied but typically include a combination of generalized lymph node enlargement and a variety of mucocutaneous lesions. The lesions of secondary syphilis are very variable in location and result from systemic dissemination of T. pallidum with infection of multiple organs. Important sites of these lesions include: ①Skin. The lesions are usually symmetrically distributed and may be maculopapular, scaly, or pustular. Involvement of the palms of the hands and soles of the feet is common. In moist skin areas, such as the anogenital region, inner thighs, and axillae, broad-based, elevated lesions termed condylomata lata may occur. Pustular destructive lesions occur on the soles of the feet or palms of the hands. ②Mucous membranes. Superficial mucosal lesions resembling condylomata lata can occur anywhere, but they are particularly common in the oral cavity, pharynx, and external genitalia. These lesions are highly infectious because they contain numerous micro-organisms. Mucous patches are termed as grey white membranes with a dull-red margin, found in the mouth, pharynx and larynx. The ulcer also can be called as Snail-track ulcers. Histologic examination reveals the characteristic proliferative endarteritis, accompanied by a lymphoplasmacytic inflammatory infiltrate. ③Lymphadenitis. Lymph node enlargement is most common in the neck and inguinal areas. Biopsy of enlarged nodes reveals nonspecific hyperplasia of germinal centers accompanied by increased numbers of plasma cells or, less commonly, granulomas or neutrophils. There are numerous spirochetes. The lymphoid follicles are hyperplastic with many lymphocytes, plasma cells, and macrophages. The blood vessels may show typical syphilitic vasculitis. ④Other organs. Less common manifestations of secondary syphilis include hepatitis, renal disease, eye disease (iritis), and gastrointestinal abnormalities. The mucocutaneous lesions of secondary syphilis resolve over a period of several weeks, at which point the patient enters the early latent phase of the disease, which lasts approximately 1 year. Lesions may recur at any time during the early latent phase, during which the disease may still be spread.

(3) Tertiary Syphilis

The lesions of tertiary syphilis are the result of chronic infection at the sites which were involved during the secondary stage of the disease. Tertiary syphilis is often detected many years after the secondary stage. The characteristic lesion is the gumma. The lesions of tertiary syphilis can involve almost any organ system.

This phase of syphilis is divided into three major categories: cardiovascular syphilis, neurosyphilis, and so-called benign tertiary syphilis. The various forms may occur singly or in combination in a given patient.

1) Cardiovascular syphilis: It accounts for more than 80% of cases of tertiary disease and it is much more common in men than in women. The fundmental lesion is an endarteritis of the vasa vasorum of the proximal aorta. Occlusion of the vasa vasorum results in scarring of the media of the proximal aortic wall, with consequent loss of elasticity. The aortic disease is characterized by slowly progressive dilation of the aortic root and arch, with resultant aortic insufficiency and aneurysms of the proximal aorta. These are characteristically located in the ascending aorta which becomes markedly dilated. The aortic valves are usually involved, causing incompetence(leaking) of the aortic valve. In some cases there is narrowing of the coronary artery ostia caused by subintimal scarring with secondary myocardial ischemia.

2) Neurosyphilis: It accounts for only about 10% of cases of tertiary syphilis. Variants of neurosyphilis include chronic meningovascular disease, tabes dorsalis, and a generalized brain parenchymal disease termed general paresis. Lesions can involve the meninges, spinal cord, or cerebral cortex. An increased frequency of neurosyphilis has been noted in patients with concomitant HIV infection.

3) The so-called benign tertiary syphilis: It is a relatively uncommon form of tertiary syphilis and characterized by the development of gummas in various sites. These lesions are probably related to the development of delayed hypersensitivity. Once common, gummas have become exceedingly rare thanks to the development of effective antibiotics such as penicillin. They are reported now mostly in patients with AIDS.

16.8   Deep Mycosis

A mycosis(plural: mycoses) is a fungal infection of animals, including humans. Diseases caused by fungi are called mycoses. They can infect the skin or deeper tissues, including the major organ systems. Mycoses are classified as superficial, cutaneous, subcutaneous, or systemic (deep) infections depending on the type and degree of tissue involvement and the host response to the pathogen. Skin infections are defined as superficial mycoses(dermatophytoses). Deep mycosis usually affects deep layer of skin and internal organs, causing more destructive disease. The deep or systemic mycoses include: candidiasis, cryptococcosis, aspergillosis, and mucormycosis. We will briefly describe the pathology of deep mycosis in this chapter.

16.8.1   Etiology and Pathogenesis

Fungi are weak pathogens and generally do not produce toxins. Fungi cause tissue damage primarily by a hypersensitivity reaction by the host to the parasitic proteins. Growth of the fungus can cause physical injury to tissue. Fungal metabolic products or enzymes can also contribute to tissue damage. The fungi are usually saprophytes that become opportunistic pathogens only under special circumstances: ①Large, long-term or multiple use of broad-spectrum and efficient antibiotics: Such treatment can cause disordered bacterial equilibrium. Iatrogenic factors, such as major surgery. ②Use of hormone or immunosuppressant; ③Elderly patients; ④Severe basic diseases, such as leukemia, lung cancer and liver cancer and other malignant tumors, chronic nephritis, uremia, renal transplantation, chronic obstructive pulmonary disease, pemphigus, cerebral hemorrhage, diabetes and AIDS; ⑤Organ transplantation; ⑥Organ intubation and catheter, catheter interventional therapy; ⑦Radiotherapy, chemotherapy. Deep fungal infections usually heal or remain latent in normal hosts; in immunocompromised hosts, however, they can spread systemically and invade tissues, destroying vital organs.

16.8.2　Pathology

Mycoses usually cause necrosis accompanied by a mixed acute and chronic inflammatory reaction. Most lesions do not have characteristic histopathological changes as listed below:

1) Acute suppurative inflammation with neutrophils and macrophages. Some fungal infections form pseudomembranes. Others cause endocarditis with lesions on the heart valves.

2) Chronic suppurative inflammation with micro-abscesses, infiltrates of lymphocytes and plasma cells, granulation tissue with fibroblasts.

3) Granulomatous inflammation Some granuloma lesions are similar to tuberculous granuloma. But massive neutrophil cells aggregate in the granuloma center.

4) Gangrenous inflammation Some necrotic lesions have different sizes and accompany with conspicuous hemorrhage.

5) Fungous septicemia Septicemia occurs when fungous infection enters the bloodstream. Untreated septicemia can quickly progress to sepsis, which is a serious complication of an infection characterized by inflammation throughout the body. This inflammation can cause blood clots and block oxygen from reaching vital organs, resulting in organ failure and death in some cases.

16.8.3　Diagnosis

Diagnosis of the deep mycoses is based on:

1) The clinical presentation of disease;

2) Visualization of the micro-organisms in smears or tissue sections;

3) Growth of the fungus in culture;

4) Detection of anti-fungal antibodies or cell-mediated immune reactions;

5) Molecular methods to detect fungal nucleic acid sequences.

16.8.4　Candidiasis

Candidiasis is a common fungal infection caused by Candida albicans which has over 20 species of yeasts. Candida albicans can be found in normal human skin, oral, vaginal and gastrointestinal candidiasis. Candidiasis is an autogenous infection and can occur in all parts of the body. There are three common presentations of candidiasis:

1) Lesions of skin and mucous membranes. Skin and mucosal superficial candidiasis arecommon. Warm, moist environment is conducive to the growth of fungi, so skin candidiasis occurres in the armpits, groin and finger(toe), around the anus. Vaginal candidiasis may occur in patients with diabetes and pregnant women because blood glucose and diabetic and urine increases. In the esophagus, candidiasis is almost always associated with one of the risk factors identified above. Skin and mucosa albicans infection often form white flaky, irregular pseudomembrane in the skin and mucosal surfaces. Candidiasis of the mucous membrane of the mouth is known as thrush.

2) Infections of deep tissue. Deep candidiasis is commonly secondary to chronic wasting disease, severe malnutrition and malignant tumor. Infection often occurs in the digestive tract, respiratory tract, heart(endocardium), kidney, brain, spleen, or other major visceral organ. There are multiple microscopic abscesses composed of fungal organisms(yeasts and hyphae), necrotic debris, with neutrophilic infiltrates. Uncommonly, a granulomatous reaction can be seen.

3) Systemic candidiasis. It results from dissemination of the organism in the blood stream. It can be

life-threatening or fatal. In internal organ, candidiasis is characterized by conspicuous tissue necrosis, micro-abscess, and subsequent granuloma.

Diagnosis: Candidiasis is diagnosed by identifying the fungus on microscopic examination or culture. In tissue sections, blastospore and pseudohyphae of Monilia is a diagnosis feature of candidiasis. These spores and hyphae are blue in the HE staining. By using gram or silver staining, spores and hyphaerule can be seen more clearly.

16.8.5   Cryptococcosis

Cryptococcosis is a systemic fungal infection, caused by Cryptococcus neoformans. It usually infects the central nervous system, lung, skin, and bone. Cryptococcus neoformans can not only be isolated from soil, pigeon droppings and fruit, but also can be isolated from healthy human skin, mucosa and feces. Environmental pathogens mainly transmit through respiratory tract into the body to cause disease. Majority of cryptococcosis is secondary, especially in patients with Hodgkin's disease and leukemia. Heathy people with cryptococcosis are rare.

Cryptococcosis is associated with chronic inflammation with a chronic granulomatous reaction. The lesions vary with the stage of disease. In the early stage, the lesion is jelly like because pathogens produce a lot of capsular substance, which can inhibit granulocyte tendency and phagocytosis. Thus, inflammation is mild in lesions. Neutrophil are rare and only a small number of lymphocytes and histiocytes infiltrate. In the late stage, granuloma formed. Fibrous tissue proliferate and there is a great deal of macrophage, foreign body giant cells and lymphocytes infiltration. The majority of macrophages and foreign body giant cell cytoplasm may have cryptococcal. Fungi invade vessels leading to hematogenous spread and thrombosis.

Over 95% of cryptococcal infections involve the meninges and the brain. Meninges become thick in the base of the brain and jelly like substance fill the subarachnoid space. In late period, there are more cellular exudation and granuloma form. Meninges are adhesion with brain tissue, which can affect cerebrospinal fluid circulation. Along the perivascular space, the infection also can invade brain tissue (mainly in the gray matter and basal ganglia) and form many small cavities. Microscopically the cystic cavity is the enlargement of perivascular space. Cavities are filled with cryptococcal and glue like substance excretion. Sometimes vascular inflammation and thrombosis can occur in small vessels, which lead to the surrounding brain tissue ischemia and softening. Glial cells may have mild hyperplasia. Later, granulomatous lesions can occur in the meninges, brain and spinal cord. The onset of cryptococcal meningitis is slow. Clinically, its symptoms are similar to tuberculous meningitis and it is easy to be misdiagnosed. Brain parenchymal lesions can confuse together. Cerebrospinal fluid examination for pathogens may confirm the diagnosis.

Diagnosis: The organism has a prominent capsule that can be seen on microscopic examination. In HE staining tissue sections, cryptococcal is pale red and is not easy to be seen. The PAS or silver stains can demonstrate the yeasts but fail to stain the polysaccharide capsule. As a result, the organism appears to be surrounded by a halo. This appearance is helpful for diagnosis.

16.8.6   Aspergillosis

Aspergillosis is an opportunistic infection, caused by the fungus *Aspergillus fumigates*. This is a common environmental fungus that grows in the soil and is present in the air. Aspergillus spores enter the body through the respiratory tract. In most cases, Aspergillus is a conditioned pathogen and pathogenicity is only based on lower body resistance. Aspergillus can cause disease in many parts of the body, such as skin, ears, eyes, nasal cavity, heart, brain, kidney, respiratory tract, gastrointestinal tract. Lung disease is the most common. Aspergillosis occurs in three relatively distinct forms:

Allergic bronchopulmonary aspergillosis occurs when fungal spores are inhaled and initiate an immune response in the airways. Bronchi and bronchioles contain fungal organisms and show chronic inflammation of the walls of the airways. Allergic bronchopulmonary aspergillosis is similar to clinical manifestations of bronchial asthma. The pathogenesis maybe related to allergic reaction induced by aspergillus antigen, which can cause the bronchial spasm and secretion of sticky sputum. Serum IgE, and precipitation of antibody against aspergillus antigen can be detected.

Aspergilloma(fungus ball)occurs in people with pre-existing lung disease. The fungal infection creates a cavity 1-7 cm in diameter, filled with a dense mass of fungal hyphae, and surrounded by fibrous tissue. The wall of the cavity is composed of collagenous connective tissue, infiltrated by lymphocytes and plasma cells.

Invasive aspergillosis occurs most often in the lungs of patients with impaired neutrophil function. In this situation, aspergillus tends to invade vessels, causing thrombosis, pulmonary infarction, and hematogenous spread of the infection. The lesions are associated with suppurative inflammation, microabscesses, and granulomas. Hyphae can be observed in the small abscesses and necrotic focus. Aspergillus often causes thrombosis, vascular obstruction, ischemia and necrosis of the tissue. The chronic lesions are fibrous tissue proliferation, including a large number of lymphocytes and mononuclear cell infiltration, and miscellaneous most macrophages and foreign body giant cells. A large number of mycelium can be observed in the lesions. The infection may spread to other organs such as the brain, kidney, or heart. Aspergillosis of the heart valve usually produces vegetations.

Diagnosis: Aspergillus showed blue purple by HE staining. With the PAS staining, aspergillus is clearly visible.

16.8.7   Mucormycosis

Mucormycosis is a fungal infection caused by fungi Mucor, Rhizopus, or Absidia species organisms. They cause serious sporadic opportunistic infections in patients with underlying diseases, such as diabetic acidosis and acute leukemia. Mucormycosis also occurs in patients treated with corticosteroids or cytotoxic drugs.

Mucormycosis is an acute suppurative inflammation, which spreads rapidly and causes disseminated diseases. The fungi vascular invasion causes thrombosis and infarction. This disease is often characterized by hyphae growing in and around vessels. Vascular invasion allows hematogenous spread of the fungus. Mucormycosis frequently involves the sinuses, brain, or lungs as the areas of infection. Cerebral mucormycosis is the most common type of the disease and can cause death in the short term.

Mucorales initially invade nasal mucosa and then diffuse around, involving the eyeball, soft tissue, blood vessels and nerves. Mucorales invasion causes eyelid infarction and local skin gangrene. Then it can spread into the cranial cavity and cause orbital, internal carotid artery cavernous sinus thrombosis, fungal meningitis and cerebral necrosis. The development is rapid and the early diagnosis is very important.

Diagnosis: In the lesions, there are generally no spores, but hyphae in HE staining by hematoxylin stain can be easily observed. PAS or silver stains show non septate wide fungal hyphae with marked right angle branching.

Chapter 17

Parasitosis

Parasitosis refers to a disease resulting from parasitic infestation. Three necessary conditions for the prevalence of parasitosis are source of infection(person or animal infected by parasite), route of transmission(living environment that is suitable for parasite, route of infestation and vulnerable group(individuals who are lack of immunity against parasitic infestation or individuals with low immunity). Therefore, the spread of parasitosis from humans to humans, animal to animal or humans to animal will be not only affected by biological factors, but also natural factors and social factors. The prevalence of parasitosis is also featured by territoriality, distinct seasonality, parasitic zoonosis, and other natural focus.

Parasitosis can be divided into acute and chronic type, and chronic type is frequently seen. Some hosts infected by parasite but showed no symptoms are called recessive infection or parasite carriers; in some cases, parasites will lodge in tissues and organs other than the common sites, and this phenomenon is called ectopic parasitism. When human body is infected by parasite, different symptoms may present according to the difference of parasite virulence and host's resistance. The main influence and damage of parasite on the host are as follows. ①Mechanical injury: parasite will lead to local damage, oppression or obstruction during the course of lodging in the host's body, migration, growth and reproduction, and removal from the body; ②toxic effect: the metabolite and secretion of parasite, and the decomposition product of dead parasite will produce toxic effect on the host; ③immunologic injury: the antigenicity possessed by the secretion, excrement of parasite and the decomposition product of parasite could induce the immune response of host, presenting protective immunity or leading to immunopathological changes; ④nutrition taking: parasite absorbs the nutrition from the host. If the nutrient substance is absorbed, the host will be in lack of nutrient, and the immunity will weaken.

Parasitosis is widespread around the world, especially in areas with poor economy and living condition. It is commonly seen in the developing countries in tropical and subtropical areas. Some parasitic diseases are very rampant at present, severely harming people's health. This chapter will only cover amoebiasis, schistosomiasis, clonorchiasis sinensis, pulmonary type paragonimiasis(paragonimiasis), and echinococcosis(hydatid disease).

17.1 Amoebiasis

Amoebiasis is an infection caused by any of amoebas of entamoeba histolytica. The amoeba mainly lodges in the colon, and from blood circulation it can also reach to the liver, brain, lung and skin where it can cause amoebic ulcer or amoebic abscesses. Also, amoebiasis may become a systemic disease after affecting various tissues and organs. Amoebiasis is usually transmitted by the fecal-oral route, and the source of infection is the cyst form of the parasite found in feces. It is often epidemic in regions of the world, especially in tropical and sub-tropical areas, with an infection rate of 0.37% –30%.

17.1.1 Intestinal Amoebiasis

17.1.1.1 Etiologyand Pathogenesis

Intestinal amoebiasis, also known as amoebic dysentery, is caused by entamoeba histolytica's infection in colon. Symptoms may include abdominal pain, diarrhea or tenesmus. The life cycle of entamoeba histolytica can be divided into cystic stage and trophozoite stage. In the infection stage, there are four mature cysts, while the pathogenic stage belongs to trophozoite stage. Cyst is usually seen in the feces of patient with amoebiasis, and taking food and water contaminated by cysts is the main route of human infection. When the cyst enters the digestive tract and reaches to the ieocecal junction, excystation will occur under the digestion of alkaline intestinal juice and trophozoite will come into being, with a size of about 10–60 μm. Trophozoite obtains nutrition at the upper end of colon and starts proliferation, and gradually becomes the early stage of cystica. Trophozoite can swallow red blood cell and tissue fragments, leading to ulcer after invading and damaging tissue of intestinal wall.

17.1.1.2 Pathological Change and Clinical Manifestation

Cecum and ascending colon are the main parts of pathological change, followed by sigmoid colon and rectum. Basic pathological changes include alterative inflammation based on histolysis and liquefaction. It is characterized by flask-shaped ulcer and can be divided into acute stage and chronic stage.

(1) Pathological Change of Acute Stage

Gross finding: multiple bullate necrosis or ulcers, which are grayish with needle shape surrounded by congestion and hemorrhage belt, are noted on the surface of intestinal mucosa in the earlier stage. The necrosis focus enlarges, presenting round button shape. Trophozoite obtains nutrition from the necrotic tissue and red blood cells of human body, breeding in the mucous layer of intestine and entering into the submucous layer after destructing the mucosal muscular layer. Tissues in the submucous layer are loose, and thus it is good for amoeba to spread around. Flask-shaped ulcer with sneak margin(Figure 17–1, Figure 17–2) will take shape when the necrosis tissue is liquefied and falls off. The mucous membranes of the ulcer are normal or manifest mild catarrhal inflammation. If the focus continues to expand, large ulcer with sneak margin will come into being. Some severe ulcers may affect intestinal wall, or even the serosal layer, leading to intestinal perforation and triggering peritonitis.

Under the microscope, pathological changes are mainly characterized by necrosis, dissolution and liquefaction of the tissues. The inflammatory reaction is mild in the surrounding area of focus, and only congestion, hemorrhage as well as infiltration of few lymphocytes, plasmacytes, and macrophagocytes are noted. Amoeba trophozoite(Figure 17–3) can be observed at the junction of ulcer margin and normal tissue, also in the venule of intestinal wall. Trophozoite on the tissue slice is usually round in shape and larger than the macrophagocyte in terms of volume. There is a spherical vesicular nucleus in the trophozoite with a diameter of 4−7 μm. The cytoplasm usually contains glycogen vacuole or swallows red blood cell, lymphocyte and fragment of tissues.

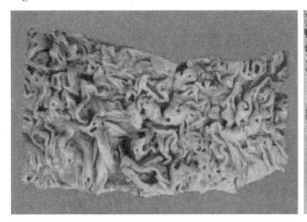

Figure 17−1　**Acute amebic dysentery of colon**
round ulcers with different sizes are scattering on the intestinal mucosa. The edge is slightly bulging)

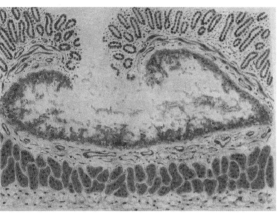

Figure 17−2　**"Flask ulcer" mode of acute amebic dysentery of colon**
ulcer reaches to the submucosa. It is in flask shape. Mucous membrane surrounding the ulcer covers the ulcer

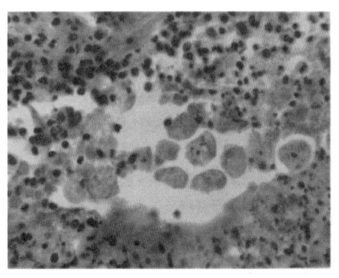

Figure 17−3　**Entamoeba histolytica trophozoite**

（2）Pathological Change of Chronic Stage

Due to the co-existence of new and old pathological change, necrosis, ulcer, granulation tissue, proliferation and scar occur repeatedly and alternatively, resulting in the formation ofhyperplastic polyp in mucous. In the end, the intestinal mucosa may loss its normal shape completely. The intestinal wall will probably be hardened because of the proliferation of fibrous tissue, which may even give rise to lumen stenosis. Sometimes, amoeboma will come into being if there is too much proliferation of granulation tissue. Such symptom is frequently seen in cecum.

The complications of amebic dysentery are intestinal perforation, intestinal hemorrhage, lumen stenosis, appendicitis, amoeba anal fistula, etc. It will also give rise to pathological change in liver, lung, brain and organs other than the intestine. Intestinal hemorrhage is common as the small vessels of the intestinal wall are destructed by the pathological change.

17.1.2   Extraintestinal Amoebiasis

Amoebic liver abscess is the most important and common complication of intestinal amoebiasis, which usually occur in amebic dysentery. The amoeba trophozoite under the intestinal mucosa or muscular layer invades the small vein of intestinal wall and reaches to the liver via portal vein. It is rarely seen that it will infect the liver directly. Amoebic liver abscess is usually in single state and is generally located in the right lobe of the liver(80%).

Gross findings: Abscesses differ in size, with the larger one as big as a fetal head. The abscess content is in brown jam shape, composed of liquefactive necrosis substance and obsolete blood. The connective tissue, blood vessel and bile duct of the portal area of the necrosis that are not completely liquefied with flocculent shape attached on the abscess wall.

Microscopic findings: Liquefactive necrosis, the light red structureless substance, is inside the intracavity. Incompletely liquefactive necrosis tissues, such as inflammatory cell infiltration, are noted in the abscess wall. Trophozoite is revealed at the junction of necrosis tissue and normal tissue, and granulation tissue and fibrous tissue are accumulated at the surrounding area of chronic abscess.

17.2   Schistosomiasis

Schistosomiasis is a parasitosis caused by the infection of cercaria via human skin or mucous membrane when human body is in contact with the infected water of schistosome cercaria. The main pathological change is the formation of granuloma triggered by the ovum. This section will briefly introduce diseases caused by Schistosoma japonicum.

17.2.1   Cause of Disease and Route of Infection

The life cycle of Schistosoma japonicum can be divided into ovum, miracidium, sporocyst, cercaria, schistosomlum and adult. Adult invades human body or other mammal such as dog, cat, pig, cattle as a host, while oncomelania as an intermediate host. The development and reproduction stage of miracidium and cercaria are completed in oncomelania. Three conditions are necessary for schistosomiasis transmission, which include ovum's feces in water, breeding of oncomelania and human body's contact with infected water.

Adult isdioecious and lodges in the portal vein and the mesenteric vein system. Female produces eggs in the vein of mesenterium, where some ova flow to the liver via the blood flow; some ova enter the intestinal cavity via intestinal wall and are excreted out of the body along with the patient or diseased animal's feces; ova deposited in the local tissues without being excreted will be gradually die andbe calcified. When the excreted ova enter the water, miracidium will be hatched. Miracidium meets oncomelania, the medium host, in water, and invades the soft tissue of breech block. After the stage of mother sporocyst-daughter sporocyst, miracidium will develop into cercaria and leave oncomelania again to the water. The cercariae of Schistosoma japonicum are mainly distributed on the water surface. When human or animal is in contact with the infected water, cercaria, based on the action of tissue plasminogen activator excreted by the cephalic gland as well as the mechanical motion of its muscle contraction, develops into schistosomlum after drilling in the skin or mucous membrane, and removing the tail. Schistosomlum enters the venule or lymph vessel, reaching to the lung along with blood flow via the right heart, and spreading to the whole body via blood circulation. Schistosomlum that has entered into the mesenteric vein will be able to develop as adult, and the rest of them are die on the way. It mainly takes about three weeks for cercaria to develop into adult. Female and male adults produce eggs after mating, which will develop into mature ovum containing miracidium after about 11 days. When the ovum matures in the intestinal wall, it will destruct the intestinal mucosa and enter the intestinal cavity and will be discharged out of the body along with the feces. This is the complete life cycle of Schistosoma japonicum. The lifespan of ovum in tissue is about 21 days, while the adult in human body is about 4.5 years on average.

17.2.2 Basic Pathological Change and Pathogenesis

During the process of Schistosoma japonicum infestation, cercaria, schistosomlum, adult and ovum will do harm to the host, among which the ovum's damage is the greatest. The antigen released by schistosome in different stage induces the host's immune response, and this is the main reason and mechanism leading to the damage.

17.2.2.1 Cercaria

Cercarial dermatitis will occur within 3 days when cercaria drills in the skin which presenting small papule with itching in the invading area. It will fade away automatically. The microscopic findings show dermis congestion, edema and hemorrhage, with infiltration of neutrophils and eosinophils in the early stage, and cellular infiltration in the later stage.

17.2.2.2 Schistosomlum

Schistosomlum may cause vasculitis and perivascular inflammation when moving in the body. The damage to lung tissue is the most obvious, presenting lung tissue congestion, edema, punctuate hemorrhage and leukocyte infiltration, but lesion is generally mild and short.

17.2.2.3 Adult

Adult's mouth and ventral sucker adsorb on the vascular wall, leading to the damage of vascular wall at the lodging position, as well as endophlebitis and periphlebitis; its metabolite, secretion-excretions and other antigen stimulate the host to produce corresponding antibody, forming antigen-antibody compound and inducing type Ⅲ allergic reaction. Mononuclear phagocyte proliferation is noted in the liver and spleen. The dark brown schistosoma pigment, which is always swallowed, is a heme-like pigment formed after hemoglobinolysis under the action of globinase in the adult body. Similar pigment is also seen in the adult's intestinal tract. The surrounding tissues of dead adult will become necrotic. With a large number of eosinophil granulocytes in infiltration, eosinophilic abscess will come into being.

17.2.2.4 Ovum

Ovum deposition causes main lesion. Ovum mainly deposits in sigmoid colon, rectum, and liver, and it is also seen in the terminal ileum, appendix, ascending colon, lung and brain. A deposited ovum can be divided into immature egg and mature egg. Mature ovum contains mature miracidium, which secretes soluble ovum antigen and thus leads to the formation of characteristic ovum nodule(schistosomal granuloma). According to the development of the pathological change, this nodule can be divided into acute ovum nodule and chronic ovum nodule.

(1)Acute Ovum Nodule

Acute ovum nodule is a kind of acute necrosis and exudative focus caused by mature ovum. Gross findings: small grayish nodule with a size of chestnut grain to green bean. Microscopic findings: 1-2 mature ova are noted in the central area of nodule. Sometimes, radial and acidic clava is attached on the ovum surface. It is the antigen-antibody composite formed by the corresponding antibody produced when the soluble egg antigens (SEA) released by ovum miracidium stimulates the B-lymphocyte system. The surrounding area is a combination of structureless granular necrosis substance and a large number of eosinophil infiltrations. It is in abscess shape and thus is known as acidophilia abscess. Rhombus or multi-faceted and refractive protein crystal, as well as charcot-leyden crystal, can be seen inside, as they are composed of acidophil granules of eosinophils. Later, the ovum generates granulation tissue layer at the surrounding area, where lymphocyte, macrophagocyte and eosinophils are in infiltration. Eosinophils account for the main proportion. As the course of disease progresses, the granulation tissue layer gradually develops toward the center of ovum nodule, and epithelioid cell layer in radiate array will come into being at the surrounding area of the nodule. Eosinophils decline significantly, constituting acute ovum nodule of later stage. This is the transition stage developing toward ovum nodule.

(2) Chronic Ovum Nodule

After about 10 days, miracidium will be dead in the egg, and the antigen substance it secretes will disappear. The necrosis substance inside the focus will gradually be eliminated by macrophagocyte, and the ovum will be disintegrated and ruptured. The macrophagocyte inside the focus will become epithelioid cell and few foreign body giant cells. Lymphocytes infiltration and granulation tissue proliferation are noted in the surrounding area of focus. It looks like tuberculoid granulation tumor, thus known as pseudotubercle or chronic ovum (Figure 17-4). In the end, the nodule will be in fibrosis hyaline change. The central fragment of egg shell and calcified dead egg will be retained for a long time.

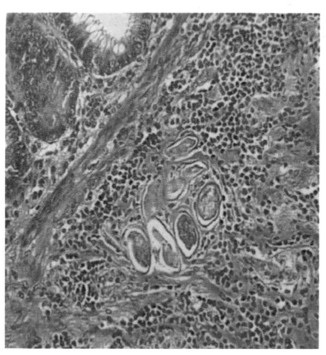

Figure 17-4   Chronic ovum nodule of schistosoma

there are several rupture and calcified ova in the central nodule, forming fake tubercle

17.2.3   Pathological Change of Main Organs

17.2.3.1   Colon

As adult usually lodges in the inferior mesenteric vein and superior vein of hemorrhoid, the symptom is most obvious in rectum, sigmoid colon and descending colon. Gross findings: intestinal mucosa with congestion and edema as well as flat but bullate focus which is yellow in granular shape with a diameter of 0.5-1 cm, is noted. Necrosis falls off from the central focus, forming superficial ulcer with uneven size and irregular edges. Ovum may fall into the intestinal cavity and appear in the feces.

In chronic phase, due to the repeated depositing of ovum, ulcer and intestinal fibrosis will occur again and again in the intestinal mucosa, leading to the thickening and hardening of intestinal wall, stenosis of intestinal cavity, or even intestinal obstruction. Due to the hyperplasia of connective tissues in intestinal wall, it is hard to secrete ovum into the intestinal cavity. This is the reason why ovum is not easily observed in the feces of patients with advanced disease. In addition, in some cases, the atrophy of intestinal mucosa is noted with disappeared plica. Some of them are in polypus hyperplasia (Figure 17-5).

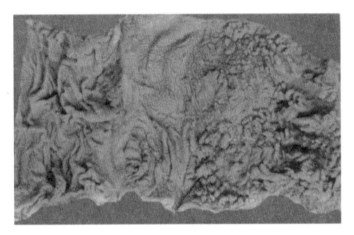

Figure 17-5   Colon of chronic schisto soma

the intestinal wall thickens, harden the bowel is narrow; the mucous
membrane is rough and uneven, with the formation of polyp and ulcer

17.2.3.2   Liver

In acute stage, the liver is slightly enlarged, and multiple small grayish white or grayish yellow nodules, in a size of chestnut grain or green bean, are noted on the surface and section. Microscopic findings: Many acute ovum nodules are revealed near the portal area. Liver cells will be atrophied because of pressure, and the possibility of degeneration and small focus necrosis also exist. The symptoms include congestion of hepatic sinusoid, Kupffer cell proliferation, and swallowing of schistosoma pigment.

In chronic stage, chronic ovum nodule and fibrosis are noted in the liver. In cases of long-term serious infection, there are a large number of fibrous tissue proliferations near the portal area. The liver will gradually be harder and smaller, turning into schistosoma-type liver cirrhosis because of severe fibrosis. The liver surface is not smooth and is divided into several upheaval areas of different sizes by shallow grooves. In serious cases, thick and large nodule will come into being. In terms of section, the hyperplastic connective tissues are distributed like branches of trees toward the portal vein. Thus, it is known as pipe stem cirrhosis (Figure 17-6). Microscopic finding shows a large number of chronic ovum nodules in the portal area, accompanied with lots of proliferation of fibrous tissue. The hepatic lobule is not seriously destructed, and the pseudo lobule is not obvious, different from portal cirrhosis.

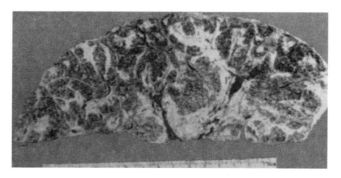

Figure 17–6   Schistosomiasis cirrhosis of liver

from the section, it can be seen that a large number of connective tissues are proliferating along the portal vein branch, splitting the liver tissue

17.2.3.3   Spleen

Gross findings: the spleen is strong but pliable in texture with thickened envelope. The section is dark red with brown siderotic nodule on the surface. It is mainly composed of old hemorrhage focus accompanied with irony and calcareous deposit as well as proliferation of fibrous tissue. Infarction tissues are occasionally found. Microscopic findings: Atrophy of splenic corpuscle reduces and schistosome pigment deposit is seen in the mononuclear macrophage. Ovum nodule is occasionally found in the spleen.

17.3   Clonorchiasis Sinensis

Clonorchiasis sinensis, or clonorchiasis, is a parasitosis caused by the adult of clonorchis sinensis, which inhabits human intrahepatic ducts. This disease is common in Asia.

17.3.1   Cause of Disease and Route of Infection

The development process of Clonorchiasis sinensis includes adult, ovum, miracidium, sporocyst, redial, cercarial, encysted metacercaria, metacercaria, etc. The adult usually lodges in the intrahepatic ducts of human, dog, cat and pig. When adult produces eggs, the ovum will be discharged via the intestinal tract with bile. Ovum containing miracidium could be swallowed by freshwater snail, the first intermediate host, and from its digestive tract, miracidium will be hatched. Miracidium develops into sporocyst in the snail body and generates many rediae and cercariae via vegetative proliferation. Mature cercaria leaves the snail to the water, invading freshwater fish or freshwater shrimp, the second intermediate host, and develops into encysted metacercaria in the second intermediate host's muscle. When human or animal ingests fish or shrimp containing encysted metacercaria without being cooked, encysted metacercaria breaks out its cyst after the action of digestive juice in the gastrointestinal tract. The cercaria reversely flows to the intrahepatic bile duct along the bile and lodges in and develops into adult. It takes about 1 month from the intake of encysted metacercaria to the appearance of ovum in feces.

17.3.2   Pathological Change and Complications

Clonorchiasis sinensis mainly lodges in the intrahepatic bile ducts. In less severe cases, there are few worms. Ovum is found in the feces. Adult lodges in the intrahepatic duct and mucosa epithelium exfoliates from the bile duct. The appearance of liver and bile duct is normal. In severely infected cases, the pathological change may cause cholangitis, cholecystitis, calculus of bile duct, cirrhosis, and atypical hyperplasia of biliary epithelia, or even cholangiocellular carcinoma.

Liver intrahepatic bile duct dilation is the most significant lesion. In cases with severe infection, the liver is slightly swollen with increased weight in the gross findings. Bile duct branches are dilated because of the mechanical blockage of adult is seen below the envelope. Such pathological change is common in the left lobe as the bile duct of the left lobe is flat and will be easily invaded by the schistosomlum. The intrahepatic large and middle bile duct with varying degrees of dilation and tube wall thickening are noted on the section. The lumen is full of bile and countless adults. According to the microscopic findings, intrahepatic bile duct dilation is noted, and the epithelial cell and submucosal glands show different degree of hyperplasia. In severe cases, papillary, adenomatous or atypical hyperplasia (Figure 17-7) will occur, which may lead to canceration. Lymphocyte, plasmocyte, and eosinophilia infiltration are found in the tube wall. In chronic disease, significant fibrous connective tissue is noted.

Adult lodges in the intrahepatic bile duct, leading to cholestasis in the bile duct and causing secondary infection easily. The dead polypide, ovum and deciduous bileepithelia can also become the core of gallstone, which is good for the gallstone formation.

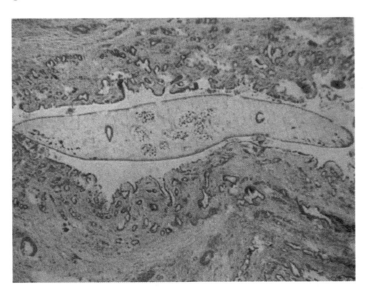

Figure 17-7   **Clonorchiasis**

Adult worm of clonorchis sinensis is noted in the hepatic bile duct)

17.4   Pulmonary-type Paragonimiasis

Paragonimiasis is a disease caused by the schistosomlum spreading in the tissue and lodging of adult worm. The worm mainly lodges in the lung, which causes pulmonary type paragonimiasis, also known as paragonimiasis. The feature of pathological change is formation of sinus and multilocular small cysts in organs and tissues. This disease is prevalent around the world, especially rampant in summer and autumn.

17.4.1   Pathogeny and Route of Transmission of Infection

This chapter will introduce how pulmonary-type paragonimiasis is caused by paragonimus westermani. The symptoms of pulmonary-type paragonimiasis are coughing, coughing with rusty sputum, hemoptysis, etc.

The adult worm of paragonimus lodges in the lung of human body and other mammals, such as cat, dog, pig etc. Ovum is usually coughed out with the sputum ordischarged with the feces. Ovum entering into water will hatch into miracidium, and then drill in the freshwater nail, which is the first host. The ovum will develop into cercaria from sporocyst, mother redia and daughter redia. The cercaria could invade into the body of freshwater stone crab or crayfish, the second host, and develop into encysted metacercaria when it leaves the nail within two days. Encysted metacercaria is the type of lung fluke infection. If people feed on stone crab or crayfish containing encysted metacercaria, which will enter the digestive tract and develop into schistosomlum after the action of digestive juice and excystation. Schistosomlum, which has strong ability in daily living, is able to enter the abdominal cavity via the intestinal wall by action of excreted enzyme. Most schistosomlums spread along the peritoneum, move upward via the surface of liver, spleen, and stomach. The schistosomlums can reach the thoracic cavity directly after passing through the diaphragm, and finally invade the lung and develop into adult, which produces cysts and ovums. A few of schistosomlum retain at the abdominal cavity and continue to grow and develop mostly into cercariae after penetrating the superficial layer of the liver or greater omentum. It takes about two months from entering into the body as encysted metacercaria to producing ovums as cercariae.

17.4.2　Pathogenesis and Basic Pathological Changes

The mechanical injury schistosomlum's spreads in tissue and adult's lodging on local tissues is the main pathogenic effect of paragonimus. In addition, immunopathological effects caused by antigen substance, such as metabolite of polypide, and the formation of foreign body granuloma induced by ovum have also played a certain role in the pathogenic effect.

17.4.2.1　Serositis

Polypide may lead to fibrinous or serous fibrinous peritonitis or pleuritis when it travels or lodges in the body cavity.

17.4.2.2　Tissue Destruction and Sinus Tract Formation

Polypide spreads in the tissue with forming tortuous sinus tract, necrosis and hemorrhage could been happen. Eosinophils and lymphocytes infiltration are noted in the sinusoidal wall under the microscope. Ovum can be developed into fibrosis.

17.4.2.3　Formation of Abscess, Cyst and Fibrous Scar

Schistosomlum or adult will lead to tissue necrosis and hemorrhage, and to severe inflammatory reaction when it lodged in the organ. Apart from eosinophils, there are a large number of neutrophil granulocytes forming abscess. The exudative inflammatory cells and necrosis tissues will disintegrate and liquefy. The abscess content formed are brown viscous liquid, with necrosis tissues, polypide, ovum and Charcot-Leyden crystal noted under the microscope. At the same time, granulation tissue hyperplasia surrounding the abscess is noted, and fibrous membrane is taking shape. Worm cysts got its name because of the existence of polypide in the cyst(Figure 17-8). Ovum entering the cyst and tissue which surrounding the cyst could lead to form foreign matter granuloma. Due to the migration characteristic, polypide could leave the original cyst and continue to destroy other tissues nearby and form new cyst. Cysts linked with sinus tracts are called multilocular cysts.

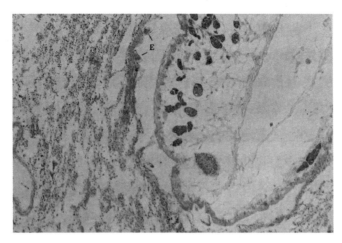

Figure 17-8   **Pulmonary-type Paragonimiasis Cyst**

polypide and ovum are noted in the cyst. The cyst wall is a thin fibrous
tissue, and the surrounding tissue of cyst is collapsed because of compression

17.4.3   Pathological Change and Clinical Manifestation of Main Organs

Pleural thickens accompanied by extensive adhesion. The diaphragmatic surface is the heaviest. Worm cysts, larvae or adults, scattered or in group, are found in the lung. Polypide and ovum could be found in the cyst(Figure 17-9). The worm cyst of lung often invades the bronchial wall, connecting the cyst and forming pulmonary cavity. If there is secondary bacterial infection, pneumothorax, empyema or even hemothorax will be happen. Obvious pulmonary fibrosis is noted in chronic cases.

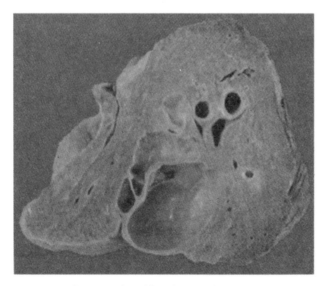

Figure 17-9   **A piece of multilocular cyst is noted below the lung**

17.5 Hydatidosis

Echinococcosis, also known as hydatid disease, is a parasitosis caused by the larva (hydatid cyst) of tapeworms.

17.5.1 Pathogeny and Route of Infection

The adult of echinococcus granulosus lodges mainly in the small intestine of definitive host, such as dog, wolf and other carnivorous animals. The polypide is small, 2-7 mm in length and hermaphrodite. It is composed of scolex and three somites (immature proglottid, mature proglottid and gravid proglottid). Gravid proglottid contains infectious ovum, and the gravid proglottid will contaminate pasture, vegetable, soil and water when it is mature in the small intestine of definitive host, split away off the polypide, and expelled in the feces. The ovum and gravid proglottid hatch in the stomach or duodenum when they are taken by the intermediate host like goat, cattle, pig, rabbit, camel or other live-stock and human. Oncosphere will break out from the shell, attaching on the mucous membrane and then drilling in the blood vessel of the intestinal wall. It will finally reach the liver via the blood flow of portal vein. Therefore, liver hydatid disease is commonly seen. Few can reach the lung from the liver and right heart.

17.5.2 Pathogenesis and Basic Pathological Change

The damages of hydatid cyst on organs can be divided into three parts, but mechanical damage is the key part: ①for the space-occupying growth of hydatid cyst, oppression and damage to the surrounding tissue, the degree of damage depends on the volume, quantity, time of lodging and position of hydatid cyst; ②when the hydatid cyst fractures, the foreign protein contained in the cyst fluid will lead to allergic reaction inside the body, or anaphylactic shock leading to death; ③hydatid cyst will take in the nutrition from host during its growth and development process, affecting the body health to some extent.

Hydatid cyst is composed of cyst wall and cyst content. The cyst wall can be divided into inner layer and outer layer. The outer layer is cuticle layer, which is white and semi-transparent. For instance, vermicelli, about 1mm in thickness, is characterized by absorbing nutrient substance and protecting the germinal layer; lamellar structure with paralleled red staining is noted below the microscope. The inner layer is germinal layer, or germ layer, with a thickness of about 20 μm. It is composed of single layer or multi-layer germinal cell with significant multiplication capacity. Inclusions are produced from this layer to the cyst. Cyst inclusion includes cyst fluid (or hydatid cyst liquid), protoscolex, brood capsule, daughter cyst, granddaughter cyst, etc. The germinal cell grows toward the internal bud and can form countless papule in the cyst inner wall, where brood capsule will gradually come into being (Figure 17-10). Brood capsule, a small cyst with only one germinal layer, contains many protocolizes inside. Brood capsule falls off and becomes daughter cyst. The cyst is able to produce protoscolex, brood capsule and granddaughter cyst that has the similar structure of daughter cyst. In older hydatid cyst, there could be hundreds of daughter cysts. Sometimes, germinal layer grows buds externally and forms cysts.

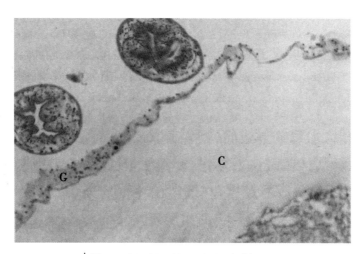

Figure 17-10   **Hepatic hydatid cyst**

The outer layer of cyst wall is lamellar cuticular layer with light red parallel
arrangement. The inside is germinal layer, with protoscolex in the cavity

17.5.3   Pathological Change of Main Organ and Its Consequence

17.5.3.1   Liver

Frequently seen in the right lobe. It is single but sometimes multiple. The cyst is located at the diaphragmatic surface, extruding toward the abdominal cavity. Hepatic hydatid cyst grows slowly, and could lead to pressure atrophy, degeneration or necrosis when it enlarges gradually. Its proliferation of fibrous tissue forms a layer of fibrous external cyst. The intrahepatic small bile duct and blood vessel will be often shifted because of compression or encapsulated in the cyst wall.

17.5.3.2   Lung

Pulmonary hydatid cyst is caused by oncosphere when it reaches the heart from liver and blood, or burrows through the lung from the organs nearby. Cyst is commonly seen in the right lung, developed in the middle lobe, and located in the surrounding area of lung. It is usually single. Affected by loose lung tissue, rich blood circulation and negative pressure suction, pulmonary hydatid cyst develops rapidly and is able to oppress the surrounding lung tissue, inducing lung atrophy and fibrosis.

Chapter 18

Pathological Techniques

> *Introduction*

The pathology technology is formed and developed on the basis of pathology, which embodies the development and application of the cross penetration and the new technology of the frontier. The contents of pathology technology include general pathological anatomy and fixed production techniques for general specimens, which are the important basis of pathology, basic knowledge, principles and techniques for preparation of cell and tissue specimens.

18.1 General Tissue and Cell for Pathological Techniques

18.1.1 General Specimen Preparation

18.1.1.1 Requirement of Material Delivery Organization

The biopsy specimen should be immediately placed in 10% formaldehyde fixation after surgical incision or biopsy.

18.1.1.2 Materials

Based on the detailed examination of the tissue specimens, the location and number of the materials shall be determined according to the needs of the diagnosis. For Multi-cut material, the same tissue "ice pair" and the remaining tissue "ice remnants" must be further compared with routine paraffin sections, especially in the "ice pair" is important. The biopsy tissue should be well preserved because it is always small and usually needs further examination, such as HE staining, special staining, immunohistochemical staining and electron microscopy analysis.

18.1.2 Tissue Fixation

The volume of the fixed liquid should be at least 4−5 times that of the tissue blocks. General fixed liquid can not penetrate more than 2−3 cm solid tissue or 0.5 cm porous tissue in 24 h. The tissue thickness of less than 3mm is more appropriate. The fixed time of the organization is usually 3−24 h. The fixed temperature is mostly room temperature. The fixed container should be relatively large, so that the fixed liquid can be well infiltrated into the blocks.

18.1.3   Tissue Dehydration Optical Clearing and Waxdip

The tissue contains a lot of water after fixed. It must be dehydrated before immersion and embedding because water and paraffin wax cannot be mixed. Ethanol is most commonly used as a tissue dehydrator which has strong dehydration capacity. To make paraffin can be immersed into the tissue, after dehydration, the tissue must go through a solvent medium, xylene, which is can mixed with ethanol and dissolve paraffin. (Table 18-1).

Table 18-1   Tissue dehydration clearing and wax dipping time

processing step	processing time(min)
70% ethanol	30-60
80% ethanol	120-300
95% ethanol Ⅰ and ethanol Ⅲ	120-300
absolute ethyl alcohol Ⅰ, ethanol Ⅱ and ethanol Ⅲ	30
absolute ethyl alcohol Ⅲ	60-120
Xylene Ⅰ, ethanol Ⅱ	30
Xylene Ⅲ	60
56-58 ℃ paraffin wax Ⅰ	30
56-58 ℃ paraffin wax Ⅱ	60-120
56-58 ℃ paraffin wax Ⅲ	120-180

18.1.4   Tissue Paraffin-Embedded

Conventional paraffin embedding method: The tissue is immersed into the melting paraffin wax with warm tweezers. The buried surface must be flat and the fragmentized tissue should be assembled The biopsy tissue should be well preserved because it is always small and usually needs further examination, such as HE staining, special staining, immunohistochemical staining and electron microscopy analysis. Generally, 56 ℃ paraffin may be used for embedding. When the embedding is ending, the wax block can be moved into the refrigerator to accelerate the solidification. The contents of the gastroscope specimen are vertically embedded. At last, the tissue is embedded into a wax block.

18.1.5   Paraffin Section

18.1.5.1   General Paraffin Section Process

The process of cutting the tissue block into thin slices(generally 4-6 μm)is called paraffin section. The tissue blocks are firstly cooled in the refrigerator and then mounted on a slicer fixture. The specimen should be repaired until all the tissue is exposed and the tissue section should be flattened before the next step.

18.1.5.2   Frozen Section Method

Frozen sections are mostly used in fresh tissue and cold storage tissue blocks. A small amount of OCT or carboxymethyl cellulose is used to cover the tissue. In the temperature of 25 ℃ below zero, the tissue becomes a frozen block which can be sliced.

18.1.6 Hematoxylin and Eosin Staining of Tissue and Cell Sections

18.1.6.1 Basic Principle

Hemalum colors nuclei of cells(and a few other objects, such askeratohyalin granules and calcified material)into blue. The staining of nuclei by hemalum is ordinarily due to binding of the dye-metal complex to DNA. Most of the cytoplasm is eosinophilic which is stained into red by Eosin. Red blood cells are stained intensely red. T The terminology of basophilic or eosinophilic is based on the affinity of cellular components for the dyes. Other colors, e. g. yellow and brown, can be present in the sample; they are caused by intrinsic pigments, e. g. melanin. Some structures do not stain well. Basal laminae need to be handled by PAS stain or some silver stain. Reticular fibers also require silver stain(Table 18-2).

Table 18-2 Harris' hematoxylin and eosin(H&E)staining protocol and time

processing step	processing time(min)	
	LEICA AUTO STAINER XL	Frozen section
Xylene Ⅰ	10	
Xylene Ⅱ	10	
absolute ethyl alcohol Ⅰ	1	
absolute ethyl alcohol Ⅱ	1	
95% ethanol Ⅰ and ethanol Ⅱ	1	
95% ethanol Ⅰ and ethanol Ⅱ	1	
90% ethanol	1	
80% ethanol	1	
Water	1	1
Hematoxylin	1-5	1-2
Water	1	20 s
1% hydrochloric acid alcohol	30 s	20 s
Water	5	30 s
aqueous solution of ammonia	1	30 s
Water	5	20 s
Eosin	30 s-5	20 s-2
Water	5	10 s
85% ethanol	20 s	20 s
95% ethanol Ⅰ	30 s	1
95% ethanol Ⅱ	1	1
absolute ethyl alcohol Ⅰ	2	1
absolute ethyl alcohol Ⅱ	2	1
Xylene Ⅰ	2	1
Xylene Ⅱ	2	2
Xylene Ⅲ	2	2
Sealing	YES	YES

The frozen section is fixed for 1 min with 95% ethanol 95 ml and 5 ml glacial acetic acid mixture before the program.

18.1.6.2   Application for HE Staining

HE staining is the most basic and widely used technical method in the teaching and scientific research of histology, embryology and pathology.

18.1.7   Connective Tissuestaining

18.1.7.1   Masson Trichromatic Staining

The collagen fiber is blue or green, muscle fiber cytoplasm and red cell red, and the nucleus is blue. Connective tissue staining is used to determine the degree of pathological changes and repair of various tissues on pathomorphology. The origin for tumor of spindle cell soft tissue is fibrous, muscular or neurogenic.

18.1.8   Collagen Fiber Staining

Collagen fibers are bright red, muscle fiber cytoplasm and red cell yellow. The pathological diagnosis of collagen fiber is mainly used in the differential diagnosis of muscle fibers. The spindle cell tumor of the soft tissue can be fibrous or myogenic. In HE dyeing, it is sometimes difficult to distinguish. The fibrotic tumor is red with the VG method, and the myogenic tumor is yellow.

18.1.9   Rhabdomyosus Tissue Staining

Rhabdomyolysis fiber, cellulose, nucleus, nucleolus and neuroglia fiber are blue, collagen fiber, reticular fiber, cartilage matrix brown red, and elastic fiber purple. If the tumor is striated muscle differentiation, blue stripes can be found in the tumor cytoplasm.

18.1.10   Carbohydrate Staining

18.1.10.1   Periodic Acid-Schiff Stain(PAS)

The positive PAS is red and the nucleus is blue. ①In diabetes, a large number of glycogen appears in the liver cells. ②Differentiate malignant lymphoma of bone and Ewing's sarcoma of bone. Glycogen granules were found in the cytoplasm of the bone's Ewing's sarcoma cells and PAS was positive; the malignant lymphoma of bone was not glycogen and PAS was negative. ③Congenital glycogen accumulation disease, it can be seen a large amount of glycogen deposit in liver, the trial, myocardium or skeletal muscle, etc.

18.1.10.2   Alcian Blue-periodic Acid Schiff(AB-PAS)

The neutral mucus is red, the acid mucus is green and blue, the compound is purple and red, the nucleus is gray-blue. Intestinal type gastric cancer cells secrete acid mucus, which is blue. Gastric phenotype gastric cancer cells secrete acid mucus, which is red.

18.2   Techniques of Histochemistry and Immunohistochemistry

Immunohistochemistry and immunocytochemistry examination is derived from tissue and cytochemical methods. IIts basic principle is to use the antigen and the antibody contact can form "antigen-antibody complex" chemical reaction to detect tissue or intracellular antigen(or antibody)technology. Immunohistochemistry and immunocytochemistry examination are invaluable for identifying disease and predicting response to therapy, and are used considerably in fundamental scientific research. At present, the immunohistochemistry autostainer is widely used(Figure 18-1).

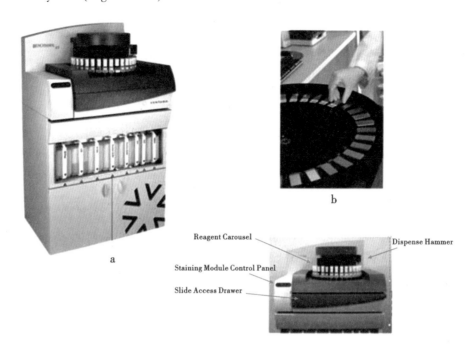

Figure 18-1 Immunohistochemistry Autostainer

18.2.1 Immunohistochemical Staining Procedure

1) Extract antigen(immune-ogen);

2) Monoclonal antibodies were prepared by hybridoma using immunogenicity(rabbit)to prepare antiserum(polyclonal antibody)or immune animal(mouse);

3) Purified antibodies;

4) Antibody marker tissue section(Figure 18-2);

5) Dyeing reaction;

6) Observe the results.

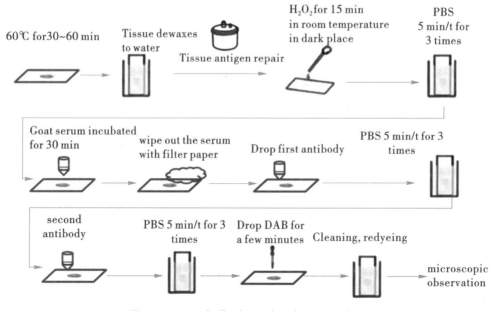

Figure 18-2 Antibody marker tissue section

18.2.2　Common Marker

18.2.2.1　Enzymes

The most commonly used markers. The enzyme that is labeled should have the following conditions: the substrate is specific and easy to display; The enzyme reaction product is stable and not easy to diffuse. It is easy to obtain a pure enzyme molecule and stable. The enzyme-labeled antibody should not affect the activity of the two. There should be no endogenous enzyme or substrate in the tissue. The commonly used markers are horseradish peroxidase(HRP), alkaline phosphatase(AKP), glucose oxidase(GOD), etc.

18.2.2.2　Fluorescein

It is a substance that produces fluorescence under the excitation of high energy light waves. Commonly used isothiocyanate fluorescein(FITC), tetramethyl isothiocyanate rhodamine(TRITC).

18.2.2.3　Biotin

The affinity of biotin and lecithin is significantly higher than that of antigen antibody.

18.2.2.4　Metal Markers

Ferritin and colloidal gold are used in immune electron microscopy.

18.2.3　Common Immunohistochemical Staining Method

The relative sensitivities of the various antigen-detection methods are well known(Figure 18−3).

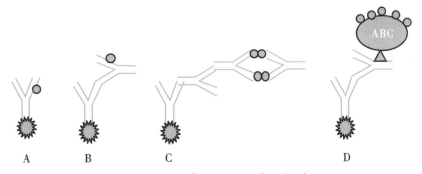

Figure 18−3　**Comparison of methods**
A. Direct; B. Indirect; C. PAP; D. ABC

18.2.3.1　Direct Method

The fluoresxein(immunofluorescence) or enzyme is directly labeled on the first antibody to examine the corresponding antigen. The direct method has the advantages of specificity, but the sensitivity is poor and the antibody is much more.

18.2.3.2　Indirect Method

The second antibody was labeled with a fluorescein or enzyme, a specific antibody, and only racial specificity. The features of this method include: ①It is convenient to pre-bid the two reactance. ②It is more sensitive than direct, but still poor.

18.2.3.3　Peroxidase Antiperoxidase Complex Method andbothway PAP

The peroxidase (HRP) immune rabbit/sheep/mouse is first made into rabbits/sheep/mice against HRP; Then, it is combined with HRP to form a stable polygon structure(PAP). The features of this method include: ①High sensitivity. ②Low background staining(relative). ③The sensitivity of the two PAP is higher, but the background is relatively heavy.

18.2.3.4 Avidin Biotin-peroxidase Complex Method

The Avidin biotin-peroxidase Complex (ABC) using avidin-biotin with high affinity, biotin and first form biotin enzyme HRP, again with biotin HRP mixed with avidin according to certain proportion, and form a compound; Also, the biotinylation was first. ①Replace the Avidin with Streptomycin, which is SABC method: Strept Avidin Biotin-peroxidase Complex. ②Link streptomycin and biotin first, which is the LSAB method: Labeled Streptavidin-Biotin. ③Streptomycin antibiotic protein linked horseradish peroxidase, which is a S-P method: Streptavidin-Peroxidase conjugated method. If alkaline phosphatase is used to mark the streptomycin, which is the SAP method. the alkaline phosphatase and horseradish peroxidase are used to mark the streptomycin, which is the DS method. The features of this methods include: ①High sensitivity (8−40 times higher than that of PAP). ②Background light, streptavidin is better. ③Method is simple, time is short. ④Wide range of applications, but also can be used for in situ hybridization and immune electron microscopy.

18.2.4 Attention in the Process of Immunohistochemical Staining

18.2.4.1 Set the Correct Control of Immunohistochemistry

Control principle: compare the first antibody. The same principle should be noticed in the substitution control; Positive results have negative control; the negative result has positive control; the staining is clear and the location is accurate. The negative control includes: ①blank control: First antibody is replaced with PBS. ②the replacement of the serum control: with the normal serum of the same animal instead of the first antibody. ③inhibition of the control: Unlabeled antibody combined with the corresponding antigen first. ④absorbable control: The purified antigen Is used to absorb the antibody. Positive control: a tissue that is known or proved to be positive. Self-control: the use of various tissue components within the tissue section as a control.

18.2.4.2 False Positive Reactions

Non-specific reactions: edge phenomena, creases and knife marks, bleeding and necrosis, etc. Endogenous peroxidase: erythrocyte, inflammatory cells, degeneration necrotic cells and certain glandular epithelial secretions, and some tissues rich in peroxidase, such as brain, liver, etc. The cross-reaction of the antibodies: the antibody itself contains the components of the cross-reaction with the human tissue. The concentration of the reagent is too high or ineffective.

18.2.4.3 False Negative Reactions

①The organization is not fixed or fixed for a long time. ②Low antibody titer is too low or too long. ③The antigen in the tissue is blocked by a viscous matrix or secretion. ④The concentration of DAB or H_2O_2 is improper.

18.2.5 Immunocytochemistry Scoringmethods

The simplest scoring system distinguishes between a positive(+) and a negative(−) result. Such a system however does not distinguish between different levels of positivity. For this, the degree of staining can be graded and given a rating of positivity −, +, + +, +++. Positivity can also be based on the number of positive cells, which is then usually expressed as a percentage of the total cell population or relevant cell type. Several systems for manually assessing both staining intensity and positive cell number have been proposed. The systems that grades weak, moderate and strong are categovised into 1, 2 and 3, respectively, multiplied by the percentage of cells stained(1% −100%), with the final result being a score range between 1 and 300

(weak,1×1%,to strong,3×100%). These scoring methods have been further refined,for example,for ER scoring,which not only takes the intensity into account but groups together the percentages of positive cells (Table 18-3).

Table 18-3　scoring methods for both the staining intensity and the number of cells staining positive

Score for percentage staining	Score for intensity
0 = No cell staining	-
1 = <1% cell staining	+
2 = 1% -10% cell staining	++
3 = 11% -33% cell staining	+++
4 = 34% -66% cell staining	
5 = 67% -100% cell staining	

18.2.6　Quality Assurance for Immunohistochemistry

ICC is constantly evolving,with the introduction of new antibodies,better detection systems,new instrumentation and so on,such that the expected levels of staining may change. The feedback given from quality-assurance schemes should be used to troubleshoot any problems that a laboratory may have with its methods and protocols. Each QA programme normally consists of a panel of expert assessors made up of health-care scientists and pathologists,who give individual participating laboratories feedback in the form of a report outlining what is and what is not acceptable for a preselected antigen. This may include the intensity of staining,poor localization,excessive background,nonspecific staining.

18.2.7　The Application of IHC in Tumor Diagnosis and Differential Diagnosis

The reasons for the application of immunohistochemical staining in the diagnosis of tumor includes: ①In conventional biopsy,5% -10% of the most difficult cases are not clearly diagnosed. ②Tumors with similar morphologic structures are difficult to identify for different tissue sources,such as undifferentiated and malignant lymphoma,hence are difficult to be treated. ③Some metastatic tumors often lack specific histologic features and are unable to determine the primary lesions(such as thyroid cancer and prostate cancer). ④Through some markers that reflect the proliferation of cells and the malignancy of the tumor,it helps to identify the benign and malignant tumors.

18.2.8　Biomarkers Predictive of Response to Therapy for Breast

Hormonal influence on tumor growth has been known about since the late nineteenth century. With the introduction of the use of the hormone receptor to estrogen(ER)inhibitor,the establishment of methods to assess receptor status,the clinical need for a cost-effective reproducible method was identified. HER-2 gene encodes for a membrane tyrosine kinase receptor. It is a member of the epidermal growth-factor receptor (EGFR) family,a family of receptor tyrosine kinases which form homo-or hetero-dimers and transmits growth signals from the external cellular environment in response to receptor-ligand activation. This family comprises at least four members and is a target for therapy using kinase inhibitors or monoclonal antibodies (Figure 18-4).

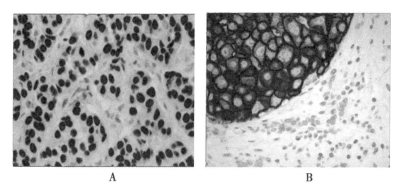

Figure 18-4   Breast carcinoma sections showing(A) ER; (B) HER-2

18.3   Electron Microscope Technology

Electron microscope , referred to as electron microscope , is based on the principle of electron optics. Instead of beam and optical lens , electron beam and electron lens are used to imaging the fine structure of matter at very high magnification. High-speed electronics than the wavelength of visible light with short wavelength(the wave-particle duality) , and the resolution of the microscope by the restrictions on the use of wavelength. In 1970s , the resolution of transmission electron microscopy was about 0. 3 nanometers(the resolution of the human eye was about 0. 1 millimeters). High speed electronics than the wavelength of visible light with short wavelength(the wave-particle duality) , and the resolution of the microscope by the restrictions on the use of wavelength , so the resolution of electron microscopy(about 0. 1 nm) is far higher than the resolution of optical microscopy(about 200 nm) , so by electron microscope can be observed by naked eyes to neat atoms lattice atoms of some heavy metals and crystals.

18.3.1   Related Technology of Electron Microscope

18.3.1.1   The Discernable Ability of the Electron Microscope

The resolution of electron microscopy is represented by the minimum distance between two adjacent points that it can distinguish , which is an important indicator of electron microscopy. The resolution of the microscope can be obtained by 0. 6 lambda/sin alpha , where alpha is half of the cone angle of the electron beam through the sample , and lambda is the wavelength.

18.3.1.2   The Composition of the Electron Microscope

The electronic source is a cathode that releases free electrons , and an annular anode accelerates the electrons. The voltage difference between the cathode and the anode must be very high , usually between thousands of volts and 3 million volts.

A detector used to collect electronic signals or secondary signals.

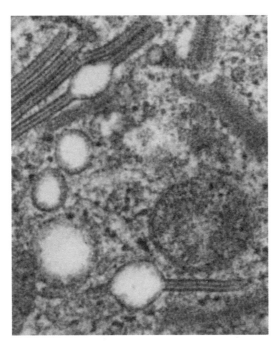

Figure 18-5   Electron microscope

※ *Source*

Book number: ISBN 978-4557-5155-6

Title of book: Review of Pathology

Chief editor: Edward. C. Klatt, Vinay. Kumar. MBBS

Revision: Fourth Edition

Page number and graph number: Page 193, appendix figure 53, electron micrograph

18.3.2   The Type of Electron Microscope

The electron microscope can be divided into transmission electron microscope, scanning electron microscope, reflective electron microscope and emittance electron microscope according to its structure and use.

Transmission electron microscopy (TEM), which is named after the electron beam that penetrates the sample, is amplified with an electronic lens. Its optical path is similar to that of the optical microscope. In this electric mirror, the contrast of the image details is formed by the scattering of the atoms in the sample to the electron beam. The thin or low-density parts of the electron beam are less scattered, so that more electrons are involved in the imaging through the optical column of the objective lens and appear brighter in the image.

The digital electron microscope is also called the video microscope, it is the physical image that the microscope can see through digital to analog conversion, and make it imaged on the screen or computer that the microscope brings. Digital electron microscope (SEM) is a high-tech electronic product which is perfectly integrated with elite optical microscope technology, advanced photoelectric conversion technology and LCD screen technology. Thus, we can improve the work efficiency by observing the microsphere from the traditional eyes to the display on the display. Three-dimensional digital microscope images can produce upright when observing an object.

18.3.3　The Insufficiency of the Electron Microscope

In the electron microscope, the sample must be observed in the vacuum, so the live sample can not be observed. The difficulty in analyzing the image is exacerbated by the possibility that the sample will not have the original structure when the sample is processed. Because the projective electron microscope can only observe very thin samples, it is possible that the structure of the surface of the material is different from the internal structure of the material. In addition, the electron beam may destroy the sample by collision and heating.

In addition, the price of electronic microscope purchase and maintenance is relatively high.

18.3.4　Comparison of Performance Between Electron Microscope and Optical Microscope

Resolution is an important index of the electron microscope. The resolving power of the electron microscope is expressed by the minimum distance between two adjacent points that it can identify. It is related to the incident cone angle and wavelength of the electron beam passing through the sample. The wavelength of the visible light is about 300－700 nanometers, and the wavelength of the electron beam is related to the acceleration voltage. So we can directly observe some atoms and crystals arranged orderly in some heavy metals by electron microscope. Although the resolving power of electron microscope is far better than that of optical microscope, the electron microscope is difficult to observe living organisms because of its need to work in vacuum. And the irradiation of electron beam will also cause damage to biological samples. Other problems, such as the luminance of the electronic gun and the improvement of the quality of the electronic lens, are still to be studied.

The advantages gained:

Extensible, future oriented platform;

Improve efficiency and reduce reporting time;

Continuous supply of captured cells to expert analysis;

Automatic record storage and data storage.

18.4　Microdissection Technology

18.4.1　What is Microdissection

Microdissection technology is based on microscope or microscope to cut and separate materials to be selected(tissue, cell group, cell component or chromosome band) through micromanipulation system and collecting technology for subsequent research. Microdissection technology is actually a technology of separating and collecting materials for research in the micro field. Therefore, applying this technology is often an important step in many in-depth research works.

18.4.2　Selection and Labelling of Probes

In the study of molecular pathology, two difficult problems are often encountered: First, the selected research materials need to have the same characteristics in a certain aspect, that is, to a certain degree of homogeneity. The vast majority of human tissues are heterogeneous cell clusters, which are made up of many different cells. This homogeneity problem is often encountered in deep research of human tissues, but it is not easy to solve.

18.4.3　The Material of Microdissection

The material of Microdissection can be attached to the solid phase in a variety of ways to support a variety of tissue cell component material, its origin is very extensive, paraffin sections and frozen sections, cell preparations, cell smear, cell smears, cell culture and conventional chromosome preparation can be used.

18.4.4　The Way of Microdissection

According to its development process, it can be divided into four kinds: manual direct microdissection, mechanical assisted microdissection, hydraulic control microdissection and laser capture microdissection (Laser Capture Microdissection).

18.4.5　Technology Combined with Microdissection

What kind of cells to choose exactly depends on the purpose of the research. However, how to identify the cells that are to be cut and how to analyze the cut cells need to be combined with other methods. It is precisely because it can be combined with a variety of molecular biology, immunology, genetics and pathology technology to make microdissection technology to show vigorous vitality. According to the needs of the research in micro cutting immunohistochemistry using histochemical, chemistry, in situ hybridization and in situ end labeling in situ, PCR, FISH, special staining methods to mark the need to cut the tissue components, micro cutting after the material can be used for extraction of protein, DNA and RNA for correlation analysis Western Blot, Southern Blot, Northern Blot, PCR protein and nucleic acid.

18.4.6　Influence Factors of Microdissection

Because microdissection is often used in combination with a variety of methods, the factors that affect the final results of microdissection are varied. So we need to grasp a principle in the process of experiment, that is, all the factors that influence the technology of microdissection should be listed as the influencing factors of the final result of microdissection experiment, which should be considered in the process of experiment. With different methods determining the need for different treatment to the microdissection materials using microdissection technique should be separated by how many cells or subcellular can meet the need of experimental research, it is influenced by many factors.

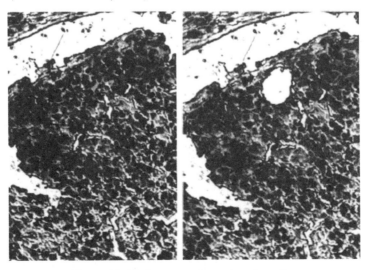

Figure 18-6　**Laser capture microdissection**

>> *Source*

Book number:ISBN 978-7-117-13102-5

Title of book:Pathology

Chief editor:Jie Chen,Gandi Li

Revision:Second Edition

Page number and graph number:Page 515,appendix Figure 2-6,Laser capture microdissection

18.4.7　The Latest Development of Microdissection

With the help of this revolutionary technology,we can quickly and accurately identify the specific separation of individual or group of cells for cellular and molecular biology research in the next step,the precise identification is based on cell morphology,immunohistochemical staining and histochemical staining methods under the microscope and computer aided realization,and specific separation is realized by low energy laser and infrared special cell transfer film. Laser capture microdissection is realized by laser microcell separation system. The system consists of inverted microscope,infrared laser transmitter,vacuum pump,cell transfer film and computer. Through the microscope in vacuum pump fixed slide,by centrifugal tube attached to the cover bottom of the ultra-thin cells separated by infrared laser transfer film will pick out the cells into the centrifuge tube,and can directly extract the centrifuge tube by dissolution and extraction,the extraction of liquid according to your cell group from the points of discretion,and all of the cell separation process, whether the transfer operation or the preservation of samples,without any manual operation,can achieve cell separation without pollution.

18.5　Laser Scanning Confocal Microscopy Technology

Laser scanning confocal microscopy(LSCM)is a set of observation,analysis and output system that uses laser as light source. It adopts the principle of confocal focusing and device based on the traditional optical microscope,and it uses the computer to process the observed objects. LSCM is one of the most important developments in modern biomedical image analysis instruments. The main components of LSCM are laser light source,automatic microscope,scanning mode(including confocal light path channel and pinhole, scanning mirror,detector),digital signal processor computer etc. Confocal imaging using the illumination point and the detection point conjugate of this feature can effectively inhibit the same focal plane of the non-measurement point of stray fluorescence and non-focal plane fluorescence from the sample to obtain ordinary optical microscope. It can not reach the resolution of both depth identification capability(maximum depth of 200-400 μm typically)and vertical resolution enable you to see details in thicker biological samples. The LSCM enables non-invasive tomography and imaging of samples to be visualized and analyzed in the three-dimensional spatial structure of cells. Combined with other technologies,dynamic observation of live cells, multiple immunofluorescence labeling or ion-fluorescent labeling can be carried out to study living cells Function and metabolic process.

18.5.1　Main functions of LSCM

1)Tissue,cell optical section. This function is also referred to as "cell CT" or "microscopic CT" (Figure 18-7).

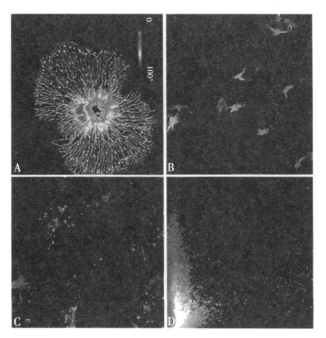

Figure 18-7　This function is also referred to as "cell CT" or "microscopic CT"

　　A. Fluorescent labeled dendritic cells with anti MHC-Ⅱ molecular antibody staining; B. Actin microfilaments(Rhodamin labeled, red) and microtubules (FITC labeled, green) of cytotoxic T lymphocytes; C. Double labelled staining showed that cathepsin D(FITC labeled. green) in the cytoplasm of fibroblast and wheat germ agglutinin in cell membrane(Texae Red labeled, red) D. Double fluorescence staining of fluorescence intensity analysis

❉ Source

Book number: ISBN 978-7-117-13102-5

Title of book: Pathology

Chief editor: Jie Chen, Gandi Li

Revision: Second Edition

Page number and graph number: Page 516, appendix Figure 2-7, laser confocal microscopy

2) Three-dimensional image reconstruction.

3) Long-term dynamic observation of living cells.

4) Quantitative determination of intracellular acidity and alkalinity.

5) Research on intercellular communication, cytoskeleton formation, biofilm structure and macromolecular assembly by FRAP.

　　FRAP irradiated a region of cells with high intensity pulse laser to cause the bleaching of fluorescent molecules in the region, and the unbleached fluorescent molecules around the region would diffuse to the irradiated area at a certain rate. The diffusion rate of the fluorescence molecules could be detected directly.

6) Measurement of cell membrane fluidity.

7) Photoactivation technology.

18.5.2　Requirements and Limitations of LSCM for Samples

Samples for LSCM are preferably samples of cultured cells, such as cell smears or crawlers, or frozen tissue sections. Paraffin-embedded tissue sections are not suitable for this technique. LSCM mainly uses direct or indirect immunofluorescence staining and fluorescence in situ hybridization. The cost of fluorescent labeled probes or antibodies is also high. In selecting this method, we should take full advantage of the advantages of LSCM and avoid using it as an advanced fluorescence microscope.

18.6　In Situ Hybridization(ISH)

In situ hybridization(ISH)is a part of nucleic acid molecular hybridization. It is a technique that combines histochemistry with molecular biology to detect and locate nucleic acids. ISH uses nucleotide fragments of labeled known sequences as probes to detect and locate a specific target DNA or RNA by hybridization on tissue sections, cell smears or culturing directly. The biochemical basis of ISH is DNA denaturation, renaturation and base complementary pairing binding. According to the selected probe and the target sequence to be detected, there are DNA-DNA hybridization, DNA-RNA hybridization and RNA-RNA hybridization.

18.6.1　Selection and Labeling of Probes

The probes used for in situ hybridization include double-stranded cDNA probes, single-stranded cDNA probes, single-stranded cRNA probes and synthetic oligo-nucleic acid probes. In general, the length of the probe is 50−300 bases, and the probe for chromosome in situ hybridization can be 1.2−1.5 kb. The probe markers have radioisotopes, such as H,35S and 33P, which are highly sensitive, but it has a high half-life and radioactive contamination, high cost and it is time-consuming. Therefore, its use is limited. The non-radioactive probe markers have fluorescein, digoxin and biotin, although its sensitivity is lower than the radiolabeled probe, because of its stable performance, simple operation, low cost and short time consuming, it is being used more and more widely. The double-stranded cDNA probe can be labeled by gap translation or random primer method, and single strand cDNA probe can be labeled by transcription. The synthetic oligonucleotide probe can be labeled with 51 terminal-labeling methods, that is a tail-labeling method.

18.6.2　Main Procedure of in Situ Hybridization

The experimental materials of in situ hybridization can be routine paraffin-embedded tissue sections, frozen tissue sections, cell smears and culturing cell climbing slices, etc. The main procedures include preparation before hybridization, pretreatment, hybridization, cleaning after treatment of hybridization and detection of hybrids, etc.

18.6.3　Application of in Situ Hybridization

In situ hybridization can be used to: ①Localize the cell-specific mRNA transcription in the use of researching gene mapping, gene expression and genome evolution. ②Detection and localization of viral DNA/RNA in infected tissues, such as EB virus mRNAs, human papillomavirus and cytomegalovirus DNA. ③The expression and changes of oncogene, tumor suppressor gene and various functional genes were detected at the transcriptional level. ④The location of genes on a chromosome. ⑤Detection of chromosome changes, such as chromosome quantity abnormality and chromosome translocation etc. ⑥The study of interphase cytogenetics, such as prenatal diagnosis of genetic diseases and the determination of some genetic carriers of genetic diseases, diagnosis of some tumors and biological dosimetry etc.

18.6.4　Recent Developments and Future Directions in Tissue ISH

Over the last decade, ISH has emerged as a powerful clinical and research tool for the assessment of DNA and RNA within interphase nuclei in tissue sections. Improved hybridization protocols, along with extensive probe availability resulting from the Human Genome Project. It has have shifted the focus from a morphology-based diagnostic approach to one which incorporates both morphologic and molecular characteristics. However, new and improved methodologies are constantly being described, such as Dual-colour chromogenic ISH, Fiction, the Allen Brain Atlas etc.

18.6.4.1　Dual-colour Chromogenic ISH

Although dual-probe FISH is gaining in popularity as a clinical diagnostic tool, it has yet to be completely embraced by the pathology community as it is time-consuming and requires specialized equipment and expertise. The enzymatic detection of two separate probe-target hybrids is now a viable alternative to fluorescent dye detection in DNA in situ hybridization. The method, known as dual-color chromogenic in situ hybridization(dcCISH), is based on peroxidase-or alkaline phosphatase-labeled reporter antibodies that are detected using a standard immunohistochemical enzymatic reaction. The advantage of CISH over FISH is that it allows the simultaneous examination of tissue morphology and hybrid signals under bright field microscopy. In addition, CISH-stained slides can be stored at room temperature with minimal loss of signal intensity over time.

The dcCISH technique is a modification of the standard dual-probe FISH technique where hybridization is followed by immunohistochemical detection of the hybrid signals(Figure 18.6.2). Probes can be labeled with biotin or digoxigenin, or with fluorochromes such as FITC or Texas red. Following hybridization the probe labels are detected with enzyme-conjugated mouse and rabbit antibodies and an enzymatic reaction with appropriate chromogens and substrates leads to the formation of strong permanent colors(usually red and green)that can be visualized using an ×40 objective.

18.6.4.2　Fiction

The Fiction(Fluorescence Immunophenotyping and Interphase Cytogenetics as a tool for the Investigation of Neoplasms)technique was developed in 1992 to allow the simultaneous detection of immunophenotypic markers and genetic aberrations in cell preparations. The original technique was restricted by the number of fluorescent dyes available and the quality of digital imaging. However, improvements in tissue pretreatment methods and the availability of many new fluorescent dyes have seen it used on FFPE material for the analysis of lymphoma and detection of the presence of minimal residual disease.

18.6.4.3　The Allen Brain Atlas

The Allen Brain Atlas(ABA)is a genomic-scale ISH project that has generated a cellular-level gene-expression proflle of the adult C57BL/6J mouse brain and spinal cord. This project has used high-throughput CISH with DIG-labelled riboprobes and tyramide amplification to detect mRNA transcripts in tissue sections and map them to the different regions of the mouse CNS. Automated image capture and analysis have provided quantitative expression data that can be directly compared with available microarray data sets. The annotated results for over 2,000 genes from this project are freely available. Other similar projects are underway and this approach to genome-wide transcriptional analysis using ISH and correlation with other genome-scale expression-proflling platforms will provide valuable insights into the organization and function of normal and abnormal cells and tissues.

18.7 In Situ PCR

The basic principle of in situ PCR is to directly amplify the target DNA or RNA fragments without changing the target location, and to detect the amplification products in situ. The specimens in situ PCR technology are usually fixed by chemistry to maintain the good morphology and structure of the tissue cells. Both cell membrane and nuclear membrane have some permeability. When PCR is amplified, all kinds of components, such as primers, DNA polymerase, nucleotides, etc. , can enter into cells or nuclei, and can be amplified in situ by RNA or DNA immobilized in cells or nuclei. The amplified products are generally large, or interwoven, and are not easy to pass through the cell membrane or diffuse inside and outside the membrane, and are retained in situ. In this way, the single or low copy specific DNA or RNA sequences in the cell are amplified exponentially in situ, and the products amplified are easily detected by in situ hybridizations(Figure 18-8).

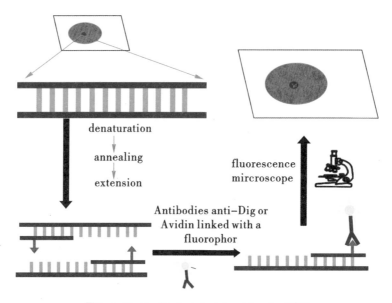

Figure 18-8　Basic principle of in situ PCR

18.8 Flow Cytometry

Flow cytometry(FCW) is a modern analytical technique for measuring suspended cells or particles in a liquid phase by flow cytometer. Flow cytometry can accurately and rapidly perform multiple parameter and quantitative analysis of individual cells in the flow of cells when the cells remain intact. Moreover, with the help of monoclonal antibody technology and fluorescent dye labeling technology, flow cytometry can not only detect multiple characteristic parameters from a cell, but also can sort a subset of cells with the same characteristics based on a certain parameter for further study. Flow cytometry has three main components: cell flow chamber and fluid flow drive system, optical system and signal detection system and data analysis system. The three systems are perpendicular to each other. The X-axis is the axis of the laser. The Y axis is the axis of detected by the fluorescence signal. The Z axis is the axis of the cell flow. It is the detection area of the FCM that intersection of three perpendicular axes(Figure 18–9).

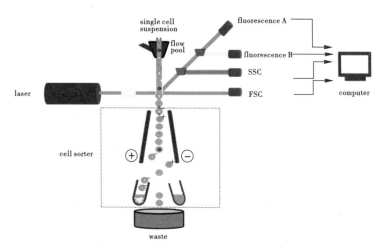

Figure 18–9　The basic structure of flow cytometry

18.9　Image Acquisition and Analysis Technology

Telemedicine(where Telepathology can be considered to be a subdiscipline), a general definition of this process would be the acquisition, storage and transmission of microscope images from a local site to a remote site for a specific reason. The initial concept was probably driven by researchers in disciplines outside those of pathology or microscopy. The first telepathology system was developed in the United States in the 1960s, and then 1980s with the advent of readily-available computer equipment. the technology would be unable to deliver a high enough image resolution for diagnostic accuracy comparable to that being achieved by traditional microscopy diagnosis.

However, the rapid growth in high-speed Internet connections, imaging and computing technology has provided a substantial backbone for the provision of a telepathology infrastructure. There have been two main types of telepathology to understand the advantages/disadvantages of these systems. The first is the Static Imaging Telepathology. This is an asynchronous technology in that there is no simultaneous interaction with the microscope slide. The second type of telepathology is Dynamic Telepathology, which is also known as Real-time Video Imaging. a microscope is used in conjunction with a PC to send images to a remote computer. This form can be subdivided into two systems: passive-dynamic and active-dynamic.

18.9.1　Digital(Virtual) Microscopy

Automated microscopes represent a form of hybrid technology in that they bring together various components within the industry to form a device capable of creating virtual slides without being dedicated to that purpose. High-specification microscopes(CCD) and computational techniques to produce the device. Due to the microscopes used in these systems, they have the capability to produce very high-quality images.

The CCD chip acquires the center of the field given by the objective, thus reducing optical aberration to a point considered negligible. When the picture is taken, the slide-moving mechanism puts the slide in the next position for image acquisition while refocusing the slide.

18.9.1.1 Olympus DotSlide

The Olympus DotSlide system is essentially an automated microscope (Olympus upright BX research microscope) that is computer-driven over the slide to form an image from a Peltier-cooled 1379×1032 pixel camera. The manufacturer quotes a figure of fewer than three minutes per slide with a X20 objective for a sample of tissue measuring 10 mm$\times$10 mm. However, many tissues that are regularly found in the average slide tray are significantly larger than this. Histology specimens may be this size, but can be 25 mm$\times$20 mm, and traditional cytology specimens can occupy the whole cover slip(50 mm$\times$25 mm), liquid-based cytology (LBC) specimens, depending on manufacturer, can be less than 25 mm diameter.

18.9.1.2 Scanners

①Progressive scan CCD systems: The Nikon COOLSCOPE Ⅱ is not truly a virtual slide scanner. It should be more correctly referred to as a digital microscope. It has the capability for slide observation and allows digital image capture. It additionally has Internet communications capabilities. ②Zeiss Mirax system: This system was developed in Hungary by a team from Semmelweis university in Budapest and is now marketed under the name Mirax by Zeiss. Mirax DESK is a semi-automatic tool for scanning a single slide using a X20 objective. Mirax SCAN is the largest machine in the family, it can be upgraded with a fluorescence module, giving it automated fluorescence slide-scanning capabilities. ③Aperio ScanScope system: The ScanScope GL system from Aperio is an entry-level device allowing small laboratories or university schools to implement a virtual microscopy programme. The machine only offers single-slide scanning on a manual basis. This is suitable for lower-volume environments provided with a X20 objective but with the capability of a final magnification of X400(via a X2 magnification changer). ④Hamamatsu NanoZoomer system: NanoZoomer Digital Pathology(NDP) is a high-throughput slide-scanning system. It is not offered as a low-throughput machine. It has been recognized that most applications will require batch processing, which is an integral part of the system. This machine does currently have two distinct advantages, namely true 3D z-stack scanning and an option to add fluorescence scanning. NanoZoomer's 3–CCD TDI camera allows the observation of low-light-level fluorescence tissue samples at high resolution. ⑤D-Metrix DX-40 imaging system: The DX-40 slide scanner has been developed by D-MetrixInc. (TucsonAZ), which could serve as a digitalimaging engine for a very rapid virtual-slide scanner.

18.9.2　The Virtual Slide Format

Virtual microscopy, from its inception, has been growing in strength significantly. However, one area in this domain that requires optimization is that of image format. When the slide has gone through the scanning process the end result is the virtual slide. This is what could be considered an image file; however, because of the file size, all the manufacturers have taken different approaches as to how this is represented and stored on hardware. TIFF or JPEG or JPEG2000 are general frameworks on which to hang the virtual slide. Virtual slides produced by scanning instrumentation are generally recorded in TIFF format with a suffix appropriate to the manufacturer. The JPEG image-compression standard is currently in worldwide use, and has become the industry standard in photography today. Initially this format was appropriate for the acquisition and efficient storage of images captured from the traditional optical microscope.

18.9.3　Image Serving and Viewing

Two applications that are core to the delivery of any virtual microscopy system are the image server and the image viewer. Image serving is going to be a central issue for digital microscopy. Pathologists/scientists can be demanding in their acceptance of any new technology and reasons not to use it tend to come easily to their minds. Buffering the image is potentially a method for significantly increasing the speed of delivery.

18.9.4 Applications of Virtual Microscopy

Quantification of biological and medical analysis is a major concern in standardizing and improving the efficiency and objectivity of the studies. Virtual microscopy in combination with sophisticated image analysis offers a great opportunity. With virtual slides, the operator can define accurate protocols and run efficient algorithms on whole slides or specified areas.

There are many limiting factors in any pathology or molecular clinical-analysis study of tissues due to: ①the non-optimization of slide-preparation procedures; ②the limited availability of diagnostic reagents used inprocessing; ③the usually less-than-optimal patient sample size. The technique of using tissue microarray (TMA) was developed to alleviate these issues.

18.10 Comparative Genomic Hybridization

Oncogenes and tumour-suppressor genes are critical for both cell proliferation and cell fate determination (differentiation, senescence and apoptosis), with cell type and context-specific effects; overexpression of a specific oncogene can enhance proliferation in one cell type but induce apoptosis in another.

Microarray techniques are subject to considerable data variability, due in part to variations in methods of DNA extraction, probe labeling and hybridization, the type of microarray platform used, the number and biological characteristics of samples analyzed, the methods used for microarray and statistical analysis, and results in validation.

18.10.1 Principles of Array CGH

Array CGH is based on the same principles as metaphase CGH, a technique that has been extensively used for the genomic characterization of a number of solid tumors. Array CGH, or matrix CGH, was first described in 1997. aCGH allows high-resolution mapping of amplicon boundaries and smallest regions of overlap, and improvement in the localization of candidate oncogenes and tumor suppressor genes, and is only limited by the insert size and density of the mapped sequences used.

18.10.2 aCGH Platforms

A wide variety of aCGH platforms are currently available and it should be emphasized that at the moment there is no ideal method for array CGH analysis. Ordered arrays are manufactured by spotting (using pins) or synthesizing individual probes in an organized pattern on a planar surface. Random arrays are constructed by immobilizing individual probes on to beads, which are then pooled and assembled on to a patterned planar surface.

18.10.2.1 BAC Arrays

Bacterial artificial chromosomes (BACs), P1−derived artificial chromosomes (PACs) and yeast artificial chromosomes (YACs) are large insert genomic clones that have been widely used in aCGH studies. The resolution of each BAC array is defined by the number of unique probes it contains. The probe content of genome-wide BAC arrays ranges from a few hundred to-32,000 unique elements (tilingpatharray). These platforms provide sufficiently intense signals for the detection of single-copy-number changes, can be readily applied to DNA extracted from archival formalin-fixed paraffin-embedded(FFPE)tissue as well.

18.10.2.2 cDNA Array

Initial studies on genome-wide approaches to aCGH were performed using cDNA microarrays, which were originally designed for expression profiling. cDNA microarray analysis enables only the detection of aberrations in known genes and ESTs, since cDNA probes are the only representative of expressed genes on a chromosome. In terms of maximal achievable resolution, cDNA arrays can not compete with currently available alternatives and have already become obsolete in aCGH studies.

18.10.2.3 Oligonucleotide Arrays

Oligonucleotide arrays CGH(OaCGH)platforms consist of single-stranded 25−85 mer oligonucleotide elements. Different types of oligonucleotide array have different labeling and hybridization protocols and can provide high-resolution measurements of copy number. There are two main types of oligonucleotide array: single-nucleotide polymorphism(SNP)arrays and non-SNP arrays.

18.10.2.4 Solexa Sequencing Technology

The Illumina Genome Analyzer(Solexa), which uses four proprietary fluorescently-labeled modified nucleotides to sequence the millions of clusters of genomic DNA present on a flow-cell surface. Following fragmentation, test DNA is ligated to adapters that facilitate the binding of the single-stranded DNA fragments to the flow-cell surface. This allows the sequence of bases in a given DNA fragment to be acquired a single base at time. From a molecular genetics perspective, this technology has the potential of solving several longstanding controversies, such as the mechanism leading to amplification, and rearrangements involved in the genesis of amplified regions.

18.10.2.5 Molecular Inversion Probe Arrays

Molecular inversion probes(MIPs)are single oligonucleotides with two flanking inverted recognition sequences that recognize and hybridize to specific genomic DNA sequences ranging between 41 and 61 bp in length. Each MIP oligonucleotide has a unique sequence barcode tag, which can be assayed via a tag microarray once it anneals to its specific complementary genomic sequence and is circularized.

18.10.3 Choosing the Right Platform

The choice of platform is dependent on the types of sample available as this has a direct impact on the quantity, quality and purity(i. e. the proportion of DNA belonging to the cells of interest)of extractable DNA for analysis. Extracted DNA from FFPE is often heavily cross-linked, degraded, fragmented and heterogeneous and is therefore suboptimal for microarray analysis.

18.10.4 Analysis and Validation

Analysis of microarray data always poses the statistical problem of false discovery given that thousands of variables(probes/genomic regions)are being investigated using a relatively small number of biological replicates(sample size)due to cost and availability of material.

Whichever method is utilized in the analysis of aCGH data, it is vitally important that the invariably and often excessively large volume of data generated is appropriately curated and validated with in situ or other molecular methods.

18.10.5 Finding the Target

There are two distinct ways: through top-down and bottom-up studies. Apart from detailed and diligent aCGH analysis, this process requires overlaying of array CGH and expression array data (or another type of Relatively high-throughput expression profiling), protein profiling or RNA interference (RNAi) analysis. After identifying a specific amplicon and its possible/likely driver(s), the next step is to identify a model to test whether cancer cells of similar phenotype depend on any of those genes for their survival (i. e. if the genes to be studied would elicit an oncogene addiction' phenomenon in a specific model that resembles cancer initially studied). It is of utmost importance to identify models that not only harbor the amplicon of interest, but also have a phenotype that is similar to that of cancer studied, as the functions and biological importance of a significant number of oncogenes appear to be context-and cell-type-dependent.

18.10.6   Clinical Applications

In parallel with and perhaps as a necessary corollary to the search for therapeutic targets, there is now widespread recognition of the essential requirement for biological or biochemical features, i. e. biomarkers, which can be used to measure or predict the effects of treatment. The availability of companion diagnostic assays for biomarkers that are inexpensive and easily performed.

18.11   Biochip Technology

Biochip technology is a high-tech emerging in the early 1990s with the Human Genome Project. It refers to the micro-processing and microelectronics technology, solid-phase matrix surface integration of thousands of densely arranged molecular microarray in order to achieve the organization, cells, nucleic acids, proteins and other biological molecules for efficient, accurate, high-throughput Detection. Commonly used biochips are divided into gene chips, protein chips, tissue chips, liquid-phase chips and micro-chip labs (Figure 18–10).

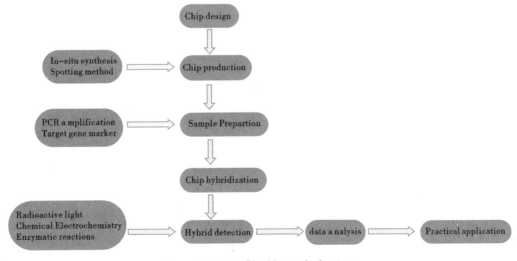

Figure 18–10   **Biochip analysis steps**

18.11.1   Gene Chip

Gene chips, also known as DNA chips, DNA microarray; a large number of gene fragments ordered, high-density fixedly arranged on the carrier made of lattice, called gene chip. The principle is that after the labeled DNA to be tested is hybridized with the probe at a specific position on the chip according to the principle of base pairing, the chip is scanned by a laser confocal fluorescence detection system and the like, and the intensity of the hybridization signal is detected to obtain the sample molecule Quantity and sequence information, using computer software for data comparison and analysis, so that the gene sequence and function of large-scale, high-throughput research. Gene chip is the first development in the field of biochips, the most mature and the first to enter the commercial application of technology.

18.11.1　Gene Chip Application

In recent years, gene chip technology has brought many revolutionary innovations in fields such as basic research, clinical diagnosis, drug screening, and guidance of clinical medication and treatment, with the advantages of multiple samples processing in parallel, high speed of analysis, small sample amount and less pollution.

（1）Gene Function Study

1）Gene expression and regulation. Gene expression analysis is the most widely used field of gene chip. It analyzes cell gene expression status as a whole, provides a powerful tool for understanding the gene expression related to certain life phenomena, and discusses the gene regulation and the mechanism of gene interaction.

2）detection of gene mutation and polypeptide. Genetic sequence variation is a major cause of intraspecific and intraspecific differences and is also a genetic basis of disease phenotypes and phenotypic differences under normal conditions. The use of gene chip technology is to locate, confirm and classify these mutations is the basis for the diagnosis of genetic diseases.

3）DNA sequencing. DNA hybridization in the chip sequence and adjacent hybridization sequencing is a new type of efficient and rapid sequencing method. The rationale is that any linear DNA or RNA single strand can be broken down into a series of oligonucleotide fragments, or sub-sequences, that have a fixed number of bases and overlapped.

4）Genome and gene research. Recently, some scholars have used this characteristic to study the replication activity of the yeast genome because of the high sensitivity and high accuracy of the gene chip. By comparing the DNA copy number of the yeast genome at 1,000 loci in S phase, the origin of replication was found. At the same time The relationship between replication fork movement in the genome and S-phase replication and transcriptional activity was also studied.

（2）Disease Diagnosis

①Infectious disease diagnosis；②diagnosis of genetic diseases；③tumor diagnosis and classification；④drug resistance test.

18.11.2　Protein Chip

18.11.2.1　Principles of Protein Chips

The basic principle of a protein chip is to immobilize a polypeptide, protein, enzyme, antigen or antibody on a solid support to form a molecular lattice by means of mechanical spotting or covalent binding and incubate the protein to be tested with the chip, and then the fluorescent labeled protein is reacted with the chip-protein complex.

18.11.2.2　Application of Protein Chips

1）Disease diagnosis and efficacy evaluation.

2）Research and development of new drugs.

3) Biomolecular interaction studies: ① antigen-antibody interaction; ② protein-protein interactions; ③small molecule-protein interaction; ④protein-nucleic acid interaction; ⑤enzyme-substrate interaction.

18.11.3　Tissue Chips

It can effectively use some precious lesions or puncture specimens to study the expression of specific genes and their corresponding proteins as well as the relationship between the disease.

18.11.4　Liquid Chip

Liquid-phase chip, also known as a suspended array, flow fluorescence technology, is based on xMAP technology, a new biochip technology platform is the rise of the mid-1990s, a new detection technology. ①Immunological analysis; ②pathogen detection; ③SNP test; ④other.

18.11.5　Microreactor Lab

The microchip lab has the advantages of highly integrated analysis process, automation, high throughput, fast analysis, less sample required, less cross pollution, low cost, small size, light weight, easy to carry and so on. Its future development trend can even become a personal bioinformatics analysis card or micromolecular biology laboratory devices, together with the corresponding computer software, as long as the sample drops on the chip, into the computer, the computer will interpret the test result. Its emergence will bring a revolution in such fields as molecular biology, disease diagnosis, curative effect monitoring, development of new drugs, forensic science, and food hygiene supervision.

18.12　Bioinformatics Technology

18.12.1　Introduction to Bioinformatics

18.12.1.1　Introduction

Bioinformatics is a new science that combines biological and informatics methods and uses computers and internet technologies to analyze vast amounts of rapidly accumulated biological data to gain new insights into biological sciences. Bioinformatics analysis includes several steps: biological information access, processing, storage, analysis and interpretation. The development of bioinformatics is the inevitable result of the development of life science and information science. It semergence and rapid development are triggering a revolution in the research methods of biological sciences. It will also have a tremendous impact on the development of life sciences and medical examinations.

Since the 1950s, the rapid development of molecular biology has enabled people's understanding of the nature of life to advance to the material basis of life activities-the two major types of biological macromolecules such as nucleic acids and proteins, resulting in a large amount of biological data. A great deal of biological data has been accumulated in the research on the structure, function and interaction of these two kinds of biological macromolecules. Especially with the completion of the Human Genome Project and the development of high-throughput genomic analysis techniques, the output of large-scale and high-throughput biological data has exceeded human's existing analytical capabilities. The use of computer technology and information technology to manage and analyze these massive biological data has become the inevitable trend of development of life science, which led to the biological sciences and information science combined with the cross-cutting edge of the discipline-bioinformatics.

18. 12. 1. 2 Bioinformatics Research Areas

1) Establishment, maintenance and management of various biological databases. It involves the basic knowledge and the classification and application of biological information in the establishment, maintenance and management of a database in information technology.

2) It is an important task of bioinformatics to study efficient statistical tools, analyze algorithms and develop convenient and fast analytical procedures. With the completion of the human genome project, the development of large-scale genome sequencing and high-throughput analysis technology, the longevity of massive biological data has come up but raised new unprecedented requirements for the collection and processing of information. The bottleneck of the speed of computer operation restricts the biological information, The study of science will inevitably require the development of efficient algorithms and procedures to achieve higher analytical capabilities under the existing computing power.

3) Discovering new knowledge from massive amounts of raw biological data. Including sequencing DNA sequences, identifying the coding protein genes, finding regulatory sequences for gene expression, predicting the function of new genes, locating new genes, predicting the structure and function domains of proteins, the expression profile based on accumulated data and knowledge and biochemical metabolic pathways.

18. 12. 1. 3 The Main Task of B ioinformatics

1) Genome-related information collection, storage, management and provision;

2) Discovery and identification of new genes;

3) Non-coding region information structure analysis;

4) Biological evolution;

5) Comparative study of the completed genome;

6) Genome information analysis methods;

7) Large-scale gene function expression profiling;

8) Protein end sequences, molecular space prediction, simulation and molecular design;

9) Drug design.

18. 12. 2 Bioinformatics Database

Researchers from around the world bring together biological data from various experiments into several international or national bioinformatics centers, which are important data institutions for bioinformatics research. This section mainly introduces a group of more important international bioinformatics centers.

References

[1]KUMAR V,ABBAS A K,FAUSTON N,et al. Bobbins and Cotran Pathologic Basis of Disease[M].8th Ed Philadelphia:Saunders Elsevier,2009.

[2]COLBY T V. Bronchiolitis:Pathologic consideration[J]. Am J Clin Pathol,1998,109(1):101-109.

[3]TURATO G,ZUIN R,SACTTA M. Pathogenesis and pathology of COPD[J]. Respiration,2001,68(2):117-128.

[4]TRAVIS W D. Pathology of Lung cancer[J]. Clin Chest Med,2002,23(1):65-81.

[5]ZANDER D Z,POOPER H H,JAGIRDAR J,et al. Molecular Pathology of Lung Diseases[M]. New York:Springer,2008:169-469.

[6]陈杰,周桥. 病理学[M].3 版. 北京:人民卫生出版社,2015.

[7]KURMAN R J,CARCANGIU M L,HERRINGTON C S,et al. WHO Classification of Tumours of the Female Reproductive Organs[M].4th Ed. Lyon:IARC Press,2014.

[8]周庚寅. 生殖系统和乳腺疾病[M].//李玉林. 病理学. 北京:人民卫生出版社,2013:288-294.

[9]张雅贤. 生殖系统及乳腺疾病[M].//王连唐. 病理学. 北京:高等教育出版社,2012:198-203.

[10]KUMAR V,ABBAS A K,ASTER J C,et al. Robbins Basic Pathology[M].9th ed. PA:Elsevier/Saunders,2011.

[11]李玉林. 病理学[M].8 版. 北京:人民卫生出版社,2013.

[12]KUMAR V,ABBAS A K,ASTER J C. Robbins Basic Pathology[M].9th ed. Philadelphia:Saunders Elsevier,2013.

[13]KUMAR V,ABBAS A K,FAUSTON N,et al. Robbins Basic Pathology[M].8th ed. Philadelphia:Saunders Elsevier,2007.

[14]LAKHANI S R,ELLIS I O,SCHNITT S J,et al. WHO Classification of Tumours of the Breast[M].4th Ed. International Agency for Research on Carcer,Lyon,2012.

[15]KUMAR V,ABBAS A K,ASTER,J C. Robbins Basic Pathology[M].9th ed. Saunders,an imprint of Elsevier Inc,2012.

[16]LEONARD V. Human Disease(Pathology and pathophysiology Correlations)[M].5th ed. Jones and Bartlett Publishers International,2001.

[17]HARSH MOHAN. Textbook of Pathology[M].7th ed. Jaypee Brothers Medical Publishers(P)Ltd,2015.

[18]翟启辉. 病理学(双语教材)[M]. 北京:北京大学医学出版社,2009.

[19]陈晓蓉,徐晨. 组织学与胚胎学[M].2 版. 合肥:中国科学技术大学出版社,2014.

[20]LOUIS D N,OHAGAKI H,WIESTLER O D,et al. WHO classification of tumours of the central nervous system[M].4th ed. Lyon:IARC Press,2007.

[21]刘彤华. 诊断病理学[M].2 版. 北京:人民卫生出版社,2006.

[22]翟启辉. 病理学(双语教材)[M]. 北京:北京大学医学出版社,2014.

[23]陈杰,李甘地. 病理学[M].2 版. 北京:人民卫生出版社,2011.

[24]李楠,尹岭,苏振伦. 激光扫描共聚焦显微镜术[M]. 北京:人民军医出版社,1997.

[25]WADE,C A,MCLEAN M J,VINCI R P,et al. Aberration-Corrected Scanning Transmission Electron Microscope(STEM)Through-Focus Imaging for Three-Dimensional Atomic Analysis of Bismuth Segregation on Copper[001]/33° Twist Bicrystal Grain Boundaries[J]. Microsc Microanal,2016,22(3):

679-689.

[26] XU W, DYCUS J H, SANG, X, et al. A numerical model for multiple detector energy dispersive X-ray spectroscopy in the transmission electron microscope[J]. Ultramicroscopy, 2016, 164(1):51-61.

[27] SCHORB M, GAECHTER L, AVINOAM O, et al. New hardware and workflows for semi-automated correlative cryo-fluorescence and cryo-electron microscopy/tomography[J]. J Struct Biol, 2017, 197(2):83-93.

[28] MATTAROZZI M, MANFREDI E, LORENZI A, et al. Comparison of Environmental Scanning Electron Microscopy in Low Vacuum or wet mode for the investigation of cell biomaterial interactions[J]. Acta Biomed, 2016, 87(1):16-21.

[29] CASTRO N P, MERCHANT A S, SAYLOR K L, et al. Adaptation of Laser Microdissection Technique for the Study of a Spontaneous Metastatic Mammary Carcinoma Mouse Model by NanoString Technologies[J]. PLoS One, 2016, 11(4):e0153270.

[30] KANG L, GEORGE P, PRICE D K, et al. Mapping Genomic Scaffolds to Chromosomes Using Laser Capture Microdissection in Application to Hawaiian Picture-Winged Drosophila[J]. Cytogenet Genome Res, 2017, 152(4):204-212.

[31] PADDOCK S W. Confocal laser scanning microscopy[J]. Biotechniques, 1999, 27(5):992-996.

[32] GALL J G, PARDUE M L. Formation and detection of RNA-DNA hybrid molecules in cytological preparations[J]. Proc Natl Acad Sci USA, 1969, 63(2):378-383.

[33] LAWRENCE J B, SINGER R H. Quantitative analysis of in situ hybridization methods for the detection of actin gene expression[J]. NucleicAcidsRes, 1985, 13(5):1777-1799.

[34] PRINGLE J H, RUPRAI A K, PRIMROSE L, et al. Close P, Lauder I. In situ hybridization of immunoglobulin light chain mRNA in paraffln sections using biotinylated or hapten-labelled oligonucleotide probes[J]. J Pathol, 1990, 162(3):197-207.

[35] LAAKSO M, TANNER M, ISOLA J. Dual-colour chromogenic in situ hybridization for testing of HER-2 oncogene ampliflcation in archival breast tumors[J]. J Pathol, 2006, 210(1):3-9.

[36] KORAC P, JONES M, DOMINIS M, et al. Application of the FICTION technique for the simultaneous detection of immunophenotype and chromosomal abnormalities in routinely fixed, paraffin wax embedded bone marrow trephines[J]. J Clin Pathol, 2005, 58(12):1336-1338.

[37] LEIN E S, HAWRYLYCZ M J, AO N, et al. Genomewide atlas of gene expression in the adult mouse brain[J]. Nature, 2007, 445(7124):168-176.

[38] WEINSTEIN I B. Cancer: addiction to oncogenes-the Achilles heel of cancer[J]. Science, 2002(297):63-64.

[39] WEINSTEIN I B, JOE A K. Mechanisms of disease: oncogene addiction-a rationale for molecular targeting in cancer therapy[J]. Nat Clin Pract Oncol, 2006(3):448-457.

[40] KALLIONIEMI A, KALLIONIEMI OP, SUDAR D, et al. Comparative genomic hybridization for molecular cytogenetic analysis of solid tumors[J]. Science, 1992(258):818-821.

[41] TAN D S, LAMBROS M B, NATRAJAN R, et al. Getting it right: designing microarray (and not 'microawry') comparative genomic hybridization studies for cancer research[J]. Lab Invest, 2007(87):737-754.

[42] JOHNSON N A, HAMOUDI R A, ICHIMURA K, et al. Application of array CGH on archival formalin-fixed paraffin-embedded tissues including small numbers of microdissected cells[J]. Lab Invest, 2006(86):968-978.

[43] FAN J B, CHEE M S, GUNDERSON K L. Highly parallel genomic assays. Nat Rev Genet, 2006(7):

632-644.

[44]JI H,KUMM J,ZHANG M,et al. Molecular inversion probe analysis of gene copy alterations reveals distinct categories of colorectal carcinoma[J]. Cancer Res,2006(66):7910-7919.

[45]尹一兵.分子诊断学[M].北京:高等教育出版社,2006.

[46]杜卫东.组织芯片技术应用新进展[J].临床与实验病理学杂志,2006,22(3):357-360.

[47]陈茹,刘林琳,许如苏.液相蛋白芯片技术及在免疫诊断和分析领域的应用进展[J].国际检验医学杂志,2007,28(3):232-234.

[48]王蕾,吴英松,李明.液相芯片分析技术及其应用简介[J].热带医学杂志,2005,5(4):562-564.

[49]吕建新,尹一兵.分子诊断学[M].北京:中国医药科技出版社,2004.

[50]陈鸿英,朱永智.生物信息学在医学上的应用[J].天津药学,2003,15(3):54-56.

[51]石鸥燕,杨文万.生物信息数据库及其利用[J].包头医学院学报,2006(3):319-320.

[52]吴耀生.生物信息数据库资源查寻及共享[J].广西医科大学学报,2003,20(A1):194-196.